A Clinician's Guide to Allergic Diseases

A Clinician's Guide to Allergic Diseases

Edited by **Kevin Parker**

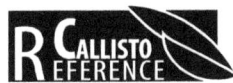

R CALLISTO REFERENCE

New York

Published by Callisto Reference,
106 Park Avenue, Suite 200,
New York, NY 10016, USA
www.callistoreference.com

A Clinician's Guide to Allergic Diseases
Edited by Kevin Parker

International Standard Book Number: 978-1-63239-660-0 (Hardback)

Printed in the United States of America.

Contents

Preface

Allergic diseases or allergy is the uneasiness caused due to the presence of some allergens like pollens, food items, grasses, dogs, cat fur etc. Generally allergic people are more sensitive to these substances which may cause swelling, sneezing, red eye and itching. Sometimes a long exposure to these materials may be life threatening. Accurate diagnosis and identification of the allergen responsible is quite crucial for clinicians to provide the curative measures. This book brings forth some of the most innovative concepts and elucidates the unexplored aspects of allergic diseases. It strives to provide a fair idea about potential allergy causing substances and treatments already available and new entrants to the list. It aims to serve as a resource guide for students and experts alike and contribute to the growth of the discipline.

This book is the end result of constructive efforts and intensive research done by experts in this field. The aim of this book is to enlighten the readers with recent information in this area of research. The information provided in this profound book would serve as a valuable reference to students and researchers in this field.

At the end, I would like to thank all the authors for devoting their precious time and providing their valuable contributions to this book. I would also like to express my gratitude to my fellow colleagues who encouraged me throughout the process.

Editor

Avidity Studies in *Anisakis simplex*-Associated Allergic Diseases

Carmen Cuéllar,[1] **Ana Valls,**[2] **Consolación de Frutos,**[2]
Marta Rodero,[1] **and Alvaro Daschner**[2]

[1] *Departamento de Parasitología, Facultad de Farmacia, Universidad Complutense, 28040 Madrid, Spain*
[2] *Servicio de Alergia, Instituto de Investigación Sanitaria, Hospital Universitario de la Princesa,*
 C/Diego de León 62, 28006 Madrid, Spain

Correspondence should be addressed to Alvaro Daschner; alvarodaschner@gmail.com

Academic Editor: S. L. Johnston

Gastroallergic anisakiasis (GAA) and *Anisakis*-sensitization-associated chronic urticaria (CU+) differ with respect to specific IgE levels. We hypothesised different immunoglobulin avidities in both entities as well as their dependence on TI and fish consumption. 16 patients with GAA and 17 patients with CU+ were included, and immunoglobulin levels were analysed by CAP (Phadia). IgE and IgG avidity indexes (AvIgE and AvIgG, resp.) were also determined. IgG avidity was higher in GAA than in CU+ ($P = 0.035$), whereas there was a tendency to lower IgE avidity in GAA ($P = 0.095$). When analysing all patients, AvIgG was positively correlated with specific IgE, IgG, and IgG_4 as well as total IgE (Rho between 0.66 and 0.71; $P < 0.002$), but AvIgE was negatively correlated with specific IgE (Rho -0.57; $P < 0.001$), specific IgG_4 (Rho -0.38; $P < 0.05$), and total IgE (Rho 0.66; $P < 0.001$). In GAA, weekly fish consumption was positively associated with AvIgE (Rho 0.51; $P = 0.05$). A multivariate regression showed that time interval was the main explaining factor for AvIgE in GAA. We could show a differential behaviour of immunoglobulin isotype avidities in both entities and their dependence on fish-eating habits as well as on the time elapsed to the last parasitic episode.

1. Introduction

Anisakis simplex is a fish parasite of worldwide distribution, whose third stage larva can be present in a huge number of marine teleost fishes. Humans can therefore be accidental hosts by consuming crude or undercooked fish [1]. Whereas IgE production is an evolutionary-maintained immunologic feature in mammals and thus can also be verified in all cases of human parasitic forms by this nematode, the allergenic potential has been an emerging health concern in the last years, giving rise to a large number of studies searching for proteins able to stimulate a specific IgE response [2, 3]. Gastroallergic anisakiasis has been described as a differential entity, where an acute parasitism by *A. simplex* produces also a clinically relevant IgE-mediated hypersensitivity reaction with appearance of acute urticaria, angioedema, or anaphylaxis [4].

It is well known that, in GAA, specific as well as total IgE and other specific immunoglobulin isotype levels depend upon the time interval elapsed (TI) between the acute parasitic episode and the obtaining of the serum sample [5]. The parasite is not adapted to the human environment and neither survives nor moults to its final stage. Even if the parasitic episode is always short-lived for mainly some hours, but maximally for a few days, as has been documented by gastroscopic findings in GAA, the immune stimulation, as witnessed by its humoral response, reaches its peak after four to six weeks and IgE is detectable in human sera or can be shown by skin prick tests (SPT) for more than ten years [5].

Another clinical entity, where a previous acute parasitic episode is suspected to play at least a necessary factor in a disease of multifactorial genesis, has been proposed to be an *Anisakis* sensitization-associated chronic urticaria (CU+) and has been described as a different phenotype of urticaria with distinct clinical as well as immunologic features with respect to other chronic urticaria forms, but also compared to GAA [6–9]. Furthermore, association of chronic urticaria with *A. simplex* hypersensitivity is now reported from different geographic regions [10]. Therefore, even if current bibliography shows chronic urticaria to have a frequent autoimmune or idiopathic origin [11], the search for underlying causes or associations with infectious or parasitic disease, such as in CU+, can be of help in research and practice. One of the main differences with GAA, where the acute reaction points to the precise moment of the human immune system coming in contact with the nematode, is the finding of lower antibody levels in CU+ [8, 12].

The experience of immune features in GAA teaches us that the allergic reaction is elicited after a secondary contact with the parasite [5, 13]. The important rise in immunoglobulin levels is similar to any secondary immune reaction against invading agents. On the other hand, the exact mechanisms by which acute urticaria/angioedema or anaphylaxis is elicited in GAA, compared to other parasitic forms without cutaneous or systemic hypersensitivity reaction, are not known. Moreover, the possible pathogenesis leading to chronic urticaria in sensitized patients has not been elucidated.

Acute allergic hypersensitivity reactions have mainly been studied in the fields of food or insect allergy. Besides the necessary production of IgE induced by proteins with specific allergenic properties, several other factors are necessary to produce allergic reactions, as IgE presence is not equivalent to clinical allergy. Further measurable amounts of detectable IgE do not properly predict allergic reactions. Further relevant factors could include the production of high-affinity IgE or the ratio of other blocking immunoglobulin isotypes, such as IgG_4 [14, 15].

Affinity and avidity studies have shown that continuous or repeated contact with antigen leads to an antibody affinity maturation [16]. This knowledge has led to studies differentiating acute from chronic infections [17–21].

Therefore, one approach to get more insight into the clinical relevance of specific IgE and IgG in *A. simplex*-associated allergic diseases is to assess hypothesized differences in avidity in GAA and CU+ and to associate them with the time interval elapsed since the parasitic episode and also with fish-eating habits as a possible correlation to the probability of previous subclinical parasitic episodes.

2. Methods

Patients were recruited at our allergy service and included prospectively if they matched the inclusion criteria. The study protocol was approved by the University Hospital La Princesa Ethical Committee.

All patients had to display a positive SPT and detectable IgE antibodies against *A. simplex* at ≥ 0.7 kU/L.

GAA patients had an acute episode of acute urticaria, angioedema, or anaphylaxis of less than 48-hour duration within 24 hours after eating raw or clearly undercooked fish, and other eliciting causes have been discarded by history and allergological workup.

CU+ patients were included if they had at least twice per week recurring wheals for at least 6 weeks. Patients were not included in this study if physical stimuli were the main eliciting agents of the urticarial reaction. Other factors associated with CU were not an exclusion factor, as CU is mainly multifactorial.

Thus 16 patients with GAA and 17 patients with CU+ were included and questioned about weekly fish and monthly anchovies in vinegar sauce consumption. Further time interval was defined as the interval between serum sample and GAA episode or onset of CU symptoms.

Anti-*Anisakis* specific IgE, IgG, and IgG_4 and total IgE were analysed by CAP-FEIA (Phadia, Uppsala, Sweden) [12]. Specific IgE and IgG against *A. simplex* whole body extract were further assessed by ELISA [22].

2.1. Avidity ELISA. Avidity ELISA was based on the dissociative method using urea as a denaturing agent [23]. Plates were coated with *A. simplex* whole body extract at 10 μg/mL overnight and incubated for 30 min with 6 M urea in PBS at room temperature. Microplates were washed and blocked with BSA for 1 h. Each serum was studied in quadruplicate (2 with urea treatment and 2 without), diluted in PBS-Tween 20, BSA 0.1%, and incubated for 2 h at 37°C. After incubating and washing, two of the quadruplicate sera were treated with PBS 6 M urea for 30 min at room temperature and the remaining sera were incubated with PBS for 30 min. After washing, goat anti-human IgG and horseradish peroxidase (HRP) conjugate (BIOSOURCE, Camarillo, CA, USA) were used. For the IgE determination, a murine monoclonal antibody against an ε-human IgE chain (IgG1κ, E21A11; INGENASA, Madrid, Spain) was added and incubated, followed by a goat anti-mouse IgG (γ1), HRP conjugate (INVITROGEN, Eugene, OR, USA). The reactions were developed with *o*-phenylenediamine with hydrogen peroxide and read at 490 nm. The avidity index (AvIgG and AvIgE, resp.) was defined as the mean optical density (OD) of urea-treated wells/mean OD urea-untreated wells × 100.

2.2. Statistics. Statistical analysis was performed using SPSS ver. 15.0 for Windows.

Median values and interquartile ranges (IQR) were calculated for total and specific IgE or IgG_4 as well as for avidity indexes and compared by Mann-Whitney U test.

We performed nonparametric correlation (Spearman Rho) studies between AvIgE, AvIgG, immunoglobulins, time interval, and fish consumption.

Furthermore, a linear regression was performed separately for GAA and CU+ for IgE avidity as dependent variable. We analysed specific IgE, total IgE, IgG, IgG_4, fish intake, and time interval as possible explaining variables with stepwise exclusion of nonsignificant variables.

3. Results

Mean age of the studied patients was 52.5 ± 14.3 years. 18 patients were females and 15 were males. These data did not differ in both groups.

Mean time from the acute parasitic episode to the serum sample in GAA was 5.0 (±5.2) months and mean duration of urticaria in CU+ was 27.0 (±20.8) months.

Mean number of fish meals per week was 2.7 (±1.5) in all patients without differences in both studied groups.

As expected, total IgE as well as specific IgE, IgG, and IgG_4 was higher in GAA than in CU+ (Table 1).

TABLE 1: Immunoglobulins and avidities in GAA (gastroallergic anisakiasis) and CU+ (*Anisakis simplex* sensitization-associated chronic urticarial).

	Total IgE (kU/L)	*Anisakis* IgE (kU/L)	*Anisakis* IgG (kU/L)	*Anisakis* IgG$_4$ (kU/L)	AvIgE	AvIgG
GAA	487 (98–1142)	48.7 (9.2–326)	17.8 (12.6–42.2)	1.930 (752–15842)	78.4 (71.4–88.6)	58.2 (48.2–70.5)
CU+	288 (117–690)	5.7 (3.7–11.9)	7.8 (7.2–15.0)	0.370 (95–910)	82.4 (74.4–98.0)	49.4 (38.0–57.1)
P =	0.29	0.005	0.01	0.001	0.095	0.035

Values are given as median (± interquartill range) and statistical significance is given for comparison between both studied groups. AvIgE: avidity index of specific IgE. AvIgG: avidity index of specific IgG.

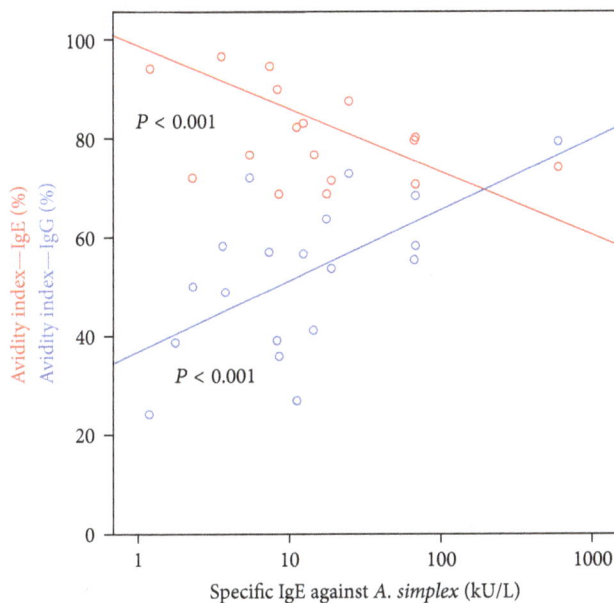

FIGURE 1: Avidity index of specific IgE and specific IgG against *Anisakis simplex* in gastroallergic anisakiasis depending on the amount of detectable specific IgE.

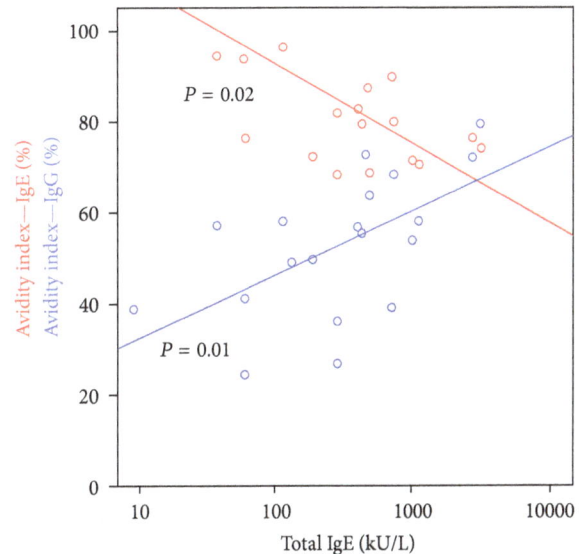

FIGURE 2: Avidity index of specific IgE and specific IgG against *Anisakis simplex* in gastroallergic anisakiasis depending on the amount of detectable total IgE.

Median AvIgE in all patients was 80.3 (interquartile range 73.2–91.8), while median AvIgG was 53.9 (37.4–91.8). Table 1 shows the results when comparing both studied groups. IgG avidity was higher in GAA than in CU+ ($P = 0.035$), whereas there was a tendency to lower IgE avidity in GAA ($P = 0.095$).

When analysing all patients, AvIgG was positively correlated with specific IgE, IgG, and IgG$_4$ as well as total IgE (Rho between 0.66 and 0.71; $P < 0.002$), but AvIgE was negatively correlated with specific IgE (Rho −0.57; $P < 0.001$), specific IgG$_4$ (Rho −0.38; $P < 0.05$), and total IgE (Rho 0.66; $P < 0.001$).

This divergent correlation depending on AvIgE or AvIgG was mainly maintained when patients with GAA were analysed (Figures 1 and 2). Here, a further negative correlation between AvIgE and time interval could be stated (Rho −0.71; $P = 0.02$). Also, in GAA weekly fish consumption was positively associated with AvIgE (Rho 0.51; $P = 0.05$).

Linear regression showed that time interval ($P = 0.015$) was the main explaining factor for AvIgE in GAA (Table 2 and Figure 3).

TABLE 2: Regression analysis for factors potentially explaining avidity index of specific IgE in gastroallergic anisakiasis.

Variable	Standardized coefficient B	Significance
Constant		**<0.001**
Total IgE	−0.28	*0.21*
Time interval	−0.59	**0.02**
Fish intake	0.27	*0.23*

Time interval explains avidity of specific IgE in gastroallergic anisakiasis. Linear regression analysis with stepwise exclusion of nonsignificant variables.

4. Discussion

Overall, we show high avidities for specific IgE and moderate avidities for specific IgG against *A. simplex* in both studied groups. Most avidity studies have been performed in order to search for differentiating recent versus chronic infections [17–19]. When analysing our patients, we have to take into account that the positive skin prick test or the presence of specific IgE denotes a past infection by the parasite, which is always self-limiting and therefore acute. Moreover, in order to have an

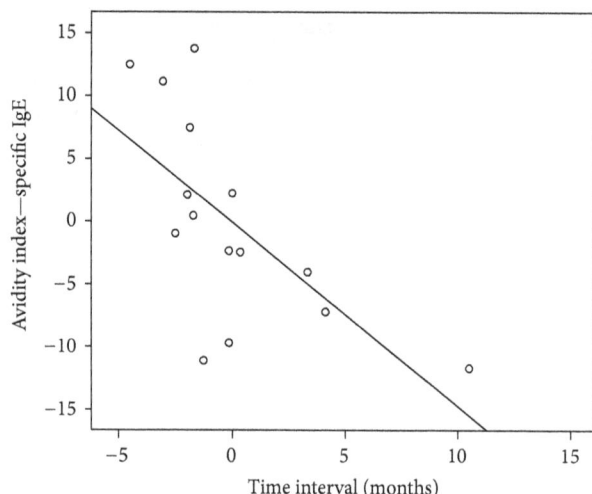

FIGURE 3: Partial regression graphic showing negative correlation of specific IgE avidity index in relationship with time interval (elapsed time from acute parasitic episode to serum sample in months).

allergic reaction accompanying the acute gastric parasitism, as in the case of our GAA patients, they obligatorily had a previous sensitizing episode [13]. In our CU+, we do not know the time of the last parasitic episode, but lower IgE values as demonstrated in the present as well as previous studies indicate a longer time interval to the last episode [8, 24]. Thus, it is to be expected that relevant antibodies had sufficient time to affinity maturation. Whereas in chronic infection, such as by *Toxocara* or *Toxoplasma*, the continuous contact with antigens facilitates affinity maturation [18, 23], there remains however the question about the source of antigen or allergen for affinity maturation in the case of rarely occurring acute episodes of parasitism such as by *A. simplex*.

In a previous *A. simplex* infection model in rats, avidity tended to exceed that at primary infection for several immunoglobulin isotypes [25]. Previous studies showed that most patients with CU+ really had a past infection with *A. simplex*, which is supported also by high IgE avidities. We have no data on avidities after a primary infection with *A. simplex* in humans, as these are expected to behave subclinically or induce only gastrointestinal, but no allergic symptoms. It may be argued that in GAA at least two episodes, as proposed above, would be sufficient to induce in the second episode a higher maturation of antibodies in the context of a secondary response [13], but the otherwise longer time interval in CU+ could be responsible for the slightly higher IgE avidities.

Whereas avidity describes the overall strength of the interaction between antibodies and their antigens, it would therefore be interesting to perform a similar study analysing affinities to already known *Anisakis* proteins or allergens. Our avidity results could be interpreted as a subset of clinically relevant IgE for the acute parasitism and a set of IgE antibodies induced by continuous fish intake (and therefore *Anisakis* contact) with possibly different avidities. In this respect, a previous study in peanut allergic subjects showed IgE : IgG avidity ratios to be higher than 1 for a total

antigenic source, whereas the opposite ratio was found when analysing avidity to a major allergen Ara h2 [26]. In our present study all but one patient showed a higher AvIgE than AvIgG (AvIgE/AvIgG ratio > 1; data not shown), a fact that does not rule out opposite findings if we would have available affinity studies with known allergens.

Whereas all immunoglobulin isotypes are known to be lower in CU+ than in GAA, a fact we could also confirm for specific IgG in our study, avidities could also be interpreted when analysing the time interval between parasitism and obtaining of the serum sample. Likewise, regression analysis showed that, in GAA, time interval was the main explaining factor for IgE avidity.

Affinity is overall expected to rise in time after infection, but this probably applies to only a few relevant allergens or epitopes [26]. A possible explanation for our results could be drawn from the correlation studies depicted in Figures 2 and 3. Polyclonal stimulation after an acute parasitic episode leads to high immunoglobulin levels, and in the case of IgE, most IgE does not recognize *Anisakis* proteins [2, 13]. Even if we only focus on specific IgE production, a mixture of high-affinity and low-affinity antibodies is to be expected. As antibody levels continuously fall again after a peak at about one month, low-affinity IgE antibodies seem here to turn up over high-affinity antibodies resulting in overall lower avidity. There is still controversy about the beneficial role of low-affinity IgE antibodies. According to Xiong et al. these can compete with high-affinity IgE for binding to high-affinity IgE receptors and prevent anaphylaxis in atopic allergy [14]. Otherwise this possibility has been stated unlikely because very high levels of IgE are needed to adequately saturate IgE receptors [27].

Again, the time interval seems to be the main explaining factor. Also in this case we could speculate that, once a sensitization process has occurred, following continuous contact with *Anisakis* proteins of other specificities than those leading to the allergic episode, leads to maintaining lower affinity antibodies. This would be an explanation to the fact that patients sensitized to *Anisakis* do not react with acute type 1 hypersensitivity reactions in provocation tests with non viable *Anisakis* larvae [28, 29]. Furthermore, blocking antibodies, such as IgG_4 included in the IgG compartment, with confirmed higher avidities in GAA could, by competing with the same epitopes recognized by IgE, prevent mast cell activation and the subsequent allergic episode, when *Anisakis* contaminated fish (nonviable or inactivated larvae) is well tolerated by patients with previous GAA.

Interestingly, if we look at the diverging correlation of AvIgG and AvIgE with specific IgE, we can also postulate that avidity is not only the outcome of an affinity maturation process of antibodies *within* an antibody isotype, but also the outcome of a mechanism, in which probably outcompeting of an immunoglobulin isotype over another could have been resulted by high-affinity antibodies in the maturation process [30].

A possible drawback of these results is of methodological concern, as there could be some controversy about the influence of IgG antibodies on an ELISA assay in avidity studies. However, previous studies with using thiocyanate as denaturing agent showed independence of immunoglobulin levels and avidity and lack of independence between avidity indexes and immunoglobulin concentrations [26, 31]. Therefore, our finding of a negative correlation of specific IgE with avidity is not expected to be influenced by a methodological constraint.

We did not show a direct negative correlation between AvIgE and AvIgG, but this could be due to the fact that we did not measure differential epitope affinity and the high variation of binding capacities and maturation process of antibodies between individuals [17]. In this respect it is interesting to note that differences in the generation of high-affinity IgE antibodies could be due to differences in sequential class switching versus direct class switching from IgM, although animal models and application in human allergic disease are still a matter of debate [14, 27]. The specific affinity maturation in Anisakis-associated allergic disease has not been studied so far, but our results could lead to a testable hypothesis, where clinically different CU+ and GAA after parasitism could be motivated by distinct class switching of specific antibodies.

5. Conclusions

In this first study on immunoglobulin avidities in humans affected by A. simplex parasitism, we could thus show a differential behaviour of immunoglobulin isotype avidities in GAA and CU+ and their dependence on fish-eating habits as well as on the time elapsed to the last parasitic episode. Further studies should address avidity studies against excretory-secretory proteins as well as affinity studies against known allergens.

Abbreviations

GAA: Gastroallergic anisakiasis
CU+:   Anisakis simplex
        sensitization-associated chronic
        urticaria
AvIgE: Avidity index for specific IgE
        against A. simplex
AvIgG: Avidity index for specific IgG
        against A. simplex.

Acknowledgments

The study was funded by grants from Fundación Sociedad Española de Alergología e Inmunología Clínica (SEAIC) 2009 and Fundación Mutua Madrileña 2009. The authors thank Raquel Barbero, Laura Fernández Gámez, and Duarte-Miguel de Sousa Teixeira for technical support.

References

[1] P. H. van Thiel and H. van Houten, "The herring worm Anisakis marina as a human parasite outside the wall of the gastrointestinal tract," Nederlands Tijdschrift voor Geneeskunde, vol. 110, no. 35, pp. 1524–1528, 1966.

[2] A. Daschner, C. Culléar, and M. Rodero, "The Anisakis allergy debate: does an evolutionary approach help?" Trends in Parasitology, vol. 28, pp. 9–15, 2012.

[3] J. F. Urban, K. B. Madden, A. Svetić et al., "The importance of Th2 cytokines in protective immunity to nematodes," Immunological Reviews, no. 127, pp. 205–220, 1992.

[4] A. Daschner, A. Alonso-Gómez, R. Cabañas, J. M. Suarez-de-Parga, and M. C. López-Serrano, "Gastroallergic anisakiasis: borderline between food allergy and parasitic disease—clinical and allergologic evaluation of 20 patients with confirmed acute parasitism by Anisakis simplex," Journal of Allergy and Clinical Immunology, vol. 105, no. 1, pp. 176–181, 2000.

[5] A. Daschner, A. Alonso-Gómez, T. Caballero, J. M. Suarez-de-Parga, and M. C. López-Serrano, "Usefulness of early serial measurement of specific and total immunoglobulin E in the diagnosis of gastro-allergic Anisakiasis," Clinical and Experimental Allergy, vol. 29, no. 9, pp. 1260–1264, 1999.

[6] C. Cuéllar, M. Rodero, and A. Daschner, "Inhibition of cytokine production in Gastro-allergic Anisakiasis and Anisakiasis simplex sensitization-associated chronic urticaria," Parasite Immunology, vol. 32, no. 7, p. 528, 2010.

[7] C. Cuéllar, A. Daschner, A. Valls et al., "Ani s 1 and Ani s 7 recombinant allergens are able to differentiate distinct Anisakis simplex-associated allergic clinical disorders," Archives of Dermatological Research, vol. 304, pp. 283–288, 2012.

[8] A. Daschner, V. Fernández-Fígares, A. Valls et al., "Different fish-eating habits and cytokine production in chronic urticaria with and without sensitization against the fish-parasite Anisakis simplex," Allergology International, 2013.

[9] A. Daschner, C. De Frutos, A. Valls, and F. Vega de la Osada, "Different clinical presentation of Anisakis simplex associated urticaria is dependent on the frequency of raw fish intake," Allergologia et Immunopathologia, vol. 38, no. 3, pp. 166–167, 2010.

[10] M. T. Ventura, S. Napolitano, R. Menga, R. Cecere, and R. Asero, "Anisakis simplex hypersensitivity is associated with chronic urticaria in endemic areas," International Archives of Allergy and Immunology, vol. 160, pp. 297–300, 2013.

[11] M. Ferrer and A. P. Kaplan, "Progress and challenges in the understanding of chronic urticaria," Allergy, Asthma and Clinical Immunology, vol. 3, no. 1, pp. 31–35, 2007.

[12] A. Daschner and C. Y. Pascual, "Anisakis simplex: sensitization and clinical allergy," Current Opinion in Allergy and Clinical Immunology, vol. 5, no. 3, pp. 281–285, 2005.

[13] A. Daschner, C. Cuéllar, S. Sánchez-Pastor, C. Y. Pascual, and M. Martín-Esteban, "Gastro-allergic anisakiasis as a consequence of simultaneous primary and secondary immune response," Parasite Immunology, vol. 24, no. 5, pp. 243–251, 2002.

[14] H. Xiong, J. Dolpady, M. Wabl, M. A. Curotto de Lafaille, and J. J. Lafaille, "Sequential class switching is required for the generation of high affinity IgE antibodies," The Journal of Experimental Medicine, vol. 209, pp. 353–364, 2012.

[15] M. E. Devey, S. R. Lee, D. Richards, and D. M. Kemeny, "Serial studies on the functional affinity and heterogeneity of antibodies of different IgG subclasses to phospholipase A2 produced in response to bee-venom immunotherapy," Journal of Allergy and Clinical Immunology, vol. 84, no. 3, pp. 326–330, 1989.

[16] M. Wabl and C. Steinberg, "Affinity maturation and class switching," Current Opinion in Immunology, vol. 8, no. 1, pp. 89–92, 1996.

[17] H. T. Gonzaga, V. S. Ribeiro, N. D. Feliciano et al., "IgG avidity in differential serodiagnosis of human strongyloidiasis active infection," *Immunology Letters*, vol. 139, no. 1-2, pp. 87–92, 2011.

[18] S. Fenoy, M. Rodero, E. Pons, C. Aguila, and C. Cuéllar, "Follow-up of antibody avidity in BALB/c mice infected with Toxocara canis," *Parasitology*, vol. 135, no. 6, pp. 725–733, 2008.

[19] J. Nedeljkovic, T. Jovanovic, and C. Oker-Blom, "Maturation of IgG avidity to individual rubella virus structural proteins," *Journal of Clinical Virology*, vol. 22, no. 1, pp. 47–54, 2001.

[20] A. Sensini, "*Toxoplasma gondii* infection in pregnancy: opportunities and pitfalls of serological diagnosis," *Clinical Microbiology and Infection*, vol. 12, no. 6, pp. 504–512, 2006.

[21] T. Lazzarotto, B. Guerra, L. Gabrielli, M. Lanari, and M. P. Landini, "Update on the prevention, diagnosis and management of cytomegalovirus infection during pregnancy," *Clinical Microbiology and Infection*, vol. 17, pp. 1285–1293, 2011.

[22] R. Gutiérrez-Ramos, R. Guillén-Bueno, R. Madero-Jarabo, and C. C. del Hoyo, "Digestive haemorrhage in patients with anti-*Anisakis* antibodies," *European Journal of Gastroenterology & Hepatology*, vol. 12, pp. 337–343, 2000.

[23] K. Hedman, M. Lappalainen, I. Seppala, and O. Makela, "Recent primary toxoplasma infection indicated by a low avidity of specific IgG," *Journal of Infectious Diseases*, vol. 159, no. 4, pp. 736–740, 1989.

[24] A. Daschner, C. De Frutos, A. Valls, and F. Vega, "*Anisakis simplex* sensitization-associated urticaria: short-lived immediate type or prolonged acute urticaria," *Archives of Dermatological Research*, vol. 302, no. 8, pp. 625–629, 2010.

[25] T. Cho, H. Park, S. Cho et al., "The time course of biological and immunochemical allergy states induced by *Anisakis simplex* larvae in rats," *Clinical & Experimental Immunology*, vol. 143, pp. 203–208, 2006.

[26] F. El-Khouly, S. A. Lewis, L. Pons, A. W. Burks, and J. O. Hourihane, "IgG and IgE avidity characteristics of peanut allergic individuals," *Pediatric Allergy and Immunology*, vol. 18, no. 7, pp. 607–613, 2007.

[27] J. M. Davies, T. A. Platts-Mills, and R. C. Aalberse, "The enigma of IgE$^+$ B-cell memory in human subjects," *Journal of Allergy and Clinical Immunology*, vol. 131, pp. 972–976, 2013.

[28] A. Alonso, A. Moreno-Ancillo, A. Daschner, and M. C. López-Serrano, "Dietary assessment in five cases of allergic reactions due to gastroallergic *Anisakiasis*," *Allergy*, vol. 54, no. 5, pp. 517–520, 1999.

[29] M. L. Baeza, A. Rodríguez, V. Matheu et al., "Characterization of allergens secreted by *Anisakis simplex* parasite: clinical relevance in comparison with somatic allergens," *Clinical and Experimental Allergy*, vol. 34, no. 2, pp. 296–302, 2004.

[30] D. R. Jackola, C. L. Liebeler, C. Y. Lin, Y. K. Chiu, M. N. Blumenthal, and A. Rosenberg, "Evidence that negative feedback between antibody concentration and affinity regulates humoral response consolidation to a non-infectious antigen in infants," *Molecular Immunology*, vol. 42, no. 1, pp. 19–30, 2005.

[31] G. R. Pullen, M. G. Fitzgerald, and C. S. Hosking, "Antibody avidity determination by ELISA using thiocyanate elution," *Journal of Immunological Methods*, vol. 86, no. 1, pp. 83–87, 1986.

Anaphylaxis Preparedness among Preschool Staff before and after an Educational Intervention

Ashley A. Foster,[1] Ronna L. Campbell,[2] Sangil Lee,[3] and Jana L. Anderson[2]

[1]Department of Emergency Medicine, University of California, San Francisco, San Francisco, CA, USA
[2]Department of Emergency Medicine, Mayo Clinic, Rochester, MN, USA
[3]Department of Emergency Medicine, Mayo Clinic Health System in Mankato, Mankato, MN, USA

Correspondence should be addressed to Jana L. Anderson; anderson.jana@mayo.edu

Academic Editor: Hugo Van Bever

Introduction. Children with severe food allergies may spend many hours in the preschool setting. Little is known about anaphylaxis recognition and management preparedness among preschool staff. The objective of this study was to assess anaphylaxis preparedness among preschool staff. *Methods.* Anonymous questionnaires were administered before and after a 40-minute educational seminar on anaphylaxis recognition and management. *Results.* In total, 181 individuals participated in the preintervention survey and 171 participated in the postintervention survey. The comfort level with recognizing anaphylaxis and administering an epinephrine autoinjector significantly increased after the intervention ($P < .001$ for both). Of the 5 steps needed to administer an epinephrine autoinjector, staff named a mean (SD) of 3 (1.3) steps in the correct order compared with 4.2 (1.1) steps after the educational intervention ($P < .001$). *Conclusion.* This study shows that a brief education intervention can significantly increase caregiver comfort regarding identifying anaphylaxis and administering an epinephrine autoinjector.

1. Introduction

Anaphylaxis is defined as a rapid-onset, potentially fatal allergic reaction [1]. Food allergy remains the most common cause of anaphylaxis in children [2]. Although the true incidence and prevalence rates of pediatric anaphylaxis are unknown because of differing clinical definitions of anaphylaxis, a recent population-based study in Rochester, Minnesota, by Decker et al. [3] showed the highest age-specific incidence in children aged 0 to 9 years. Accidental exposure to an allergen is frequent in the pediatric population, with up to 50% of children with a known food allergy having an accidental exposure in a 1-year period [4]. Because children spend much of their time in a school environment, potential exposure to allergens and subsequent anaphylactic reactions are anticipated at many preschools and schools [5]. Nevertheless, recent studies have shown that few preschool staff are trained to administer epinephrine, and those who have received training are still often unable to properly administer the appropriate therapy [6, 7].

Although preventing allergic reactions to known triggers remains the best management strategy, in the case of severe allergy or anaphylaxis, epinephrine is the first-line treatment [8]. Anaphylaxis requires quick action to prevent complications and potential fatality [9]. Studies show that delayed treatment with epinephrine is a major risk factor for death from anaphylaxis [9–11]. Although the universally recommended method of treating anaphylaxis is intramuscular injection of epinephrine, it still is uncommonly used as therapy for food-induced anaphylaxis in the prehospital setting or emergency department [12].

Because children with severe food allergies can spend many hours in the preschool setting, childcare staff must be proficient in recognizing anaphylaxis and using an epinephrine autoinjector [13]. Currently, many preschools do not have a nurse on staff who could quickly treat a child in anaphylaxis; thus, classroom teachers are responsible for taking action and administering an epinephrine autoinjector when needed. However, deficits exist in staff education regarding recognition of symptoms of food allergy and knowledge about the correct use of an epinephrine autoinjector during anaphylaxis [7, 14]. Although recognition and management of anaphylaxis has been studied in preschool directors [13, 15], little is known about whether preschool teachers and other staff members can recognize anaphylaxis and properly use an epinephrine autoinjector. Thus, the objective of this study was to assess anaphylaxis preparedness among preschool staff members, including school directors, teachers, teaching assistants, and ancillary staff, before and after an educational intervention.

2. Methods

This project was approved by our institutional review board.

2.1. Participants. We identified preschools with children aged 6 years and under in the community. Directors were contacted via telephone and invited to participate in the study between September 2011 and May 2012.

Participating staff included preschool directors, teachers, assistants, teaching aides, and home visitors. Participation was voluntary. Staff who could not attend the educational session completed only the preintervention questionnaire. Consent was obtained from all preschool directors via telephone, and consent from the remaining staff was obtained before survey administration.

2.2. Intervention and Questionnaire. Preschool staff attended a 40-minute educational seminar (presented by Ashley A. Foster) that included an overview of recognition and immediate management of anaphylaxis, a hands-on demonstration, and practice session with an epinephrine autoinjector training device.

Anonymous questionnaires were administered to staff before and after the educational session to assess baseline characteristics and the effectiveness of the intervention (the same questionnaires were used both times). The postintervention questionnaire was administered immediately after the educational seminar.

The survey assessed staff characteristics, educational experience and responsibilities, training in and comfort level associated with anaphylaxis recognition, competence and comfort level of epinephrine autoinjector administration, and barriers to epinephrine administration. Comfort levels associated with recognizing anaphylaxis and administering an epinephrine autoinjector were evaluated on a scale of 1 to 10, with 1 indicating not comfortable and 10 indicating very comfortable. Participants were asked to sequentially order the steps of epinephrine autoinjector administration in the setting of anaphylaxis. Steps included (1) make a fist around the epinephrine autoinjector; (2) remove the protective cap; (3) push the injector firmly against child's anterior-lateral thigh; (4) hold for 10 seconds; and (5) discard epinephrine autoinjector in the proper container. Potential barriers to successful recognition and administration of epinephrine were assessed.

2.3. Statistical Analysis. Data are presented as mean (SD). Categorical data are presented as percent frequency of

TABLE 1: Staff characteristics.

Characteristic	Number (%)
Years of providing care ($n = 169$)	
0–5	87 (51)
>5–10	26 (15)
>10–20	30 (18)
>20–30	18 (11)
>30	8 (5)
Ages of children under care[a] ($n = 168$)	
<6 mo.	50 (30)
6 mo.–2 y	68 (40)
>2–4 y	112 (67)
>4–6 y	98 (58)
>6 y	30 (18)
Children currently under care ($n = 168$)	
0–5	7 (4)
6–10	18 (11)
11–19	89 (53)
20–29	11 (7)
>30	43 (26)

[a]More than 1 response possible. For example, a participant could be caring for children younger than 6 months and children 6 months to 2 years old.

occurrence. Comparisons between features of interest were evaluated using Spearman rank correlation coefficients and the Kruskal-Wallis, Wilcoxon rank sum, χ^2, and Fisher exact tests.

3. Results

We contacted 24 preschools and 10 (42%) agreed to participate. The preintervention survey was completed by 181 staff members, and 171 participated in the educational seminar and postintervention survey. Staff characteristics, educational experience, and responsibilities are summarized in Table 1. Eighty-seven participants (51%) had fewer than 5 years of teaching experience. Although 120 participants (70%) reported prior training using an epinephrine autoinjector, only 98 (57%) reported prior training on anaphylaxis recognition. The majority of those who answered the survey ($n = 151$ (90%)) indicated wanting more anaphylaxis education.

Survey responses, stratified by participant educational role, are summarized in Table 2. We observed no significant differences in preintervention comfort level with recognizing anaphylaxis or with administering an epinephrine autoinjector on the basis of educational role. Potential barriers to successful recognition and administration of epinephrine were identified before the educational intervention (Table 2). The most common perceived barriers were uncertainty about anaphylaxis recognition (91/132 (69%)) and uncertainty about using the epinephrine autoinjector (71/132 [54%]).

The 5 steps to administering an epinephrine autoinjector were assessed (Table 3). Before the educational intervention, staff ordered a mean (SD) of 3 (1.3) steps correctly, whereas they correctly ordered 4.2 (1.1) steps correctly after the educational intervention ($P < .001$). Overall, 98 staff

TABLE 2: Staff characteristics, perceived barriers to epinephrine administration, and preintervention assessment.

Characteristic, barrier, or assessment	Overall ($n = 171$)	Director ($n = 11$)	Teacher ($n = 91$)	Assistant ($n = 33$)	Other ($n = 26$)	Unspecified ($n = 10$)
Staff characteristic, number (%)						
Currently caring for a child with severe allergies	15/168 (9)	4 (36)	6 (7)	3 (9)	2 (8)	0 (0)
Previous EAI administration	6/170 (4)	1 (9)	4 (4)	0 (0)	1 (4)	0 (0)
Prior EAI training	120 (71)	9 (82)	73 (80)	17 (52)	16 (62)	5/9 (56)
Prior anaphylaxis recognition training	98/171 (57)	9 (82)	58 (64)	13 (39)	12 (46)	6 (60)
Desire for more anaphylaxis education	151/168 (90)	10 (91)	84 (92)	29/32 (91)	24 (92)	4/8 (50)
Perceived barriers to epinephrine administration, number (%)	Overall ($n = 132$)	Director ($n = 10$)	Teacher ($n = 73$)	Assistant ($n = 23$)	Other ($n = 19$)	Unspecified ($n = 7$)
Uncertainty about anaphylaxis recognition	91 (69)	8 (80)	51 (70)	14 (61)	16 (84)	2 (29)
Uncertainty about EAI use	71 (54)	8 (80)	38 (52)	13 (57)	10 (53)	2 (29)
Uncertainty about EAI location	15 (11)	1 (10)	10 (14)	2 (9)	1 (5)	1 (14)
Not allowed to administer EAI	17 (13)	0 (0)	14 (19)	1 (4)	1 (5)	1 (14)
Other	12 (9)	1 (10)	7 (10)	1 (4)	1 (5)	2 (29)
Preintervention staff assessment, mean (SD)						
Anaphylaxis recognition comfort level ($n = 166$)	5.1 (2.4)	4.4 (2.8)	5.2 (2.0)	5.0 (2.3)	4.8 (3.1)	6.5 (2.7)
EAI administration comfort level ($n = 169$)	5.4 (2.8)	5.3 (3.2)	5.7 (2.4)	4.9 (2.8)	5.0 (3.4)	4.7 (3.0)
Number of correctly sequenced steps for EAI administration ($n = 161$)	2.0 (2.1)	1.0 (2.2)	2.3 (2.1)	1.6 (2.2)	1.6 (2.0)	2.0 (2.2)

EAI: epinephrine autoinjector.

TABLE 3: Participant comfort level regarding procedure for EAI administration, before and after the educational intervention.

EAI procedure	Before intervention, mean (SD)	After intervention, mean (SD)	P value
Anaphylaxis recognition comfort level ($n = 166$)	5.1 (2.4)	8.7 (1.2)	<.001
EAI administration comfort level ($n = 169$)	5.4 (2.8)	8.8 (1.3)	<.001
Number of correctly sequenced steps for EAI administration ($n = 161$)	3.0 (1.3)	4.2 (1.1)	<.001

EAI: epinephrine autoinjector.

members (57%) ordered all 5 steps correctly after the intervention compared with only 28 (15%) before the intervention. The number of correctly identified epinephrine autoinjector administration steps was weakly but positively correlated with comfort level with epinephrine administration (Spearman rank correlation coefficient, 0.16; $P = .04$).

Comfort levels with recognizing anaphylaxis and administering an autoinjector were evaluated, and responses before and after the educational intervention are summarized in Table 3. Comfort level with recognizing anaphylaxis significantly increased after the education session (mean (SD), 5.2 (2.4) versus 8.7 (1.2); $P < .001$). Two participants (1%) indicated that they were less comfortable recognizing anaphylaxis after the seminar, 19 participants (11%) had the same level of comfort, and the remaining 150 participants (88%) had a higher level of comfort. Additionally, the comfort level with administering an epinephrine autoinjector significantly increased after the intervention (mean (SD) increase, 3.7 (2.3); $P < .001$). Almost all participants (99%) believed that they benefited from the seminar, with 126 (76%) endorsing education annually.

Prior training affected preintervention comfort levels regarding preparedness. Individuals who received prior anaphylaxis recognition training had significantly higher preintervention anaphylaxis recognition comfort levels compared with participants who had not received such training (mean: 5.7 versus 4.3; $P < .001$). Similarly, participants who received prior training in epinephrine autoinjector administration had a significantly higher comfort level with administering an autoinjector in the event of anaphylaxis than those without previous training (mean: 5.9 versus 4.0; $P < .001$).

4. Discussion

An increasing incidence of food allergies and anaphylaxis, especially in children aged 5 years and younger, has been reported in multiple countries, including the United States, United Kingdom, and Australia [16]. Because intramuscular epinephrine is the definitive therapy for anaphylaxis, it is imperative to establish a knowledge base and increase preparedness among preschool staff regarding recognition of anaphylaxis and the use of an epinephrine autoinjector

[7, 13, 15, 17]. To our knowledge, this is the first study to assess anaphylaxis recognition and epinephrine administration preparedness among multiple categories of preschool staff (e.g., school directors, teachers, teaching assistants, ancillary staff).

Because teachers are more likely to be directly supervising the students throughout the day, teachers specifically must be able to rapidly recognize and appropriately manage anaphylaxis. Our results showed that although 64% of all teachers reported previous training in anaphylaxis recognition and 80% had prior training on epinephrine autoinjector administration, 70% were uncertain about recognizing anaphylaxis and considered it a barrier to epinephrine administration. Further, more than half were uncertain about how to administer epinephrine.

Because the ability to recognize a severe allergic reaction is the critical first step in managing anaphylaxis, health care providers should focus attention not only on education about proper autoinjector technique but also on the clinical signs and symptoms of a child in anaphylaxis. A study by Bansal et al. [13] reported that approximately 50% of preschool directors had prior training on identification and treatment of an allergic reaction. Overall, 57% of our participants had received prior training on recognizing anaphylaxis and 71% reported prior training in administering an epinephrine autoinjector.

An important outcome of anaphylaxis education is assessment of the comfort level of preschool staff who will be administering the epinephrine autoinjector in the event of pediatric anaphylaxis. We reported a significant increase in comfort level of recognizing anaphylaxis and administering an epinephrine autoinjector ($P < .001$ for both) when comparing questionnaire responses before and after the education seminar. In our study, one of the most common barriers to autoinjector administration was the lack of comfort in knowing how to use the autoinjector. To our knowledge, no previous study has specifically assessed comfort levels in a preschool staff population and showed a significant increase in comfort for both the recognition of anaphylaxis and the technique for administering epinephrine. Our study indicates that staff had similarly improved comfort levels after the education seminar, regardless of their prior training.

Two participants noted decreased comfort in recognition of anaphylaxis in the postintervention questionnaire. Possible explanations include an overwhelming amount of information in the seminar or a need for different educational mediums to better communicate the information included in the seminar.

Finally, participants in this study showed an increase in correctly sequenced steps for epinephrine autoinjector administration after the intervention. These findings are similar to those of Bansal et al. [13], who reported that, after an allergy seminar, 77% of center directors surveyed would administer intramuscular epinephrine correctly compared with only 24% before the educational seminar.

5. Limitations

Preschools in the area were approached and asked to participate, irrespective of the number of students and faculty,

public versus private status, or prior anaphylaxis training. Consequently, those who agreed to participate in the study may have had a special interest in anaphylaxis in children. The issue with selection bias needs to be considered carefully, as reported by Nguyen Luu et al. [18]. Additionally, although personal demographics of participants were not collected, the participant population was relatively homogenous (e.g., white, middle aged, predominantly female).

Limitations of this study were consistent with limitations inherent in a survey study (e.g., ambiguous or undefined terms within the questionnaire, no demographic assessment of participants, and incomplete surveys). Also, many data points were based on subjective answers from participants.

6. Conclusion

Because of the rise of food allergies in the pediatric population, particularly in children aged 5 years and younger, preschool staff preparedness to recognize and manage anaphylaxis should be regularly assessed and reinforced. This study illustrates a need and desire among preschool staff for more consistent anaphylaxis education and underscores a significant increase in the comfort level of identifying anaphylaxis and administering an epinephrine autoinjector after a brief educational seminar. Further studies are needed to determine the appropriate interval for and most effective means of education to ensure knowledge retention and sufficient anaphylaxis preparedness.

Disclosure

Portions of this paper have been published in abstract form: *Annals of Emergency Medicine*, 2012; 60 Suppl S101.

Conflict of Interests

The authors declare that there is no conflict of interests regarding the publication of this paper.

Acknowledgment

The authors thank Christine M. Lohse for her contributions and statistical support.

References

[1] H. A. Sampson, A. Muñoz-Furlong, R. L. Campbell et al., "Second symposium on the definition and management of anaphylaxis: summary report—second National Institute of Allergy and Infectious Disease/Food Allergy and Anaphylaxis Network symposium," *Annals of Emergency Medicine*, vol. 47, no. 4, pp. 373–380, 2006.

[2] S. A. Rudders, A. Banerji, M. F. Vassallo, S. Clark, and C. A. Camargo, "Trends in pediatric emergency department visits for food-induced anaphylaxis," *Journal of Allergy and Clinical Immunology*, vol. 126, no. 2, pp. 385–388, 2010.

[3] W. W. Decker, R. L. Campbell, V. Manivannan et al., "The etiology and incidence of anaphylaxis in Rochester, Minnesota: a report from the Rochester Epidemiology Project," *Journal of Allergy and Clinical Immunology*, vol. 122, no. 6, pp. 1161–1165, 2008.

[4] S. A. Bock and F. M. Atkins, "The natural history of peanut allergy," *The Journal of Allergy and Clinical Immunology*, vol. 83, no. 5, pp. 900–904, 1989.

[5] H. A. Sampson, "Food-induced anaphylaxis," *Novartis Foundation Symposium*, vol. 257, pp. 161–171, 2004.

[6] A. Nowak-Wegrzyn, M. K. Conover-Walker, and R. A. Wood, "Food-allergic reactions in schools and preschools," *Archives of Pediatrics and Adolescent Medicine*, vol. 155, no. 7, pp. 790–795, 2001.

[7] P. Joshi, C. H. Katelaris, and B. Frankum, "Adrenaline (epinephrine) autoinjector use in preschools," *Journal of Allergy and Clinical Immunology*, vol. 124, no. 2, pp. 383–384, 2009.

[8] K. A. DeMuth and A. M. Fitzpatrick, "Epinephrine autoinjector availability among children with food allergy," *Allergy and Asthma Proceedings*, vol. 32, no. 4, pp. 295–300, 2011.

[9] H. A. Sampson, L. Mendelson, and J. P. Rosen, "Fatal and near-fatal anaphylactic reactions to food in children and adolescents," *The New England Journal of Medicine*, vol. 327, no. 6, pp. 380–384, 1992.

[10] S. A. Bock, A. Muoz-Furlong, and H. A. Sampson, "Fatalities due to anaphylactic reactions to foods," *Journal of Allergy and Clinical Immunology*, vol. 107, no. 1, pp. 191–193, 2001.

[11] S. A. Bock, A. Muñoz-Furlong, and H. A. Sampson, "Further fatalities caused by anaphylactic reactions to food, 2001–2006," *Journal of Allergy and Clinical Immunology*, vol. 119, no. 4, pp. 1016–1018, 2007.

[12] T. J. Gaeta, S. Clark, A. J. Pelletier, and C. A. Camargo Jr., "National study of US emergency department visits for acute allergic reactions, 1993 to 2004," *Annals of Allergy, Asthma and Immunology*, vol. 98, no. 4, pp. 360–365, 2007.

[13] P. J. Bansal, R. Marsh, B. Patel, and M. C. Tobin, "Recognition, evaluation, and treatment of anaphylaxis in the child care setting," *Annals of Allergy, Asthma and Immunology*, vol. 94, no. 1, pp. 55–59, 2005.

[14] G. S. Rhim and M. S. McMorris, "School readiness for children with food allergies," *Annals of Allergy, Asthma and Immunology*, vol. 86, no. 2, pp. 172–176, 2001.

[15] B. M. Patel, P. J. Bansal, and M. C. Tobin, "Management of anaphylaxis in child care centers: evaluation 6 and 12 months after an intervention program," *Annals of Allergy, Asthma and Immunology*, vol. 97, no. 6, pp. 813–815, 2006.

[16] J. J. Koplin, P. E. Martin, and K. J. Allen, "An update on epidemiology of anaphylaxis in children and adults," *Current Opinion in Allergy and Clinical Immunology*, vol. 11, no. 5, pp. 492–496, 2011.

[17] K. Sasaki, S. Sugiura, T. Matsui et al., "A workshop with practical training for anaphylaxis management improves the self-efficacy of school personnel," *Allergology International*, vol. 64, no. 2, pp. 156–160, 2015.

[18] N. U. Nguyen Luu, L. Cicutto, L. Soller et al., "Management of anaphylaxis in schools: evaluation of an epinephrine autoinjector (EpiPen) use by school personnel and comparison of two approaches of soliciting participation," *Allergy, Asthma and Clinical Immunology*, vol. 8, article 4, 2012.

3

The Differences and Similarities between Allergists and Non-Allergists for Penicillin Allergy Management

Nayot Suetrong[1] and Jettanong Klaewsongkram[2]

[1] *Department of Medicine, Faculty of Medicine, Chulalongkorn University, Bangkok 10330, Thailand*
[2] *Division of Allergy and Clinical Immunology, Department of Medicine, Faculty of Medicine,*
 and Allergy and Clinical Immunology Research Group, Chulalongkorn University, Bangkok 10330, Thailand

Correspondence should be addressed to Jettanong Klaewsongkram; jettanong.k@chula.ac.th

Academic Editor: William E. Berger

The purpose of this study was to compare the management of patients with a history of penicillin allergy between allergists and non-allergists in Thailand. A questionnaire was distributed to Thai physicians by online survey. The answers from 205 physicians were analyzed. The discrepancy of penicillin allergy management between allergists and non-allergists was clearly demonstrated in patients with a history of an immediate reaction in the presence of penicillin skin test ($P < 0.01$) and in patients with a history of Stevens-Johnson syndrome ($P < 0.05$) from penicillin. Allergists are more willing to confirm penicillin allergic status, more likely to carefully administer penicillin even after negative skin test, but less concerned for the potential cross-reactivity with 3rd and 4th generation cephalosporins, compared to non-allergists. The lack of penicillin skin test reagents, the reliability of penicillin allergy history, and medicolegal problem were the main reasons for prescribing alternate antibiotics without confirmation of penicillin allergic status. In summary, the different management of penicillin allergy between allergists and non-allergists was significantly demonstrated in patients with a history of severe non-immediate reaction and in patients with a history of an immediate reaction when a penicillin skin test is available.

1. Introduction

Penicillin allergy is one of the most commonly reported drug allergies worldwide. About 10% of the general population report suspected allergic reactions to penicillin [1]. However, only a minority of patients with such a history are actually allergic to penicillin(s), based on the results of allergological work-up [2]. In real life, most physicians prefer to prescribe alternate antibiotics to these patients, unless a penicillin allergic status can be excluded [3, 4]. Since the prescription of alternate antibiotics may have undesirable consequences in terms of antibiotic susceptibility, adverse reactions, and health economics, the confirmation of penicillin allergic status would be beneficial in patients with a suspected history of penicillin allergy.

In clinical practice, the confirmation of penicillin allergic status is not always feasible, which results in unnecessary avoidance of beta-lactam antibiotics in patients who are over-diagnosed [5]. It is well recognized nowadays that the cross-reactivity rate among beta-lactams is lower than previously expected [6]. However, the consensus recommendation of antibiotic selection in these "suspected" penicillin allergic patients has yet to be established [7–9]. Allergists, physicians specialized in managing allergy and immunology disorders, are responsible for confirming penicillin allergic status, preventing overdiagnosis, and determining appropriate alternative antibiotics. In reality, the number of certified allergists in many countries may not be sufficient to manage this common problem. This task is particularly difficult in Thailand, as there are only 148 certified allergists (28 adult allergists and 120 pediatric allergists), among a total of 45,124 medical doctors, or an equivalent of 0.3% registered medical doctors in the country [10]. As a result, the selection of antibiotics in these patients is often decided by doctors of other specialties in real life before they can seek help from allergists. Even among Thai allergists themselves, penicillin skin test is mainly performed by using penicillin G alone and the use of penicilloyl-polylysine and minor determinant mixture is mostly limited for research purposes. The confirmation of drug allergy status has not been emphasized in medical school curriculum resulting in inadequate knowledge for non-allergists to handle this problem. The potential role of pharmacists in conducting penicillin skin testing in these patients has also been suggested but rarely implemented [11].

It is understandable that doctors in other specialties may have limited knowledge and different perspectives about managing allergic disorders, as compared to allergists [12]. Their perspectives and fundamental knowledge on penicillin allergy might have an impact on how they manage these patients in clinical practice.

The lack of allergists and standard skin test reagents for the diagnosis of penicillin allergy makes the confirmation of penicillin allergic status not always possible [13–17]. Types of medical practice settings and clinical practice duration may also influence the selection of antibiotics in patients with a history of penicillin allergy. The selection of antibiotic prescription in patients with different types of previous penicillin reactions could be influenced by several factors such as the availability of skin test reagents and medicolegal risk. It would be interesting to know how patients with a history of penicillin allergy are mainly managed in the real life by non-allergists where certified allergists may not always be available.

The purpose of this study was to comparatively survey the management of penicillin allergy between allergists and non-allergists in Thailand in patients with different patterns of penicillin-induced suspected allergic reactions. The awareness of cross-reactivity among beta-lactam antibiotics as well as the knowledge and attitudes towards penicillin allergy management was also determined. The impacts of areas of expertise, types of medical practice settings, and duration of clinical practice on penicillin allergy management were also analyzed.

2. Methods and Materials

This study was a cross-sectional survey on the management of patients with a suspected history of penicillin allergy in Thailand. After approval by the Ethics and Research Committee of Faculty of Medicine at Chulalongkorn University, the web-based questionnaire was created by using Google Docs and e-mailed to 1,000 Thai physicians (57 allergists and 943 non-allergists in various fields) throughout the country. The questionnaire was focused on four aspects: (1) the management of patients with a history of penicillin-induced immediate reactions in the presence and absence of penicillin skin test reagents, (2) the management of patients with a history of penicillin-induced non-immediate reactions, (3) the prescription of other beta-lactams in patients with a history of penicillin allergy, and (4) the fundamental knowledge of penicillin allergy skin testing and attitudes towards the management of patients with a history of penicillin allergy in

TABLE 1: Characteristics of Thai physicians participating in this survey.

Physicians	Total ($N = 205$)
Area of expertise	
General practitioners	54 (26.3%)
Internists and pediatricians	83 (40.5%)
Allergists	29 (14.1%)
Other specialists	39 (19.0%)
Medical practice settings	
Primary care hospitals	39 (19.0%)
General hospitals/provincial hospitals	47 (22.9%)
Academic institutes	94 (45.9%)
Private practice	25 (12.2%)
Medical practice duration	
Less than 5 years	94 (45.9%)
5–10 years	62 (30.2%)
More than 10 years	49 (23.9%)

Thailand. Details of the web-based questionnaire are available in Supplemental Appendix A in Supplementary Material available online at http://dx.doi.org/10.1155/2014/214183).

The online survey responses were automatically collected and subsequently analyzed using SPSS 17.0 for Windows (SPSS, Chicago, Il, USA). The actual rates of penicillin allergy in patients with a suspected history estimated by physicians were calculated by using class interval arithmetic means. Chi-square test and multinomial logistic regression were used for univariate and multivariate analysis. P values < 0.05 were considered statistically significant.

3. Results

3.1. Characteristics of Thai Physicians Participating in This Survey. A total of 205 completed surveys were received (a 20.5% response rate) from the online questionnaire. 14.1% were adult or pediatric allergists, while 26.3%, 40.5%, and 19.0% were general practitioners, internists or pediatricians (excluding allergists), and other specialists, respectively. Almost half (45.9%) of the responders worked for an academic institute (university hospital or research center) and 19.0% worked in a primary care hospital, 22.9% in a general/provincial hospital, and 12.2% in the private practice sector. About 45.9% of the responders have less than 5-year experience in clinical practice, while 30.2% and 23.9% of them have 5–10 years and more than 10 years of practice experience, respectively (Table 1).

3.2. The Management of Patients with a History of Penicillin-Induced Immediate Reaction according to the Availability and Result of Penicillin Skin Testing. When penicillin administration was indicated, the different management between allergists and non-allergists in patients with a history of penicillin-induced immediate reaction was not statistically different if skin testing was positive (P value = 0.06) but was clearly

(a)

(b)

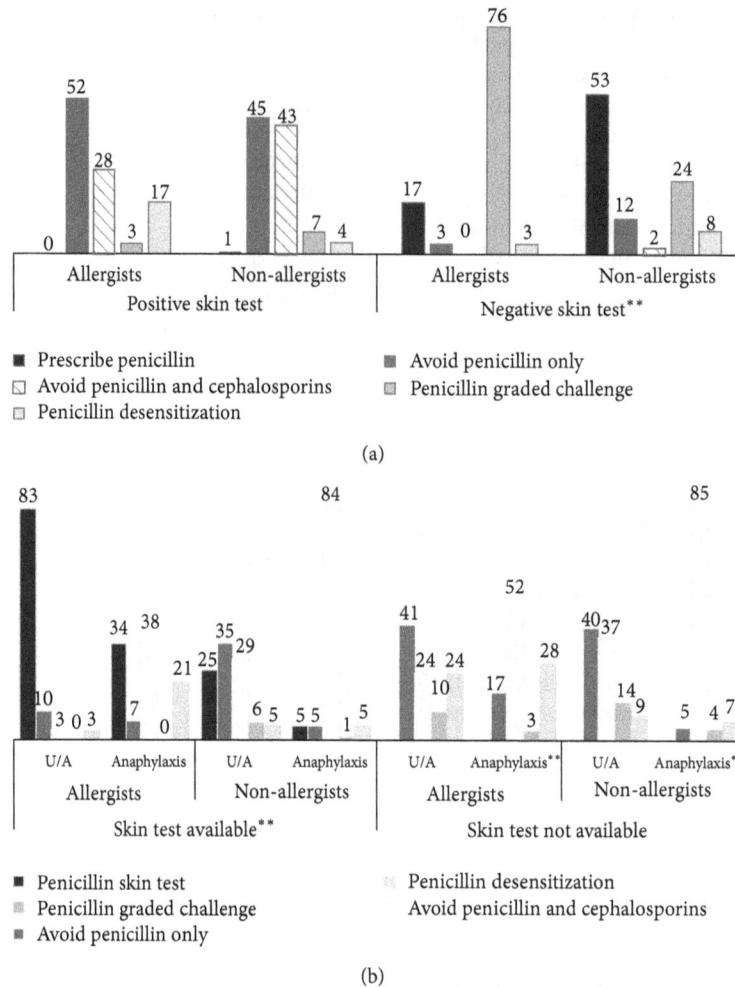

FIGURE 1: Management of patients with a history of penicillin-induced immediate reaction. The difference in penicillin allergy management between patients with mild and severe immediate allergic reactions was clearly demonstrated regardless of skin test availability and depending on penicillin skin test results (data represent percentages of each group, ∗∗ represents P values < 0.01 between allergists and non-allergists, and U/A: urticaria and/or angioedema).

demonstrated if the penicillin skin test was negative (P value < 0.01) (Figure 1(a)). 79.3% of allergists and 88.1% of non-allergists would avoid penicillin or both penicillin and cephalosporins if penicillin skin testing yielded a positive result. In contrast, 75.9% of allergists would use graded challenge first if penicillin skin test was negative, while 53.4% of non-allergists would prescribe penicillin normally.

A question was addressed whether the severity of the immediate reaction influenced patient management in the presence or absence of penicillin skin test reagents (Figure 1(b)). The difference of decision making between allergists and non-allergists was observed in patients for whom penicillin was indicated regardless of clinical severity and who had been skin-tested with penicillin reagents (P values < 0.01). If a penicillin skin test was not available, the management of patients with a history of penicillin-induced severe immediate reaction (anaphylaxis) between allergists and non-allergists was still different (P value < 0.01), but no longer different (P value = 0.12) in patients

with a history of penicillin-induced mild immediate reaction (urticaria and/or angioedema).

In patients with a history of anaphylaxis, 83.5–84.7% of non-allergists would avoid both penicillin and cephalosporins regardless of skin testing availability. In contrast, 34.5% of allergists would perform a penicillin skin test if available, and 20.7% considered prescribing penicillin using a desensitization technique in patients requiring penicillin therapy. In patients with a history of penicillin-induced urticaria or angioedema, 82.8% of allergists would perform penicillin skin testing first, while only 25.0% of non-allergists would do so. However, if the penicillin skin test was not available, the majority of physicians (65.5% of allergists and 77.3% of non-allergists) would avoid both penicillin and cephalosporins.

3.3. The Management of Patients with a History of Penicillin-Induced Non-Immediate Reaction. Regarding the management of patients with a history of penicillin-induced non-immediate reaction, the prescription pattern between

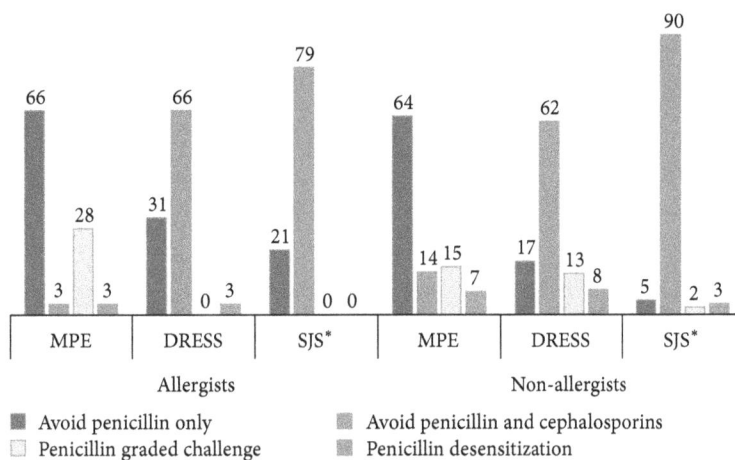

FIGURE 2: Management of patients with a history of penicillin-induced non-immediate reactions. Antibiotic prescription among Thai physicians in patients with various manifestations of penicillin-induced non-immediate reaction (data represent percentages of each group, * represents P value < 0.05 between allergists and non-allergists, MPE: maculopapular exanthema, DRESS; drug reaction with eosinophilia and systemic symptoms, SJS: Stevens-Johnson syndrome).

allergists and non-allergists was significantly different in Stevens-Johnson syndrome (SJS, P value = 0.03), borderline different in drug reaction with eosinophilia and systemic symptoms (DRESS, P value = 0.05), but not statistically different in maculopapular exanthema (MPE, P value = 0.20) (Figure 2). Only 3.4% of allergists would readminister penicillin with graded challenge or desensitization methods in patients with a history of DRESS, while 21.1% of non-allergists considered doing so. Some of non-allergists (5.7%) still considered prescribing penicillin with graded challenge or desensitization methods in patients with a history of SJS, while none of allergists would do it. In contrast, the majority of both allergists (65.5%) and non-allergists (63.6%) would avoid only penicillin in patients with a history of penicillin-induced MPE.

3.4. Patterns of Beta-Lactam Prescription in Patients with Unconfirmed Allergic Reaction to Penicillin.

When penicillin skin test reagents are not available, the decision making between allergists and non-allergists in terms of beta-lactam prescription in patients with an unconfirmed history of an immediate reaction to penicillin was different in the case of first generation and third/fourth generation cephalosporins (P values < 0.01) but not with other drugs (Figure 3). Aminopenicillins were completely avoided by more than 60% of all Thai physicians, while about half of them considered carbapenem and monobactam "prescribable." First generation cephalosporins would be completely avoided by 48.3% of allergists or prescribed with precaution by 41.4%. In contrast, only 18.8% of non-allergists would completely avoid these drugs, while 58.0% of non-allergists indicated that they would prescribe them with precaution. For third and fourth generation cephalosporins, 62.1% of allergists said that they could be prescribed, while only 29.5% of non-allergists agreed so.

3.5. Knowledge and Attitudes of Thai Physicians towards the Management of Patients with a History of Penicillin Allergy.

Regarding basic knowledge of penicillin skin testing for diagnosis of an immediate reaction, less than half of non-allergists (29.1%) have accurate knowledge on the appropriate recommended skin test reagents (penicilloyl-polylysine and minor determinants) and only 5.1% of them know how to correctly interpret penicillin skin test results according to the ENDA recommendation (an increase in wheal diameter greater than 3 mm read 15–20 minutes after the test compared to the initial wheal size) [18]. It is worth noting that only 48.3% of trained allergists in Thailand could properly interpret the result of penicillin skin tests as well (Figure 4). The actual rate of penicillin allergy in patients with a suspected history estimated by allergists was significantly lower than that estimated by non-allergists (18.9% to 35.6%, resp., P value = 0.02).

A difference in opinion between allergists and non-allergists was observed. The preferred approach to manage patients with a history of an immediate reaction to penicillin was significantly different between allergists and non-allergists (P value = 0.04). While the majority of allergists (69.0%) favored penicillin skin tests over penicillin avoidance (24.1%), both approaches were equally elected by the non-allergist group (39.2–40.3% each). The reasons for prescribing an alternate drug without confirming penicillin allergy status were not statistically different between allergists and non-allergists (P value = 0.50). The easy availability of alternate antibiotics was the main reason, followed by a convincing drug allergy history. Interestingly, the medicolegal problem was another main concern for Thai physicians, especially among non-allergists.

3.6. Multivariate Analysis of Factors Influencing Penicillin Allergy Management among Thai Physicians.

Factors possibly influencing penicillin allergy management were analysed

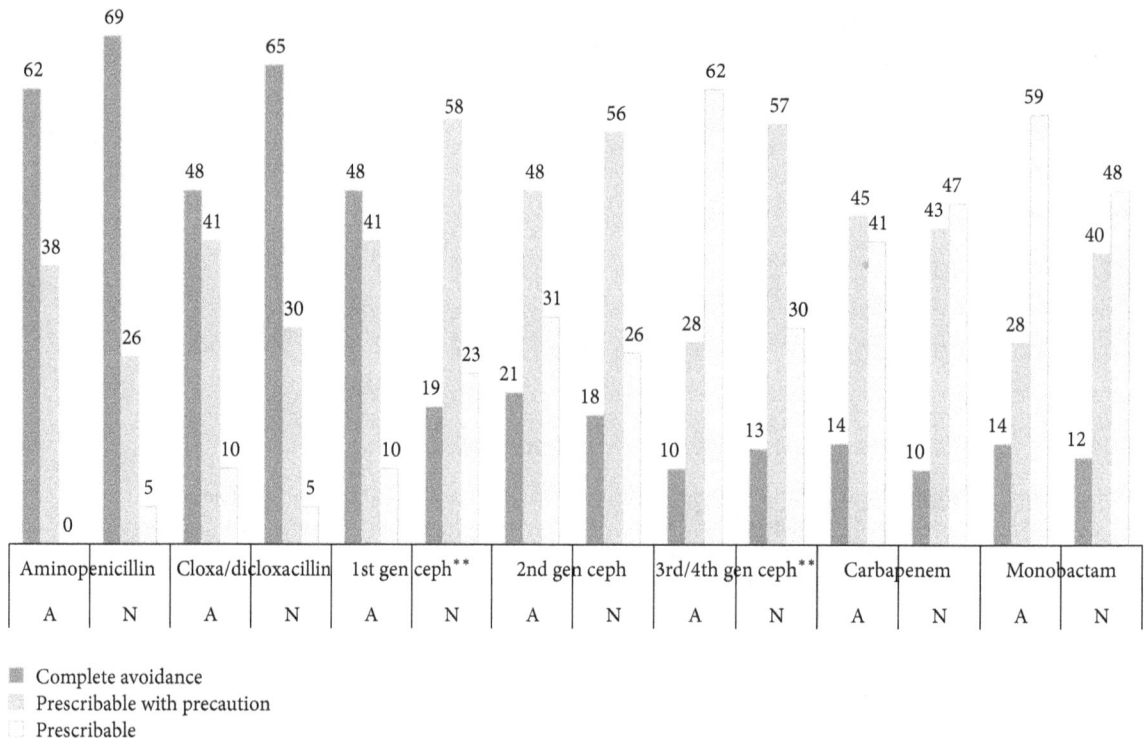

FIGURE 3: Patterns of beta-lactam prescription in patients with unconfirmed allergic reactions to penicillin. The cross-reactivity between penicillin and other beta-lactams was mainly concerned among Thai physicians when prescribing aminopenicillin and the different decision making between allergists and non-allergists was significantly observed when prescribing first or third/fourth generations of cephalosporins (data represent percentages of each group, ∗∗ represents P values < 0.01 between allergists and non-allergists, gen ceph: generations of cephalosporin, A: allergists, and N: non-allergists).

based on physician's area of expertise, medical practice setting, and clinical practice duration. The results indicated that the most important factor determining the management of penicillin allergy was the area of expertise (see Supplemental Appendix B). After multivariate analysis, penicillin allergy management by allergists was significantly different from non-allergist counterparts (Figure 5).

Non-allergists preferred to confirm an allergic history by means of skin tests in patients with a history of penicillin-induced urticaria and anaphylaxis, much less than allergists would do (0.07- and 0.10-fold, resp.), and less likely to administer penicillin with graded challenge technique (0.10-fold) in patients with a suspected history of penicillin allergy after negative skin test, compared to allergists. In contrast, non-allergists were more likely to avoid not only penicillin but also cephalosporins in patients with a history of penicillin-induced anaphylaxis and SJS than allergists would do so (6.62- and 5.15-fold, resp.). Interestingly, they avoided first generation cephalosporins much less than allergists (0.17-fold) in patients with a history of penicillin allergy. Probably due to limited knowledge in penicillin skin test procedure and interpretation, non-allergists rather preferred to avoid penicillin (7.29 folds) than to confirm allergic status (0.14 fold), as compared to their allergist counterparts.

Clinical practice duration also had some influence since physicians with less than 5 years of experience in practice

were more in favor of penicillin allergy confirmation (4.65-fold) than those practicing medicine longer than 10 years and were less likely to avoid cephalosporins in patients with a history of penicillin-induced DRESS (0.11-fold).

4. Discussion

Although allergists are primarily responsible for the management of patients with a history of a drug allergy, in the real life, these patients are often cared for by doctors in other specialties due to the shortage of certified allergists in some areas. This study surveyed how the problem of penicillin allergy in different circumstances was managed by allergists and non-allergists, including their knowledge and attitudes towards this problem.

Our study shows that allergists are more willing to confirm the status of penicillin allergy and more inclined to use a desensitization procedure in patients with a history of penicillin-induced immediate reaction, as compared to non-allergists. The study also shows that the limited availability of penicillin skin tests clearly impacts their clinical judgment. If the penicillin skin testing was not available, the discrepancy of patient management between allergists and non-allergists in patients with a history of penicillin-induced urticaria or angioedema would no longer be observed, since allergists

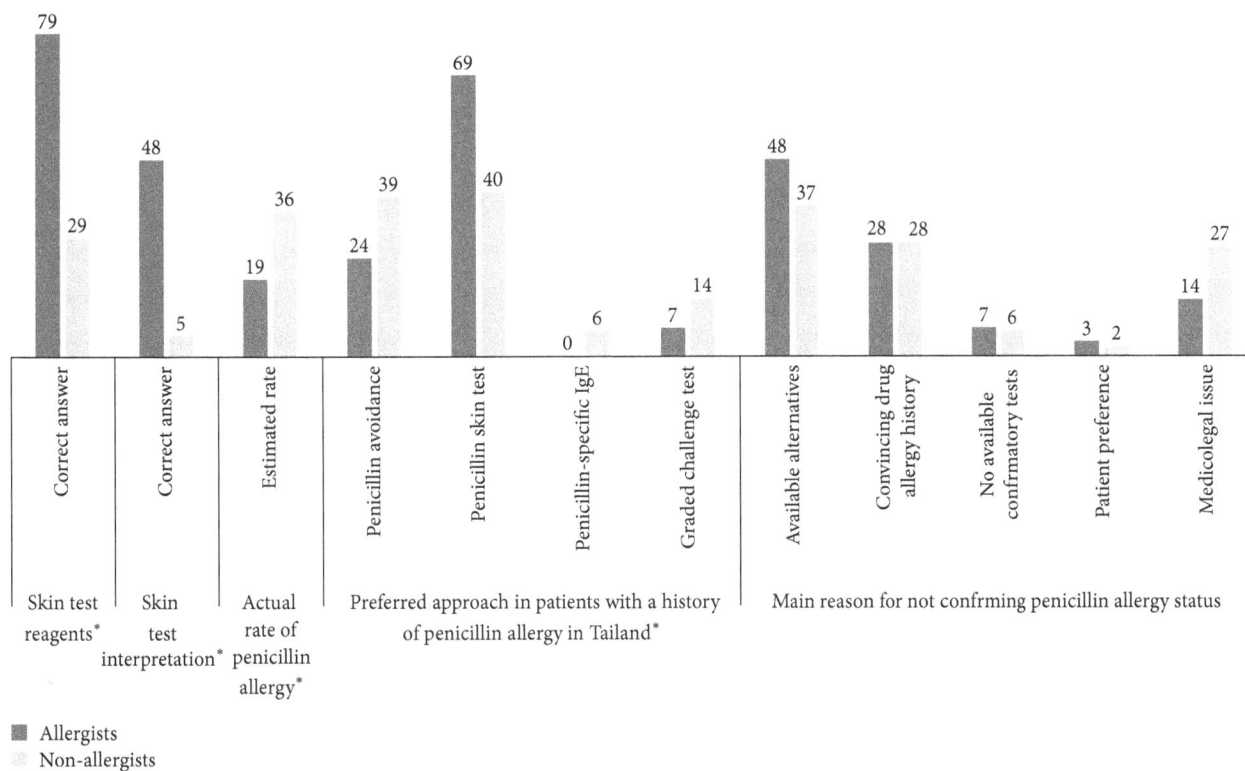

FIGURE 4: Knowledge and attitudes towards the management of patients with a history of penicillin-induced immediate reactions. Non-allergists have limited knowledge concerning penicillin skin test reagents and interpretation. Different opinions between allergists and non-allergists were demonstrated regarding the reasons for not confirming penicillin allergy status and the preferred approach to confirm penicillin allergy (data represent percentages of each group; * represents P values < 0.05 between allergists and non-allergists).

also avoided penicillin ± cephalosporins in these cases. Interestingly, the majority of allergists were very cautious when prescribing penicillin in patients with a suspected history even after a negative penicillin skin test, while half of non-allergists would prescribe penicillin normally in a similar circumstance.

Different views on beta-lactam cross-reactivity between allergists and non-allergists were noted. Interestingly, allergists were more reluctant to prescribe first generation cephalosporins in penicillin allergic patients while being less concerned about third/fourth generation cephalosporins, as compared to their non-allergist counterparts. Current data indicates that the potential cross-reactivity with penicillin is noteworthy only in first generation cephalosporins [19]. In terms of non-immediate reactions, more non-allergists considered avoiding cephalosporins in patients with a history of penicillin-induced SJS, as compared to allergists. No statistical difference was observed between allergists and non-allergists in the management of penicillin-induced MPE and DRESS. However, allergists seemed less likely to perform graded challenge or desensitize patients with previous DRESS.

Regarding knowledge and attitudes towards penicillin allergy management, it was clear that non-allergists have limited knowledge regarding penicillin skin test reagents and interpretation as compared to certified allergists. Even

though both allergists and non-allergists agreed that majority of patients with a history of penicillin allergy are not truly allergic, the allergists' estimated rate of penicillin allergy in these patients was significantly lower than that of their non-allergist counterparts. Surprisingly, less than half of Thai allergists could correctly interpret penicillin skin test results as well. A refresher course for allergists on drug allergy testing should be organized. The appropriate modalities of allergological work-up in patients with suspected beta-lactam hypersensitivity should be finalized. The lack of penicillin metabolites (penicilloyl-polylysine and minor determinant mixture) could potentially be replaced by the soluble forms of the suspected beta-lactams or other beta-lactams from the same classes, along with benzylpenicillin and aminopenicillin, as skin test reagents since they are more easily available and have good predictive values in clinical practice [20].

While penicillin skin testing was more favoured among allergists, many non-allergists still preferred penicillin avoidance. The availability of alternate drugs and the convincing drug allergy history were the main factors for prescription of alternate antibiotics instead of the confirmation of penicillin allergy status. It is worth mentioning that the medicolegal problem from harmful reactions, which are possible after a drug rechallenge, was one of the major concerns for not confirming the status of penicillin allergy particularly among non-allergists. The launch of a national standard practice

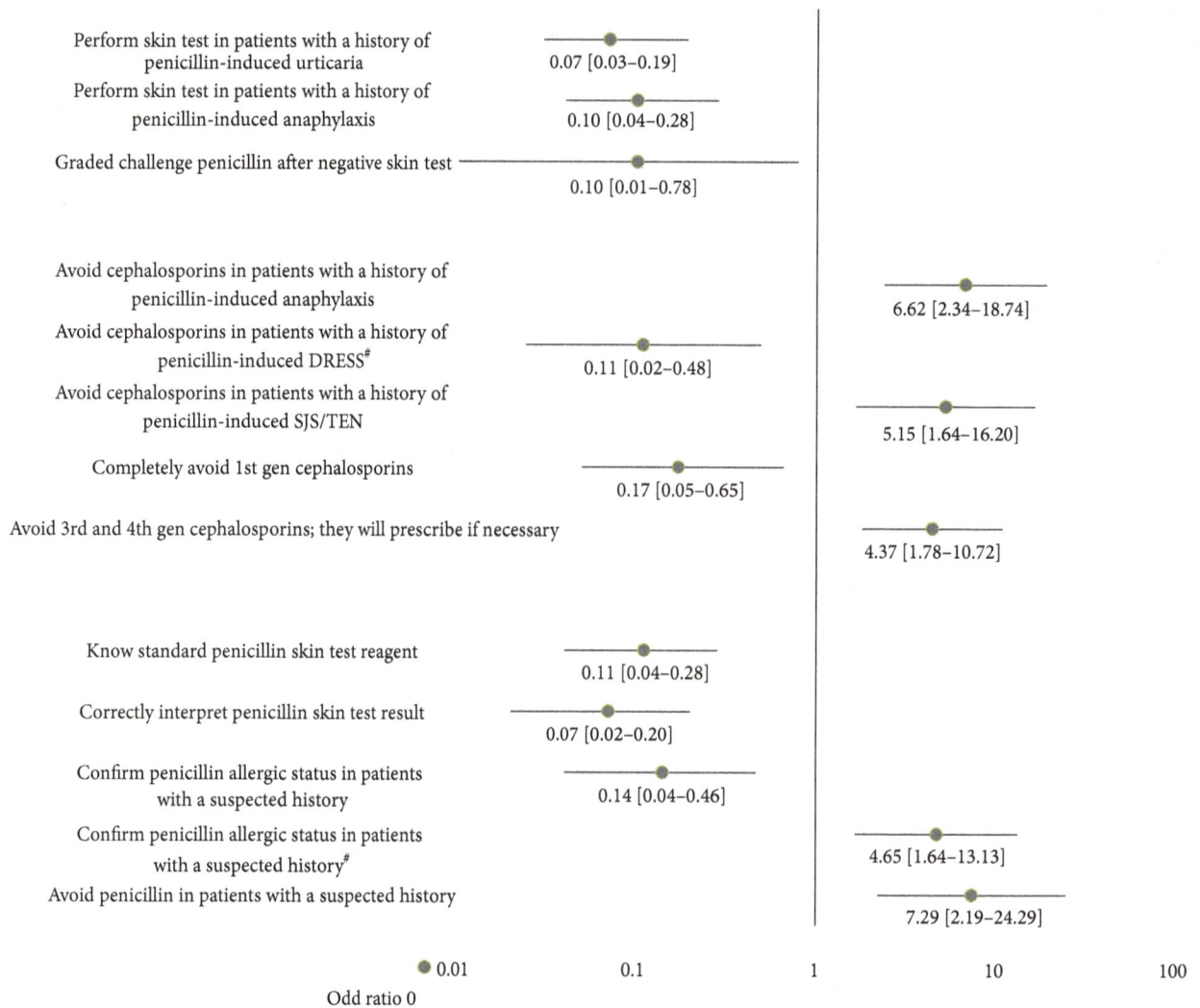

FIGURE 5: Factors affecting penicillin allergy management. Multivariate analysis by using multinomial logistic regression demonstrates that area of expertise was the main factor determining penicillin allergy management. Data represent the odds ratio with 95% confidence intervals of how non-allergists manage penicillin allergy compared to allergists except #, which represent the odds ratio with 95% confidence intervals of how physicians who have less than 5 years' clinical experience manage penicillin allergy compared to those who have longer than 10 years' clinical experience.

guideline to manage patients with a history of penicillin allergy would be helpful to prevent medicolegal problems. Health economics and outcome research regarding the confirmation of penicillin allergy in patients with a suspected history should be carefully investigated.

The study demonstrates the diversity of management in patients with a history of penicillin allergy among Thai physicians, although most of them knew that only a minority of these patients are truly allergic. Although the duration of medical practice may also play a role, the results of our study emphasize that the area of expertise was the most important factor determining penicillin allergy management. As the different opinions between allergists and non-allergists were statistically significant in patients with a history of severe non-immediate reaction and in patients with a history of mild immediate reaction if penicillin skin test reagents are

available, we recommend that these patients are managed by allergists. Nevertheless, penicillin skin test reagents should be provided to practice allergists and the accurate skin test procedure emphasized. In contrast, it might be possible that non-allergists should be allowed to handle patients with a history of penicillin-induced mild non-immediate reaction (simple MPE) if no certified allergist is available. According to our study, the current approach between allergists and non-allergists in this patient group is already similar. In fact, graded challenge test is the recommended procedure for any physicians knowledgeable in treating adverse drug reactions to manage these patients, since the risk to develop severe reaction is small [21]. In this regard, updated information about beta-lactam cross-reactivity and drug readministration by graded challenge technique should be provided to non-allergists to minimize patient risk.

There are some limitations to this study. The ratio of non-allergists to allergists was 6 : 1 due to the limited number of allergists in the country. In fact, the number of allergists who replied to this survey was already one-fifth of total certified allergists in Thailand. The response rate was rather low but still within a similar range to prior studies [3, 9]. Data from this study may not represent the views of Thai physicians as a whole since almost half of the responders worked in academia. Although medical practice setting alone did not have a significant impact on penicillin allergy management after multivariate adjustment, stratified survey in all types of medical practice could possibly be conducted to reduce response bias.

5. Conclusions

The different management of penicillin allergy between allergists and non-allergists was mainly observed in patients with a history of severe non-immediate reaction and in patients with a history of an immediate reaction, particularly in the patients who have been skin-tested with penicillin reagents. Pitfalls in penicillin allergy management by both allergists and non-allergists are addressed. The possible role of non-allergists in the management of patients with a history of penicillin-induced mild non-immediate reaction has been raised.

Conflict of Interests

The authors declare that there is no conflict of interests regarding the publication of this paper.

Acknowledgment

This study was supported by the Special Task Force for Activating Research (STAR), Chulalongkorn University.

References

[1] R. Y. Lin, "A perspective on penicillin allergy," *Archives of Internal Medicine*, vol. 152, no. 5, pp. 930–937, 1992.

[2] A. R. Salkind, P. G. Cuddy, and J. W. Foxworth, "Is this patient allergic to penicillin?: an evidence-based analysis of the likelihood of penicillin allergy," *Journal of the American Medical Association*, vol. 285, no. 19, pp. 2498–2505, 2001.

[3] R. Solensky, H. S. Earl, and R. S. Gruchalla, "Clinical approach to penicillin-allergic patients: a survey," *Annals of Allergy, Asthma and Immunology*, vol. 84, no. 3, pp. 329–333, 2000.

[4] T. C. Puchner Jr. and M. C. Zacharisen, "A survey of antibiotic prescribing and knowledge of penicillin allergy," *Annals of Allergy, Asthma and Immunology*, vol. 88, no. 1, pp. 24–29, 2002.

[5] E. J. MacLaughlin, J. J. Saseen, and D. C. Malone, "Costs of β-lactam allergies: selection and costs of antibiotics for patients with a reported β-lactam allergy," *Archives of Family Medicine*, vol. 9, no. 8, pp. 722–726, 2000.

[6] M. E. Pichichero, "A review of evidence supporting the American Academy of Pediatrics recommendation for prescribing cephalosporin antibiotics for penicillin-allergic patients," *Pediatrics*, vol. 115, no. 4, pp. 1048–1057, 2005.

[7] American Academy of Allergy, Asthma and Immunology, "Drug allergy: an updated practice parameter," *Annals of Allergy, Asthma & Immunology*, vol. 105, no. 4, pp. 259–273, 2010.

[8] B. A. Cunha, "Antibiotic selection in the penicillin-allergic patient," *Medical Clinics of North America*, vol. 90, no. 6, pp. 1257–1264, 2006.

[9] T. Prematta, S. Shah, and F. T. Ishmael, "Physician approaches to beta-lactam use in patients with penicillin hypersensitivity," *Allergy and Asthma Proceedings*, vol. 33, no. 2, pp. 145–151, 2012.

[10] The Medical Council of Thailand, http://www.tmc.or.th/pdf/Summary2555_Graph_SubSpecifically_forTMCWebsite.pdf.

[11] G. C. Wall, L. Peters, C. B. Leaders, and J. A. Wille, "Pharmacist-managed service providing penicillin allergy skin tests," *American Journal of Health-System Pharmacy*, vol. 61, no. 12, pp. 1271–1275, 2004.

[12] P. W. Ewan, "Provision of allergy care for optimal outcome in the UK," *British Medical Bulletin*, vol. 56, no. 4, pp. 1087–1101, 2000.

[13] M. Picard, P. Bégin, H. Bouchard, J. Cloutier, J. Lacombe-Barrios, J. Paradis et al., "Treatment of patients with a history of penicillin allergy in a large tertiary-care academic hospital," *Journal of Allergy and Clinical Immunology in Practice*, vol. 1, pp. 252–257, 2013.

[14] A. T. Nagao-Dias, A. C. Pereira, M. F. E. Silva, E. D. R. Néri, J. W. Accioly, and J. E. S. Lima, "Implementation of a penicillin allergy skin test," *Brazilian Journal of Pharmaceutical Sciences*, vol. 45, no. 3, pp. 567–572, 2009.

[15] P. Wangrattanasopon, K. Ruxrungtham, H. Chantaphakul, S. Buranapraditkun, and J. Klaewsongkram, "Alkali-treated penicillin G solution is a better option than penicillin G as an alternative source of minor determinants for penicillin skin test," *Allergy and Asthma Proceedings*, vol. 33, no. 2, pp. 152–159, 2012.

[16] M. J. Torres and M. Blanca, "Importance of skin testing with major and minor determinants of benzylpenicillin in the diagnosis of allergy to betalactams. Statement from the European Network for Drug Allergy concerning AllergoPen withdrawal," *Allergy*, vol. 61, no. 8, pp. 910–911, 2006.

[17] S. H. Lee, H. W. Park, S. H. Kim et al., "The current practice of skin testing for antibiotics in Korean hospitals," *Korean Journal of Internal Medicine*, vol. 25, no. 2, pp. 207–212, 2010.

[18] M. J. Torres, M. Blanca, J. Fernandez et al., "Diagnosis of immediate allergic reactions to beta-lactam antibiotics," *Allergy*, vol. 58, no. 10, pp. 961–972, 2003.

[19] J. D. Campagna, M. C. Bond, E. Schabelman, and B. D. Hayes, "The use of cephalosporins in penicillin-allergic patients: a literature review," *Journal of Emergency Medicine*, vol. 42, pp. 612–620, 2012.

[20] C. Ponvert, Y. Perrin, A. Bados-Albiero et al., "Allergy to beta-lactam antibiotics in children: results of a 20-year study based on clinical history, skin and challenge tests," *Pediatric Allergy and Immunology*, vol. 22, no. 4, pp. 411–418, 2011.

[21] A. B. Yates, "Management of patients with a history of allergy to beta-lactam antibiotics," *The American Journal of Medicine*, vol. 121, no. 7, pp. 572–576, 2008.

4

Adipokines and Cysteinyl Leukotrienes in the Pathogenesis of Asthma

Michael J. Coffey, Barbara Torretti, and Peter Mancuso

Division of Pulmonary and Critical Care Medicine, University of Michigan Medical Center, Ann Arbor, MI 48109, USA

Correspondence should be addressed to Michael J. Coffey; coffeym@umich.edu

Academic Editor: Marek L. Kowalski

Background. The prevalence of obesity has increased dramatically over the last decades, and its association with asthma is being increasingly recognized. *Aims.* Our hypothesis is that increased leptin and decreased adiponectin levels in obese subjects play a direct role in regulating inflammation in asthmatics. We wanted to examine the hypothesis that cysteinyl leukotrienes (cys-LT), inflammatory mediators that are regulated by adipokines, are involved in the pathogenesis of asthma. *Methods.* We studied a population of asthmatics and nonasthmatics, who in turn were divided into obese and nonobese categories. We examined leptin and its ratio to adiponectin, in asthmatics and nonasthmatics, with and without obesity. In addition, we measured cys-LT levels in exhaled breath condensate (EBC) and in peripheral blood monocytes (PBM) in these groups. *Results.* Leptin levels were increased in obese asthmatics compared to obese nonasthmatics. The leptin/adiponectin (L/A) ratio was higher in obese asthmatics compared to obese nonasthmatics. EBC cys-LT levels were elevated in asthmatics compared to nonasthmatics. *Discussion.* Proinflammatory adipokines, released from adipose tissue, may promote an asthma phenotype through enhanced cys-LT production that may result in more prevalent and difficult to control airway disease.

1. Introduction

Over the past 30 years there has been a dramatic increase in the prevalence in obesity in the US, from 18% in the 80s to approximately 35% in 2010 [1, 2]. In parallel, there has been an increase in the prevalence of asthma from 30.7 to 53.8 per thousand population between 1980 and 1994 [3]. A prospective epidemiologic study demonstrated a positive independent association between obesity and the incidence of adult onset asthma [4]. Likewise, using National Health and Nutrition Examination Survey data, Ma et al. have reported an independent association between obesity and atopic and nonatopic asthma [5]. Furthermore, obesity is independently associated with increased bronchial hyperresponsiveness [6]. Intervention with weight reduction improves airway narrowing and bronchial hyperresponsiveness [7]. Obesity is associated with a dose-dependent increase in the odds of incident asthma [8, 9].

Leukotrienes (LT) are potent lipid mediators of inflammation derived from arachidonic acid known to play a critical role in the pathogenesis of asthma. Arachidonic acid is acted upon by the enzyme 5-lipoxygenase to synthesize LTB_4 and cysteinyl leukotrienes (cys-LT C_4, D_4, and E_4). Both cys-LT and LTB_4 are released by neutrophils, eosinophils, mast cells, peripheral blood monocytes, and macrophages and are involved in the pathogenesis of obstructive lung disease [10]. LT synthesis has been shown to be increased in peripheral blood leukocytes [11, 12], airway macrophages, and eosinophils [13] from asthmatics compared to cells from healthy controls. Asthma with obesity is often difficult to control and manifests steroid resistance [14]. Interestingly, obese subjects that had reduced responsiveness to inhaled corticosteroids with increasing body mass index (BMI) demonstrated a stable response to treatment with the LT modifier, montelukast [15]. Therefore, LTs may play a greater role in the pathogenesis of asthma in obese subjects compared to nonobese patients.

Obesity is a proinflammatory state associated with increased systemic cytokine levels such as tumor necrosis factor α, interleukin-1β, and interleukin-6 and other classical mediators produced by adipocytes termed adipokines [16]. Adipokines are hormones that display both pro- and anti-inflammatory properties. One such adipokine is leptin, a 16 kD protein synthesized by adipocytes and involved in the regulation of food intake and energy balance [17]. Levels of plasma leptin correlate with total body fat stores, being elevated in obesity and reduced in weight loss. Leptin has been shown to enhance proinflammatory cytokine expression, specifically to upregulate Th1 cytokines [18] and the eicosanoid, LT [19, 20]. In contrast to the proinflammatory effects of leptin, adiponectin is predominantly an anti-inflammatory mediator, mainly involved in glucose control and fatty acid metabolism, that is synthesized in adipose tissue and plasma levels of adiponectin are decreased in obesity.

A role for leptin in promoting pulmonary inflammation and bronchoconstriction has been demonstrated in murine models of obesity and asthma [21, 22]. However, data supporting a role for leptin in the prevalence or severity of asthma in adult humans, independent of BMI, are inconsistent [23]. Adiponectin has also been shown to play a role in animal models of asthma but, in contrast to leptin, this adipokine attenuates pulmonary inflammation [24, 25]. The impact of reduced serum adiponectin levels in humans with asthma is, like leptin, not clearly defined [23]. Preliminary data from our laboratory demonstrate increased plasma leptin levels in obese asthmatics compared to obese nonasthmatics. Leptin levels also tended to increase in asthmatics compared to nonasthmatics whether they were obese or nonobese. In view of the positive association between leptin and LT level, we examined cys-LT levels in the exhaled breath condensate (EBC) and peripheral blood leukocytes of asthmatics compared to nonasthmatics and obese compared to nonobese subjects.

2. Methods

2.1. Recruitment. All subjects were 18–65 years old with or without asthma, male and female, with ethnicity and race distribution of the community's population seen at the University of Michigan Health Centers. The nonasthmatic subjects were healthy volunteers without a history of lung disease. Fully informed consent was obtained from each subject before entry into the study. All procedures were approved by the Institutional Review Board. BMI calculations were determined by dividing the weight by the square of the height (kg/m^2). Asthmatic and nonasthmatic subjects were studied based on BMI, (1) normal BMI (20–24.9 kg/m^2) and (2) obese BMI (>30 kg/m^2) to maximize potential differences on cys-LT synthesis. Stable asthmatics without exacerbations for 2 months were included. Diagnosis of asthma was based on history, physical exam, and pulmonary function testing including peak expiratory flow rate (PEFR) (L/min) (AsthmaCheck, Respironics, Inc., Youngwood, PA) performed within 3 months of starting the study. Approximately 50% of the asthmatics had spirometry, with forced expiratory volume in one-second (FEV$_1$) measurements. Patients with mild to moderate persistent asthma (Steps 1–3) were studied. Subjects on inhaled corticosteroids (ICS) were included [26].

Peak flow meter and BMI values were determined in all subjects on the day of the study. An asthma questionnaire was administered which includes frequency of day and night time asthma symptoms [27].

Exclusion criteria included current smokers within the past 6 months and previous smokers > 20 pack years, intercurrent infection, and treatment with LT-modifier drugs, aspirin, nonsteroidal anti-inflammatory agents, and oral steroids. Aspirin sensitive asthmatics were excluded because of their tendency to display excess cys-LT synthesis at baseline [28].

2.2. Exhaled Breath Condensate. Exhaled breath condensate (EBC) was collected with RTube to determine airway lining fluid levels of cys-LT levels [29, 30]. The subjects breathe at their normal rate and depth for 5–7 min. The exhaled air cools below the dew point by transfer of heat to a chilled condenser surface. Condensation of the aerosolized airway lining fluid occurs as EBC. Samples were frozen at −70°C to be studied in batches later. cys-LT were determined by enzyme immunoassay (EIA) (Cayman Chemicals, Ann Arbor, MI). Samples were run in duplicate, neat, and diluted, using a competitive assay based on a high-affinity monoclonal antibody measuring cys-LT. The lower range detection limit (80% B/B_0) was 34 pg/mL. Significant numbers of both male and female patients were studied because of possible greater levels of leptin [31] and LT in women than in men [32].

2.3. Blood. A volume of 5 mL of heparinized whole blood was layered over 3.5 mL of a mixture of sodium metrizoate and Ficoll (1-Step Polymorphs, Accurate Chemical & Scientific Corporation, Westbury, NY) in a 15 mL centrifuge tube. The sample was centrifuged at 450 ×g for 30 min in a swing-out rotor at 22°C. Adipokines, leptin, and adiponectin were measured in the plasma by enzyme immunoassay (EIA) according to the protocol described [33]. Plasma leptin levels were determined spectrophotometrically using commercially available colorimetric EIA kits (Millipore, MA USA) and run according to the manufacturer's instructions. The coefficient of variation for duplicate samples was 3.7% and the lower limit of detection was 0.5 ng/mL. Similarly, plasma high molecular weight adiponectin (Linco Research, a subsidiary of Millipore, St. Charles, Mo) was run in duplicate according to the manufacturer's directions (LLD: 8.1%, 0.5 ng/mL.). Blood samples were drawn from patients at the same time of the day, in the morning, and when patients were in the fasting state. Total IgE levels were determined in all subjects (Clinical Pathology Laboratory, University of Michigan).

Peripheral Blood Monocytes (PBM). We measured LT levels in PBM from subjects obese and nonobese with and without asthma. PBM were isolated from whole blood by Ficoll (One Step, Accurate Chemical & Scientific Corp, Westbury, NY) centrifugation and adherence, as previously described [34]. Cells were >90% PBM by differential staining and viability >95% by trypan blue exclusion. Isolated PBM were resuspended in lipopolysaccharide-free Dulbecco's Modified Eagle Medium at 0.5 × 10^6/mL and adhered for 1 h at 37°C in a humidified atmosphere of 5% CO_2/95% O_2 for EIA. Nonadherent cells were removed by washing twice with Dulbecco's Modified Eagle Medium.

The cells were stimulated *ex vivo* with $1\,\mu$M calcium ionophore A23187 (Calbiochem-Behring Corp., La Jolla, CA) in dimethyl sulfoxide [35]. Final concentrations of dimethyl sulfoxide (0.05%) added to cultures had no effect on either cell viability or eicosanoid synthesis. This compound liberates intracellular calcium from intact cells and releases arachidonic acid from cell membranes. It also activates lipoxygenases and stimulates LTC_4 synthase. The eicosanoid products were measured by EIA.

2.4. Statistics. Our study was designed to have 80% power with a type I error 5% to detect significant differences between asthmatics and normal subjects, as well as between obese and nonobese asthmatics. From the preliminary data, we estimate the median log LTB_4 levels in exhaled breath condensate for nonobese asthmatics as 50 pg/mL, corresponding to a median log level of 3.90. The study is powered to detect a doubling in the median LT levels for the obese compared to the nonobese groups. Based on preliminary data and to achieve the above differences 20 subjects were needed in each group, that is, 80 total for the four groups: obese asthma, nonobese nonasthma, asthma nonobese, and obese nonasthma.

Mean and standard deviations for normally distributed data were calculated and differences between groups determined by Student's *t*-test. For skewed data Mann-Whitney tests were utilized. Correlations and partial correlations were performed using Pearson's coefficient. For the evaluation of possible associations between each study variable (dependent) and BMI (independent), linear regression was performed. We log-transformed the data since it was not normally distributed. This log transformation resulted in normalization of the data. Multivariable regression analysis was performed for leptin, adiponectin, and EBC cys-LT levels, adjusting for age, gender, and asthma status. We evaluated the association with BMI categories as well as BMI as a continuous variable.

Comparison of study variables among the four groups was performed with one-way analysis of variance (ANOVA). The data were log transformed prior to ANOVA. *p* values < 0.05 were considered statistically significant. All statistics were performed on IBM SPSS version 21 statistical software.

3. Results

We set out to study four groups of subjects: obese asthmatics, nonobese asthmatics, obese nonasthmatics, and nonobese nonasthmatics. The total number of subjects studied was 82. By design the BMI of the control and obese subjects were recruited to obtain optimal separation of the groups (Table 1). Mean peak flow meter (PFM) readings of the asthmatics and nonasthmatics were also significantly different (Table 1). There was no difference in PFM between obese and nonobese (82.5 ± 21 versus 80.3 ± 12.2 L/min, *p* = ns) asthma subjects. There was also no significant difference in FEV_1 between obese and nonobese asthmatics (74.6 ± 19.4 versus 91.5 ± 12.5% predicted, *p* = 0.052). The asthma control test

TABLE 1: Demographics of the study population of obese, nonobese, asthmatic, and nonasthmatic subjects.

	Asthma	Nonasthma	*p*
n	42	40	
BMI	30.3 ± 8.6	30.4 ± 7.9	= 0.5
PFR L/min	82 ± 17.6	107 ± 16.3	= 0.01
M/F	15/27	15/25	
Subgroups			
	Obese/nonobese	Obese/nonobese	
n	21/21	21/19	
BMI	38.7 ± 5.4/23.0 ± 1.8	37.1 ± 3.6/23.1 ± 1.8	
PFR L/min	82.5 ± 21/80.3 ± 12.2	91.5 ± 14.2/89 ± 18.9	
M/F	8 : 13/7 : 14	10 : 11/5 : 14	

Note: M/F: male/female; PFR: peak flow rate % normal predicted; BMI: body mass index.

(ACT) questionnaire was lower in obese asthma (19.8 ± 11.9) compared to nonobese asthma (22.1 ± 1.6) patients, *p* = 0.01. Total IgE levels were different but quite variable in both asthmatics and nonasthmatics (326 ± 519 versus 73 ± 124 kU/L, *p* = 0.004). There was no difference in IgE levels between obese and nonobese asthmatics (315 ± 448 versus 336 ± 586 kU/L, *p* = 0.13).

The gender breakdown was 64% female (36% male), which was as close as we could get to equality in recruitment. Males (35.2 ± 12.2 years) and females (35.1 ± 12.7 years) displayed no difference in age. No significant difference occurred in BMI between the genders, obese (36.5 ± 5.7 versus 38.4 ± 4.6 years male : female) or nonobese (23.6 ± 1.3 versus 22.5 ± 1.7).

The recruitment age in the subjects, asthma versus nonasthma subjects, was not significantly different (32.7 ± 12.3 versus 37 ± 12.1 years, *p* = 0.31). Obese subjects were generally older, displaying an age-related increase in fat mass (obese 41.8 ± 11.6 versus nonobese 27.7 ± 8.4, *p* < 0.001). Obese asthmatics were on average older than nonobese asthmatics (40.6 ± 12.8 versus 25.5 ± 5.9 years, *p* < 0.001).

Comorbidities. There are a number of comorbidities that contribute to exacerbations of asthma. Twelve of the obese subjects had a diagnosis of obstructive sleep apnea (OSA). These were evenly divided among asthmatics and nonasthmatics (7/42 versus 5/40 subjects). Gastroesophageal reflux disease (GERD) was more common in obese than nonobese (8/42 versus 3/40 subjects) subjects. GERD was equally distributed between asthmatics and nonasthmatics (6/42 versus 5/40 subjects).

Medications. The asthmatics studied had mild to moderate persistent disease with all of them on ICS (42 subjects). None of the asthmatics were on leukotriene modifier therapy, since that was an exclusionary criterion for subject recruitment.

3.1. Leptin. As expected, fasting leptin levels were higher in obese subjects than nonobese subjects (32.7 ± 20.2 versus 8.5 ± 6.3 ng/mL, *p* = 0.0001). There was no significant difference in leptin levels between asthmatics and nonasthmatics

TABLE 2: Adipokine levels in obese, nonobese, asthmatic, and nonasthmatic subjects.

	Asthma	Nonasthma	p
Leptin ng/mL	24.9 ± 22.3	17.4 ± 15.3	= 0.125
Adiponectin μg/mL	10.9 ± 5.7	12.3 ± 5.9	= 0.13
L/A ratio	3.0 ± 3.8	2.1 ± 2.2	= 0.09
EBC μg/mL	70.1 ± 29.4	59.1 ± 27.8	= 0.04
Subgroups			
	Obese/nonobese	Obese/nonobese	
Leptin ng/mL	40.2 ± 21.9/9.7 ± 7.2	26.8 ± 15.8/7.1 ± 4.5	
Adiponectin μg/mL	9.0 ± 4.7/12.6 ± 6.3	9.5 ± 4.9/14.7 ± 5.6	
L/A ratio	5.5 ± 4.3/2.5 ± 0.76	2.3 ± 2.1/3.1 ± 0.3	
EBC μg/mL	72.9 ± 29.7/67.8 ± 29.7	60.8 ± 28.1/57.1 ± 28.2	

Note: L/A: leptin/adiponectin ratio; EBC: exhaled breath condensate.

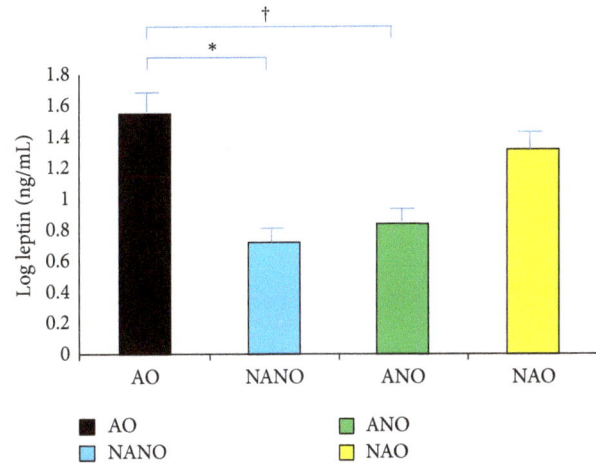

FIGURE 1: Increase in leptin levels in obese asthmatics. Serum leptin levels log mean transformed (ng/mL) in subjects with asthma obesity (AO), nonasthma nonobesity (NANO), asthma nonobesity (ANO), and nonasthma obesity (NAO). AO had significantly higher leptin levels (ANOVA $p < 0.05$), compared with NANO* and ANO[†].

(Table 2). Mean leptin levels were higher in females than in males (26.4 ± 21 versus 12.4 ± 12.3 ng/mL, $p < 0.05$). Female asthmatics had higher leptin levels than males with asthma (31.6 ± 24.1 compared to 13.1 ± 11.9 ng/mL, $p = 0.01$). Leptin levels were higher in obese female asthmatics compared to obese male asthmatics (52.1 ± 18.6 versus 20.8 ± 11.6 ng/mL, $p < 0.001$). Leptin levels in female asthmatics were 31.6 ± 24.1 compared to females without asthma 20.9 ± 3.7 ng/mL, $p = 0.03$. Leptin levels in men with and without asthma were 13.1 ± 11.9 and 11.7 ± 8.5 ng/mL, respectively ($p = 0.29$).

Leptin's correlation with weight is 0.77 which was significant ($p < 0.0001$). When it was adjusted for asthma, it is 0.78 ($p < 0.0001$). The correlation of leptin with asthma is 0.17 ($p = 0.119$). When adjusted for BMI, the correlation was 0.27 ($p = 0.14$).

Linear regression demonstrated a positive correlation between leptin and obesity. There was also a positive correlation between leptin and the female gender ($p = 0.001$). Using multiple linear stepwise regression only weight and gender (female) had a positive correlation, when the variables age, gender, weight, and asthma were considered. There was no correlation between leptin and ICS or OSA.

Using ANOVA, leptin was significantly different between the four groups: obese asthmatics, nonasthma nonobese, asthma nonobese, and nonasthma obese. Obese asthmatics had significantly higher levels than both nonobese asthmatics and nonobese nonasthmatics ($p < 0.0001$) (Figure 1). The only groups that were not statistically different were the obese asthmatics and obese nonasthmatics ($p = 0.27$).

3.2. Adiponectin. Adiponectin was decreased overall in the obese versus nonobese subjects (mean 9.3 ± 4.7 versus 14.1 ± 20 μg/mL, $p < 0.05$), as expected. There was no difference in adiponectin levels between asthmatics compared to nonasthmatics (Table 2). As noted for leptin, mean adiponectin levels were higher in females than in males (14.1 ± 5.5 versus 7.2 ± 3.1 μg/mL, $p < 0.05$) especially in nonobese. This was also

true for obese females who had higher mean levels compared to obese males (11.3 ± 4.8 versus 6.4 ± 2.7 μg/mL, $p < 0.05$). Males with asthma display lower mean levels of adiponectin than those seen in females with asthma (6.9 ± 2.8 versus 13.3 ± 5.6 μg/mL $p < 0.05$).

Adiponectin's correlation with weight is −0.44 which was significant ($p < 0.0001$). When adjusted for asthma it was −0.44 ($p < 0.0001$). The correlation of adiponectin with asthma was −0.10 but was not significant ($p = 0.36$). When adjusted for BMI the correlation was −0.134 ($p = 0.22$). There was a positive correlation between adiponectin and ACT (0.35) which did reach significance ($p = 0.002$). When adjusted for asthma it was a positive correlation (0.36) and was significant ($p = 0.001$).

Linear regression demonstrated a negative correlation between adiponectin and obesity. Using multiple linear stepwise regression, there was a negative correlation with weight and a positive correlation with gender when the variables age, gender, weight, and asthma were considered. There was no correlation between adiponectin and ICS or OSA.

ANOVA demonstrated that adiponectin was significantly different between the four groups: obese asthmatics, nonasthma nonobese, asthma nonobese, and nonasthma obese. Obese asthmatics had lower adiponectin levels than nonobese nonasthmatics ($p < 0.008$) (Figure 2). Obese nonasthmatics also had lower adiponectin than nonobese nonasthmatics ($p = 0.017$).

3.3. Leptin/Adiponectin Ratio. Since both leptin and adiponectin are increased in women compared to men, we next examined the leptin/adiponectin ratio as a method to better compare genders with regard to the role of adipokines in the pathogenesis of asthma in obesity. The mean leptin/adiponectin ratio was 2.8 ± 3.6 in women compared to 2.1 ± 1.9 in men ($p = 0.15$). Obese subjects had a significantly higher mean ratio than nonobese subjects (4.3 ± 3.5 versus

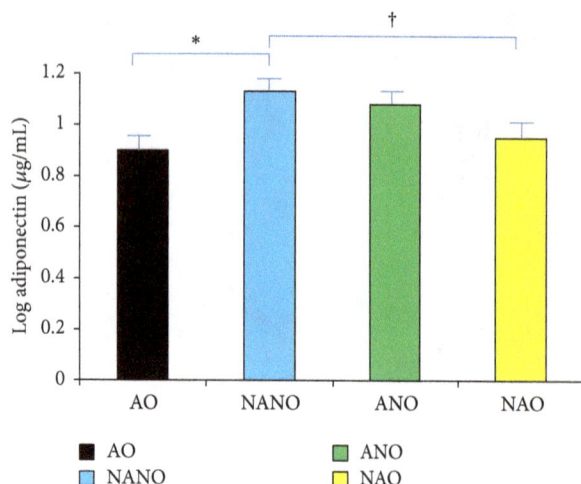

FIGURE 2: Lower adiponectin levels in obese asthmatics. Serum adiponectin levels log mean transformed (μg/mL) in subjects with asthma obesity (AO), nonasthma nonobesity (NANO), asthma nonobesity (ANO), and nonasthma obesity (NAO). AO had significantly lower adiponectin levels (ANOVA $p < 0.05$) compared with NANO*. NAO also had significantly lower adiponectin than NANO[†].

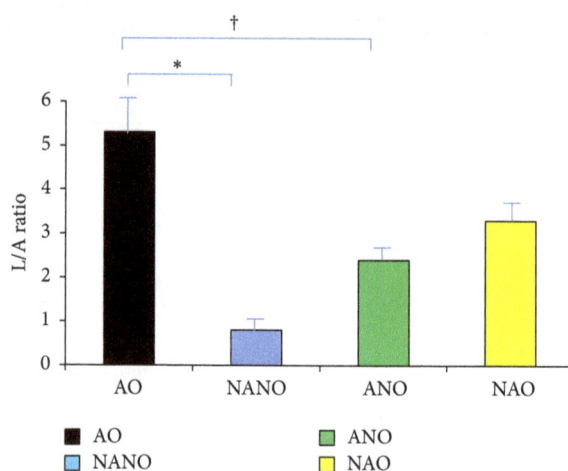

FIGURE 3: Elevated leptin/adiponectin ratio in obese asthmatics. Serum leptin/adiponectin (L/A) ratio in subjects with asthma obesity (AO), nonasthma nonobesity (NANO), asthma nonobesity (ANO), and nonasthma obesity (NAO). AO had significantly higher L/A ratio (ANOVA $p < 0.05$) compared with NANO* and ANO[†].

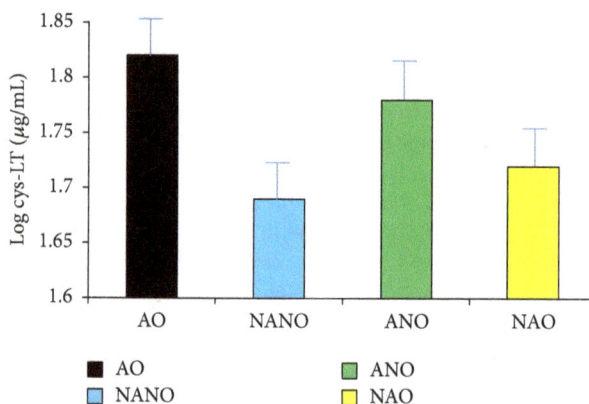

FIGURE 4: Exhaled breath condensate cysteinyl leukotriene levels in obesity and asthma. Exhaled breath condensate (EBC) cys-LT levels log mean transformed (μg/mL) in subjects with asthma obesity (AO), nonasthma nonobesity (NANO), asthma nonobesity (ANO), and nonasthma obesity (NAO). There was no significant difference between the groups with ANOVA testing.

0.78 ± 0.8, $p < 0.01$). Asthmatics did not have a significantly higher mean ratio compared to nonasthmatics (Table 2). Although the mean leptin/adiponectin ratio trended to be higher in patients with worse airway obstruction (PFR < 80% predicted), it did not reach statistical significance ($p = 0.26$).

Linear regression demonstrated a positive correlation between leptin/adiponectin ratio and weight ($p = 0.0001$), as well as age ($p = 0.0001$). Using multiple linear stepwise regression, there was a correlation with weight ($p = 0.0001$). There was no correlation with gender, asthma, ICS, or OSA.

ANOVA demonstrated that leptin/adiponectin ratio was significantly different between the four groups: obese asthmatics, nonasthma nonobese, asthma nonobese, and nonasthma obese. Obese asthmatics had higher leptin/adiponectin ratios than nonobese nonasthmatics (5.3 ± 4.3 versus 0.75 ± 0.9, $p < 0.0001$) and nonobese asthmatics ($p < 0.0001$) (Figure 3), but not obese nonasthmatics ($p = 0.16$). This was mainly accounted for by female obese asthmatics (6.3 ± 4.9 versus 3.3 ± 1.7 for males, $p = 0.03$).

3.4. *EBC cys-LT Levels.* Exhaled breath concentrate (EBC) cys-LT levels were higher in all asthmatics compared to nonasthmatics (Table 2). There was no difference in EBC cys-LT levels between obese and nonobese subjects (66.1 ± 29.00 versus $62.8 \pm 29.1 \mu$g/mL, $p = 0.3$). Obese asthmatics had higher EBC cys-LT levels than nonobese nonasthmatic subjects (73 ± 29.7 versus $57 \pm 28.1 \mu$g/mL, $p = 0.05$).

The correlation of EBC with obesity was 0.11 ($p = 0.34$). When it was adjusted for asthma it was 0.13 ($p = 0.26$). EBC correlation with asthma was 0.23 which is significant ($p = 0.04$). When this is adjusted for BMI it was 0.24 ($p = 0.03$).

Multiple regression analysis revealed a significant correlation between EBC cys-LT and asthma ($p = 0.04$). There was no correlation with weight, age, gender, ICS, or OSA.

ANOVA demonstrated no difference between four groups, likely due to the variability of the samples. The greatest difference was between obese asthmatics and nonobese nonasthmatics but only reached a p value of 0.3 (Figure 4).

3.5. *Peripheral Blood cys-LT.* PBM cys-LT production was higher in females than males (222 ± 132 versus $142 \pm 116 \mu$g/mL, $p < 0.05$). PBM cys-LT levels were comparable in the asthmatic versus nonasthma subjects (197 ± 148 versus $190 \pm 115 \mu$g/mL, $p = 0.4$). However, in view of the increased variability of the PBM cys-LT levels, there were no significant increased values in obese asthmatics compared to nonobese nonasthmatics.

4. Discussion

The main findings of this study are the following: (1) plasma leptin levels are increased in obese asthmatics compared to obese nonasthmatics. This was mainly accounted for by higher leptin levels in females, and especially obese female asthmatics. (2) Adiponectin levels were lower in obese asthmatics compared to nonobese nonasthmatics. (3) The leptin/adiponectin ratio was significantly higher in obese asthmatics compared to nonobese nonasthmatics. (4) EBC cys-LT levels were higher in asthmatics than in nonasthmatics. (5) PBM cys-LT levels were higher in women than in men, irrespective of asthma or obesity.

An important finding in our study was the association between leptin and asthma, and specifically in obese asthmatics. This was especially true in obese female asthmatics. Leptin levels are thought to be higher in females because of increased percentage body fat in women [31] as well as increased secretion of leptin from adipose tissue. The latter may be related to increased estradiol levels and its effect of increased leptin secretion from adipose tissue [36]. Leptin has been noted to be a proinflammatory adipokine driving the immune system towards a predominant Th1 phenotype [37]. Leptin may also have an impact on the airway milieu in asthmatics with obesity. Leptin may increase proinflammatory phenotype in macrophages [38], augmenting the response to LPS. Leptin receptors have been described in the airway and investigators have shown a correlation between plasma and BAL levels [38]. Leptin deficient mice display reduced LT synthesis, and exogenous leptin augments LT production in macrophages from these animals [19]. Obesity has also been associated with an alteration in adipokines that predispose to neutrophilic inflammation [39]. However, other investigators have demonstrated decreased inflammation in the airways of obese asthmatics [40], which is reversed by weight loss. They propose that adipokines may augment airway bronchial reactivity without increasing airway inflammation. Recently, it has also been shown that leptin may also affect the airway diameter through noninflammatory pathways by inhibiting the cholinergic pathway [22]. Although we have shown an association between leptin and asthma, population studies by Sutherland et al. have shown no such association [41]. Sampling of nonfasting subjects, some of whom smoked, can affect leptin levels and may explain the differences in conclusions of these studies.

Adiponectin is another adipokine formed in adipose tissue. In contrast to leptin, adiponectin levels are decreased in obesity and tend to increase in starvation. It has a number of metabolic actions including increasing insulin sensitivity, diminishing atherosclerosis, and being generally anti-inflammatory [24]. Although adiponectin receptors have been detected in the lungs, serum levels do not consistently correlate with BAL fluid levels. This finding may be explained by the fact that active transport of adiponectin, which is a large molecule (full length form), may be necessary for penetration into the airways [42]. Higher adiponectin levels have been associated with lower asthma prevalence rates in women [43]. In our population, obese asthmatics had lower adiponectin levels than nonobese nonasthmatics. We also demonstrated a positive correlation between adiponectin and asthma symptoms (ACT). However, the higher levels of adiponectin in women compared to men, as was noted for leptin, may be the confounding variable, which detracts from the association of lower adiponectin levels in obese asthmatics compared to other groups. Other investigators have questioned the association between adiponectin and asthma. Cross-sectional analysis of an asthmatic population, who were nonfasting and smokers, did not demonstrate an association between adiponectin and asthma [41].

An increased leptin/adiponectin ratio is associated with asthma compared to control subjects without asthma. The increased leptin/adiponectin ratio is also associated with severe asthma compared to mild to moderate asthma [44]. In our study, leptin/adiponectin ratios were significantly elevated in obese asthmatics compared to nonobese nonasthmatics. Obese asthmatic women had the highest leptin/adiponectin ratio. However, in our study the leptin/adiponectin ratio was not associated with asthma or increased airway obstruction.

The reduced responsiveness to inhaled corticosteroids with increasing BMI, with a relatively stable response to montelukast, has been previously described [15]. Sutherland et al. also examined the comparative effects of BMI in response to asthma controller medication [45]. By contrast, they demonstrated that inhaled corticosteroids were superior to LT modifiers at all BMI levels, in patients who were underweight compared to those with morbid obesity. In our study we demonstrated that EBC cys-LT levels correlated with asthma, being higher in asthmatics than in nonasthmatics. The trend was greater in obese asthmatics compared to nonobese asthmatics. Other investigators have demonstrated an association between BMI and urine cys-LT in obese asthmatics [46]. Obese patients had significantly higher values of LTE_4/creatinine in urine compared to subjects who were preobese and in the normal range. In a linear regression model, the only significant associations were those between BMI and LTE_4/creatinine in urine. Using the same model, log leptin and log adiponectin presented positive and negative associations, respectively, with LTE_4/creatinine in urine. Notably, there was no association between BMI and EBC LTE_4 levels [46]. This was because of the increased variability noted with EBC samples, which may also explain the marginal increase in EBC cys-LT levels in obese asthmatics in our study. The other problem is the inability to adequately standardize dilution factors for EBC across subjects. An alternative explanation is that alveolar cys-LT synthesis may not be as important as airway levels. A recent study demonstrated elevated submucosal but not sputum eosinophil levels in obese subjects with severe asthma [47, 48]. This may explain the elevated urine cys-LT levels in obese subjects compared to EBC measurements [46].

In our cohort subjects with the older obese women phenotype trended to have increased leptin and EBC cys-LT levels with worse pulmonary function. Obese female asthmatics had higher leptin levels than obese male asthmatics. Recently, investigators have demonstrated that BMI was associated with the incidence of asthma in women but not in men [49]. Furthermore, adult onset nonatopic asthma has become the most common type of asthma in women [50]. Investigators have demonstrated that both testosterone (negative) and estrogen (positive) were associated with alterations in adipokines, specifically leptin levels [51]. We detected no significant difference between premenopausal obese women with asthma compared to nonobese patients. There was no decline in leptin levels in asthma with age, in postmenopausal compared to premenopausal subjects matched for BMI. Similarly, there was no change in adiponectin levels. The increase in BMI with age may have offset the effect of any change in estrogen/testosterone levels on adipokine levels as subjects increased in years. We did document that PBM from female subjects had higher cys-LT levels than that of male subjects. This has been noted by other investigators and may in part be due to suppression of 5-LO enzymatic activity by testosterone [52]. Although PBM cys-LT levels were trending higher in asthmatics than nonasthmatics, this did not reach significance. Increased plasma leptin levels in women may be associated with the elevated PBM cys-LT production noted in females [20].

We documented comorbidities of OSA and GERD in asthmatics and nonasthmatics. Poorly controlled OSA has been shown to worsen asthma control, in part through increased release of proinflammatory mediators during episodes of hypoxia and disrupted sleep [53]. Nocturnal GERD may exacerbate asthma with aspiration of acid, during inhalation against a closed airway, following episodes of upper airway obstruction. Like OSA, the incidence of GERD is also increased in obese subjects and may exacerbate airway disease after eating. GERD can result in reflex bronchospasm from irritation of the esophagus or directly spilling into the airway with gross reflux. Although both OSA and GERD were more common in obese than nonobese subjects in our study, the incidence was equally distributed in the asthmatic and nonasthmatic groups.

There are a number of potential limitations with this study. It is a relatively small study number-wise, examining the role of obesity in the pathogenesis of asthma. Furthermore, it is an observational study, with no interventions. Although the diagnosis of asthma was made by a physician with history, physical examination, and pulmonary function testing, spirometry or methacholine challenge testing was not performed. Spirometry with FEV_1 measurements was only obtained in ~50% of the asthma subjects. Instead PFM readings were obtained during the study visit. In addition, a number of variables to assess the role of EBC cys-LT readings limited the interpretation of results. Inhaled corticosteroids can result in ~18% reduction in EBC cys-LT levels, but we wanted to include asthmatics that were with mild to moderate severity [54]. Although adipokines can be affected by the gender and the menstrual cycle, we did not determine the reproductive hormone concentrations in our premenstrual patients. Despite these issues, the study has a number of strengths. In recruiting subjects, there was good characterization and separation of subjects between the control group and obese subject group. In addition, the asthmatics were well characterized compared to the nonasthmatics with peak flow rates and asthma control test questionnaires. Furthermore, the significance of the study was improved since we studied predominantly moderate persistent asthmatics all on inhaled corticosteroid therapy. None of the asthmatics were on LT modifier medications.

In summary, we have demonstrated that leptin levels and the leptin/adiponectin ratio are increased in obese asthmatics compared to obese nonasthmatics. Proinflammatory mediators, cys-LT, were increased in obese asthmatics compared to nonobese nonasthmatics. Adipokines, especially in obese female asthmatics, may promote an asthma phenotype that has become more prevalent and results in difficult to control airway disease.

Conflict of Interests

The authors declare that there is no conflict of interests regarding the publication of this paper.

Acknowledgment

This work was supported by a Grant from the General Clinical Research Center at the University of Michigan (HUM00005182).

References

[1] K. M. Flegal, D. Carroll, B. K. Kit, and C. L. Ogden, "Prevalence of obesity and trends in the distribution of body mass index among US adults, 1999-2010," *The Journal of the American Medical Association*, vol. 307, no. 5, pp. 491–497, 2012.

[2] K. R. Fontaine, D. T. Redden, C. Wang, A. O. Westfall, and D. B. Allison, "Years of life lost due to obesity," *The Journal of the American Medical Association*, vol. 289, no. 2, pp. 187–193, 2003.

[3] L. Akinbami, J. E. Moorman, C. Bailey et al., "Trends in asthma prevalence, health care use, and mortality in the United States, 2001–2010," *NCHS Data Brief*, no. 94, pp. 1–8, 2012.

[4] C. A. Camargo Jr., S. T. Weiss, S. Zhang, W. C. Willett, and F. E. Speizer, "Prospective study of body mass index, weight change, and risk of adult-onset asthma in women," *Archives of Internal Medicine*, vol. 159, no. 21, pp. 2582–2588, 1999.

[5] J. Ma, L. Xiao, and S. B. Knowles, "Obesity, insulin resistance and the prevalence of atopy and asthma in US adults," *Allergy*, vol. 65, no. 11, pp. 1455–1463, 2010.

[6] A. A. Litonjua, D. Sparrow, J. C. Celedon, D. DeMolles, and S. T. Weiss, "Association of body mass index with the development of methacholine airway hyperresponsiveness in men: the Normative Aging Study," *Thorax*, vol. 57, no. 7, pp. 581–585, 2002.

[7] K. Hakala, B. Stenius-Aarniala, and A. Sovijarvi, "Effects of weight loss on peak flow variability, airways obstruction, and lung volumes in obese patients with asthma," *Chest*, vol. 118, no. 5, pp. 1315–1321, 2000.

[8] D. A. Beuther and E. R. Sutherland, "Overweight, obesity, and incident asthma: a meta-analysis of prospective epidemiologic studies," *American Journal of Respiratory and Critical Care Medicine*, vol. 175, no. 7, pp. 661–666, 2007.

[9] M. Yigla, N. Tov, A. Solomonov, A.-H. E. Rubin, and D. Harlev, "Difficult-to-control asthma and obstructive sleep apnea," *Journal of Asthma*, vol. 40, no. 8, pp. 865–871, 2003.

[10] W. R. Henderson Jr., "Eicosanoids and lung inflammation," *American Review of Respiratory Disease*, vol. 135, no. 5, pp. 1176–1185, 1987.

[11] F. Mitsunobu, T. Mifune, Y. Hosaki et al., "Enhanced peripheral leukocyte leukotriene production and bronchial hyperresponsiveness in asthmatics," *European Respiratory Journal*, vol. 16, no. 3, pp. 504–508, 2000.

[12] O. Abrahamsen, H. Haas, J. Schreiber, and M. Schlaak, "Differential mediator release from basophils of allergic and non-allergic asthmatic patients after stimulation with anti-IgE and C5a," *Clinical and Experimental Allergy*, vol. 31, no. 3, pp. 368–378, 2001.

[13] T. R. Martin, "Arachidonic acid metabolism in lung phagocytes," *Seminars in Respiratory Infections*, vol. 1, no. 2, pp. 89–98, 1986.

[14] E. R. Sutherland, E. Goleva, M. Strand, D. A. Beuther, and D. Y. M. Leung, "Body mass and glucocorticoid response in asthma," *American Journal of Respiratory and Critical Care Medicine*, vol. 178, no. 7, pp. 682–687, 2008.

[15] M. Peters-Golden, A. Swern, S. S. Bird, C. M. Hustad, E. Grant, and J. M. Edelman, "Influence of body mass index on the response to asthma controller agents," *European Respiratory Journal*, vol. 27, no. 3, pp. 495–503, 2006.

[16] R. S. Ahima and J. S. Flier, "Leptin," *Annual Review of Physiology*, vol. 62, pp. 413–437, 2000.

[17] J. M. Friedman and J. L. Halaas, "Leptin and the regulation of body weight in mammals," *Nature*, vol. 395, no. 6704, pp. 763–770, 1998.

[18] L. Steinman, P. Conlon, R. Maki, and A. Foster, "The intricate interplay among body weight, stress, and the immune response to friend or foe," *Journal of Clinical Investigation*, vol. 111, no. 2, pp. 183–185, 2003.

[19] P. Mancuso, A. Gottschalk, S. M. Phare, M. Peters-Golden, N. W. Lukacs, and G. B. Huffnagle, "Leptin-deficient mice exhibit impaired host defense in Gram-negative pneumonia," *Journal of Immunology*, vol. 168, no. 8, pp. 4018–4024, 2002.

[20] P. Mancuso, C. Canetti, A. Gottschalk, P. K. Tithof, and M. Peters-Golden, "Leptin augments alveolar macrophage leukotriene synthesis by increasing phospholipase activity and enhancing group IVC iPLA2 (cPLA 2γ) protein expression," *American Journal of Physiology—Lung Cellular and Molecular Physiology*, vol. 287, no. 3, pp. L497–L502, 2004.

[21] S. A. Shore, I. N. Schwartzman, M. S. Mellema, L. Flynt, A. Imrich, and R. A. Johnston, "Effect of leptin on allergic airway responses in mice," *Journal of Allergy and Clinical Immunology*, vol. 115, no. 1, pp. 103–109, 2005.

[22] E. Arteaga-Solis, T. Zee, C. W. Emala, C. Vinson, J. Wess, and G. Karsenty, "Inhibition of leptin regulation of parasympathetic signaling as a cause of extreme body weight-associated asthma," *Cell Metabolism*, vol. 17, no. 1, pp. 35–48, 2013.

[23] N. Ali Assad and A. Sood, "Leptin, adiponectin and pulmonary diseases," *Biochimie*, vol. 94, no. 10, pp. 2180–2189, 2012.

[24] S. A. Shore, R. D. Terry, L. Flynt, A. Xu, and C. Hug, "Adiponectin attenuates allergen-induced airway inflammation and hyperresponsiveness in mice," *Journal of Allergy and Clinical Immunology*, vol. 118, no. 2, pp. 389–395, 2006.

[25] B. D. Medoff, Y. Okamoto, P. Leyton et al., "Adiponectin deficiency increases allergic airway inflammation and pulmonary vascular remodeling," *American Journal of Respiratory Cell and Molecular Biology*, vol. 41, no. 4, pp. 397–406, 2009.

[26] S. Zanconato, S. Carraro, M. Corradi et al., "Leukotrienes and 8-isoprostane in exhaled breath condensate of children with stable and unstable asthma," *Journal of Allergy and Clinical Immunology*, vol. 113, no. 2, pp. 257–263, 2004.

[27] National Asthma Education and Prevention, *Practical Guide for the Diagnosis and Management of Asthma. Expert Panel Report 2*, US Department of Health and Human Services, Public Health Service, National Institute of Health, National Heart, Lung and Blood Institute, Bethesda, Md, USA, 1997.

[28] M. Sanak, M. Pierzchalska, S. Bazan-Socha, and A. Szczeklik, "Enhanced expression of the leukotriene C_4 synthase due to overactive transcription of an allelic variant associated with aspirin-intolerant asthma," *American Journal of Respiratory Cell and Molecular Biology*, vol. 23, no. 3, pp. 290–296, 2000.

[29] J. Hunt, "Exhaled breath condensate: an evolving tool for non-invasive evaluation of lung disease," *Journal of Allergy and Clinical Immunology*, vol. 110, no. 1, pp. 28–34, 2002.

[30] P. Montuschi and P. J. Barnes, "Exhaled leukotrienes and prostaglandins in asthma," *Journal of Allergy and Clinical Immunology*, vol. 109, no. 4, pp. 615–620, 2002.

[31] L. Hellström, H. Wahrenberg, K. Hruska, S. Reynisdottir, and P. Arner, "Mechanisms behind gender differences in circulating leptin levels," *Journal of Internal Medicine*, vol. 247, no. 4, pp. 457–462, 2000.

[32] C. Pergola, G. Dodt, A. Rossi et al., "ERK-mediated regulation of leukotriene biosynthesis by androgens: a molecular basis for gender differences in inflammation and asthma," *Proceedings of the National Academy of Sciences of the United States of America*, vol. 105, no. 50, pp. 19881–19886, 2008.

[33] E. V. Kotidis, G. G. Koliakos, V. G. Baltzopoulos, K. N. Ioannidis, J. G. Yovos, and S. T. Papavramidis, "Serum ghrelin, leptin and adiponectin levels before and after weight loss: comparison of three methods of treatment—a prospective study," *Obesity Surgery*, vol. 16, no. 11, pp. 1425–1432, 2006.

[34] M. J. Coffey, S. E. Wilcoxen, S. M. Phare, M. R. Gyetko, M. Peters-Golden, and R. U. Simpson, "Reduced 5-lipoxygenase metabolism in macrophages from 1,25-dihydroxyvitamin D3-deficient rats," *Prostaglandins*, vol. 48, no. 5, pp. 313–329, 1994.

[35] M. J. Coffey, C. S. Wheeler, K. B. Gross, W. L. Eschenbacher, P. H. S. Sporn, and M. Peters-Golden, "Increased 5-lipoxygenase metabolism in the lungs of human subjects exposed to ozone," *Toxicology*, vol. 114, no. 3, pp. 187–197, 1996.

[36] X. Casabiell, V. Piñeiro, R. Peino et al., "Gender differences in both spontaneous and stimulated leptin secretion by human omental adipose tissue in vitro: dexamethasone and estradiol stimulate leptin release in women, but not in men," *The Journal of Clinical Endocrinology & Metabolism*, vol. 83, no. 6, pp. 2149–2155, 1998.

[37] F. Malli, A. I. Papaioannou, K. I. Gourgoulianis, and Z. Daniil, "The role of leptin in the respiratory system: an overview," *Respiratory Research*, vol. 11, article 152, 2010.

[38] N. L. Lugogo, J. W. Hollingsworth, D. L. Howell et al., "Alveolar macrophages from overweight/obese subjects with asthma demonstrate a proinflammatory phenotype," *American Journal of Respiratory and Critical Care Medicine*, vol. 186, no. 5, pp. 404–411, 2012.

[39] J. Cao, J.-H. Chen, and S.-Y. Zhu, "Effects of leptin on airway inflammation and the expression of Th1/Th2 cytokines in asthmatic rats," *Zhonghua Jie He He Hu Xi Za Zhi*, vol. 32, no. 3, pp. 171–176, 2009.

[40] O. Sideleva, B. T. Suratt, K. E. Black et al., "Obesity and asthma: an inflammatory disease of adipose tissue not the airway," *American Journal of Respiratory and Critical Care Medicine*, vol. 186, no. 7, pp. 598–605, 2012.

[41] T. J. T. Sutherland, M. R. Sears, C. R. McLachlan, R. Poulton, and R. J. Hancox, "Leptin, adiponectin, and asthma: findings from

a population-based cohort study," *Annals of Allergy, Asthma and Immunology*, vol. 103, no. 2, pp. 101–107, 2009.

[42] F. Holguin, M. Rojas, L. A. Brown, and A. M. Fitzpatrick, "Airway and plasma leptin and adiponectin in lean and obese asthmatics and controls," *Journal of Asthma*, vol. 48, no. 3, pp. 217–223, 2011.

[43] A. Sood, X. Cui, C. Quails et al., "Association between asthma and serum adiponectin concentration in women," *Thorax*, vol. 63, no. 10, pp. 877–882, 2008.

[44] A. Tsaroucha, Z. Daniil, F. Malli et al., "Leptin, adiponectin, and ghrelin levels in female patients with asthma during stable and exacerbation periods," *Journal of Asthma*, vol. 50, no. 2, pp. 188–197, 2013.

[45] E. R. Sutherland, C. A. Camargo Jr., W. W. Busse et al., "Comparative effect of body mass index on response to asthma controller therapy," *Allergy and Asthma Proceedings*, vol. 31, no. 1, pp. 20–25, 2010.

[46] P. Giouleka, G. Papatheodorou, P. Lyberopoulos et al., "Body mass index is associated with leukotriene inflammation in asthmatics," *European Journal of Clinical Investigation*, vol. 41, no. 1, pp. 30–38, 2011.

[47] D. Desai, C. Newby, F. A. Symon et al., "Elevated sputum interleukin-5 and submucosal eosinophilia in obese individuals with," *American Journal of Respiratory and Critical Care Medicine*, vol. 188, no. 6, pp. 657–663, 2013.

[48] D. Wu, A. B. Molofsky, H.-E. Liang et al., "Eosinophils sustain adipose alternatively activated macrophages associated with glucose homeostasis," *Science*, vol. 332, no. 6026, pp. 243–247, 2011.

[49] N. Assad, C. Quails, L. J. Smith et al., "Body mass index is a stronger predictor than the metabolic syndrome for future asthma in women. The longitudinal CARDIA study," *American Journal of Respiratory and Critical Care Medicine*, vol. 188, no. 3, pp. 319–326, 2013.

[50] A. Sood, C. Quails, M. Schuyler et al., "Adult-onset asthma becomes the dominant phenotype among women by age 40 years. The longitudinal CARDIA study," *Annals of the American Thoracic Society*, vol. 10, no. 3, pp. 188–197, 2013.

[51] A. M. Isidori, F. Strollo, M. Moré et al., "Leptin and aging: correlation with endocrine changes in male and female healthy adult populations of different body weights," *Journal of Clinical Endocrinology and Metabolism*, vol. 85, no. 5, pp. 1954–1962, 2000.

[52] C. Pergola, A. Rogge, G. Dodt et al., "Testosterone suppresses phospholipase D, causing sex differences in leukotriene biosynthesis in human monocytes," *The FASEB Journal*, vol. 25, no. 10, pp. 3377–3387, 2011.

[53] M. Teodorescu, F. B. Consens, W. F. Bria et al., "Predictors of habitual snoring and obstructive sleep apnea risk in patients with asthma," *Chest*, vol. 135, no. 5, pp. 1125–1132, 2009.

[54] C. Mondino, G. Ciabattoni, P. Koch et al., "Effects of inhaled corticosteroids on exhaled leukotrienes and prostanoids in asthmatic children," *Journal of Allergy and Clinical Immunology*, vol. 114, no. 4, pp. 761–767, 2004.

5

Noninterventional Open-Label Trial Investigating the Efficacy and Safety of Ectoine Containing Nasal Spray in Comparison with Beclomethasone Nasal Spray in Patients with Allergic Rhinitis

Uwe Sonnemann,[1] Marcus Möller,[2] and Andreas Bilstein[3]

[1] Private Health Centre, Institute for ENT Elmshorn, Hermann-Ehlers-Weg 4, 25337 Elmshorn, Germany
[2] Joint Practice for ENT, Willy-Brandt Straße 2, 21335 Lüneburg, Germany
[3] Bitop AG, Stockumer Straße 28, 58453 Witten, Germany

Correspondence should be addressed to Andreas Bilstein; bilstein@bitop.de

Academic Editor: Ralph Mösges

Objectives. The current study aimed to compare the efficacy and safety of a classical anti-inflammatory beclomethasone nasal spray in comparison to a physic-chemical stabilizing ectoine containing nasal spray in the treatment of allergic rhinitis. *Design and Methods.* This was a noninterventional, open-label, observational trial investigating the effects of beclomethasone or ectoine nasal spray on nasal symptoms and quality of life. Over a period of 14 days, patients were asked to daily document their symptoms. Efficacy and tolerability were assessed by both physicians and patients. *Results.* Both treatments resulted in a significant decrease of TNSS values. An equivalence test could not confirm the noninferiority of ectoine treatment in comparison with beclomethasone treatment. Although clear symptom reduction was achieved with the ectoine products, the efficacy judgment showed possible advantages for the beclomethasone group. Importantly, tolerability results were comparably good in both groups, and a very low number of adverse events supported this observation. Both treatments resulted in a clear improvement in the quality of life as assessed by a questionnaire answered at the beginning and at the end of the trial. *Conclusion.* Taken together, it was shown that allergic rhinitis can be safely and successfully treated with beclomethasone and also efficacy and safety were shown for ectoine nasal spray.

1. Introduction

Allergic rhinitis is a common disease with estimated 600 million patients suffering from this disease worldwide [1]. According to a large scale investigation, about 20% of the European population suffers from allergic rhinitis [2] and numbers are increasing, particularly in industrial states. Although not being a life-threatening disease, allergic rhinitis has a considerable impact on general well-being and work/school performance, and particularly its impact on comorbidities such as, for example, asthma reflects the need for good treatment options.

A number of pharmacological treatments against allergic rhinitis exist, such as antihistamines, leukotriene receptor agonists, mast cell stabilizing agents, and glucocorticosteroids. According to the ARIA (Allergic Rhinitis and its Impact on Asthma) guidelines, intranasal glucocorticosteroids are recommended as pharmacological treatment of allergic rhinitis and should be prescribed preferable to intranasal antihistamines and oral leukotriene receptor agonists [1]. However, many patients have reservations to use corticosteroids, and phobia of their usage can result in bad compliance [3]. This together with the fact that patients often seek alternative treatments to pharmacological options reflects the need for new treatment strategies.

The current noninterventional trial compared efficacy and safety of treatment of allergic rhinitis patients with intranasal spray containing either the glucocorticoid beclomethasone or the natural, nonpharmacological substance ectoine. Overview of the results are shown in Figure 9.

Ectoine is a compatible solute which is produced by microorganisms living under harsh environmental conditions such as extreme salinity or dryness [4–6]. In those microorganisms, ectoine acts as natural cell protectant. Halophilic microorganisms living in habitats of high ionic strength cope with hyperosmotic stress by changing the composition of membrane lipids and by regulating the intracellular concentration of low molecular weight solutes such as the compatible solute Ectoine. As a result of the latter response, the cells are able to maintain proper osmotic balance under conditions of hyperosmotic stress, which is crucial to prevent the cell from leaking water, hence avoiding irreversible plasmolysis and dehydration, and to generate turgor pressure within limits necessary for growth [7, 8]. Ectoin is industrially produced via the "bacterial milking process" using the gram negative bacterium *Halomonas elongata* [9, 10]. It is known that ectoine works via an entropy-driven mechanism called "preferential exclusion" or "preferential hydration" during which ectoine influences the characteristics of the water shell surrounding biomolecules like membranes. By excluding osmolytes from the direct hydrate shell of proteins and membranes, a preferential hydration of such proteins or membranes occurs, thereby stabilizing their native confirmation and making them less vulnerable to external stressors [11, 12]. Preclinical studies have demonstrated that the beneficial effects of ectoine can be transferred to human or animal models, and they have also shown that ectoine possesses membrane-stabilizing and inflammation-reducing properties [13–16]. Additional experiments on human nasal epithelial cell lines have confirmed the protective action of ectoine against osmotic stress (data not published). Recent developments have demonstrated that this attribute can be successfully transferred to a number of application forms such as ectoine containing creams, nasal sprays, or eye drops which can be used on humans for treatment of rhinosinusitis and atopic dermatitis [11, 12] and also congress reports point towards efficacy when applied to patients with allergic rhinitis [17–20].

This study assessed development of nasal symptoms, changes in quality of life, and judgment of efficacy and tolerability upon treatment with either the well-known steroid beclomethasone or barrier stabilizing, physically acting ectoine nasal spray in order to compare the effect levels of these different treatment concepts in patients with allergic rhinitis.

2. Materials and Methods

2.1. Treatment and Study Design. This was a controlled, open-labelled, noninterventional, multicenter study assessing the efficacy and safety of ectoine containing nasal spray in comparison to beclomethasone containing nasal spray. The patients could freely choose their treatment: they were treated with either ectoine nasal spray or beclomethasone containing nasal spray (0.05% beclomethasone).

According to §23b of the German medical device law, this study was carried out with the CE-marked medical device ectoine nasal spray without changes in its intended use; therefore, §§20–23a of the MPG had not been complied with. Open observational trials are health authority accepted in Germany for nonpharmaceutical treatment options. According to a general statement by ethical committees, this type of study does not allow for a placebo group, because this would involve a lack of benefit for patients.

Ectoine nasal spray is an isotonic solution containing 2% ectoine, natural salt, and water. According to the instructions for use, one puff of the spray had to be applied into each nostril three times daily. The beclomethasone spray was used in accordance with the instructions for use: two puffs of the spray had to be applied into each nostril twice a day. Each puff of the nasal spray contains 0.05 mg beclomethasone diproprionate. Further ingredients are benzalkonium chloride (preservative), polysorbate, glucose, cellulose, sodium carmellose, water, sodium hydroxide, and hydrochloric acid for pH adjustment.

Male and female patients aged 18–70 years with documented diagnosed seasonal allergic rhinitis were eligible for the study, based on the discretion of the investigator. In order to be sure of the allergic symptoms, the nasal symptom score (TNSS) at study start had to be ≥ 6.

Patients had to attend two site visits (V1 on day 0 and V2 on day 14 ± 2). During the entire treatment period, patients were asked to document their symptoms in patient diaries once daily. Assessments of symptoms by physicians were carried out during site visits V1 and V2.

The medication was handed over to the patients by the physician. After completion of the study, no drug accountability was performed.

For simplification reasons, patients of the ectoine group will be termed group 1 in this paper, and patients of the beclomethasone group will be termed group 2.

2.2. Endpoints. Primary endpoints were changes in the single symptoms nasal obstruction, rhinorrhea, nasal itching, and sneezing as well as changes in the sum of nasal symptoms (TNSS). Secondary endpoints were the assessment of the symptom itchy ear/palate and assessment of efficacy and tolerability as well as analysis of safety data.

2.3. Scoring of Nasal Symptoms. Single nasal symptoms as well as ear/palate itching were assessed with a score described as follows: 0 (no symptoms), 1 (slight symptoms), 2 (moderate symptoms), and 3 (severe symptoms). Patients assessed their symptoms reflectively, and scores describing the symptoms within the last 24 h were documented in the patients' diaries. Physicians scored the current symptoms during both patient visits (V1 and V2).

In order to account for the influence of pollen intensity on the nasal symptoms, the quotient TNSS/pollen count score was calculated. Pollen count scores were derived from online available daily pollen counts for the relevant local area. The scoring of pollen counts was as follows: no pollen count was scored with 0.1, low pollen count with 1, moderate pollen count with 2, and strong pollen count with 3.

2.4. Scoring of Efficacy and Tolerability. At the end of the study, patients assessed both efficacy and tolerability with a score of 0 (no efficacy, bad to tolerate), 1 (moderate efficacy, moderate tolerability), 2 (good efficacy, good tolerability), and 3 (very good efficacy, very good tolerability).

2.5. Quality of Life Questionnaire. A modified, nonvalidated quality of life questionnaire based on the RQLQ from Juniper et al. was used in this study. During both site visits (V1 and V2), patients were asked to fill out the questionnaire. It contained 14 questions covering three topics (daily life activities, general wellbeing, and emotional status) which were to be answered on a score from 0 (none) to 6 (very/always).

2.6. Data Management and Statistics. Data of this open-label trial were collected by the physicians in an anonymized paper CRF and by the patients in diaries and questionnaires. Proper data management was monitored during the study. A SAP was set up before study closure and the data were analyzed according to the SAP. Source data from the CRFs, diaries, and questionnaires were transferred to digital data format by the physicians. The statistical analysis was carried out with SPSS Statistics 20 and SigmaPlot version 12. The primary endpoint TNSS was summarized descriptively for both V1 and V2, and differences between V1 and V2 were documented. Noninferiority of the ectoine product versus the beclomethasone containing spray was assessed with an equivalence range of 15%. Analysis of secondary parameters was done descriptively. In addition, changes during the period of the study were analyzed via Bowker's test of symmetry. Group comparisons were analyzed via Chi-square test or Fisher's exact test. All significance levels were set to 5%. Unavailable data were treated as "missing values."

3. Results

The current study was conducted in accordance with the Declaration of Helsinki. All investigations were carried out with the understanding and consent of all participants. The study took part at two German ear nose throat (ENT) practices starting in May 2011 and being completed at the end of June 2011. In total, 50 patients (34 women, 16 men) diagnosed with seasonal allergic rhinitis were included in the study. Mean age of the patients was 33.3 years. Of the 50 patients, 25 received ectoine and 25 patients received beclomethasone nasal spray. All patients completed the study. Distribution of patients is shown in Figure 1.

3.1. Total Nasal Symptom Score (TNSS). The development of the total nasal symptom score (sum of nasal obstruction, rhinorrhea, sneezing, and nasal itching) was judged by both patients and the investigators.

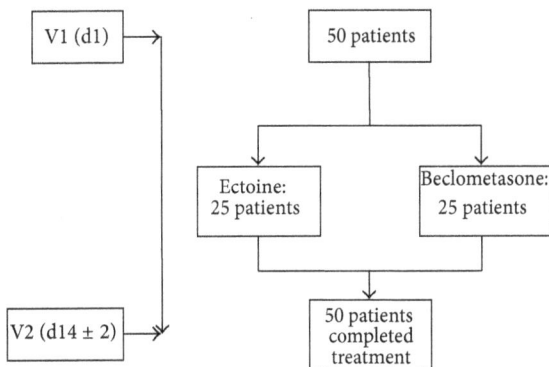

FIGURE 1: Patient flow during the study. On day 1 (V1), patients were asked to participate in the study. 25 patients received ectoine nasal spray, and 25 patients received beclomethasone nasal spray for a treatment period of 14 ± 2 days. All 50 patients finished the study with the final study visit V2.

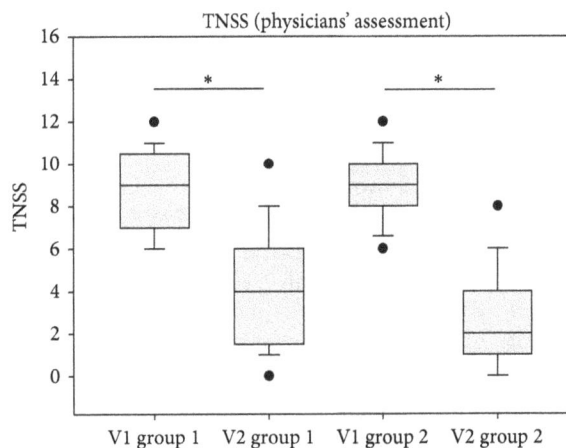

FIGURE 2: TNSS development during the study based on the physicians' assessment of symptoms. $^*P < 0.001$. Lines within the box mark the median; the upper and lower ends of the box indicate the 75th and 25th percentiles, respectively. Whiskers above and below the box indicate the 90th and 10th percentiles. Dots (•) represent outlying points.

Results of the investigators' assessment are shown in Figure 2. TNSS values decreased significantly in both groups ($P < 0.001$). In the ectoine group, values decreased from 8.76 ± 1.79 (V1) to 4.04 ± 2.75 (V2) corresponding to a total decrease of −4.72 (−51.20%), whereas values in the beclomethasone group decreased from 9.04 ± 1.53 (V1) to 2.52 ± 2.22 (V2) corresponding to a total decrease of −6.52 (−71.49%).

According to the patients' assessment (see Figure 3(a)), TNSS values decreased clearly in the ectoine group ($P = 0.072$, decrease by −12.86%) and a significant decrease was observed in the beclomethasone group ($P < 0.001$, decrease by 39.69%).

In order to consider the influence of pollen on the strength of nasal symptoms, quotients of TNSS values and pollen count scores were calculated. Those confirmed the statistically significant decrease of TNSS values from V1

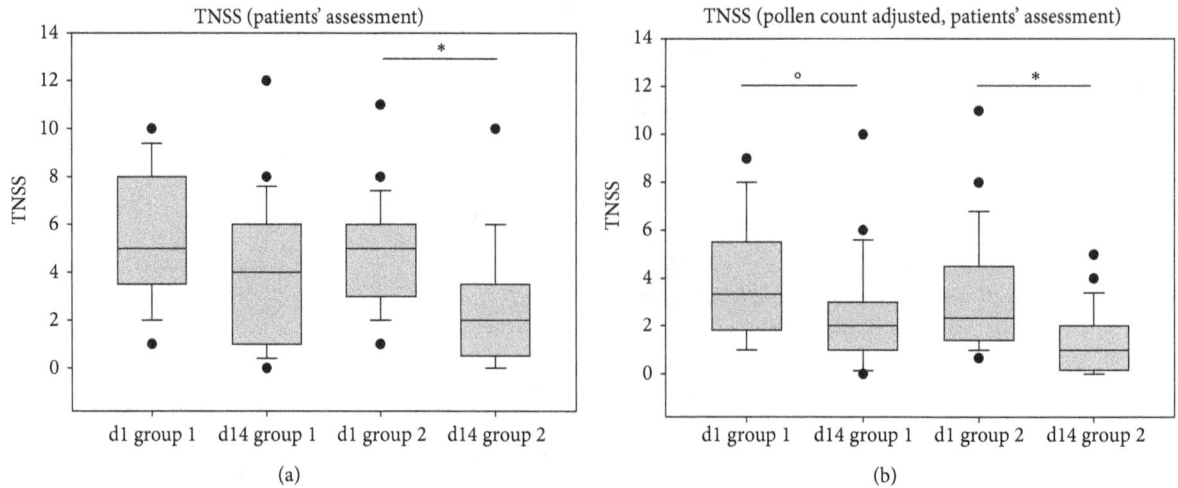

FIGURE 3: TNSS development during the study based on the patients' assessment of symptoms. (a) TNSS values on day 1 (d1) and day 14 (d14); (b) TNSS values adjusted for pollen counts, $^*P < 0.001$, $^\circ P = 0.043$. Lines within the box mark the median; the upper and lower ends of the box indicate the 75th and 25th percentiles, respectively. Whiskers above and below the box indicate the 90th and 10th percentiles. Dots ($\bullet$) represent outlying points.

to V2 as assessed by investigators ($P < 0.001$ for both groups, details not shown). When patients' TNSS values were normalized to the pollen count scores, TNSS decreased in both groups and reached statistical significance ($P = 0.043$ for group 1, $P < 0.001$ for group 2; see Figure 3(b)).

3.2. Equivalence Test. An equivalence test was carried out to investigate the hypothesis that ectoine nasal spray is not inferior to beclomethasone containing nasal spray. As shown in Table 1, no significant differences could be shown. Thus, noninferiority of the ectoine nasal spray could not be confirmed.

3.3. Comparison of TNSS Values from V1 until the End of the First Treatment Day. In order to study the time of onset of both treatments, TNSS value development within the first 12 hours of treatment was analyzed. As shown in Figure 4, both groups showed a significant decrease of TNSS values from the first site visit until the first patient assessment at the end of the first day of treatment ($P < 0.001$ for both groups). This indicates that a comparably quick reduction of allergic symptoms was achieved within the first day of treatment in both groups.

3.4. Development of Single Symptom Scores. In order to correlate group affiliation and development of single symptoms, data were further analyzed with Fisher's exact test. Table 2 lists the number of patients with reduced, unchanged, or deteriorated symptoms as assessed by patients themselves or by the physicians. The analysis of data demonstrated that only the patients' assessment of the symptom sneezing revealed a statistically significant correlation ($P = 0.039$), indicating that this symptom improved significantly better in the patient group treated with beclomethasone nasal spray.

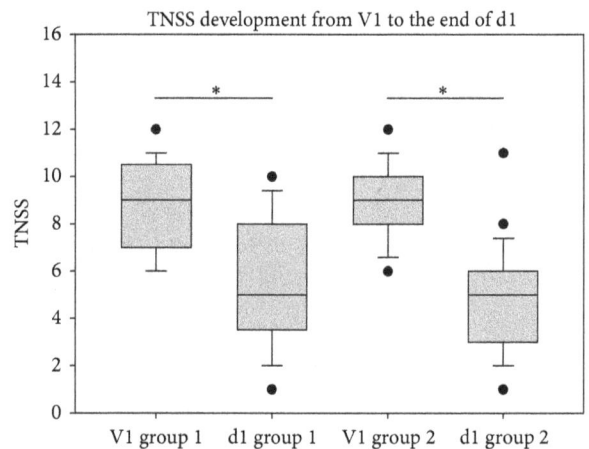

FIGURE 4: TNSS development from site visit 1 (V1) until the end of the first treatment day (d1). $^*P < 0.001$.

3.5. Ear/Palate Itching. In addition to the assessment of nasal symptoms, development of ear/palatal itching was assessed both by investigators and by patients. Results are depicted in Table 3 showing that there was no significant correlation between symptom development and group affiliation detectable neither in accordance with the investigators' nor in accordance with the patients' assessment.

3.6. Results of the Quality of Life Questionnaire. At the beginning and at the end of study participation, patients were asked to fill out a quality of life questionnaire which consisted of 14 questions. In order to investigate a correlation between changes in life quality and group affiliation, all single parameters of the questionnaire were analyzed via Fisher's exact test. A comparison of the patients' evaluation of quality of life both at d1 and d14 did not show statistical differences

TABLE 1: TNSS differences from treatment day 1/site visit 1 (d1/V1) to treatment d14/V2, respectively. Values are given as absolute value differences (abs) or as percentage differences (%).

TNSS difference variable	Equivalence range	TNSS difference of mean values			P value
		Value	SD	95% CI	
d14 (abs)	−2.32 ± 0.35	−1.10	0.92	[−2.64; 0.44]	P = 0.939
d14 [%]	−39.69 ± 5.95	−26.84	20.86	[−61.96; 8.29]	P = 0.938
V2 (abs)	−6.52 ± 0.98	−1.80	0.87	[−3.26; −0.34]	P = 0.999
V2 [%]	−71.49 ± 10.72	−20.29	8.91	[−35.25; −5.32]	P = 0.999

SD: standard deviation, CI: confidence interval.

TABLE 2: Development of single nasal symptoms during the study. Improvement, deterioration, or unchanged status of single symptoms was assessed by patients and investigators.

	Patients' assessment		Total	Physicians' assessment		Total
	Group 1	Group 2		Group 1	Group 2	
Rhinorrhoea						
Reduced	11 (47.8%)	12 (48.0%)	23 (47.9%)	17 (68.0%)	22 (88.0%)	39 (78.0%)
Unchanged	9 (39.1%)	11 (44.0%)	20 (41.7%)	6 (24.0%)	3 (12.0%)	9 (18.0%)
Deteriorated	3 (13.0%)	2 (8.0%)	5 (10.4%)	2 (8.0%)	0 (0.0%)	2 (4.0%)
Total	**23 (100.0%)**	**25 (100.0%)**	**48 (100.0%)**	**25 (100.0%)**	**25 (100.0%)**	**50 (100.0%)**
Fisher's exact test		**P = 0.919**			**P = 0.221**	
Nasal itching						
Reduced	7 (30.4%)	12 (48.0%)	19 (39.6%)	20 (80.0%)	22 (88.0%)	42 (84.0%)
Unchanged	13 (56.5%)	10 (40.0%)	23 (47.9%)	4 (16.0%)	2 (8.0%)	6 (12.0%)
Deteriorated	3 (13.0%)	3 (13.0%)	6 (12.5%)	1 (4.0%)	1 (4.0%)	2 (4.0%)
Total	**23 (100.0%)**	**25 (100.0%)**	**48 (100.0%)**	**25 (100.0%)**	**25 (100.0%)**	**50 (100.0%)**
Fisher's exact test		**P = 0.440**			**P = 0.830**	
Nasal obstruction						
Reduced	11 (47.8%)	10 (40.0%)	21 (43.8%)	18 (72.0%)	22 (88.0%)	40 (80.0%)
Unchanged	7 (30.4%)	13 (52.0%)	23 (41.7%)	6 (24.0%)	2 (8.0%)	8 (16.0%)
Deteriorated	5 (21.7%)	2 (8.0%)	7 (14.6%)	1 (4.0%)	1 (4.0%)	2 (4.0%)
Total	**23 (100.0%)**	**25 (100.0%)**	**48 (100.0%)**	**25 (100.0%)**	**25 (100.0%)**	**50 (100.0%)**
Fisher's exact test		**P = 0.258**			**P = 0.347**	
Sneezing						
Reduced	5 (21.7%)	12 (48.0%)	17 (35.4%)	18 (72.0%)	23 (92.0%)	41 (82.0%)
Unchanged	10 (43.5%)	11 (44.0%)	21 (43.8%)	3 (12.0%)	2 (8.0%)	5 (10.0%)
Deteriorated	8 (34.8%)	2 (8.0%)	10 (20.8%)	4 (16.0%)	0 (0.0%)	4 (8.0%)
Total	**23 (100.0%)**	**25 (100.0%)**	**48 (100.0%)**	**25 (100.0%)**	**25 (100.0%)**	**50 (100.0%)**
Fisher's exact test		**P = 0.039**			**P = 0.115**	

TABLE 3: Development of ear/palate itching during the study (d1 to d14 or V1 to V2) as assessed by patients and investigators. The total number of patients (% given in brackets) where symptoms were reduced, unchanged, or deteriorated is shown.

Ear/palate itching	Patients' assessment		Total	Physicians' assessment		Total
	Group 1	Group 2		Group 1	Group 2	
Reduced	4 (17.4%)	12 (48.0%)	16 (33.3%)	12 (48.0%)	14 (56.0%)	26 (52.0%)
Unchanged	14 (60.9%)	9 (36.0%)	23 (47.9%)	12 (48.0%)	8 (32.0%)	20 (40.0%)
Deteriorated	5 (21.7%)	4 (16.0%)	9 (18.8%)	1 (4.0%)	3 (12.0%)	4 (8.0%)
Total	**23 (100.0%)**	**25 (100.0%)**	**48 (100.0%)**	**25 (100.0%)**	**25 (100.0%)**	**50 (100.0%)**
Fisher's exact test		P = 0.088			P = 0.357	

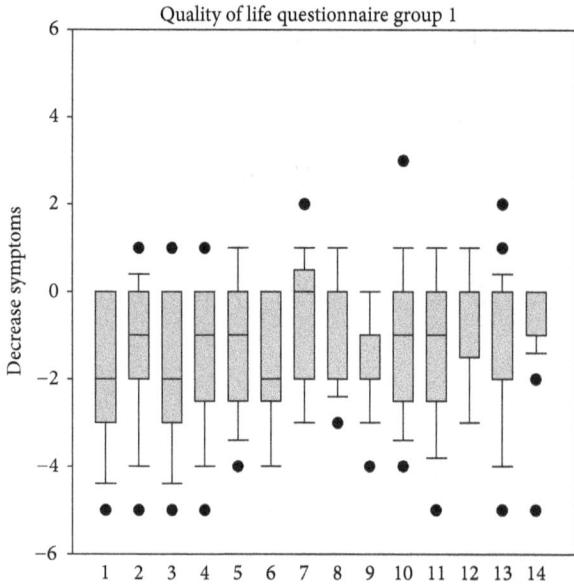

FIGURE 5: Reduction of scores of the quality of life questionnaire from V1 to V2 in group 1. 1 = frequency of tissue use, 2 = rubbing eyes and nose, 3 = frequency of brushing of nose, 4 = bad sleep, 5 = bad work performance, 6 = fatigue, 7 = thirst, 8 = lack of concentration, 9 = general well-being, 10 = headache, 11 = bad temper, 12 = general disconcertment, 13 = frustration, and 14 = reactions of others to the allergy.

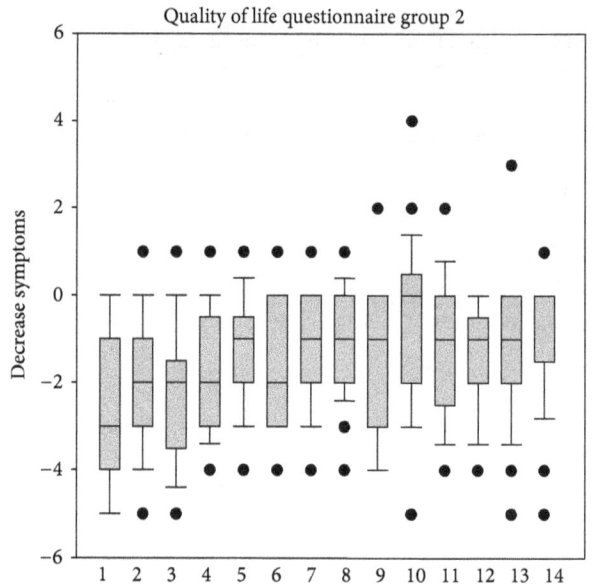

FIGURE 6: Reduction of scores of the quality of life questionnaire from V1 to V2 in group 1. 1 = frequency of tissue use, 2 = rubbing eyes and nose, 3 = frequency of brushing of nose, 4 = bad sleep, 5 = bad work performance, 6 = fatigue, 7 = thirst, 8 = lack of concentration, 9 = general well-being, 10 = headache, 11 = bad temper, 12 = general disconcertment, 13 = frustration, and 14 = reactions of others to the allergy.

between groups 1 and 2 in any of the questions asked (details not shown). Analysis of the results of the quality of life questionnaire as assessed by the investigators only showed a statistical significance ($P = 0.008$) for the parameter "frequency of brushing the nose" indicating that this parameter improved significantly better in the beclomethasone group (for details, see Table 4).

In addition to the analysis described above, total decreases of scores of the quality of life questionnaires were analyzed. As depicted in Figures 5 and 6, treatment resulted in decreases of all questioned parameters, thus indicating that all bothersome points which were covered in the questionnaire of life had improved during treatment.

3.7. Efficacy and Tolerability. Patients and investigators evaluated both the efficacy and tolerability of treatments during the study. Judgment of patients was given on a daily basis, whereas the investigators assessed those parameters at the end of the study (V2). As shown in Figure 7, patients judged the tolerability of both products similarly, and mean values of 2.42 ± 0.72 (group 1) and 2.53 ± 0.55 (group 2) corresponded to good to very good tolerability. No significant differences were detectable between groups. Similarly, assessment by the investigators during V2 confirmed a good tolerability of the treatments which was comparable between groups (see Figure 8).

The results of the assessment of efficacy of both treatments are depicted in Figures 10 and 11. As shown in Figure 10, efficacy assessment was similar during the first two days of treatment but increased over the treatment period of 14 days in the beclomethasone group compared to the ectoine group.

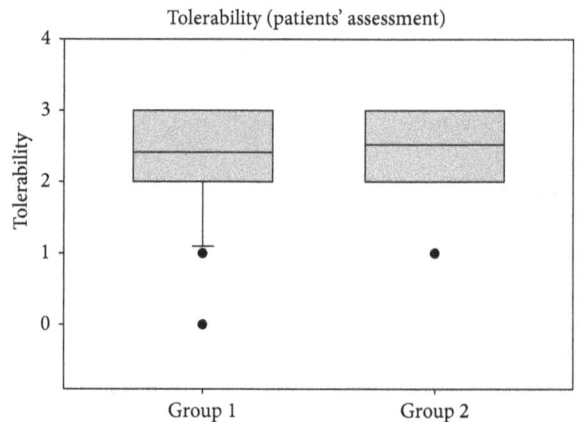

FIGURE 7: Tolerability assessments of patients during the entire study period of 14 days. Lines within the box mark the median; the upper and lower ends of the box indicate the 75th and 25th percentiles, respectively. Whiskers below the box indicate the 10th percentiles. Dots (•) represent outlying points.

In group 1, mean values of 1.09 ± 0.78 (mean values of entire study period) reflected moderate efficacy assessed by patients and a value of 1.44 ± 1.00 showed similar judgment by the physicians. In group 2, the efficacy was judged as good by patients (1.73 ± 0.94) and as very good by investigators (2.60 ± 0.58).

3.8. Adverse Events (AEs). In total, 3 adverse events were reported. Details are given in Table 5. No serious adverse

TABLE 4: Results (changes from V1 to V2) of the quality of life questionnaire documented by physicians.

		Group 1	Group 2	Total
	Frequency of tissue use			
	Reduced	12 (48.0%)	15 (60.0%)	27 (54.0%)
$P = 0.568$	Unchanged	11 (44.0%)	7 (28.0%)	18 (36.0%)
	Increased	2 (8.0%)	3 (12.0%)	5 (10.0%)
	Total	**25 (100.0%)**	**25 (100.0%)**	**50 (100.0%)**
	Rubbing eyes and nose			
	Reduced	14 (56.0%)	14 (56.0%)	28 (56.0%)
$P = 0.999$	Unchanged	8 (32.0%)	7 (28.0%)	15 (30.0%)
	Increased	3 (12.0%)	4 (16.0%)	7 (14.0%)
	Total	**25 (100.0%)**	**25 (100.0%)**	**50 (100.0%)**
	Frequency of brushing of nose			
	Reduced	12 (48.0%)	21 (84.0%)	33 (66.0%)
$P = 0.008$	Unchanged	8 (32.0%)	4 (16.0%)	12 (24.0%)
	Increased	5 (20.0%)	0 (0.0%)	5 (10.0%)
	Total	**25 (100.0%)**	**25 (100.0%)**	**50 (100.0%)**
	Bad sleep			
	Reduced	15 (60.0%)	17 (68.0%)	32 (64.0%)
$P = 0.878$	Unchanged	9 (36.0%)	7 (28.0%)	16 (32.0%)
	Increased	1 (4.0%)	1 (4.0%)	2 (4.0%)
Gesamt	Total	**25 (100.0%)**	**25 (100.0%)**	**50 (100.0%)**
	Bad work performance			
	Reduced	15 (60.0%)	20 (80.0%)	35 (70.0%)
$P = 0.328$	Unchanged	7 (28.0%)	4 (16.0%)	11 (22.0%)
	Increased	3 (12.0%)	1 (4.0%)	4 (8.0%)
	Total	**25 (100.0%)**	**25 (100.0%)**	**50 (100.0%)**
	Fatigue			
	Reduced	16 (64.0%)	15 (60.0%)	31 (62.0%)
$P = 0.690$	Unchanged	8 (32.0%)	7 (28.0%)	15 (30.0%)
	Increased	1 (4.0%)	3 (12.0%)	4 (8.0%)
	Total	**25 (100.0%)**	**25 (100.0%)**	**50 (100.0%)**
	Thirst			
	Reduced	10 (40.0%)	14 (56.0%)	24 (48.0%)
$P = 0.178$	Unchanged	8 (32.0%)	9 (36.0%)	17 (34.0%)
	Increased	7 (28.0%)	2 (8.0%)	9 (18.0%)
	Total	**25 (100.0%)**	**25 (100.0%)**	**50 (100.0%)**
	Lack of concentration			
	Reduced	10 (40.0%)	15 (60.0%)	25 (50.0%)
$P = 0.389$	Unchanged	13 (52.0%)	8 (32.0%)	21 (42.0%)
	Increased	2 (8.0%)	2 (8.0%)	4 (8.0%)
	Total	**25 (100.0%)**	**25 (100.0%)**	**50 (100.0%)**
	General well-being			
	Reduced	20 (80.0%)	16 (64.0%)	36 (72.0%)
$P = 0.462$	Unchanged	4 (16.0%)	6 (24.0%)	10 (20.0%)
	Increased	1 (4.0%)	3 (12.0%)	4 (8.0%)
	Total	**25 (100.0%)**	**25 (100.0%)**	**50 (100.0%)**
	Headache			
	Reduced	16 (64.0%)	10 (40.0%)	26 (52.0%)
$P = 0.081$	Unchanged	8 (32.0%)	9 (36.0%)	17 (34.0%)
	Increased	1 (4.0%)	6 (24.0%)	7 (14.0%)
	Total	**25 (100.0%)**	**25 (100.0%)**	**50 (100.0%)**

TABLE 4: Continued.

		Group 1	Group 2	Total
	Bad temper			
	Reduced	13 (52.0%)	17 (68.0%)	30 (60.0%)
P = **0.549**	Unchanged	8 (32.0%)	6 (24.0%)	14 (28.0%)
	Increased	4 (16.0%)	2 (8.0%)	6 (12.0%)
	Total	**25 (100.0%)**	**25 (100.0%)**	**50 (100.0%)**
	General disconcertment			
	Reduced	12 (48.0%)	19 (76.0%)	31 (62.0%)
P = **0.099**	Unchanged	11 (44.0%)	6 (24.0%)	17 (34.0%)
	Increased	2 (8.0%)	0 (0.0%)	2 (4.0%)
	Total	**25 (100.0%)**	**25 (100.0%)**	**50 (100.0%)**
	Frustration			
	Reduced	10 (40.0%)	16 (64.0%)	26 (52.0%)
P = **0.195**	Unchanged	14 (56.0%)	8 (32.0%)	22 (44.0%)
	Increased	1 (4.0%)	1 (4.0%)	2 (4.0%)
	Total	**25 (100.0%)**	**25 (100.0%)**	**50 (100.0%)**
	Reactions of others to the allergy			
	Reduced	7 (28.0%)	10 (40.0%)	17 (34.0%)
P = **0.377**	Unchanged	18 (72.0%)	14 (56.0%)	32 (64.0%)
	Increased	0 (0.0%)	1 (4.0%)	1 (2.0%)
	Total	**25 (100.0%)**	**25 (100.0%)**	**50 (100.0%)**

In addition to the analysis described above, total decreases of scores of the quality of life questionnaires were analyzed. As depicted in Figure 5 and Figure 6, treatment resulted in decreases of all questioned parameters, thus indicating that all bothersome points which were covered in the questionnaire of life had improved during treatment.

TABLE 5: Adverse events during the study.

Description AE	Treatment group	Relationship
Headache	Ectoine	Highly unlikely
Headache	Ectoine	Highly unlikely
Burning of nose	Beclomethasone	Probably

events (SAEs) occurred during the study. Both AEs occurring in the ectoine group were assessed as highly unlikely by the investigators, whereas the correlation of the AE "burning of nose" with the study medication was judged as probable in the beclomethasone group.

4. Conclusions

The current noninterventional, open-label study investigated treatment of allergic rhinitis comparing the intranasal glucocorticoid beclomethasone with that of ectoine containing nasal spray. Within the study, different mode of action, on the one hand the glucocorticoid, was compared to a physical, membrane stabilizing molecule. Importantly, it was shown that nasal symptom scores of both treatment groups improved significantly over the study period of 14 days. Although advantages of the beclomethasone spray in comparison with the ectoine spray were shown, results of the ectoine group showed its potential clinical efficacy. Glucocorticoids bind to specific glucocorticoid receptors which are present on almost all cells of the body. Following binding,

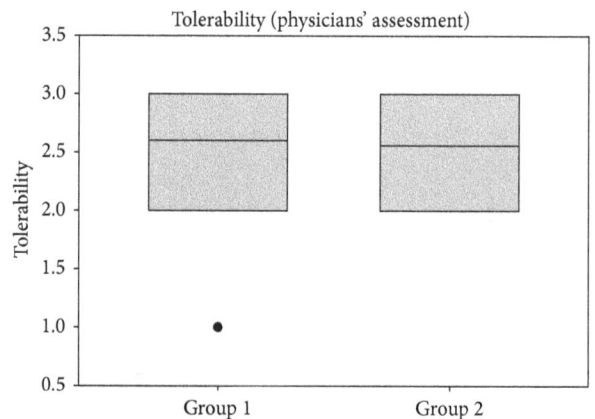

FIGURE 8: Assessment of tolerability at V2 assessed by the physicians. Lines within the box mark the median; the upper and lower ends of the box indicate the 75th and 25th percentiles, respectively. Dots (•) represent outlying points.

transcription of a number of inflammatory cytokines and chemokines can be modulated, which in turn results in decreased recruitment and activation of inflammatory cells [21]. In allergic rhinitis, this results in a quick improvement of inflammatory symptoms which was confirmed in the results of the beclomethasone group. Oppositely, ectoine acts physically via a mechanism called "preferential exclusion." In the presence of ectoine, membranes and lipids are protected indirectly. As ectoine is expelled from the surface of proteins

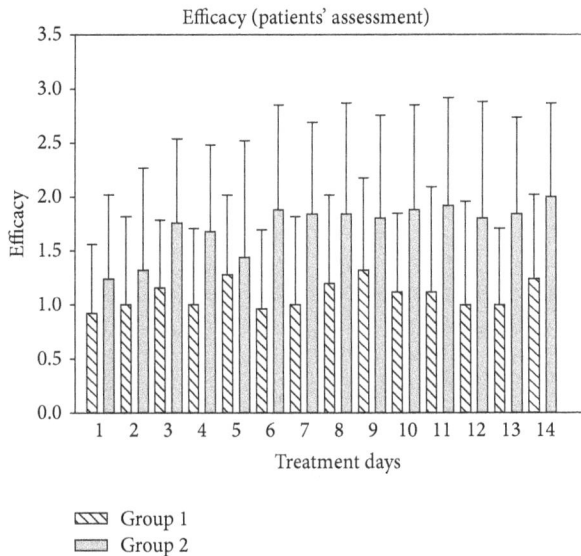

FIGURE 9: Efficacy assessment of treatments assessed by patients over a study period of 14 days. Mean values ± SD are depicted.

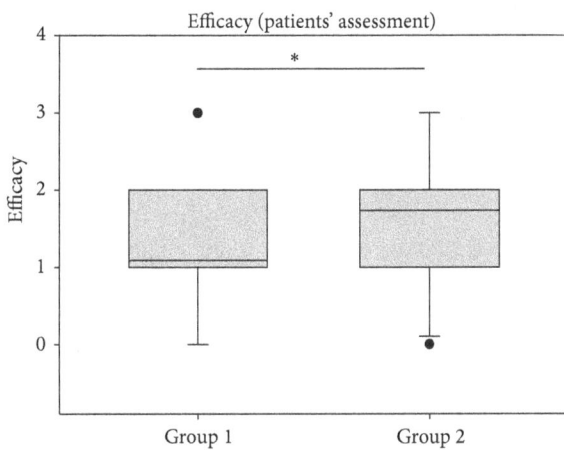

FIGURE 11: Assessment of efficacy of both treatments at site visit 2 (V2) by investigators. $°P = 0.009$. Lines within the box mark the median; the upper and lower ends of the box indicate the 75th and 25th percentiles, respectively. Whiskers above and below the box indicate the 90th and 10th percentiles. Dots (•) represent outlying points.

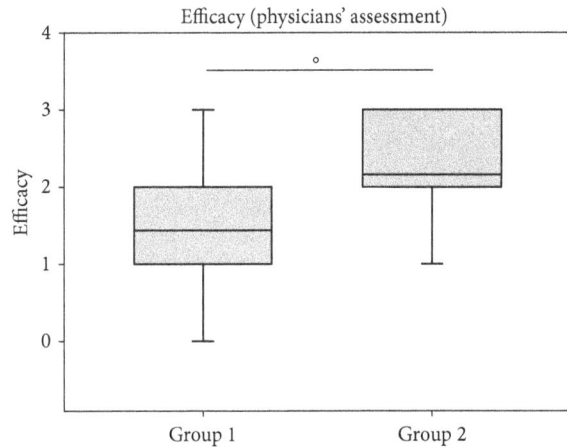

FIGURE 10: Assessment of efficacy of treatments in groups 1 and 2 over a period of 14 days (mean). $^*P < 0.001$. Lines within the box mark the median; the upper and lower ends of the box indicate the 75th and 25th percentiles, respectively. Whiskers above and below the box indicate the 90th and 10th percentiles. Dots (•) represent outlying points.

and lipids, those are protected by a water shell, thereby increasing the fluidity of membranes and resulting in the preferential formation of the native conformation of proteins [8, 16, 22–25]. This might stabilize mucous membranes such as lining epithelia of the nose, thereby protecting those from invading allergens and reducing allergen-induced inflammations as shown in different model systems [13, 26, 27] and as reported in congress report [28, 29]. It is understood that many allergens which cause allergic rhinitis symptoms have protease activities which act by impairing epithelial barrier function. This in turn results in increased penetration of allergens into nasal mucosa [30]. The barrier stabilizing properties of ectoine may counteract this scenario by improving the epithelial barrier and stabilizing membranes. In allergic rhinitis, this might protect the nasal mucosae from invading allergens, resulting in improvement of symptoms.

The study was intentionally performed as noninterventional study, reflecting the most realistic standard clinical practice and German law. However, this study design forbids randomization of patients, use of placebo, and blinding of study medication. Thus, patients were included independently of their prior medication and no wash-out period had to be kept. All patients had to show a certain degree of symptoms, measured by a minimum TNSS, at study start. Although we believe that valuable results can be drawn from noninterventional trials, one drawback of this study design is the fact that one cannot include a placebo group into the study population. On the other hand, it has been demonstrated that double-blind randomized placebo-controlled trials clearly have their limitations and disadvantages; for example, a comparison of open and controlled study designs in neuroleptic studies indicated that results of well performed open studies can earn more attention. The study design, however, reduces the grade of evidence delivered by the study data from Ib to IIa. On the other hand, it presents a realistic view of the most common clinical practice. Importantly, patient parameters in the current trial seemed to be well balanced between the two groups, with no major differences existing in terms of baseline values at the beginning, demography, history, and symptoms/health status before treatment.

As confirmed in the current study, beclomethasone acts rather quickly, and reduction of nasal symptoms was already observed within the first 12 hours of treatment. Surprisingly, the ectoine nasal spray seems to work comparably quick and results in a clear improvement of symptoms within the same time period of 12 h. Although the percentage of symptom decline was slightly larger in the beclomethasone group (decrease by −47.35%) in comparison to the ectoine group (decrease by −37.44%), decreases were both statistically significant ($P < 0.001$). Within the following treatment days, nasal symptoms decreased further, and at the final visit, TNSS values had decreased by −51.20% in the ectoine group and by 71.49% in the beclomethasone group. The degree of improvement following treatment with nasal corticosteroids corresponds to comparable data from the literature, describing decreases of total nasal symptoms of about 40–85% [31–33]. All those studies reported that corticosteroid treatment of allergic rhinitis worked significantly better than placebo treatment, and although the current study does not include a placebo group, it allows bringing the current results into a broader context.

The decreases of TNSS as assessed by the physicians were confirmed by the patients, with stronger decreases documented in the beclomethasone group in comparison with the ectoine group. In total, patients' baseline TNSS values were lower than the physicians' scores, whereas TNSS values at the end of the study were comparable between physicians and patients assessments. This difference can be explained with the fact that physicians' assessment of baseline values took part prior to treatment, whereas the first patients' documentations of TNSS values were performed at the end of the first treatment day and confirmed the quick onset of action of both treatments.

The aim of the current study was to investigate if ectoine nasal spray is as equally effective as treatment with a glucocorticoid nasal spray. As evaluated with an equivalence test of TNSS values assessed both by physicians and by patients, noninferiority of ectoine versus beclomethasone could not be confirmed. It is noteworthy that the safety profile of both treatments was assessed as good to very good both by investigators and by patients which was underlined by the very low number of adverse events. This goes in line with reports confirming that intranasal glucocorticosteroids can be applied safely [34], even in children and for chronic rhinitis [35]. Positive treatment effects of the current study were also reflected by the results of the quality of life questionnaire which demonstrated improvements in all questioned areas covering daily life activities, general well-being, and the emotional status of patients.

Additional support to the potential efficacy of the ectoine nasal spray comes from similar studies. In a single center, double-blind, placebo-controlled cross-over study consisting of 5 visits involving patients suffering from allergic rhinoconjunctivitis, it could be demonstrated that ectoin nasal spray and eye drops relieved all of the hallmark symptoms of allergic rhinoconjunctivitis with minimal side-effects thereby showing a statistically significant effect over the placebo group. Corresponding data has been presented on a scientific congress [19]. Furthermore, additional noninterventional studies and another placebo-controlled clinical trial involving ectoine containing products in the treatment of allergic rhinitis were analyzed together. Both nasal and ocular symptoms decreased significantly upon treatment with ectoine products. The strength of effects of ectoine products was assessed by comparison of symptom scores on day 7 and baseline values on day 1 with reference products (azelastine, beclomethasone, or cromoglycic acid) or placebo treatment and showed comparable (nasal obstruction and rhinorrhea)

or better (nasal itching and sneezing) efficacy of the ectoine products in comparison to control substances ([36], congress report, paper accepted).

Taken together this study supports that allergic rhinitis can be successfully treated with beclomethasone and also it was shown that ectoine nasal spray may be a future treatment option. Whereas efficacy of the pharmaceutically active steroid beclomethasone seems to be superior to that of the natural, barrier stabilizing substance ectoine, with its nonpharmaceutical mode of action, the safety profiles of both treatment groups were comparable. Thus, after proving the hints towards efficacy with further studies, ectoine containing products might become interesting alternative treatment strategies for symptom reduction in allergic rhinitis, particularly for patients seeking nonpharmaceutical treatments, as they contain a natural substance and are free of preservatives. Those alternative treatments are highly demanded but not yet generally recommended [37] and, thus, should be evaluated in more detail in further studies.

Disclosure

Bilstein is an employee of Bitop AG, a company where medical devices, including the ectoine nasal spray, were developed and registered. Bitop AG sponsored the trial discussed in this paper. Sonnemann and Möeller received sponsorship by Bitop AG to conduct the study.

Conflict of Interests

The authors declare that there is no conflict of interests regarding the publication of this paper.

Acknowledgment

The authors thank Ulrike von Hehn for statistical analysis of data.

References

[1] J. Bousquet, N. Khaltaev, A. A. Cruz et al., "Allergic Rhinitis and its Impact on Asthma (ARIA) 2008 update (in collaboration with the World Health Organization, GA2LEN and AllerGen)," *Allergy: European Journal of Allergy and Clinical Immunology*, vol. 63, no. 86, pp. 8–160, 2008.

[2] V. Bauchau and S. R. Durham, "Prevalence and rate of diagnosis of allergic rhinitis in Europe," *European Respiratory Journal*, vol. 24, no. 5, pp. 758–764, 2004.

[3] O. Kaschke, "Auswirkungen einer steroidphobie in deutschland auf die therapie mit topischen glukokortikoiden," *MedReport*, vol. 32, no. 17, p. 10, 2011.

[4] E. A. Galinski and A. Oren, "Isolation and structure determination of a novel compatible solute from the moderately halophilic purple sulfur bacterium ectothiorhodospira marismortui," *European Journal of Biochemistry*, vol. 198, no. 3, pp. 593–598, 1991.

[5] J. M. Pastor, M. Salvador, M. Argandoña et al., "Ectoines in cell stress protection: Uses and biotechnological production," *Biotechnology Advances*, vol. 28, no. 6, pp. 782–801, 2010.

[6] K. Lippert and E. A. Galinski, "Enzyme stabilization by ectoine-type compatible solutes: protection against heating, freezing and drying," *Applied Microbiology and Biotechnology*, vol. 37, no. 1, pp. 61–65, 1992.

[7] T. Arakawa and S. N. Timasheff, "The stabilization of proteins by osmolytes," *Biophysical Journal*, vol. 47, no. 3, pp. 411–414, 1985.

[8] J. Smiatek, R. K. Harishchandra, O. Rubner, H.-J. Galla, and A. Heuer, "Properties of compatible solutes in aqueous solution," *Biophysical Chemistry*, vol. 160, no. 1, pp. 62–68, 2012.

[9] T. Sauer and E. A. Galinski, "Bacterial milking: a novel bioprocess for production of compatible solutes," *Biotechnology and Bioengineering*, vol. 57, no. 3, pp. 306–313, 1998.

[10] P. Peters, E. A. Galinski, and H. G. Truper, "The biosynthesis of ectoine," *FEMS Microbiology Letters*, vol. 71, no. 1-2, pp. 157–162, 1990.

[11] I. Yu, Y. Jindo, and M. Nagaoka, "Microscopic understanding of preferential exclusion of compatible solute ectoine: direct interaction and hydration alteration," *Journal of Physical Chemistry B*, vol. 111, no. 34, pp. 10231–10238, 2007.

[12] S. Kolp, M. Pietsch, E. A. Galinski, and M. Gütschow, "Compatible solutes as protectants for zymogens against proteolysis," *Biochimica et Biophysica Acta, Proteins and Proteomics*, vol. 1764, no. 7, pp. 1234–1242, 2006.

[13] U. Sydlik, I. Gallitz, C. Albrecht, J. Abel, J. Krutmann, and K. Unfried, "The compatible solute ectoine protects against nanoparticle-induced neutrophilic lung inflammation," *American Journal of Respiratory and Critical Care Medicine*, vol. 180, no. 1, pp. 29–35, 2009.

[14] U. Sydlik, H. Peuschel, A. Paunel-Görgülü et al., "Recovery of neutrophil apoptosis by ectoine: a new strategy against lung inflammation," *European Respiratory Journal*, vol. 41, no. 2, pp. 433–442, 2012.

[15] S. Grether-Beck, A. Timmer, I. Felsner, H. Brenden, D. Brammertz, and J. Krutmann, "Ultraviolet A-induced signaling involves a ceramide-mediated autocrine loop leading to ceramide de novo synthesis," *Journal of Investigative Dermatology*, vol. 125, no. 3, pp. 545–553, 2005.

[16] R. Graf, S. Anzali, J. Buenger, F. Pfluecker, and H. Driller, "The multifunctional role of ectoine as a natural cell protectant," *Clinics in Dermatology*, vol. 26, no. 4, pp. 326–333, 2008.

[17] A. Marini, K. Reinelt, J. Krutmann, and A. Bilstein, "Ectoine-containing cream in the treatment of mild to moderate atopic dermatitis: a randomised, comparator-controlled, intra-individual double-blind, multi-center trial," *Skin Pharmacology and Physiology*, vol. 27, no. 2, pp. 57–65, 2014.

[18] A. Eichel, J. Wittig, K. Sha-Hosseini, and R. Mösges, "Prospective, controlled study of SNS01 (ectoine nasal spray) compared to BNO-101 (phytotherapeutic dragées) in patients with acute rhinosinusitis," *CMRO Description*, vol. 29, no. 7, pp. 739–746, 2013.

[19] A. Salapatek, M. Bates, A. Bilstein, and D. Patel, "Ectoin, a novel, non-drug, extremophile-based device, relieves allergic rhinoconjunctivitis symptoms in patients in an environmental exposure chamber model," *Journal of Allergy and Clinical Immunology*, vol. 127, no. 2, 2011.

[20] A. Bilstein and U. Sonnemann, "Nasal spray and eye drops containing ectoine, a novel natural, non-drug anti-allergic substance are not less effective than azelastine nasal spray and eye drops in improving the symptoms of allergic rhinitis and conjunctivitis," in *Proceedings of the 30th Congress of the European Academy of Allergy and Clinical Immunology (EAACI '11)*, 2011.

[21] V. H. J. Van Der Velden, "Glucocorticoids: mechanisms of action and anti-inflammatory potential in asthma," *Mediators of Inflammation*, vol. 7, no. 4, pp. 229–237, 1998.

[22] R. K. Harishchandra, A. K. Sachan, A. Kerth, G. Lentzen, T. Neuhaus, and H.-J. Galla, "Compatible solutes: ectoine and hydroxyectoine improve functional nanostructures in artificial lung surfactants," *Biochimica et Biophysica Acta, Biomembranes*, vol. 1808, no. 12, pp. 2830–2840, 2011.

[23] R. K. Harishchandra, M. Saleem, and H.-J. Galla, "Nanoparticle interaction with model lung surfactant monolayers," *Journal of the Royal Society Interface*, vol. 7, no. 1, pp. S15–S26, 2010.

[24] R. K. Harishchandra, S. Wulff, G. Lentzen, T. Neuhaus, and H.-J. Galla, "The effect of compatible solute ectoines on the structural organization of lipid monolayer and bilayer membranes," *Biophysical Chemistry*, vol. 150, no. 1–3, pp. 37–46, 2010.

[25] J. Smiatek, R. K. Harishchandra, H. J. Galla, and A. Heuer, "Low concentrated hydroxyectoine solutions in presence of DPPC lipid bilayers: a computer simulation study," *Biophysical Chemistry*, vol. 180-181, pp. 102–109, 20132013.

[26] H. Peuschel, U. Sydlik, J. Haendeler et al., "C-Src-mediated activation of Erk1/2 is a reaction of epithelial cells to carbon nanoparticle treatment and may be a target for a molecular preventive strategy," *Biological Chemistry*, vol. 391, no. 11, pp. 1327–1332, 2010.

[27] H. Peuschel, U. Sydlik, S. Grether-Beck et al., "Carbon nanoparticles induce ceramide- and lipid raft-dependent signalling in lung epithelial cells: a target for a preventive strategy against environmentally-induced lung inflammation," *Particle and Fibre Toxicology*, vol. 9, no. 48, 2012.

[28] H. G. Hoymann, A. Bilstein, G. Lenzen et al., "Effects of ectoine on early allergic response, airway hyperresponsiveness and inflammation In ovalbumin-sensitized rats," *The American Journal of Respiratory and Critical Care Medicine*, vol. 181, p. A5693, 2010.

[29] A. Bilstein, F. Bernal, J. Klein et al., "Immuno-protective effects of the extremolyte Ectoine in animal models and humans," in *Proceedings of the 28th Congress of the European Academy of Allergy and Clinical Immunology*, EAACI, Warsaw, Poland, 2009.

[30] H. Wan, H. L. Winton, C. Soeller et al., "Der p 1 facilitates transepithelial allergen delivery by disruption of tight junctions," *The Journal of Clinical Investigation*, vol. 104, no. 1, pp. 123–133, 1999.

[31] W. Lumry, F. Hampel, C. LaForce, F. Kiechel, T. El-Akkad, and J. J. Murray, "A comparison of once-daily triamcinolone acetonide aqueous and twice-daily beclomethasone dipropionate aqueous nasal sprays in the treatment of seasonal allergic rhinitis," *Allergy and Asthma Proceedings*, vol. 24, no. 3, pp. 203–210, 2003.

[32] T. B. Casale, S. M. Azzam, R. E. Miller et al., "Demonstration of therapeutic equivalence of generic and innovator beclomethasone in seasonal allergic rhinitis," *Annals of Allergy, Asthma and Immunology*, vol. 82, no. 5, pp. 435–441, 1999.

[33] J. Van Bavel, W. C. Howland, N. J. Amar, W. Wheeler, and H. Sacks, "Efficacy and safety of azelastine 0.15% nasal spray administered once daily in subjects with seasonal allergic rhinitis," *Allergy and Asthma Proceedings*, vol. 30, no. 5, pp. 512–518, 2009.

[34] O. Emin, M. Fatih, D. Emre, and S. Nedim, "Lack of bone metabolism side effects after 3 years of nasal topical steroids in children with allergic rhinitis," *Journal of Bone and Mineral Metabolism*, vol. 29, no. 5, pp. 582–587, 2011.

[35] E. Ozkaya, M. Ozsutcu, and F. Mete, "Lack of ocular side effects after 2 years of topical steroids for allergic rhinitis," *Journal of Pediatric Ophthalmology and Strabismus*, vol. 48, no. 5, pp. 311–317, 2011.

[36] A. Eichel, N. Werkhäuser, A. Bilstein, and R. Mösges, "Meta-analysis of the efficacy of ectoine nasal spray and eye drops in the treatment of allergic rhinoconjunctivitis," *Allergy*, vol. 2014, Article ID 292545, 12 pages, 2014.

[37] G. Passalacqua, P. J. Bousquet, K.-H. Carlsen et al., "ARIA update: I—Systematic review of complementary and alternative medicine for rhinitis and asthma," *The Journal of Allergy and Clinical Immunology*, vol. 117, no. 5, pp. 1054–1062, 2006.

6

Treatment of Rhinitis Sicca Anterior with Ectoine Containing Nasal Spray

Uwe Sonnemann,[1] Olaf Scherner,[2] and Nina Werkhäuser[2]

[1] Private Health Centre, Institute for ENT Elmshorn, Hermann-Ehlers-Weg 4, 25337 Elmshorn, Germany
[2] Bitop AG, Stockumer Street 28, 58453 Witten, Germany

Correspondence should be addressed to Olaf Scherner; scherner@bitop.de

Academic Editor: Ralph Mösges

Objectives. The safety and efficacy of ectoine nasal spray and ectoine nasal spray with dexpanthenol in the treatment of rhinitis sicca were evaluated in two studies. *Design and Methods.* Two noninterventional observational studies were performed to evaluate the efficacy and safety of a nasal spray containing ectoine (study 1) and ectoine/dexpanthenol (study 2) over a period of two weeks including comparable numbers of patients suffering from rhinitis sicca anterior. Patients and physicians were asked to rate the efficacy in reducing symptoms and the tolerability over the treatment phase. *Results.* The treatment in both studies resulted in a clinical and statistical significant reduction of the main diagnosis parameters, nasal airway obstruction, and crust formation. There was also a significant reduction in the secondary diagnosis parameters in both studies. Importantly, the tolerability was very good. During the whole observational study, neither patients nor doctors stopped the medication due to unwanted effects. *Conclusion.* Rhinitis sicca could be successfully treated with a nasal spray containing ectoine and a nasal spray combining ectoine with dexpanthenol. The combination of both substances led to slight advantages.

1. Introduction

Rhinitis sicca or generally speaking dry nose is a rather frequent problem involving many people. The term "dry nose" has not yet been uniformly defined [1]. Otolaryngologists often use the terms "rhinitis sicca" or "dry rhinitis," although no clear definition exists. Many symptoms during dry nose could be encountered ranging from subjective sensation of the dry nose and itching up to mild burning, nasal obstruction, crusting associated with unpleasant smell, epistaxis, and diminished sense of smell. Rhinitis sicca anterior means a chronic inflammation in the region of the anterior part of the nose, affecting the anterior and caudal septum and/or the corresponding lateral nasal vestibule. Mechanical as well as environmental irritations lead to crust formation. In rare cases, patients suffer from a slight stench due to bacterial colonization of the crust formations. The treatment of rhinitis sicca involves mainly elimination of promoting factors, moistening, sufficient daily drinking amount, cleansing of the crusts, care of the mucosa and inhibition of possible infections, or in rare cases the elimination of overlarge

endonasal space [1]. The main treatment for rhinitis sicca consists of humidification of the nose, especially the mucus, focusing in a real wash-out of possible inflammatory triggers and application of a protective layer on the mucus. The market offers a huge number of different devices involving saline, oils, moisturizers, sprays, and ointments for this purpose. Nasal irrigation and nasal saline sprays wash out inflammatory triggers directly [2, 3] and achieve an improvement of mucociliary clearance by improving the ciliary beat frequency [4, 5]. Nasal ointments mostly including glycerol develop a protective moistening effect and protect the nose from water loss [6]. Low concentrated oils also have beneficial effects on nasal ciliary beat frequency [7]. The efficacy of dexpanthenol, the alcohol analog of pantothenic acid, in the treatment of rhinitis sicca is widely spread in the OTC use and has been shown clinically [8]. In addition, use of dexpanthenol has a strong tradition in the treatment of various skin diseases in which dexpanthenol is used as humidifier/ moisturizer. Also, use in wound healing has been reported [9]. Besides these different options, patients ask for alternative treatments as the current treatments often leave patients unsatisfied and a demand for other nonpharmacological treatment options exists.

Ectoine is an extremolyte, a compatible solute which is produced by microorganism living under extreme environmental conditions such as extreme salinity or dryness [10]. In those microorganisms, ectoine serves as natural cell protectant [11, 12]. Different in vitro, ex vivo, and in vivo studies have shown that ectoine can be used to protect epithelial tissues and moisturize and reduce inflammations [13–15]. Ectoine acts physically via a mechanism called "preferential exclusion." In the presence of ectoine, membranes and lipids are protected indirectly: as ectoine is expelled from the surface of proteins and lipids, those are protected by a water shell, thereby increasing the fluidity of membranes and resulting in the preferential formation of the native conformation of proteins [11]. This might stabilize mucous membranes such as lining epithelia of the nose, thereby protecting those cells from invading allergens or pathogens [16]. Recent developments have demonstrated that these cell protective attributes could be transferred into medical devices including ectoine containing creams, nasal sprays, or eye drops which can be used for human use, for example, the treatment of atopic dermatitis, allergic rhinitis, and rhinosinusitis [17–20].

The use of ectoine in a saline based nasal spray could be a useful therapeutic approach for patients suffering from dry nose syndrome. Additionally a combinatory approach could be applied, for example, of ectoine and dexpanthenol. The combined effects of ectoine and/or dexpanthenol are already used in the field of dermatology and promise a useful combination effect for the treatment of rhinitis sicca. By using an ectoine and dexpanthenol nasal spray, the moisturizing and regeneration supporting effects of both compounds could assist a possible healing of ulcers and prevent nasal obstruction in addition to the reduction of primary symptoms.

2. Materials and Methods

The current paper describes two prospective, open-label, noninterventional trials (studies 1 and 2). Restricted inclusion of patients study based on the diagnosis of rhinitis sicca and strict adherence to the principle of nonintervention allowed data to be collected for a very unselective patient population. As study designs for both studies were very similar, data are summarized and differences are only outlined where applicable.

2.1. Medication. Patients in study 1 were treated with an ectoine containing nasal spray with 0.5% ectoine and further ingredients were sodium chloride, sodium-di-hydrogen-phosphate dihydrate, di-sodium-hydrogen-phosphate, and water.

Patients in study 2 used a 0.5% ectoine nasal spray which contained 1.0% dexpanthenol, sodium chloride, sodium-di-hydrogen-phosphate dihydrate, di-sodium-hydrogen-phosphate, and water.

2.2. Treatment and Study Design. Both studies were open for all patients from 18 years on, who were identified by ENT specialist with symptoms of dry nose. Following confirmation of the diagnosis of rhinitis sicca, patients were asked by the ENT specialist whether they were interested to participate in the current trials. Upon signing a patient information and consent form, patients had to attend two more site visits: V2 on day 7 ± 2 and V3 on day 14 ± 2. During the entire treatment period of 2 weeks, patients were asked to use the nasal sprays at least five times daily.

2.3. Scoring of Symptoms. Clinical symptoms were assessed on a 12-point scale ranging from 0 (no symptoms) to 12 (very severe symptoms).

During the visits, the physician assessed the main symptoms of nasal obstruction and crusting of the nose as well as the following secondary symptoms: endonasal blood deposits, concomitant pharyngitis, cacosmia, rhinorrhea, exudate viscosity, and turbinate hyperplasia.

On days 3, 6, 9, and 12 after start of the study, patients were asked to document the severity of the following symptoms in a patient diary: nasal obstruction, dryness of the nose, nose bleeding, sore throat, cacosmia, and exudate from the nose. In addition, patients were asked to describe the consistency of exudate on a 12-point scale from 0 (fluid) to 12 (crusted).

3. Scoring of Efficacy, Tolerability, and Compliance

Both efficacy and tolerability were assessed by physicians (during V2 and V3) and by the patients (days 3, 6, 9, and 12) on a scale from 0 (very good) to 12 (none/bad).

3.1. Statistics. The statistical analysis was carried out with SPSS version 15 (study 1) or 17 (study 2), respectively. Both efficacy and safety analyses were performed on the entire study population. Descriptive statistics were used for a quantitative report of the main study population features. Continuous variables were tested for normal distribution via Kolmogorov-Smirnov test. Further analysis was carried out with the Mann-Whitney U test, Wilcoxon test, or Friedman test. The level of significance was set to $P < 0.05$ in all tests. Unavailable data were treated as "missing values" or substituted by the "last value carried forward" method.

4. Results

Both studies were conducted in accordance with the Declaration of Helsinki. All investigations were carried out with informed consent of all participants.

Study 1 was a noninterventional trial taking place from April to July 2008; study 2 took place from March to April 2009. Both studies were carried out at a German ear nose throat (ENT) practice. Distribution and demographics of patients are shown in Figures 1 and 2.

4.1. Development of Symptoms

4.1.1. Nasal Obstruction. In both studies, the investigators assessment revealed that the symptom nasal obstruction decreased significantly from V1 to V2 as well as further to V3.

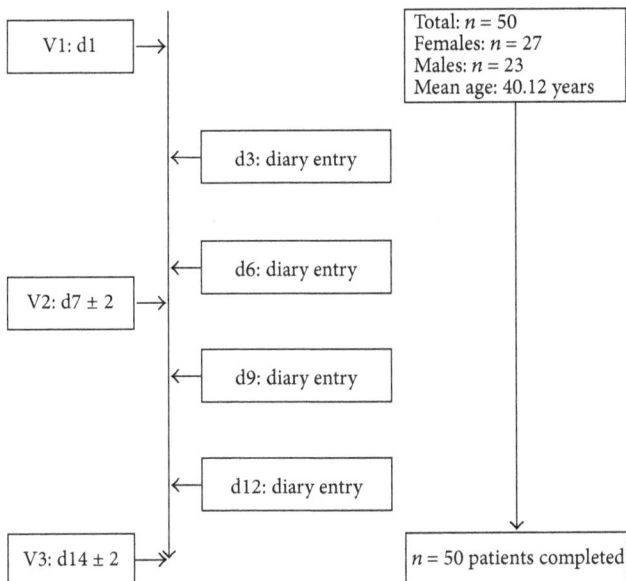

FIGURE 1: Patient flow and characteristics of demographic data in study 1.

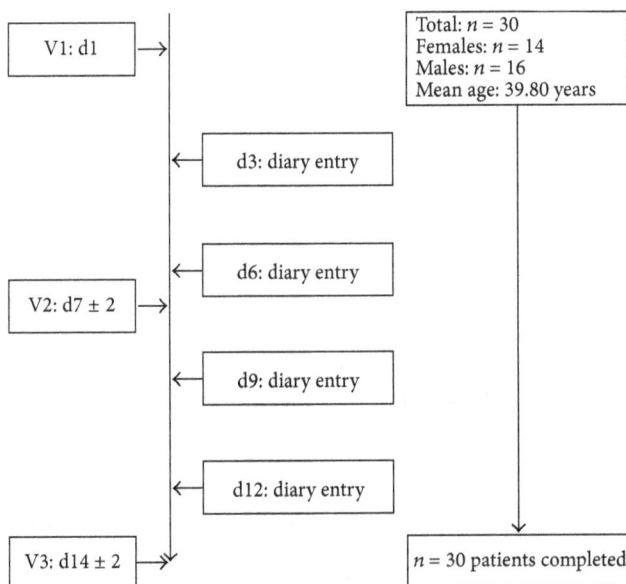

FIGURE 2: Patient flow and characteristics of demographic data in study 2.

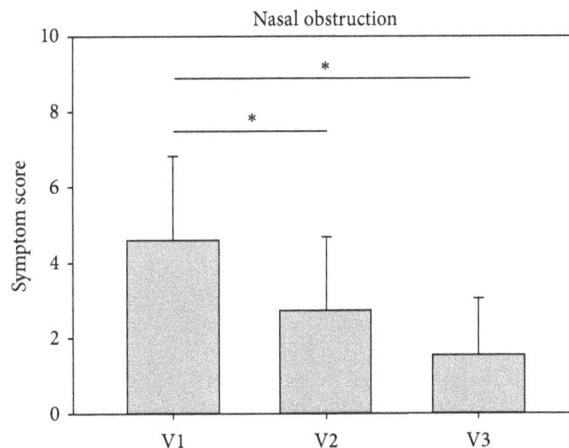

FIGURE 3: Development of nasal obstruction from V1 to V3 assessed by the investigator (study 1). The asterisks mark a statistical significance; the whiskers mark the standard deviation.

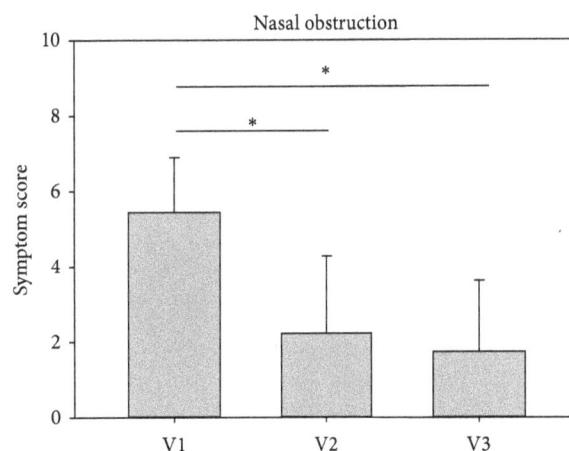

FIGURE 4: Development of nasal obstruction from V1 to V3 assessed by the investigator (study 2). The asterisks mark a statistical significance; the whiskers mark the standard deviation.

In study 1, symptom scores decreased from baseline values 4.60 ± 2.23 at V1 to 2.74 ± 1.95 at V2 and then to 1.54 ± 1.52 at V3. Values in study 2 decreased comparably from 5.43 ± 1.46 at V1 to 2.23 ± 2.05 at V2 and further to 1.73 ± 1.89 at V3 (Figures 3 and 4).

Decreases of the symptom nasal obstruction were similar and in accordance with the patients' assessments. Values are listed in Table 1.

4.1.2. Crust Formation/Nasal Dryness. The symptom nasal crust formation decreased significantly from V1 to V2 and further to V3 in both studies in the investigators assessment. Values in study 1 decreased from baseline values of 6.20 ± 1.99 to 2.16 ± 2.26 at V2 and further to 1.52 ± 1.85 at V3. Values in study 2 decreased comparably from baseline values of 6.43 ± 2.08 to 2.40 ± 1.81 at V2 and to 1.30 ± 1.24 at V3. Results are depicted in Figures 5 and 6.

Patients evaluated the decrease of the symptom dry nose in a similar way to the physician's assessments as listed in Table 2. The symptom nasal dryness decreased significantly from day 3 to day 12 in both studies.

4.1.3. Secondary Symptom Scores. In addition to the symptoms nasal obstruction and crust formation/nasal dryness, further symptoms were assessed by both investigators and patients. As depicted in Figures 7 and 8, there was a similarity between the results of both studies in the investigators assessment. The symptoms blood deposits, pharyngitis, turbinate hyperplasia, and exudate viscosity improved significantly

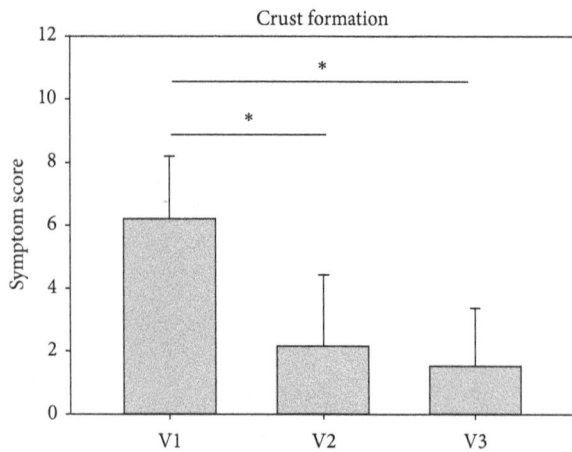

FIGURE 5: Development of crust formation from visit 1 (V1) to visit 3 (V3) in study 1. $^*P < 0.001$. The asterisks mark a statistical significance; the whiskers mark the standard deviation.

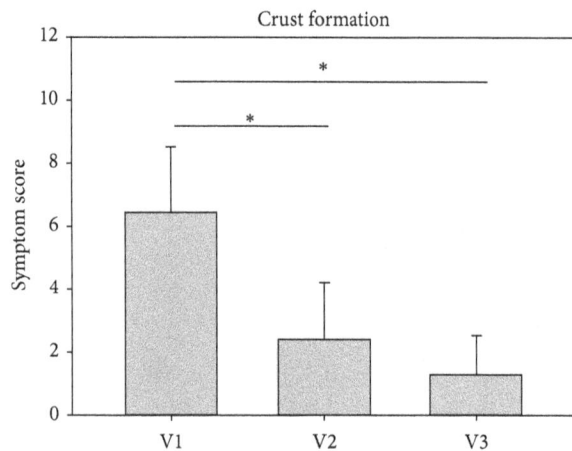

FIGURE 6: Development of crust formation from visit 1 (V1) to visit 3 (V3) in study 2. $^*P < 0.001$.

from baseline values at V1 to the final visit V3. The symptom rhinorrhea only improved significantly in study 2, whereas decreases in this symptom were nonsignificant in study 1. As only very few patients complained about the symptom cacosmia ($n = 2$ in study 1 and $n = 5$ in study 2), decreases in this symptom were negligible.

Patients' scores of secondary symptom evaluation are listed in Tables 3 and 4. In study 1, the symptom rhinorrhea improved significantly from d3 to d12. In study 2, nose bleeding, rhinorrhea, cacosmia, and exudate viscosity improved significantly over this time frame.

5. Efficacy, Tolerability, and Compliance

The physician judged both efficacy and tolerability of treatment after 7 days (V2) and after 14 days (V3). As shown in Figures 9 and 10, ectoine nasal spray treatment was considered to be both efficient and well tolerable. Mean values for efficacy at V3 were 3.5 ± 2.06 (study 1) and 1.83 ± 1.39

(study 2) meaning good to very good efficacy. Mean values for tolerability were 2.08 ± 1.21 (study 1) and 0.57 ± 0.97 (study 2), which also means good to very good tolerability.

Patients' assessments of tolerability and efficacy of treatment are depicted in Figures 11 and 12. Mean efficacy values were 3.12±3.08 at day 12 of treatment in study 1 and 2.43±2.24 in study 2 corresponding to good efficacy. Tolerability was judged as very good in both studies with mean values on day 12 of 1.40 ± 1.80 in study 1 and 1.17 ± 1.21 in study 2.

5.1. Adverse Events (AEs). In study 1, no AE occurred. In study 2, 1 AE occurred (acute rhinitis). The correlation with the treatment was judged as unlikely by the investigator. No SAE occurred in either of the two studies.

6. Conclusions

The aim of these observational studies was to gain insight into the tolerability and the extent to which the treatments influenced the severity of the patients' symptoms. An ectoine nasal spray (study 1) or an ectoine and dexpanthenol nasal spray (study 2) was tested in patients with rhinitis sicca under practical conditions. A total of 80 patients (50 patients in study 1, 30 patients in study 2) with a wide variety of disease severities participated in this postmarketing surveillance study. However, the potential flaw of these studies is their noncontrolled character, the missing randomization, or placebo control. Therefore the evidence grade of the results needs to be reduced at least to IIb.

Both nasal spray formulations showed a good tolerability and safety in the studies. No drop-out was recorded. The studies showed a significant decrease of the main symptoms nasal obstruction and crust formation from V1 to V2 as well as further to V3. The decrease of nasal obstructions assessed by the physicians was confirmed by patients in both studies, with a stronger decrease of symptoms assessed by the physicians. This is likely to be due to the timing of the patient's diary, as this was started at day three of treatment, when the first positive effect of the respective treatments had occurred already.

Apart from main symptoms, the secondary symptom scores also decreased similarly in both studies. In the investigators assessment, the symptoms blood deposits, pharyngitis, turbinate hyperplasia, and exudate viscosity improved significantly from starting values at V1 to the final visit V3. Differences in symptom reduction between both studies occurred only with respect to rhinorrhea. Treatment with the nasal spray with ectoine only did not lead to a significant improvement of rhinorrhea, whereas the improvement in with the ectoine nasal spray alone was not statistically significant. The degree of symptom reduction in the main parameter nasal obstruction seemed to be reduced more efficiently in the study with the combined nasal spray, as the score started with a higher value and dropped faster and to a higher degree as in the study with the ectoine nasal spray. In the patient assessment of study 2 symptom improvement was significant for nose bleeding, exudate viscosity, rhinorrhea, and cacosmia, whereas the patient assessment in study 1 showed only a significant reduction of the symptoms in nose

TABLE 1: Development of nasal obstruction assessed by patients on days 3, 6, 9, and 12 following treatment with ectoine nasal spray.

	d3	d6	d9	d12	P (d3 versus d12)
Study 1	2.74 ± 2.31	2.52 ± 2.18	2.10 ± 2.00	1.64 ± 1.68	<0.001
Study 2	3.67 ± 2.28	2.80 ± 1.99	2.33 ± 1.65	1.87 ± 1.33	<0.001

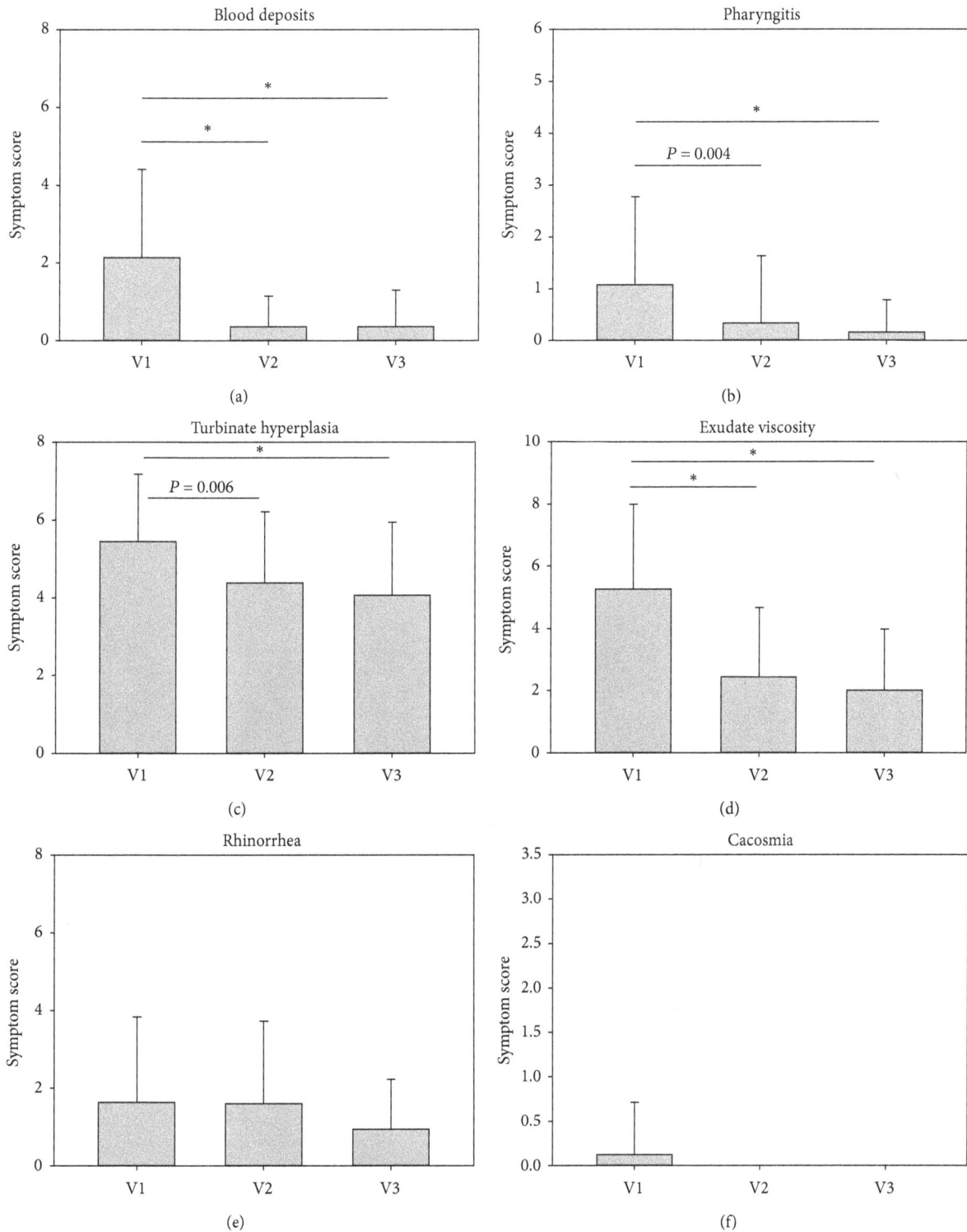

FIGURE 7: Development of secondary symptoms (ENT evaluation) during study 1. $^{*}P < 0.001$. The asterisks mark a statistical significance; the whiskers mark the standard deviation.

TABLE 2: Development of nasal dryness assessed by patients on days 3, 6, 9, and 12 following treatment with ectoine nasal spray.

	d3	d6	d9	d12	P (d3 versus d12)
Study 1	4.64 ± 2.40	3.76 ± 2.53	2.90 ± 2.48	2.42 ± 2.37	<0.001
Study 2	4.43 ± 2.49	3.30 ± 2.12	2.33 ± 1.97	1.83 ± 1.49	<0.001

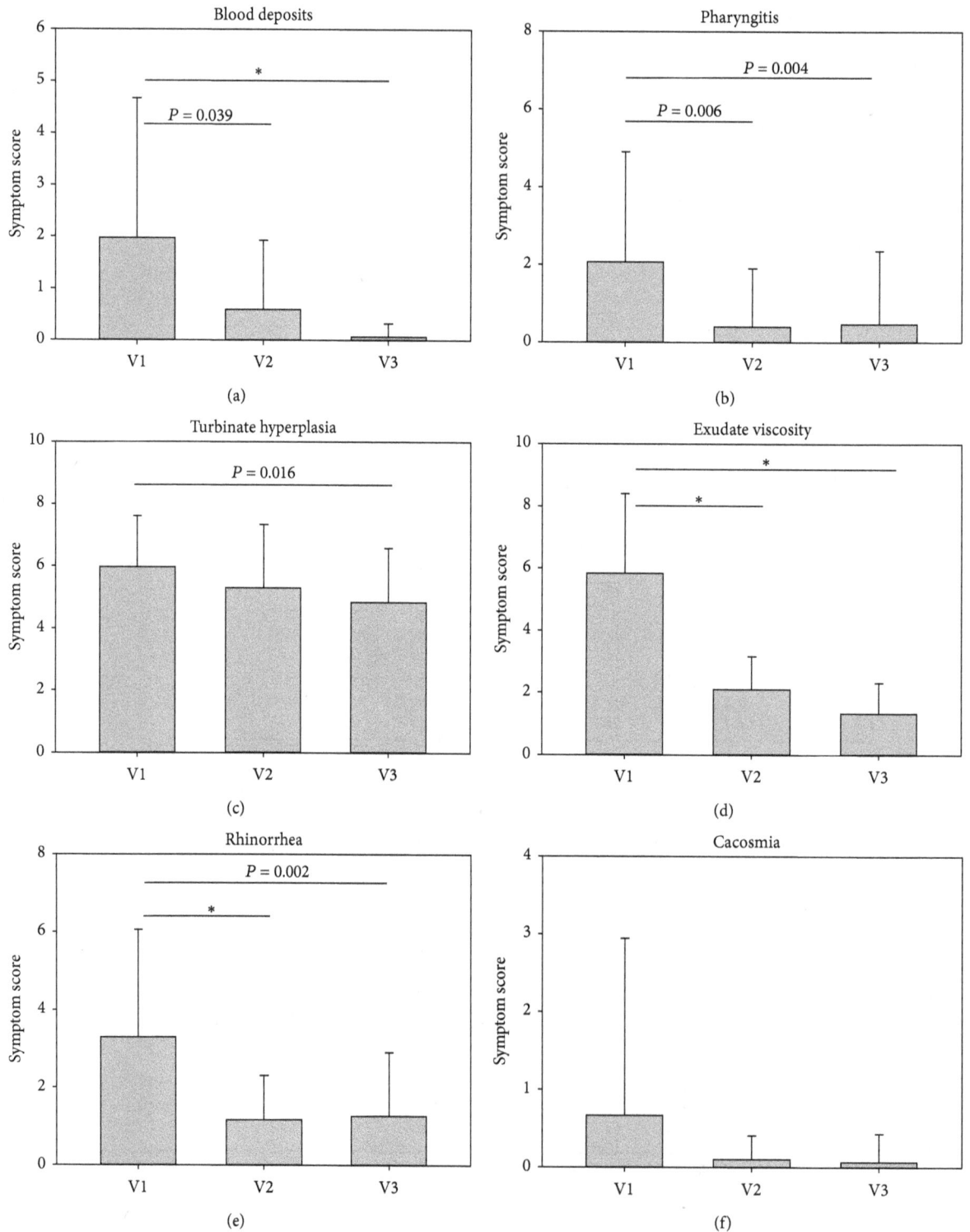

FIGURE 8: Development of secondary symptoms during study 2. $^*P < 0.001$.

TABLE 3: Patients' assessments of secondary symptom scores at days 3, 6, 9, and 12 following treatment start of study 1.

Symptoms	d3	d6	d9	d12	P value (d3 versus d12)
Nose bleeding	0.36 ± 0.85	0.46 ± 1.07	0.36 ± 0.85	0.30 ± 0.74	0.787
Pharyngitis	0.64 ± 1.77	0.62 ± 1.74	0.46 ± 1.20	0.42 ± 1.13	0.754
Exudate viscosity	3.36 ± 3.50	2.90 ± 3.03	2.38 ± 2.86	2.40 ± 2.93	0.108
Rhinorrhea	2.44 ± 2.16	2.10 ± 2.14	1.74 ± 1.88	1.42 ± 1.54	0.021
Cacosmia	0.60 ± 1.53	0.48 ± 1.31	0.42 ± 1.57	0.26 ± 0.69	0.388

TABLE 4: Patients' assessments of secondary symptom scores at days 3, 6, 9, and 12 following treatment start of study 2.

Symptoms	d3	d6	d9	d12	P value (d3 versus d12)
Nose bleeding	0.70 ± 1.60	0.73 ± 1.72	0.50 ± 1.01	0.17 ± 0.59	0.0019
Pharyngitis	1.07 ± 2.26	0.67 ± 1.63	0.57 ± 1.19	0.60 ± 1.00	0.719
Exudate viscosity	2.67 ± 2.38	2.50 ± 2.64	2.10 ± 2.23	1.67 ± 2.19	0.027
Rhinorrhea	2.57 ± 1.99	2.00 ± 1.72	1.90 ± 1.83	1.57 ± 1.45	0.025
Cacosmia	0.90 ± 2.26	0.70 ± 1.82	0.33 ± 0.99	0.30 ± 0.99	0.005

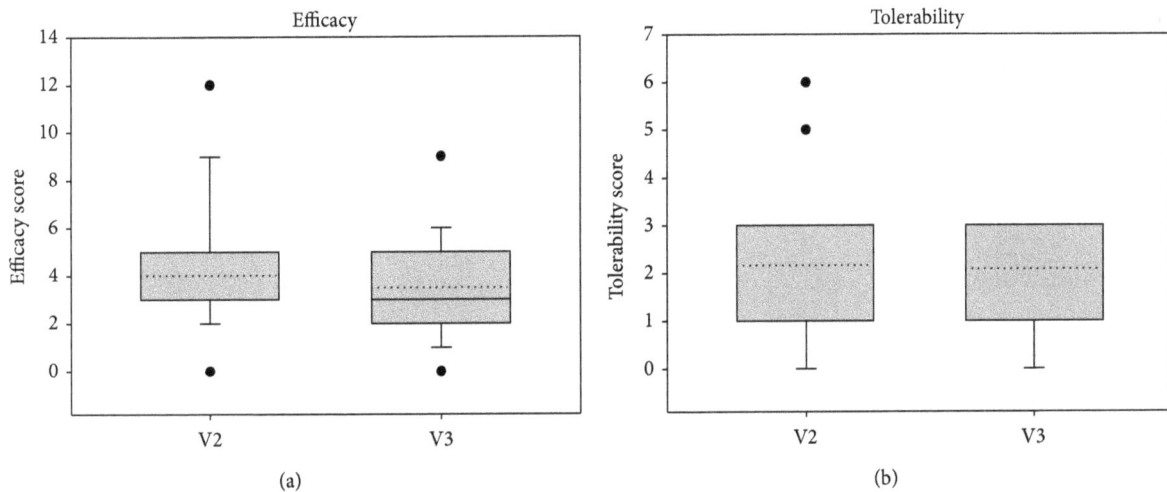

FIGURE 9: Judgment of efficacy and tolerability according to the physician's assessment in study 1.

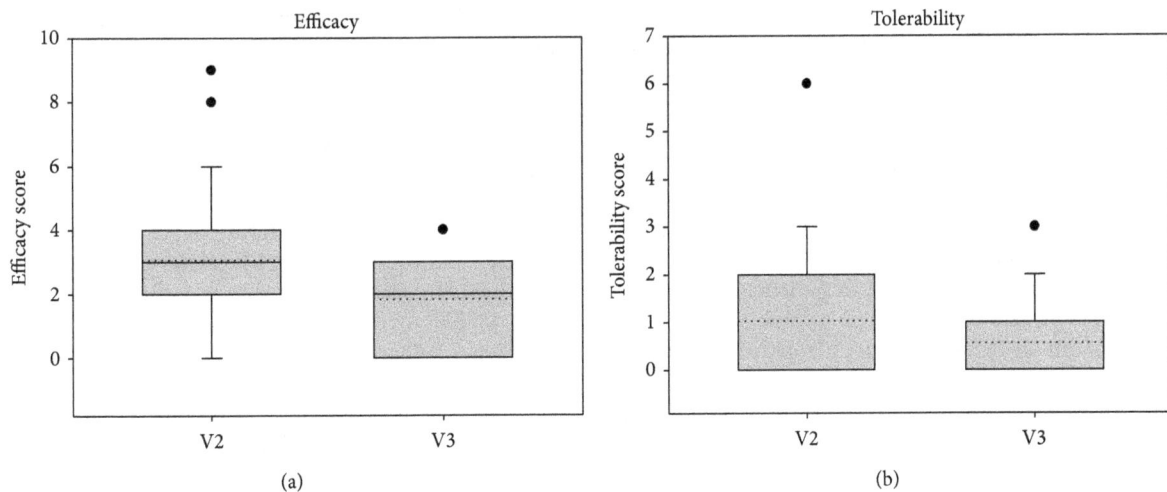

FIGURE 10: Judgment of efficacy and tolerability according to the physician's assessment in study 2.

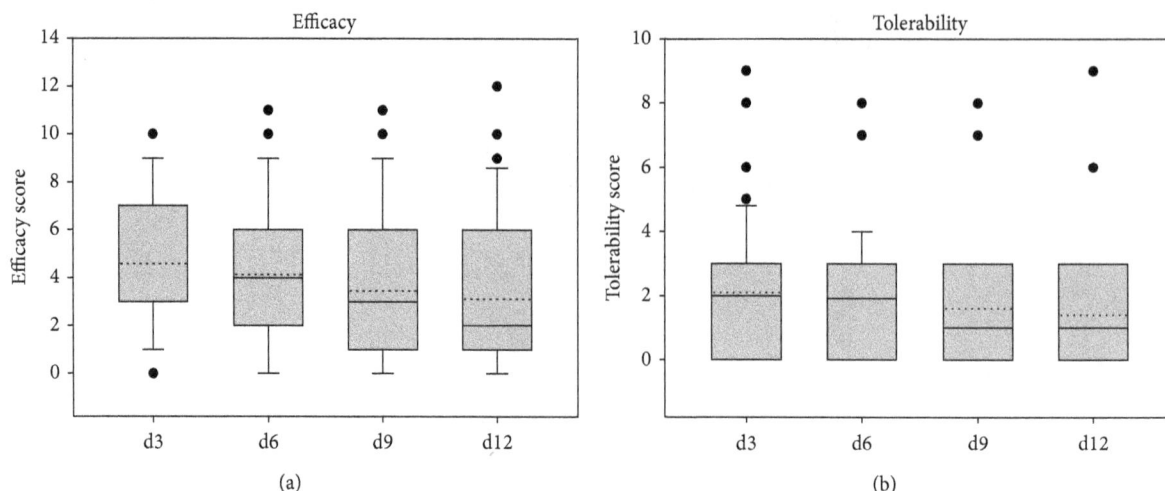

FIGURE 11: Judgment of efficacy and tolerability according to the patients' assessment in study 1.

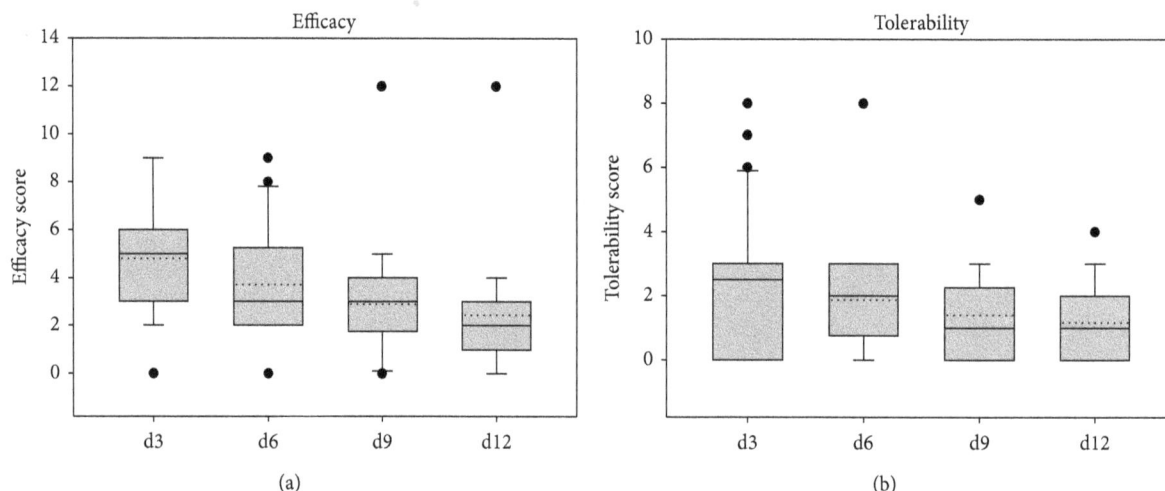

FIGURE 12: Judgment of efficacy and tolerability according to the patients' assessment in study 2.

bleeding. It can be mentioned that only a few patients in both studies suffered from cacosmia and the decreases in these symptoms were negligible for both of them.

As a summary, the ectoine nasal spray achieved in study 1 treatment success similar to that of the combination of ectoine and dexpanthenol in study 2 with respect to the main symptom scores of both studies, crust formation and nasal obstruction. Differences in treatment effect between both nasal sprays and studies were observable in the secondary parameters, both in physicians and in patients assessment, tending towards an additional effect if ectoine and dexpanthenol are combined in one product compared to ectoine alone. Both natural nonpharmacological nasal sprays showed efficacy in treatment of rhinitis sicca, which is comparable to the reported outcome for other products [21]. Data from preclinical studies also support the combination of ectoine and dexpanthenol (data not shown).

The mode of action and subsequent effect in treatment of rhinitis sicca of dexpanthenol is understood from the

literature [22]. The treatment effects of the ectoine nasal spray can be attributed to its physical action. By increasing the fluidity of the nasal epithelia, the barrier function of this membrane is increased, therefore inhibiting the potential loss of water. Experiments with ectoine on biological and artificial membranes support this thesis further, including the reduction of mechanical stress induced membrane damage [15–17]. The additional hydrating effect of ectoine is well described in the literature [15, 23, 24] as well as the capacity of reduction of inflammation in skin and respiratory epithelium [14, 17, 18, 25].

Taken together, rhinitis sicca anterior or dry nose could be successfully treated with an ectoine containing nasal spray. Therefore an interesting option of a new and safe nonpharmacological treatment of rhinitis sicca will be available in the future. The addition of the well-known and accepted dexpanthenol did not enhance the treatment regarding the major symptoms scores. The decrease of symptom over the 14-day treatment period was more pronounced for the combination of ectoine and dexpanthenol, but this difference was not significant. Slightly better improvement in different secondary symptoms revealed synergistic characteristics of the two substances in combination when compared to the ectoine nasal spray alone. However, these findings came from two independent noncontrolled trials. Therefore additional controlled trials are suggested to further prove the efficacy of ectoine nasal spray with or without dexpanthenol.

Disclosure

Dr. O. Scherner and Nina Werkhäuser are employees of Bitop AG, a company where medical devices, including the ectoine nasal spray, were developed and registered. Bitop AG sponsored the trials discussed in this paper. Dr. Uwe Sonnemann received sponsorship by Bitop AG to conduct the studies.

Conflict of Interests

The authors declare that there is no conflict of interests regarding the publication of this paper.

Acknowledgment

The authors thank Dr. T. Kottmann for statistical analysis of data.

References

[1] T. Hildenbrand, R. K. Weber, and D. Brehmer, "Rhinitis sicca, dry nose and atrophic rhinitis: a review of the literature," *European Archives of Oto-Rhino-Laryngology*, vol. 268, no. 1, pp. 17–26, 2011.

[2] C. L. Brown and S. M. Graham, "Nasal irrigations: good or bad?" *Current Opinion in Otolaryngology & Head and Neck Surgery*, vol. 12, no. 1, pp. 9–13, 2004.

[3] O. Michel, "Nasenspülung bei rhinosinusitis," *Laryngo-Rhino-Otologie*, vol. 85, no. 6, pp. 448–458, 2006.

[4] W. M. Boek, N. Keleş, K. Graamans, and E. H. Huizing, "Physiologic and hypertonic saline solutions impair ciliary activity in vitro," *Laryngoscope*, vol. 109, no. 3, pp. 396–399, 1999.

[5] A. R. Talbot, T. M. Herr, and D. S. Parsons, "Mucociliary clearance and buffered hypertonic saline solution," *Laryngoscope*, vol. 107, no. 4, pp. 500–503, 1997.

[6] M. Miwa, N. Nakajima, M. Matsunaga, and K. Watanabe, "Measurement of water loss in human nasal mucosa," *American Journal of Rhinology*, vol. 20, no. 5, pp. 453–455, 2006.

[7] A. Neher, M. Gstöttner, M. Thaurer, P. Augustijns, M. Reinelt, and W. Schobersberger, "Influence of essential and fatty oils on ciliary beat frequency of human nasal epithelial cells," *American Journal of Rhinology*, vol. 22, no. 2, pp. 130–134, 2008.

[8] W. Kehrl and U. Sonnemann, "Dexpanthenol-nasenspray als wirksames therapieprinzip zur behandlung der rhinitis sicca anterior," *Laryngo-Rhino-Otologie*, vol. 77, no. 9, pp. 506–512, 1998.

[9] M. Dohil, "Natural ingredients in atopic dermatitis and other inflammatory skin disease," *Journal of Drugs in Dermatology*, vol. 12, supplement 9, pp. S128–S132, 2011.

[10] E. A. Galinski and A. Oren, "Isolation and structure determination of a novel compatible solute from the moderately halophilic purple sulfur bacterium *Ectothiorhodospira marismortui*," *European Journal of Biochemistry*, vol. 198, no. 3, pp. 593–598, 1991.

[11] T. Arakawa and S. N. Timasheff, "The stabilization of proteins by osmolytes," *Biophysical Journal*, vol. 47, no. 3, pp. 411–414, 1985.

[12] J. Smiatek, R. K. Harishchandra, O. Rubner, H.-J. Galla, and A. Heuer, "Properties of compatible solutes in aqueous solution," *Biophysical Chemistry*, vol. 160, no. 1, pp. 62–68, 2012.

[13] J. Buenger and H. Driller, "Ectoin: an effective natural substance to prevent UVA-induced premature photoaging," *Skin Pharmacology and Physiology*, vol. 17, no. 5, pp. 232–237, 2004.

[14] U. Sydlik, I. Gallitz, C. Albrecht, J. Abel, J. Krutmann, and K. Unfried, "The compatible solute ectoine protects against nanoparticle-induced neutrophilic lung inflammation," *American Journal of Respiratory and Critical Care Medicine*, vol. 180, no. 1, pp. 29–35, 2009.

[15] R. Graf, S. Anzali, J. Buenger, F. Pfluecker, and H. Driller, "The multifunctional role of ectoine as a natural cell protectant," *Clinics in Dermatology*, vol. 26, no. 4, pp. 326–333, 2008.

[16] K. Unfried, U. Sydlik, H. Peuschel, C. Albrecht, A. Bilstein, and J. Krutmann, "The compatible solute ectoine prevents neutrophilic lung inflammation induced by environmental model nanoparticles in vivo," *Toxicology Letters*, vol. 196, p. S67, 2010.

[17] A. Marini, K. Reinelt, J. Krutmann, and A. Bilstein, "Ectoine-containing cream in the treatment of mild to moderate atopic dermatitis: a randomised, comparator-controlled, intra-individual double-blind, multi-center trial," *Skin Pharmacology and Physiology*, vol. 27, pp. 57–65, 2014.

[18] A. Eichel, J. Wittig, K. Sha-Hosseini, and R. Mösges, "A prospective, controlledstudy of SNS01 (ectoine nasal spray) compared to BNO-101 (phytotherapeutic dragées) in patients with acute rhinosinusitis," *Current Medical Research and Opinion*, vol. 29, no. 7, pp. 739–746, 2013.

[19] M. Böhm, A. Michels, and R. Mösges, "Pharmaotherapie: therapeutischer stand der allergischen rhinits," *Forum HNO*, vol. 14, pp. 156–161, 2012.

[20] A. Salapatek, M. Bates, A. Bilstein, and D. Patel, "Ectoin, a novel, non-drug, extremophile-based device, relieves allergic rhinoconjunctivitis symptoms in patients in an environmental exposure chamber model," *The Journal of Allergy and Clinical Immunology*, vol. 127, supplement 2, p. 202, 2011.

[21] C. Hahn, M. Böhm, S. Allekotte, and R. Mösges, "Tolerability and effects on quality of life of liposomal nasal spray treatment compared to nasal ointment containing dexpanthenol or isotonic NaCl spray in patients with rhinitis sicca," *European Archives of Oto-Rhino-Laryngology*, vol. 270, no. 9, pp. 2465–2472, 2013.

[22] W. Kehrl and U. Sonnemann, "Dexpanthenol nasal spray as an effective therapeutic principle for treatment of rhinitis sicca anterior," *Laryngo-Rhino-Otologie*, vol. 77, no. 9, pp. 506–512, 1998.

[23] J. Bünger, J. Degwert, and H. Driller, "The protective function of compatible solute ectoin on the skin cells and its biomolecules with respect to UV-ratiation, immunosupression and membrane damage," *IFSCC Magazine*, vol. 4, no. 2, pp. 1–6, 2001.

[24] U. Heinrich, B. Garbe, and H. Tronnier, "In vivo assessment of ectoin: a randomized, vehicle-controlled clinical trial," *Skin Pharmacology and Physiology*, vol. 20, no. 4, pp. 211–218, 2007.

[25] H. Peuschel, U. Sydlik, S. Grether-Beck et al., "Carbon nanoparticles induce ceramide- and lipid raft-dependent signalling

in lung epithelial cells: a target for a preventive strategy against environmentally-induced lung inflammation," *Particle and Fibre Toxicology*, vol. 9, article 48, 2012.

7

Possible Mechanism of Action of the Antiallergic Effect of an Aqueous Extract of *Heliotropium indicum* L. in Ovalbumin-Induced Allergic Conjunctivitis

Samuel Kyei,[1,2] **George Asumeng Koffuor,**[1,3] **Paul Ramkissoon,**[1] **Samuel Abokyi,**[2]
Osei Owusu-Afriyie,[4] **and Eric Addo Wiredu**[2]

[1]*Discipline of Optometry, School of Health Sciences, College of Health, University of KwaZulu-Natal, Durban 4041, South Africa*
[2]*Department of Optometry, School of Allied Health Sciences, University of Cape Coast, Cape Coast, Ghana*
[3]*Department of Pharmacology, Faculty of Pharmacy and Pharmaceutical Sciences,*
 Kwame Nkrumah University of Science and Technology, Kumasi, Ghana
[4]*Department of Pathology, Komfo Anokye Teaching Hospital, Kumasi, Ghana*

Correspondence should be addressed to Samuel Kyei; skyei@ucc.edu.gh

Academic Editor: William E. Berger

Heliotropium indicum is used traditionally as a remedy for conjunctivitis in Ghana. This study therefore evaluated the antiallergic potential of an aqueous whole plant extract of *Heliotropium indicum* (HIE) in ovalbumin-induced allergic conjunctivitis and attempted to predict its mode of action. Clinical scores for allergic conjunctivitis induced by intraperitoneal ovalbumin sensitization ($100 : 10\,\mu g$ OVA/Al(OH)$_3$ in phosphate-buffered saline [PBS]) and topical conjunctival challenge (1.5 mg OVA in $10\,\mu L$ PBS) in Dunkin-Hartley guinea pigs were estimated after a week's daily treatment with 30–300 mg kg^{-1} HIE, 30 mg kg^{-1} prednisolone, 10 mg kg^{-1} chlorpheniramine, or 10 mL kg^{-1} PBS. Ovalbumin-specific IgG and IgE and total IgE in serum were estimated using Enzyme-Linked Immunosorbent Assay. Histopathological assessment of the exenterated conjunctivae was also performed. The 30 and 300 mg kg^{-1} HIE treatment resulted in a significantly ($p \leq 0.001$) low clinical score of allergic conjunctivitis. Ovalbumin-specific IgG and IgE as well as total serum IgE also decreased significantly ($p \leq 0.01$–0.001). The conjunctival tissue in HIE treated guinea pigs had mild mononuclear infiltration compared to the PBS-treated ones, which had intense conjunctival tissue inflammatory infiltration. HIE exhibited antiallergic effect possibly by immunomodulation or immunosuppression.

1. Introduction

Allergic conjunctivitis is a common problem that ophthalmic practitioners have to deal with, almost on daily basis, as it affects nearly 40% of the populace in advanced nation [1, 2]. Various studies in Africa have indicated the prevalence of allergic conjunctivitis to range between 7.3 and 32% [3, 4].

The conjunctiva is a dynamic immunologic tissue that suffers lymphoid hyperplasia in reaction to a stimulant such as pollens, animal dander, and other environmental antigens [5]. Allergic conjunctivitis (AC), therefore, is clinically characterized by pruritus, hyperemia, chemosis, tearing, and photophobia [6]. These clinical symptoms are the reason for the high morbidity associated with AC and consequential impact on quality of life of AC victims [7, 8]. Due to the large burden of AC and its spate of increase all over the world and across all ages, it possesses a great challenge to the health care resources of many countries [9, 10].

Allergic conjunctivitis is prompted by IgE-mediated immediate hypersensitivity reaction. Mast cell plays an important role in these allergic inflammations [11, 12]. Available medical therapies which include antihistamines, mast cell stabilizers, corticosteroids, nonsteroidal anti-inflammatory drugs, immunomodulatory agents, and allergen-specific immunotherapy could be rendered ineffective due to discomfort associated with administration of medications, intricacy of administration guidelines, perceived lack of efficacy by users, and/or adverse effects [13].

In the light of these bottlenecks associated with effective management of AC, current studies have focused attention on plants and natural products based therapeutic strategies in the bid to broaden treatment horizon, improve efficacy, and address safety concerns [14]. *Heliotropium indicum* L. (Boraginaceae), also known as Indian heliotrope, is one such plant used in the traditional management of conjunctivitis [15, 16]. Although *H. indicum* is well-studied medicinal plant, its traditional use in treating ocular allergic inflammation is yet to be evaluated. This study therefore sought to evaluate the antiallergic effect and possible mechanism of action of whole plant aqueous extract of *Heliotropium indicum* L. in ovalbumin-induced allergic conjunctivitis in Dunkin-Hartley guinea pigs.

2. Materials and Methods

2.1. Plant Collection. Heliotropium indicum was collected from the botanical gardens of the University of Cape Coast, Cape Coast, in the Central Region of Ghana (5.1036°N, 1.2825°W) in November 2012. It was identified and authenticated by a botanist at the School of Biological Sciences, College of Agricultural and Natural Science, University of Cape Coast, Cape Coast, Ghana, where a voucher specimen with number 4873 has been deposited at the herbarium for future reference.

2.2. Preparation of the Aqueous Extract of H. indicum (HIE). Whole plants of *H. indicum* were washed thoroughly with tap water and shade-dried. The dry plants were milled into coarse powder by a hammer mill (Schutte Buffalo, New York, NY). One and half kilograms of the plant powder was mixed with one liter of water. The mixture was Soxhlet-extracted at 80°C for 24 h. The aqueous extract obtained was freeze-dried (Hull Freeze-Dryer/Lyophilizer 140 SQ, Warminster, PA). The powder (yield 12.2%), labeled as HIE, was stored at 4°C and reconstituted in normal saline to the desired concentration for dosing in this study.

2.3. Drugs and Chemicals. Ovalbumin (OVA) (Cayla-InvivoGen, Toulouse, France), aluminum hydroxide (Merck, Darmstadt, Germany), chloroform (Sigma-Aldrich, USA), cetirizine (McNeil Consumer Healthcare, Washington, USA), and prednisolone (Taizhou Baida Pharmaceutical Chemical Co., Ltd., China) were some chemicals used in this study.

2.4. Animal and Husbandry. Dunkin-Hartley guinea pigs (weight 300 ± 25 g) were kept in the Animal House of the School of Biological Sciences, University of Cape Coast, Ghana. The experimental animals were housed in aluminum cages (34 cm × 47 cm × 18 cm) with soft wood shavings as bedding, under ambient laboratory conditions (temperature 28°C ± 2°C, relative humidity 60–70%, and a normal light-dark cycle). They were fed on a normal commercial pellet diet (Agricare Ltd., Kumasi, Ghana) and had access to water *ad libitum*.

2.5. Ethical and Biosafety Considerations. The study protocols were approved by the Institutional Review Board on Animal Experimentation of the Faculty of Pharmacy and Pharmaceutical Sciences, Kwame Nkrumah University of Science and Technology, Kumasi, Ghana (Ethical Clearance number FPPS/PCOL/0030/2013). All activities performed during the studies conformed to accepted principles for laboratory animal use and care (EU directive of 1986: 86/609/EEC) and Association for Research in Vision and Ophthalmology Statement for Use of Animals in Ophthalmic and Vision Research. Biosafety guidelines for protection of personnel in the laboratory were observed.

2.6. Preliminary Phytochemical Screening. Screening was performed on HIE to ascertain the presence of phytochemicals using standard procedures described by Harborne [17] and Kujur et al. [18].

2.7. Ovalbumin-Induction Allergic Conjunctivitis (OIAC). OIAC was carried out as described by Shoji et al. [19] and Abokyi et al. [20]. Guinea pigs were sensitized by two intraperitoneal injections of 0.2 mL solution containing 100 μg OVA and 0.01 mg aluminum hydroxide in phosphate buffer saline (pH 7.4) at an interval of 2 weeks. On day 8 after the sensitization, conjunctivitis was induced by topical instillation (challenge stage) of OVA (1.5 mg OVA in 10 μL PBS) into the conjunctival sac of each eye. The topical challenge was repeated after 2 days. Physical and slit lamp (Marco II-B, Lombart Instrument, Japan) biomicroscopic ocular examinations were conducted. Hyperemia of palpebral conjunctiva, chemosis of bulbar conjunctiva, and lid swelling (clinical symptoms of AC) observed in the animal were an indication that AC had been induced.

2.8. Effect of HIE on OIAC

2.8.1. Grouping and Dosing. The animals with conjunctivitis were put into six groups ($n = 5$). Groups I–III were treated with 30, 100, and 300 mg kg^{-1} HIE, respectively, Group IV was treated with 10 mg kg^{-1} chlorpheniramine, and Group V received 30 mg kg^{-1} prednisolone, while Group VI (control group) was treated with 10 mL kg^{-1} PBS. A normal control group, Group VII (no sensitization and challenge, no interventionary treatment), was kept under experimental condition. All treatments were *per os* and were started 24 h after the last topical challenge. Treatment was twice daily (12-hour interval) for one week.

2.8.2. Clinical Assessment of HIE in OIAC. Clinical examination was performed on days 1, 3, 5, and 7 in the various groups of animals. Hyperemia of palpebral conjunctiva, chemosis of bulbar conjunctiva, and lid swelling were scored on a scale of 0–3. The total of clinical scores for hyperemia of palpebral conjunctiva, chemosis of bulbar conjunctiva, and lid swelling was also evaluated as an overall clinical score [21].

2.8.3. Determination of Ovalbumin Specific IgE, IgG, and Total Serum IgE. Twenty-four hours after the last treatment had been administered, guinea pigs were anesthetized with chloroform and whole blood was collected from the jugular vein into pyrogenic free test tube (Indigo Instrument,

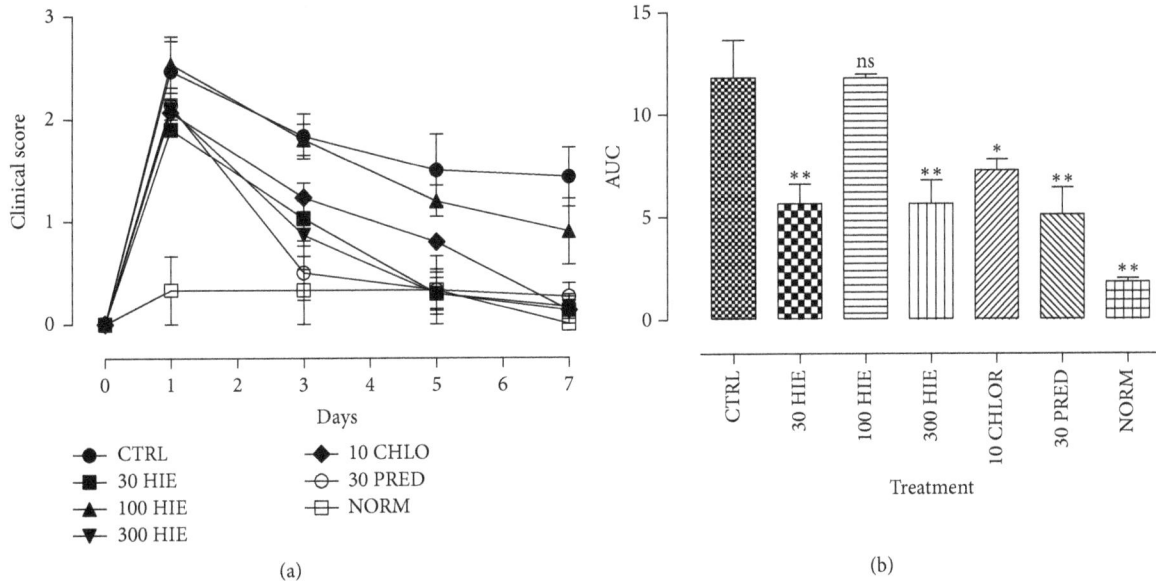

FIGURE 1: Time-course curves (a) and areas under the curve (b) for the effects of 30, 100, and 300 mg kg^{-1} of HIE and 10 mg kg^{-1} chlorpheniramine and 10 mg kg^{-1} prednisolone on OIAC in Dunkin-Hartley guinea pigs. Values plotted are mean ± SEM ($n = 5$). $^*p \leq 0.01$; $^{**}p \leq 0.001$, ANOVA followed by Dunnett's multiple comparisons test.

Waterloo, Canada). Serum was prepared by centrifuging the clotted blood (temperature 25°C, speed 3000 g) for 5 min using a Mikro 220R machine (Hettich Zentrifuge, Tuttlingen, Germany). The serum was then subjected to Enzyme-Linked Immunosorbent Assay (ELISA) (MyBioSource, San Diego, CA, USA) as per the manufacturer's instructions briefly described. This employed the double-sandwich ELISA technique. The precoated antibodies were either one of the following: guinea pig OVA sIgG, sIgE, and IgE monoclonal antibody and the detecting antibodies, a biotin labeled polyclonal antibody. In each case test samples and biotin labeled antibody were added to ELISA plate microwells. These were washed out with phosphate buffered saline (PBS). Avidin-peroxidase conjugates were then added to the ELISA wells; tetramethylbenzidine (TMB) substrate was used for coloring and washed out. TMB turned blue after intermittent incubation and finally yellow under the action of acid. The absorbances were then read at 450 nm using an URIT-660 microplate reader (URIT Medical Electronic Co., Ltd., Guangxi, China). Each determination was in triplicate.

2.8.4. Histopathological Assessment. The eyeballs together with the conjunctiva and lids of animals from the various groups were exenterated and fixed in 10% buffered formalin. Conjunctival tissue was stained with hematoxylin and eosin. Histopathological assessment was done by a specialist pathologist at Komfo Anokye Teaching Hospital, Kumasi, Ghana.

2.9. Statistical Analysis. The statistical analysis of data obtained was made using GraphPad Prism Version 5.0 (GraphPad Software, Inc., USA). Differences between treatment groups and the controls were estimated using One-Way Analysis of Variance (ANOVA) followed by Dunnett's Multiple Comparisons Test (post hoc test) at a confidence

TABLE 1: Results obtained after preliminary phytochemical screening of HIE.

Phytochemical tested for	Results obtained
Anthraquinones	−
Tannins	+
Flavonoids	+
Alkaloids	+
Sterols	+
Glycosides	+
Saponins	+
Triterpenoids	−

"+" indicates presence; "−" indicates absence.

level of 95%. Probability values less than or equal to 5% ($p \leq 0.05$) were considered significant.

3. Results

3.1. Phytochemical Screening. Preliminary phytochemistry showed that flavonoids, saponins, cyanogenic glycosides, sterols, tannins, and alkaloids were present in HIE (Table 1).

3.2. Effect of HIE on Clinical Signs of OIAC. The clinical scores for OIAC indicated a U-shaped effect of HIE in mitigating the clinical signs of allergic conjunctivitis. The 30 and 300 mg kg^{-1} significantly ($p \leq 0.001$) attenuated the clinical signs of allergic inflammation and not the 100 mg kg^{-1} (Figures 1(a) and 1(b)). Chlorpheniramine and prednisolone (reference drugs) significantly ($p \leq 0.01$–0.001) attenuated the clinical signs of AC (Figures 1(a) and 1(b)).

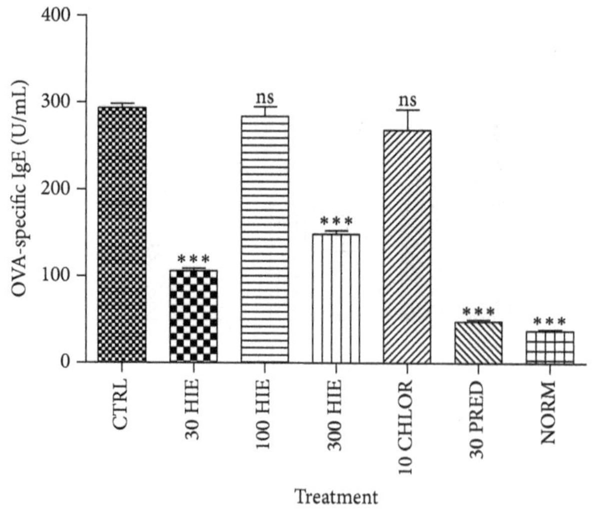

FIGURE 2: The effect of 30, 100, and 300 mg kg^{-1} HIE, 30 mg kg^{-1} prednisolone, and 10 mg kg^{-1} chlorpheniramine on OVA-specific serum IgE in OIAC in guinea pigs. $^{***}p \leq 0.001$, ANOVA followed by Dunnett's post hoc test.

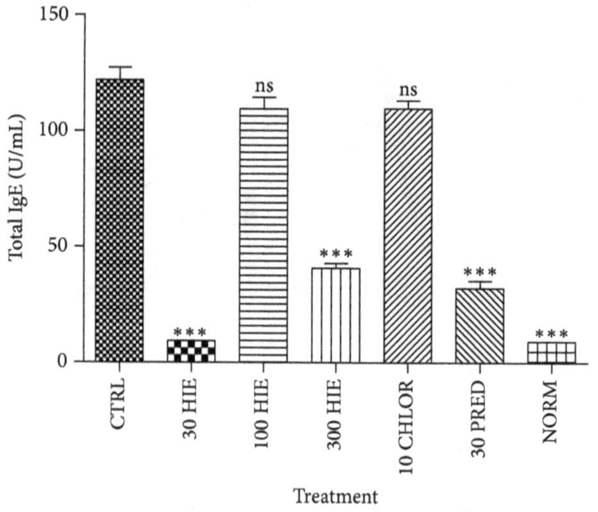

FIGURE 4: The effect of 30, 100, and 300 mg kg^{-1} HIE, 30 mg kg^{-1} prednisolone, and 10 mg kg^{-1} chlorpheniramine on total serum IgE in OIAC in guinea pigs. $^{***}p \leq 0.001$, ANOVA followed by Dunnett's post hoc test.

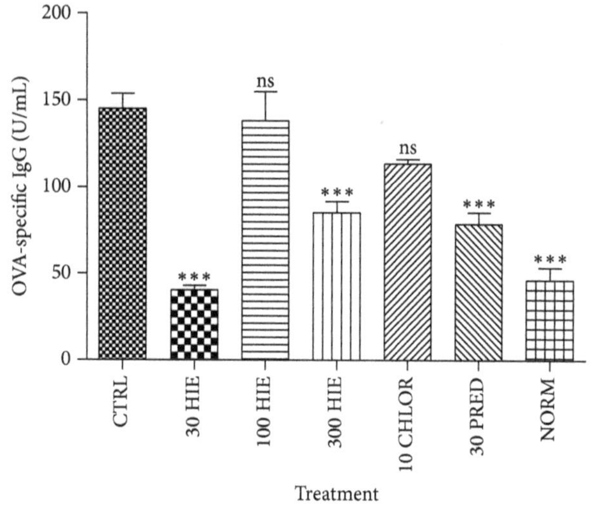

FIGURE 3: The effect of 30, 100, and 300 mg kg^{-1} HIE, 30 mg kg^{-1} prednisolone, and 10 mg kg^{-1} chlorpheniramine on OVA-specific serum IgG in OIAC in guinea pigs. $^{***}p \leq 0.001$, ANOVA followed by Dunnett's post hoc test.

3.3. HIE Effect on Sera OVA-Specific IgE, IgG, and Total IgE. HIE showed a U-shaped effect in decreasing ($p \leq 0.01$–0.001) sera OVA-specific IgE, IgG, and total IgE antibodies in serum. Prednisolone caused significant reduction ($p \leq 0.001$) in the immunoglobulin, but chlorpheniramine did not (Figures 2–4).

3.4. Histopathological Assessment. The histopathological assessment showed remarkable signs of mononuclear infiltration in conjunctival tissue of the control (PBS treated) group. Treatment with 30 and 300 mg kg^{-1} showed a reduction in mononuclear infiltrations but not the 100 mg kg^{-1} HIE

treated group. Prednisolone reduced the infiltration much more than chlorpheniramine (Figure 5).

4. Discussion

Ovalbumin-induced allergic conjunctivitis model in the guinea pig has been used in preclinical studies in screening for potential antiallergic agents [22]. It has been noted as an ideal model for both IgE mediated and non-IgE mediated allergic conjunctivitis [23]. This model of ocular allergic disease is typically related to type 1 hypersensitivity reactions. It is biphasic with the early-phase reaction driven primarily by mast cell degranulation and ensues right after exposure to the allergen; the late-phase reaction is marked by cell infiltration, mainly eosinophils, neutrophils, and lymphocytes, 6 to 24 hours after antigen application, corresponding to the clinical findings of allergic conjunctivitis [24]. Activation and conscription of inflammatory cells and the liberation of cytokines, chemokines, adhesion molecules, and proteases promote more serious chronic forms [25].

The low clinical scores obtained for the extract treated group justify the extract's potency in relieving the noisome symptoms associated with the underlying pathology of allergic conjunctivitis, the hallmark of most antiallergic agents. Although the U-shaped dose-response effect observed in clinical scores of ocular allergy remains unclear, it has been reported in several pharmacological investigations. This observation could be due to the inhibitory tendencies of the active phytochemical at that dose [26].

HIE reduced both allergen- (OVA-) specific IgG and IgE indicating a mechanistic deviation of activity from antihistaminic and mast cell stabilizing agents [20, 27]. Treatment with chlorpheniramine irrespective of the favorable clinical outcome regarding the resolution of allergic inflammation had no significant effect on allergen-specific IgG, IgE, and total sera IgE. This is because the release of histamine

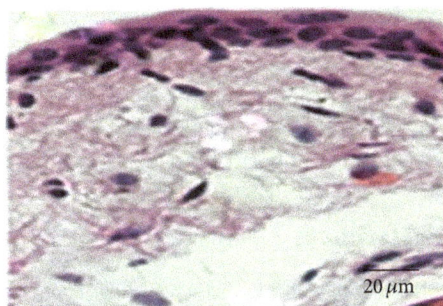

(a) Normal conjunctival tissue with normal epithelial architecture without evidence of mononuclear infiltration

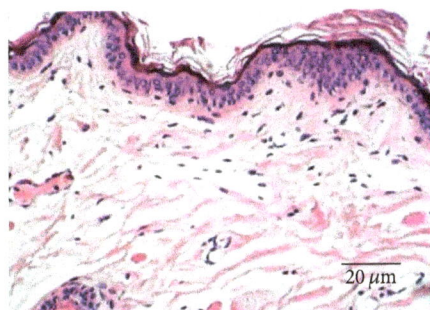

(b) 30 mg kg^{-1} prednisolone treated with mild mononuclear infiltration into the subepithelial tissue of the conjunctiva

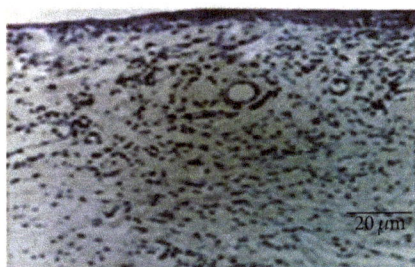

(c) PBS-treated conjunctival tissue with widespread infiltration of neutrophils and eosinophils

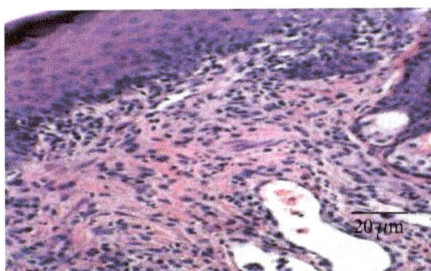

(d) 10 mg kg^{-1} chlorpheniramine treatment with remarkably unresolved inflammatory process seen as intense polymorphonuclear infiltration

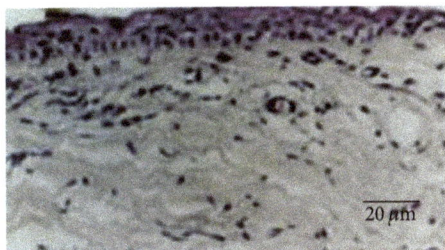

(e) 30 mg kg^{-1} HIE treated with mild infiltration of neutophilic and eosinophilic cells

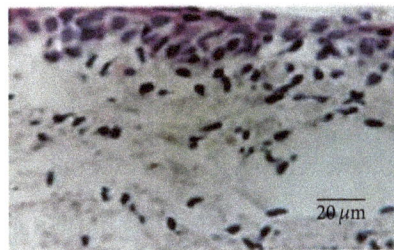

(f) 100 mg kg^{-1} HIE treated conjunctival tissue with moderately diffuse neutrophils and eosinophils exudation

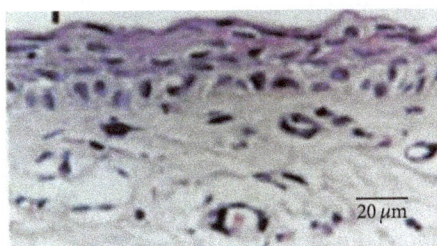

(g) 300 mg kg^{-1} HIE treated with mild neutophils and eosinophil infiltration in subepithelial conjunctival tissue

FIGURE 5: Photomicrographs of the conjunctival tissues in OIAC in guinea pigs treated with 30, 100, and 300 mg kg^{-1} HIE, 30 mg kg^{-1} prednisolone, 10 mg kg^{-1} chlorpheniramine, and PBS, compared to that of normal guinea pigs.

whose receptors are the target for antihistaminic agents lies downstream immunoglobulin production. This therefore accounts for its ability to attenuate the clinical signs of allergic inflammation [28]. The extract treatment causing relevant reduction in allergen-specific immunoglobulins was similar to the effect of the steroid treatment (prednisolone). This presupposes that the extract may have immunomodulatory and or immunosuppressive effect [13, 29].

A number of immunomodulatory compounds have been isolated from natural products [30, 31]. Antioxidant-rich extracts have been found relevant as immunomodulatory or immunosuppressive agents and have been mainly used in control of the immune response in conditions like transplantation, autoimmune disorders, and alleviation of allergic diseases [31]. Some studies have already reported the antioxidant properties of both extract and different fractions of *H. indicum* which in effect suggest that HIE's antiallergic inflammatory effect could probably be due to its rich antioxidant constituents such as flavonoids, alkaloids, and tannins [32–34].

HIE treatment reduced serum levels of IgE which is one of the necessary ingredients in the promulgation of allergic inflammatory processes [35]. When an allergen (e.g., ovalbumin) is taken up by antigen presenting cells (e.g., allergen-specific B cell), via the cell surface immunoglobulin receptor, processed fragments are then presented in the context of major histocompatibility class II (MHC class II) to Th2 cells recognizing the allergen-MHC II complex. Activation of the allergen-specific Th2 cells results in the expression of IL-4, IL-13, and CD154 and introduction of class switching to IgE. Class switching, a process involved in the biosynthesis of immunoglobulins, is driven by allergens [36]. Class switching is ushered by T cells signalling. Nevertheless, basophils express high levels of IL-4, IL-13, and CD154 after stimulation and it has been postulated to play a role in polyclonal amplification of IgE production and in the differentiation of Th2 cells [37]. These immunoglobulins bind to high-affinity IgE receptor; FcεR1 expressed on mast cells and basophils as tetramers ($\alpha\beta\gamma_2$) and on antigen presenting cells, at much lower levels, as trimers ($\alpha\gamma_2$) leading to degranulation of mast cells [38]. Studies have shown that the density of human basophil and mast cell FcεR1 expression is associated with serum IgE levels [39]. Mast cell degranulation is dependent on Syk kinase responsible for signaling proceedings subsequent to mast cells and basophils stimulation. This assertion is supported by recent finding indicating that Syk kinase deficient mast cells and basophils do not undergo degranulation after FcεR1 aggregation [40]. This therefore opens a window of opportunity for therapeutic exploration. The extract in this case indicates a mechanistic efficacy in reducing serum OVA allergen-specific and total IgE levels.

5. Conclusion

The aqueous whole plant extract of *Heliotropium indicum* exhibits antiallergic effect in ovalbumin-induced conjunctivitis in guinea pigs via a probable immunomodulating or immunosuppressive action supporting its traditional use in treatment of conjunctivitis.

Disclosure

This paper results from research towards a Ph.D. (optometry) degree in the discipline of optometry at the University of KwaZulu-Natal under the supervision of Dr. George A. Koffuor and cosupervision of Professor Paul Ramkissoon.

Conflict of Interests

The authors declare no conflict of interests whatsoever.

Acknowledgments

The authors are grateful to the management and staff of Life Science Diagnostic Centre, Cape Coast, for permitting the authors to use their facility for carrying aspects of this study. This study was partly funded by the University of Cape Coast.

References

[1] K. Singh and L. Bielory, "Ocular allergy: a national epidemiologic study," *Journal of Allergy and Clinical Immunology*, vol. 119, supplement 1, p. S154, 2007.

[2] K. Singh, S. Axelrod, and L. Bielory, "The epidemiology of ocular and nasal allergy in the United States, 1988–1994," *Journal of Allergy and Clinical Immunology*, vol. 126, no. 4, pp. 778–783.e6, 2010.

[3] S. Abokyi, G. A. Koffuor, M. Ntodie, S. Kyei, and L. Gyanfosu, "Epidemiological profile and pharmacological management of allergic conjunctivitis: a study in Ghana," *International Journal of Pharmaceutical and Biomedical Research*, vol. 3, no. 4, pp. 195–201, 2012.

[4] K. N. Malu, "Allergic conjunctivitis in Jos-Nigeria," *Nigerian Medical Journal*, vol. 55, no. 2, pp. 166–170, 2014.

[5] P. Isaacson and D. H. Wright, "Extranodal malignant lymphoma arising from mucosa-associated lymphoid tissue," *Cancer*, vol. 53, no. 11, pp. 2515–2524, 1984.

[6] S. M. Whitcup, C.-C. Chan, D. A. Luyo, P. Bo, and Q. Li, "Topical cyclosporine inhibits mast cell-mediated conjunctivitis," *Investigative Ophthalmology and Visual Science*, vol. 37, no. 13, pp. 2686–2693, 1996.

[7] A. D. Pitt, A. F. Smith, L. Lindsell, L. W. Voon, P. W. Rose, and N. J. Bron, "Economic and quality-of-life impact of seasonal allergic conjunctivitis in Oxfordshire," *Ophthalmic Epidemiology*, vol. 11, no. 1, pp. 17–33, 2004.

[8] J. Palmares, L. Delgado, M. Cidade, M. J. Quadrado, and H. P. Filipe, "Allergic conjunctivitis: a national cross-sectional study of clinical characteristics and quality of life," *European Journal of Ophthalmology*, vol. 20, no. 2, pp. 257–264, 2010.

[9] S. Bonini, "Allergic conjunctivitis: the forgotten disease," *Chemical Immunology and Allergy*, vol. 91, pp. 110–120, 2006.

[10] K. Singh and L. Bielory, "Ocular allergy: a national epidemiologic study," *Journal of Allergy and Clinical Immunology*, vol. 119, no. 1, supplement 1, p. S154, 2007.

[11] L. Bielory, "Allergic and immunologic disorders of the eye. Part I: immunology of the eye," *Journal of Allergy and Clinical Immunology*, vol. 106, no. 5, pp. 805–816, 2000.

[12] T. Tominaga, D. Miyazaki, S.-I. Sasaki et al., "Blocking mast cell-mediated type i hypersensitivity in experimental allergic conjunctivitis by monocyte chemoattractant protein-1/CCR2," *Investigative Ophthalmology and Visual Science*, vol. 50, no. 11, pp. 5181–5188, 2009.

[13] C. Córdova, B. Gutiérrez, C. Martínez-García et al., "Oleanolic acid controls allergic and inflammatory responses in experimental allergic conjunctivitis," *PLoS ONE*, vol. 9, no. 4, Article ID e91282, 2014.

[14] B. B. Cota, C. M. Bertollo, and D. M. de Oliveira, "Anti-allergic potential of herbs and herbal natural products—activities and patents," *Recent Patents on Endocrine, Metabolic & Immune Drug Discovery*, vol. 7, no. 1, pp. 26–56, 2013.

[15] M. Rahmatullah, A. K. Das, M. A. H. Mollik et al., "An ethnomedicinal survey of Dhamrai sub-district in Dhaka District, Bangladesh," *American-Eurasian Journal of Sustainable Agriculture*, vol. 3, no. 4, pp. 881–888, 2009.

[16] E. Roeder and H. Wiedenfeld, "Plants containing pyrrolizidine alkaloids used in the Traditional Indian medicine—including Ayurveda," *Pharmazie*, vol. 68, no. 2, pp. 83–92, 2013.

[17] J. B. Harborne, *Phytochemical Methods: A Guide to Modern Techniques of Plant Analysis*, Chapman and Hall, London, UK, 3rd edition, 1998.

[18] R. S. Kujur, V. Singh, M. Ram et al., "Antidiabetic activity and phytochemical screening of crude extract of Stevia rebaudiana in alloxan-induced diabetic rats," *Pharmacognosy Research*, vol. 2, no. 4, pp. 258–263, 2010.

[19] J. Shoji, N. Inada, N. Takaura, and M. Sawa, "Histological study of allergic conjunctivitis. 1. Study on the adhesion molecules to allergic conjunctivitis," *Journal of Japanese Ophthalmological Society*, vol. 99, no. 2, pp. 129–134, 1995.

[20] S. Abokyi, G. A. Koffuor, S. Kyei, E. A. Asiamah, C. N. Atobiga, and A. Awuah, "Antiallergic effect of an aqueous leaf extract of Pistia stratiotes in murine model of ovalbumin-induced allergic conjunctivitis," *Pharmacognosy Research*, vol. 6, no. 4, pp. 274–279, 2014.

[21] A. Ozaki, Y. Seki, A. Fukushima, and M. Kubo, "The control of allergic conjunctivitis by suppressor of cytokine signaling (SOCS)3 and SOCS5 in a murine model," *The Journal of Immunology*, vol. 175, no. 8, pp. 5489–5497, 2005.

[22] J. Shouji, K. Saito, N. Takaura, N. Inada, and M. Sawa, "Histological study of allergic conjunctivitis report 2. Time course of allergic conjunctival inflammation," *Nihon Ganka Kiyo*, vol. 46, no. 10, pp. 1015–1020, 1995.

[23] D. A. Groneberg, L. Bielory, A. Fischer, S. Bonini, and U. Wahn, "Animal models of allergic and inflammatory conjunctivitis," *Allergy*, vol. 58, no. 11, pp. 1101–1113, 2003.

[24] B. P. Bielory, T. P. O'Brien, and L. Bielory, "Management of seasonal allergic conjunctivitis: guide to therapy," *Acta Ophthalmologica*, vol. 90, no. 5, pp. 399–407, 2012.

[25] H. Hirai, K. Tanaka, O. Yoshie et al., "Prostaglandin D2 selectively induces chemotaxis in T helper type 2 cells, eosinophils, and basophils via seven-transmembrane receptor CRTH2," *Journal of Experimental Medicine*, vol. 193, no. 2, pp. 255–261, 2001.

[26] D. Wu, J. R. Cypser, A. I. Yashin, and T. E. Johnson, "The U-shaped response of initial mortality in Caenorhabditis elegans to mild heat shock: does it explain recent trends in human mortality?" *Journals of Gerontology—Series A Biological Sciences and Medical Sciences*, vol. 63, no. 7, pp. 660–668, 2008.

[27] Y. Ohashi, Y. Nakai, A. Tanaka et al., "Serum levels of specific IgE, soluble interleukin-2 receptor, and soluble intercellular adhesion molecule-1 in seasonal allergic rhinitis," *Annals of Allergy, Asthma & Immunology*, vol. 79, no. 3, pp. 213–220, 1997.

[28] G. M. Walsh, "The anti-inflammatory effects of levocetirizine—are they clinically relevant or just an interesting additional effect?" *Allergy, Asthma & Clinical Immunology*, vol. 5, article 14, 2009.

[29] G. R. Duddukuri, R. Y. Vasudeva, D. N. Rao, and R. A. Rao, "Immunomodulation of ovalbumin-specific IgG and other classes of antibody response by honey in mice," *Indian Journal of Clinical Biochemistry*, vol. 16, no. 1, pp. 89–94, 2001.

[30] V. P. Kurup and C. S. Barrios, "Immunomodulatory effects of curcumin in allergy," *Molecular Nutrition and Food Research*, vol. 52, no. 9, pp. 1031–1039, 2008.

[31] M.-H. Boskabady, R. Keyhanmanesh, S. Khameneh, Y. Doostdar, and M.-R. Khakzad, "Potential immunomodulation effect of the extract of Nigella sativa on ovalbumin sensitized guinea pigs," *Journal of Zhejiang University: Science B*, vol. 12, no. 3, pp. 201–209, 2011.

[32] R. M. Ammal and V. S. Bai, "Free radical scavenging activity of Heliotropium indicum leaves," *International Journal of Research in Plant Science*, vol. 4, no. 3, pp. 63–67, 2014.

[33] Y. Begum, "Antibacterial, antioxidant and cytotoxic activities of Heliotropium indicum," *The Experiment*, vol. 23, no. 1, pp. 1564–1569, 2014.

[34] R. R. Pragada, S. Rao Ethadi, B. Yasodhara, V. S. Praneeth Dasari, and T. Mallikarjuna Rao, "In-vitro antioxidant and antibacterial activities of different fractions of Heliotropium indicum L.," *Journal of Pharmacy Research*, vol. 5, no. 2, pp. 1051–1053, 2012.

[35] P. Smith and D. R. Ownby, "Clinical significance of IgE," in *Middleton's Allergy: Principles and Practice*, N. Adkinson, B. S. Bochner, W. W. Busse, S. T. Holgate, R. F. Lemanske, and F. E. R. Simons, Eds., Mosby Elsevier, 7th edition, 2009.

[36] K. D. Stone, C. Prussin, and D. D. Metcalfe, "IgE, mast cells, basophils, and eosinophils," *Journal of Allergy and Clinical Immunology*, vol. 125, supplement 2, no. 2, pp. S73–S80, 2010.

[37] H. C. Oettgen, "Immunobiology of IgE and IgE receptors," in *Middleton's Allergy: Principles and Practice*, N. F. Adkinson, B. S. Bochner, A. W. Burks et al., Eds., Mosby Elsevier, 8th edition, 2014.

[38] H. J. Gould and B. J. Sutton, "IgE in allergy and asthma today," *Nature Reviews Immunology*, vol. 8, no. 3, pp. 205–217, 2008.

[39] D. MacGlashan Jr., "IgE receptor and signal transduction in mast cells and basophils," *Current Opinion in Immunology*, vol. 20, no. 6, pp. 717–723, 2008.

[40] A. M. Gilfillan and J. Rivera, "The tyrosine kinase network regulating mast cell activation," *Immunological Reviews*, vol. 228, no. 1, pp. 149–169, 2009.

8

Exploring Low-Income Families' Financial Barriers to Food Allergy Management and Treatment

Leia M. Minaker,[1] Susan J. Elliott,[2] and Ann Clarke[3]

[1] School of Public Health and Health Systems, University of Waterloo LHN 1711, 200 University Avenue West, Waterloo, ON, Canada N2L 3G1

[2] Faculty of Applied Health Sciences, University of Waterloo BMH 3115, 200 University Avenue West, Waterloo, ON, Canada N2L 3G1

[3] Department of Medicine, McGill University, Room 101, Lady Meredith House, 1110 Pine Avenue West, Montreal, QC, Canada H3A 1A3

Correspondence should be addressed to Susan J. Elliott; elliotts@uwaterloo.ca

Academic Editor: Hugo Van Bever

Objectives. Low-income families may face financial barriers to management and treatment of chronic illnesses. No studies have explored how low-income individuals and families with anaphylactic food allergies cope with financial barriers to anaphylaxis management and/or treatment. This study explores qualitatively assessed direct, indirect, and intangible costs of anaphylaxis management and treatment faced by low-income families. *Methods.* In-depth, semistructured interviews with 23 participants were conducted to gain insight into income-related barriers to managing and treating anaphylactic food allergies. *Results.* Perceived direct costs included the cost of allergen-free foods and allergy medication and costs incurred as a result of misinformation about social support programs. Perceived indirect costs included those associated with lack of continuity of health care. Perceived intangible costs included the stress related to the difficulty of obtaining allergen-free foods at the food bank and feeling unsafe at discount grocery stores. These perceived costs represented barriers that were perceived as especially salient for the working poor, immigrants, youth living in poverty, and food bank users. *Discussion.* Low-income families report significant financial barriers to food allergy management and anaphylaxis preparedness. Clinicians, advocacy groups, and EAI manufacturers all have a role to play in ensuring equitable access to medication for low-income individuals with allergies.

1. Introduction

Food allergies affect 4–8% of people in the Western world [1–3]. Anaphylactic food allergies are rapid in onset and can be fatal if treatment is delayed [4]; thus, complete dietary avoidance of the allergen and timely access to treatment are essential. Three studies found that children from low-income families face barriers to appropriate anaphylaxis management [5–7]. Conversely, one study found that associations between allergy severity and health care utilization did not differ by poverty status [8] and another study found no conclusive associations between the epinephrine autoinjectors (EAIs) availability and sociodemographic factors [9].

A recent study on the economic impact of childhood food allergy in the United States found the overall economic cost of food allergy to be almost $25 billion annually [10]. This study found that costs borne by families affected by food allergies include lost labour productivity, out-of-pocket costs, and opportunity costs [10]. Costs associated with food allergies are described as direct, indirect, or intangible [11–13]. Direct costs are financial costs incurred as a result of the food allergy (including inpatient admissions, outpatient visits, medication costs, and the cost of suitable foods) [14]. Indirect costs reflect time spent in various activities as a result of food allergy, including lost productivity and opportunity costs. Intangible costs are losses of utility, such as experiences of pain, suffering, and grief, and can be measured by self-reported quality of life and well-being [12, 15]. One recent study on the intangible costs of food allergy in four European countries found that patients with food hypersensitivity reported lower well-being than the control group. The authors note, however, that well-being was positively related to income and, thus, income compensation might improve welfare among food hypersensitive individuals [15]. Low-income individuals are differentially affected by the costs of food allergy, since "… people with allergy who also have low incomes may have greater difficulties in access to [allergen-free] food." [11, page 999]. It is intuitive that absolute costs of allergy medication or allergen-free foods pose a disproportionate burden to low-income families. Although these costs are conventionally assessed quantitatively, exploring qualitatively assessed direct, indirect, and intangible costs of food allergies among low-income families is important for three reasons. First, low-income individuals may have poorer access to anaphylaxis treatment [5, 6] and may therefore be at high risk of allergy-related harms. Second, understanding barriers to anaphylaxis management or treatment faced by low-income individuals can facilitate the development of valid quantitative surveys intended to describe the overall scope of food allergies and treatment accessibility. Third, exploring how low-income families cope with or manage anaphylactic allergies has both clinical and policy implications.

Qualitative research has "enormous potential to make a distinctive contribution to knowledge about allergy management and to provide insights that quantitative studies cannot." [16, page 1117]. Although extant research assesses direct, indirect, and intangible costs quantitatively, this study explores these costs qualitatively from the perspective of low-income families, which is a current gap in the allergy literature. Findings from in-depth interviews with key informants and low-income families affected by food allergy begin to fill the gaps in our understanding around coping and management for this vulnerable population. The purpose of this study was to take an in-depth look at the direct, indirect and intangible costs that are particularly burdensome for low-income families in terms of anaphylactic food allergy management and treatment.

2. Methods

In-depth, semi-structured interviews with key informants (*n* = 10) and low-income individuals affected by food allergy (*n* = 13) were conducted in southwestern Ontario, Canada. In Ontario, the provincial health insurance plan covers the cost of physician and other "medically necessary" services. Of note, drugs (including EAIs) are not covered by the provincial health insurance plan. However, individuals who are receiving social assistance or are 65 years of age or older are eligible for drug coverage through the provincial government. Individuals who are not receiving social assistance either have private drug insurance through their employer or pay out of pocket for drugs. Key informants were recruited from agencies working with low-income families in a context relevant to food allergy (i.e., food procurement or medication access) (Table 1). Low-income participants were recruited via posters placed in these targeted agencies. Over half (54%) of participants were parents of allergic children;

the remainder were allergic adults. Most (77%) participants were on social assistance, which included drug benefits (Table 2). All allergic individuals had been prescribed EAIs for their food allergies. Verification of diagnosis was not requested from participants' doctors because many participants reported not having a family doctor. All participants self-identified as being low income and were using community services offered specifically to low-income people. The first author conducted all interviews, which continued until saturation was reached. Interviews were transcribed verbatim for subsequent thematic analysis using NVivo 10 [17]. Interrater reliability assessment between two transcripts achieved reliability of 0.70 [18]. After a theme code set was developed, two researchers conducted intercoder tests to determine levels of coding agreement (70% agreement or higher is considered acceptable) to ensure confidence in the coding scheme [18]. Ethical clearance was received from the University of Waterloo.

3. Results

3.1. Perceived Direct Costs

3.1.1. Medication. Over half (54%) of low-income participants and 20% of key informants noted the high cost of EAIs as a barrier to anaphylaxis treatment for low-income families. EAIs cost about USD$100, which many allergists consider to be high in relation to minimum wage and average daily earnings [19]. Participants often kept expired EAIs rather than replacing them promptly; cost also affected their decision whether to purchase at all:

> When you have an anaphylactic reaction you don't just have the fear in that whole process and then your body feeling terrible for two to five days after, you have also just lost $100 or $200. (Allergic female)

One mother, unsure of her son's EAI expiry date, spoke of the impact her financial situation had on replacing expired EAIs:

> So coming up with a hundred dollars to replace it again, that is probably one of the reasons why I haven't checked to see if it is expired. (Mother of allergic toddler)

Keeping expired EAIs was reported by 31% of low-income participants. One woman described her experience of living as a homeless youth with an anaphylactic allergy thus,

> They expire. Yeah I always carry around all of mine, and the first ones I ever try would be the expired ones, just to try… it will save… like money, while you are saving your life, right. Sounds terrible to say it that way but it is really true. Just with the cost of an EpiPen, like that is a lot of money especially if you are like fifteen and living on the street. So it is like take the expired ones first and then usually they work and if they don't take the other one. (Allergic female)

TABLE 1: Key informant sectors and job descriptions.

Number	Sector	Job description
1	Health care	Allergist
2	Health care	Allergist
3	Public health	Public health dietitian (schools)
4	Social services	Dietitian (low-income family programs)
5	Social services	Food bank
6	Social services	Food bank
7	Social services	Food bank
8	Social services	Employment support (working centre)
9	Social services	Ontario Works
10	Social services	Ontario Works

TABLE 2: Demographic data of low-income individuals or families.

Number	Child/adult	Male/female respondent	Male/female with allergy	On social support
1	Child	Female	Male	No
2	Child	Female	Female	Yes
3	Child	Female	Male	Yes
4	Child	Female	Male	Yes
5	Child	Female	Female	Yes
6	Child	Female	Female	Yes
7	Child	Male	Male	No
8	Adult	Female	Female	No
9	Adult	Female	Female	Yes
10	Adult	Female	Female	Yes
11	Adult	Female	Female	Yes
12	Adult	Female	Female	Yes
13	Adult	Male	Male	Yes
Totals	54% children	85% female	62% female	23% no

Some participants reported retaining an inadequate number of EAIs or not having one at all due to cost. When asked how many EAIs she had for her tree-nut-allergic son, a low-income mother said, "Just the one. I can only afford one."

These experiences were echoed by the perceptions of an allergist:

> I think there is a considerable amount... especially in the lower income, that will make a decision based on, "if I use that now, I am not going to have it for the next ten months." And a $100 item may be a big deal for somebody who is generating... income below the poverty line. So I think that their reliance would still be on an antihistamine and prolonged care at home. (Allergist)

This is problematic because the first line of anaphylaxis treatment is epinephrine; antihistamines are not a recommended treatment [20], although they may be perceived as a low-cost alternative. Several participants confirmed the allergist's perception. One woman said:

> ... my first initial thing is to take Benadryl. I always take Benadryl. I use liquid, so that way

it gets into your system faster, as opposed to pill form. (Allergic female)

A peanut-allergic woman who had been hospitalized numerous times for anaphylactic reactions and who considered EAIs to be a "waste of money" considered antihistamines a "life line" for treating her peanut allergy.

3.1.2. Procuring Safe Foods. Less than half (43%) of respondents perceived no price differential for allergen-free foods, while 35% did:

> I think they are more expensive... because the factories have to make sure that you know there is no allergens in it... because we had to figure out how to make this without eggs, we are going to charge you two bucks more. (Allergic female)

Five participants (22%) thought that cost was dependent on the type of allergen-free food:

> It depends what you are looking for—wheat stuff—like wheat free stuff is expensive. (Mother of an allergic child)

Beyond the direct cost of specialty food items, participants differed in their opinions of how their overall grocery bill changed subsequent to an allergy diagnosis. Participants who reported that their grocery bill remained unchanged generally referred to the allergen being a previously infrequent purchase with no overall impact on their grocery bill. Overall, no clear consensus on costs associated with procuring allergen-free foods emerged among participants.

About a quarter (23%) of low-income participants reported that their weekly grocery bill decreased since the allergy diagnosis due to a reduction in purchasing more expensive processed (and potentially cross contaminated) foods or due to the elimination of purchasing expensive, allergenic foods (e.g., cashews). Regarding prediagnosis grocery bills, one woman explained,

> Probably more, just because there were more things that I could buy. And then I had to start like making my own I guess... you know, which could be cheaper. (Mother of an allergic child)

Finally, two participants (15%) described increased grocery costs after diagnosis:

> I would say our grocery budget... I would have to estimate... 15% increase overall simply because we buy brand name. We can't buy bulk... being a low-income family that is where it affects us... (Father of an allergic child)

3.1.3. Direct Costs Resulting from Misinformation. A significant proportion (46%) of low-income participants reported misinformation related to social support programs and medical insurance coverage. Some misinformation resulted in direct costs to participants:

Ontario Works [Ontario's Welfare System] won't pay for an epi-pen. It isn't covered through their benefit program. (Allergic female)

This statement was in direct contradiction to information provided by a key informant employed by Ontario Works who noted how common misinformation was:

We can't tell each person everything that they can qualify for. You say a drug card and you hope they kind of put it all together. So with allergies and everything you hope people will come to you and say, "I have this problem." And then we can talk about just that one specific one, but it is hard to get enough of the information out there... (Social assistance key informant)

One participant who knew she required an EAI but was unaware that it would be covered by her social assistance drug plan rationalized her lack of EAI by exaggerating the direct costs,

And I haven't gotten one now, because they are like a hundred and fifty bucks a piece... Every six months you have to renew it.

Other participants who were unaware that they qualified for EIA coverage through Ontario Works spoke of "taking care of themselves" so they would not require an EIA:

And so it is sometimes like wasting money... but I think as an adult now I will take much better care of myself and I just don't eat nothing [if] I don't know who cooked it. (Allergic female)

In the event of an unintentional exposure to an allergen, two participants who did not have EAIs due to the perceived high cost reported using emergency services instead of an EAI.

3.2. Perceived Indirect Costs

3.2.1. Lack of a Consistent Family Doctor. There were few indirect costs associated with anaphylactic food allergies that were unique to low-income families. This is because indirect costs, including lost labour productivity, obtaining health care, and time spent shopping for safe foods, are actually higher for people who earn more money [10, 12]. Only one indirect cost emerged as unique to low-income individuals with anaphylactic food allergies: 17% of participants referred to low-income groups having poorer continuity of care by family doctors, which may result in increased opportunity costs in terms of being unnecessarily re-tested for allergies.

... for folks who are dependent on urgent care, which is a lot of people, they just don't have family doctors... that would be... terrible to try and navigate. (Employment centre key informant)

One woman said,

You have to have some sort of identification proving your allergies. We have a new family doctor, and I have never had a scratch test done with him, so he does not have anything really on record about my allergies... (Allergic female)

3.3. Perceived Intangible Costs

3.3.1. Stress. Almost 40% of participants (5 key informants and 4 low-income respondents) reflected on the challenge of eating an adequate, healthy diet due to a lack of money. Many participants who relied on food banks felt stress due to the additional difficulty of obtaining allergen-free foods from the food bank (48% of participants):

Well a grocery store, you can pick and choose what you are getting. When it comes to the food hamper, you have got to take what you get, right... Even though you put down specifically in a yellow highlight pencil, or whatever, that [I'm] severely allergic to nuts, I still get it. (Allergic male)

One woman further explained how reporting allergies can actually decrease the overall amount of food that can be obtained from a food bank,

... they don't give you anything extra. If you are allergic to something, you just don't get it. They don't substitute it with anything, because they can only give you what they have, right... we have never said okay we are allergic to this, and they will give us something else. No, it is just you just don't get it. You get whatever else is left in your hamper. (Allergic female)

3.3.2. Feeling Unsafe. Almost one-third of participants reported feeling less safe at discount supermarkets relative to regular supermarkets because of perceived poor food availability and cross-contamination that participants thought was worse in discount supermarkets. In terms of product availability:

I know they are going to have a wide variety of brands to choose from, so it makes it easier for me. Whereas [discount supermarket] might get stuff from the States, so it takes much longer to go through all the labels at [discount supermarket] than it would at [regular supermarket]. (Mother of allergic child)

Respondents also pointed to employees practices:

Because I don't feel that [discount supermarket] probably deals with their produce as well as [regular supermarket] does. Like at [regular supermarket] you can see that how often the employees wash their hands. At [discount supermarket] they just touch this and they go touch that. I have watched them... they will pay their employees less. You know they are less worried about what kind of produce they have, and what they're touching and what they are doing with it. (Allergic female)

These data reveal trade-offs between direct and intangible risks: participants who shopped at regular grocery stores recognized that spending more on groceries (increased direct costs) reduced their fear of cross-contamination (decreased intangible costs).

3.4. Especially "at Risk" Groups. Four distinct low-income groups were described by participants as facing substantial barriers to proper anaphylaxis management and treatment. Of note, groups identified by participants were not groups with which the participants self-identified (e.g., only Canadian-born participants identified that newcomers to Canada may face additional barriers to food allergy management). These were the working poor with no or inadequate health insurance (22% of participants), newcomers to Canada (i.e., foreign immigrants) (17%), food bank users (13%), and youth living in poverty (9%). Both allergists and several low-income participants identified the working poor as being likely unable to afford EAIs. One allergist said,

> *If you are a working poor person that is making minimum wage or a little bit more, they may not have the drug benefits that the government offers and their jobs might not be "good enough" to have a drug plan. They would fall through the cracks. So I suspect that the majority of these people will not buy themselves EpiPens because they are just too expensive.*

Newcomers to Canada were another low-income group considered to be especially at risk:

> *New Canadians would be on very limited incomes, but they might have like food sensitivities and like, "My child is very, very sick and has to go to the hospital", but anaphylactic just isn't a familiar word and allergy even is not like a familiar word. (Employment centre key informant)*

A newcomer who participated in this research had difficulty articulating her son's allergies:

> *To eggs, some of the nuts... cashews, and there is another one. I don't know what the name of that. It is, it looks similar like walnut, but it is not walnut. It is round and kind of this much big. (Mother of allergic child)*

This mother knew no one in her home country with a food allergy and had an EAI trainer device but was unsure what it was or how to use it. She did not have an EAI for her son.

Participants' stress related to the difficulty of obtaining allergen-free foods at the food bank (discussed above) explains why several participants noted that food bank users qualify as another "at risk" group. In addition to the perceived potential for cross-contamination at the food bank, one woman said,

> *It frustrates me that the food bank never says nut-free products when they are looking for food. They always advertise, "We need baby cereal. We need peanut butter. We need this." They never say peanut-free anything. (Mother of an allergic child)*

Finally, two key informants related their concerns about youth with anaphylactic allergies who lived in poverty. One key informant was concerned about youth living in poverty being embarrassed to vocalize their allergy-related concerns,

> *I think it is embarrassing for a lot of the kids. I don't want to ask for food from you, because I don't want you to know I am hungry, like that I have no money, and that my parents have kicked me out. A lot of them don't know a nice way of saying, just tell me what is in this, you know, so they don't. (Social assistance key informant)*

Another key informant shared knowledge of how a street youth with anaphylactic food allergies might cope:

> *I think too, people on the street share EpiPens or sell expired ones or like there is kind of a small black market. [EpiPens are] probably $20–40. $20 probably for an expired one. $40–60 maybe for one that is not expired. Something like that. A lot less, but pretty much 50% less. (Employment centre key informant)*

Youth in extreme poverty who have no access to drug insurance may have to rely on drastic measures to access medication—in this case, medication that is much more affordable once it has expired.

4. Discussion

The economic impact of food allergies is significant [10, 14, 15]. Out-of-pocket costs differentially impact low-income families. No studies to date have provided an in-depth exploration of how low-income families experience the direct, indirect, or intangible costs associated with food allergy management or treatment. Complementing the economic analyses that have described costs of food allergy, our qualitative study has described the *meaning* of the costs of food allergy (including how they cope with and manage the high cost of EAIs) among a group of low-income families. The qualitative approach we adopted highlighted discrepancies between low-income families' perceptions about barriers to managing food allergies and the actual availability of support (e.g., while Ontario's social assistance drug plan covers the cost of EAIs, many families perceived that the social assistance drug plan did not cover EAIs).

Low-income families and key informants perceive significant financial barriers to appropriate management and treatment of anaphylactic food allergies. These barriers can be broadly conceived as access to drugs and procuring safe foods. Our findings that low-income individuals are perceived to have low access to family doctors are contradicted by empirical evidence suggesting that, in countries where income-related inequities exist in the distribution of family doctor visits, it is often a propoor distribution [21]. That said, prorich income-related inequalities in access to specialists (such as allergists) are common [21, 22]. In terms of access to medication, in many jurisdictions, pharmaceuticals are not publicly insured. Therefore, working poor families (which comprise 25% of low-income Canadians under 65 years [23]) may be particularly at risk of having inadequate access to medication. Almost 70% of our low-income sample reported having an up-to-date EAI; in another study, 87% of a fairly well-educated sample had an up-to-date EAI [9] and 75% of children of wealthier families registered in a Peanut Allergy Registry reported having up-to-date EAIs (A. Clarke, unpublished observation). Although retaining expired EAIs is not practiced exclusively by low-income families, financial barriers to medication access should be addressed alongside educational campaigns for the broader allergic population. Indeed, the fact that some families would chance an anaphylactic reaction for themselves or their children due to the cost of an EAI is quite concerning.

Limitations of this study include the fact that all participants were from Ontario: experiences with allergy management and access to medication and allergen-free foods may differ in other jurisdictions. Although there were only 23 participants, the goal of qualitative research is to explore individuals' experiences rather than to generalize or verify hypotheses about causal relationships, and thus the small sample was not necessarily a limitation of the current study [24]. Strengths of this study are the in-depth interviews employed to gain insight into the experiences of low-income families affected by food allergies as well as the inclusion of both affected individuals and a number of key informants who represented a variety of stakeholder perspectives.

Perceived direct and intangible costs represented barriers to procuring safe foods for participants. Media reports suggest that food allergies greatly increase a family's food budget [25]; empirical evidence from the UK indicates that nut-allergic individuals pay an average of 11% more for a grocery basket than non-nut-allergic individuals [26]. These findings may explain increased grocery bills observed in Finland for families with allergic infants [13]. Moreover, the availability of suitable food options in budget supermarkets may be limited [27]. Finally, food bank use is increasing in Canada [28], the United States [29], and the UK [30]; these trends have implications for the safety of low-income individuals with anaphylactic food allergies.

The lack of robust findings around indirect costs of food allergy unique to low-income families reflects the fact that indirect costs like labour productivity are higher for people who make more money per hour relative to people who make less money per hour.

"At risk" groups, including the working poor, newcomers, food bank users, and youth in poverty, are especially important groups to target in terms of education and medication assistance. In terms of newcomers, however, it is likely that competency in the host country's language would moderate experiences of difficulty managing anaphylactic food allergies. Although many clinicians do not collect income data from participants, encouraging patients on social assistance to confirm their drug benefits to procure EAIs at low or no cost may be an important practice implication from this research. Clinicians, advocacy groups, policy makers, and EAI manufacturers all have a role to play in ensuring more equitable access to required medication for low-income individuals with anaphylactic food allergies. In addition, from a prevention perspective, securing allergen-free foods is equivalent to a "treatment." Thus, providing additional funds to families to ensure their ability to secure allergen-free foods for their families may be another potential policy option.

Abbreviations

EAI: Epinephrine auto injector.

Conflict of Interests

The authors declare that there is no conflict of interests regarding the publication of this paper.

Acknowledgment

This work was funded by AllerGen NCE Inc., the Allergy, Genes and Environment Network.

References

[1] L. Soller, M. Ben-Shoshan, D. W. Harrington et al., "Overall prevalence of self-reported food allergy in Canada," *Journal of Allergy and Clinical Immunology*, vol. 130, no. 4, pp. 986–988, 2012.

[2] M. Ben-Shoshan, E. Turnbull, and A. Clarke, "Food allergy: temporal trends and determinants.," *Current Allergy and Asthma Reports*, vol. 12, pp. 346–372, 2012.

[3] A. M. Branum and S. L. Lukacs, "Food allergy among children in the United States," *Pediatrics*, vol. 124, no. 6, pp. 1549–1555, 2009.

[4] H. A. Sampson, A. Muñoz-Furlong, R. L. Campbell et al., "Second symposium on the definition and management of anaphylaxis: summary report—second National Institute of Allergy and Infectious Disease/Food Allergy and Anaphylaxis Network symposium," *Journal of Allergy and Clinical Immunology*, vol. 117, no. 2, pp. 391–397, 2006.

[5] R. Coombs, E. Simons, R. G. Foty, D. M. Stieb, and S. D. Dell, "Socioeconomic factors and epinephrine prescription in children with peanut allergy," *Paediatrics and Child Health*, vol. 16, no. 6, pp. 341–344, 2011.

[6] D. W. Frost and C. G. Chalin, "The effect of income on anaphylaxis preparation and management plans in Toronto primary schools," *Canadian Journal of Public Health*, vol. 96, no. 4, pp. 250–253, 2005.

[7] R. S. Gupta, E. E. Springston, M. R. Warrier et al., "The prevalence, severity, and distribution of childhood food allergy in the United States," *Pediatrics*, vol. 128, no. 1, pp. e9–e17, 2011.

[8] A. M. Branum, A. E. Simon, and S. L. Lukacs, "Among children with food allergy, do sociodemographic factors and healthcare use differ by severity?" *Maternal and Child Health Journal*, vol. 16, supplement 1, pp. 44–50, 2012.

[9] M. Ben-Shoshan, R. Kagan, M.-N. Primeau et al., "Availability of the epinephrine autoinjector at school in children with peanut allergy," *Annals of Allergy, Asthma and Immunology*, vol. 100, no. 6, pp. 570–575, 2008.

[10] R. Gupta, D. Holdford, L. Bilaver, A. Dyer, J. L. Holl, and D. Meltzer, "The economic impact of childhood food allergy in the United States," *JAMA Pediatrics*, vol. 167, no. 11, pp. 1026–1031, 2013.

[11] S. Miles, R. Fordham, C. Mills, E. Valovirta, and M. Mugford, "A framework for measuring costs to society of IgE-mediated food allergy," *Allergy*, vol. 60, no. 8, pp. 996–1003, 2005.

[12] J. Voordouw, M. Fox, J. Cornelisse-Vermaat, G. Antonides, M. Mugford, and L. Frewer, "Household costs associated with food

allergy: an exploratory study," *British Food Journal*, vol. 112, no. 11, pp. 1205–1215, 2010.

[13] S. Alanne, A. Maskunitty, M. Nermes, K. Laitinen, and M. Pekurinen, "Costs of allergic diseases from birth to two years in Finland," *Public Health*, vol. 126, pp. 866–872, 2012.

[14] D. A. Patel, D. A. Holdford, E. Edwards, and N. V. Carroll, "Estimating the economic burden of food-induced allergic reactions and anaphylaxis in the United States," *Journal of Allergy and Clinical Immunology*, vol. 128, no. 1, pp. 110–115, 2011.

[15] J. Voordouw, G. Antonides, M. Fox et al., "Subjective welfare, well-being, and self-reported food hypersensitivity in four European countries: implications for European policy," *Social Indicators Research*, vol. 107, no. 3, pp. 465–482, 2012.

[16] M. Gallagher, A. Worth, and A. Sheikh, "Clinical allergy has much to gain from engagement with qualitative research," *Allergy*, vol. 64, no. 8, pp. 1117–1120, 2009.

[17] QSR International Pty Ltd., "NVivo qualitative data analysis software," 2012.

[18] M. B. Miles and A. M. Huberman, *Qualitative Data Analysis: An Expanded Sourcebook*, Sage, Thousand Oaks, Calif, USA, 1994.

[19] F. E. R. Simons, "Epinephrine auto-injectors: first-aid treatment still out of reach for many at risk of anaphylaxis in the community," *Annals of Allergy, Asthma and Immunology*, vol. 102, no. 5, pp. 403–409, 2009.

[20] D. A. Andreae and M. H. Andreae, "Should antihistamines be used to treat anaphylaxis?" *British Medical Journal*, vol. 339, article b2489, pp. 290–291, 2009.

[21] E. Van Doorslaer, C. Masseria, and X. Koolman, "Inequalities in access to medical care by income in developed countries," *Canadian Medical Association Journal*, vol. 174, no. 2, pp. 177–183, 2006.

[22] L. McLeod, "Income-related horizontal inequities in physician use by asthmatics and diabetics: evidence using linked administrative data from Ontario," RDC Research Paper 22, 2011.

[23] Human Resources and Skills Development Canada, "Financial security—low income incidence," 2013, http://www4.hrsdc.gc.ca/.3ndic.1t.4r@-eng.jsp?iid=23.

[24] J. W. Creswell, *Qualitative Inquiry and Research Design: Choosing among Five Designs*, Sage, Thousand Oaks, Calif, USA, 1998.

[25] W. Konrad, "Food allergies take a toll on families and finances," 2010, http://www.nytimes.com/2010/05/15/health/15patient.html?_r=0&adxnnl=1&adxnnlx=1369318008-CKJYKLh5/g5xXT9A2bmMBg.

[26] Food Standards Agency, "'May Contain' labelling—the consumer's perspective," 2002, http://www.food.gov.uk/multimedia/pdfs/maycontainreport.pdf.

[27] J. Singh and K. Whelan, "Limited availability and higher cost of gluten-free foods," *Journal of Human Nutrition and Dietetics*, vol. 24, no. 5, pp. 479–486, 2011.

[28] Food Banks Canada, "Hunger count: a comprehensive report on hunger and food bank use in Canada, and recommendations for change," 2011.

[29] Feeding America, "Hunger study 2010," 2013, http://feedingamerica.org/hunger-in-america/hunger-studies/hunger-study-2010.aspx.

[30] The Trussell Trust, "Biggest ever increase in UK foodbank use," 2013, http://www.trusselltrust.org/stats.

Omega-3 Fatty Acids Supplementation in Children to Prevent Asthma: Is It Worthy?—A Systematic Review and Meta-Analysis

Prasad Muley,[1] **Monali Shah,**[2] **and Arti Muley**[3]

[1]*Department of Paediatrics, S.B.K.S MIRC, Sumandeep Vidyapeeth, Vadodara, Gujarat 391760, India*
[2]*Department of Periodontics, K.M.S DCH, Sumandeep Vidyapeeth, Vadodara, Gujarat 391760, India*
[3]*Department of Medicine, S.B.K.S MIRC, Sumandeep Vidyapeeth, Vadodara, Gujarat 391760, India*

Correspondence should be addressed to Prasad Muley; muleyprasad123@gmail.com

Academic Editor: Stephen P. Peters

Asthma is one of the most common respiratory diseases affecting all age groups. The world is now trying to identify some dietary factors which can play a preventive role. We performed this systematic review and meta-analysis of RCTs to assess the effect of intake of polyunsaturated fatty acid (PUFA) in infancy and/or childhood on incidence of asthma or wheezing episodes. We searched MEDLINE, EBSCO, Trip, and Google Scholar up to January 31, 2015. All RCTs where infants or children who were given omega-3 fatty acid supplementation and which reported incidence of asthma and/or wheezing episodes as dichotomous outcomes were included in this review. Random effects model was used for pooling the risk estimates. Total five articles were included. Most of them were from Australia. On meta-analysis, the pooled estimate of odds ratios by random effects model showed no significant change in incidence of asthma after supplementation of omega-3 FA in infancy or childhood (OR 0.974; CI 0.646, 1.469; $p = 0.900$). We concluded that a multicentric RCT is required to assess the effect of omega-3 FA supplementation exclusively to infants or children to predict the best time of omega-3 FA supplementation to prevent asthmatic or wheezing episodes later in life.

1. Introduction

Asthma is one of the most common respiratory diseases affecting all age groups. Around 300 million people are suffering from this disease worldwide [1]. The increasing prevalence of asthma over the years is an important cause of concern all over the globe. Inhaled corticosteroids are used for the management of asthma, but 5–10% of asthma patients are resistant to this therapy, leading to difficulties in managing the disease [2]. Hence, the world is now focusing on environmental factors and genetic susceptibility to identify the reason for this surge so that some effective strategy to prevent the disease can be developed. For the same reason, there has been increase in studies to find some dietary factors which can play a preventive role.

Omega-3 fatty acids are essential nutrients that cannot be synthesized in the body and must be obtained from the diet. Dietary omega-3 fatty acids are incorporated into cellular membranes of all tissues and are naturally enriched in fatty fish like salmon and tuna and in fish oil supplements. There have been reports that omega-3 fatty acids (omega-3 FA), docosahexaenoic acid (DHA), and eicosapentaenoic acid (EPA) have protective role against coronary artery diseases, hypertension, and dyslipidemia [3]. Their preventive role has also been reported in diabetes [4] and chronic inflammatory diseases including chronic obstructive pulmonary disease (COPD), rheumatoid arthritis, and inflammatory bowel disease [5, 6]. Molecular mechanisms have been revealed to support efficacy of omega-3 fatty acids in prevention of asthma and allergic diseases in part by the identification of fatty acid bioactive metabolites. It has been proposed that in severe asthma specialized proresolving mediators (SPM: protectins, resolvins, and maresins) production is impaired. Thus, by generating SPM, omega-3 fatty acids such as EPA and DHA counterregulate airway eosinophilic inflammation and promote the resolution of inflammation in vivo [7].

Fish oil contains two main omega-3 fatty acids, docosahexaenoic acid (DHA) and eicosapentaenoic acid (EPA).

Many epidemiological studies have reported reduction in incidence of allergic or atopic outcomes in infants or children of those pregnancies as an effect of maternal fish intake during pregnancy [8–12]. Some questionnaire based studies have also reported a protective effect of fish intake during infancy or childhood on allergic outcomes [13–19] paving the way for the question whether long-chain omega-3 FA have any significant role in prevention of asthma. A systematic review and meta-analysis assessed the relation of omega-3 FA supplementation (both in mothers and children) with the incidence of asthma or allergic or wheezing episodes; however it did not include RCTs [20]. So, we performed this systematic review and meta-analysis of RCTs to assess the effect of intake of polyunsaturated fatty acid (PUFA) in infancy and/or childhood on the incidence of asthma or wheezing episodes. Our research question was "In children (P) does omega-3 fatty acid supplementation (I) as compared to no intervention (C) help in primary prevention of asthma (O)?"

2. Methodology

2.1. Searching. A comprehensive search was performed using search terms (Omega 3 fatty acids OR PUFA OR fish oil) AND (Asthma OR wheezing episodes). We used medical subject headings (MeSH or MH) as search terms when available or key words when appropriate and searched four electronic databases, namely, MEDLINE, EBSCO, Trip, and Google Scholar up to January 31, 2015. Limits used were "humans," "children," and "0–18 years." We searched only for RCTs. Additional information was retrieved through hand search of the references from relevant articles. Three authors independently reviewed all titles retrieved and abstracts were screened where title was unclear. The abstracts thus found relevant were selected for full text reading. The articles selected for full text reading were read by the three reviewers independently for assessing the risk of bias and retrieving the information relevant for the review and meta-analysis. All discrepancies were solved by group discussion.

2.2. Study Eligibility Criteria. Inclusion criteria were all RCTs where only infants or children were given omega-3 fatty acid supplementation and which reported change in FEV1 or asthma severity scores or incidence of asthma and/or wheezing episodes as dichotomous outcomes. Exclusion criteria were all non-RCTs, studies where mothers were also given experimental supplementation, and studies which did not report the outcome in terms of incidence of asthma or wheezing episodes after supplementation.

2.3. Data Extraction and Assessment of Quality of Trial. Data was extracted individually by two authors (Prasad Muley and Arti Muley) and any disagreement was resolved by opinion of the third author (Monali Shah). The details of place, sample size, age, intervention, comparator, follow-up, and outcome monitored were recorded from included studies. Risk of bias was assessed according to Cochrane assessment of risk of bias tool based on randomization, blinding, allocation concealment, loss to follow-up, and intention to treat analysis. Quality of included trials was categorized as high risk,

moderate risk, and low risk if more than two, two, or one criterion were not fulfilled, respectively.

2.4. Statistical Analysis. We used comprehensive meta-analysis version 2 for pooling the results. We used odds ratio as the outcome measure. In the studies in which outcome was presented as relative risk or ARR (absolute risk reduction), we derived information of number of episodes of wheezing or asthma and calculated odds ratio from it to get uniform measure of outcome as odds ratio for all included studies. I^2 was used as a measure of heterogeneity. $I^2 > 50\%$ was considered significant heterogeneity. Random effects model was used for pooling the risk estimates when heterogeneity among the studies was more than fifty percent and fixed effects model when it was less than fifty percent. A sensitivity analysis was also carried out to find if there was any study which had grossly impacted the overall pooled result. We did not exclude any study on the basis of risk of bias.

3. Results

3.1. Searching. Fourteen relevant RCTs were identified for full text reading after comprehensive search of published literature and, thereafter, exclusion of irrelevant titles and abstracts (Figure 1). Twelve articles were retrieved from electronic database and two from hand searching. After full text reading, nine [17, 21–28] were excluded for various reasons (Table 1) while five articles were included (Table 2) in the meta-analysis [29–33].

3.2. Design and Quality of Included Studies (Table 3). All the included trials reported adequate randomization and blinding while allocation concealment was done in all except one. One trial mentioned doing intention to treat analysis also. Using Cochrane tool for assessing risk of bias, one study showed moderate risk of bias while others had low risk of bias.

3.3. Study Characteristics. Total 2415 children were randomized in the studies and outcome was available for 1932 (80%) children. Average age of administration of supplements was 0–12 months. Longest duration of supplementation was up to five years of age in the study by Ng et al. [33]. Average duration of follow-up was 3.5 years ranging from 6 months [32] to as long as 8 years [33]. Almost all of them gave fish oil capsules as supplementation of omega-3 FA. The content of omega-3 FA was 60% in only one study [32] while the content in all other studies was about 37%. All the RCTs which reported the results as relative risk or hazard ratio or odds ratio were included in the meta-analysis.

3.4. Heterogeneity and Pooled Result. The included studies did not show significant heterogeneity amongst them ($I^2 = 52.20$, Tau$^2 = 0.109$, $p = 0.07$). On meta-analysis, the pooled estimate of odds ratios by random effects model showed no significant change in incidence of asthma after supplementation of omega-3 FA in infancy or childhood (OR 0.974; CI 0.646, 1.469; $p = 0.900$) (Figure 2).

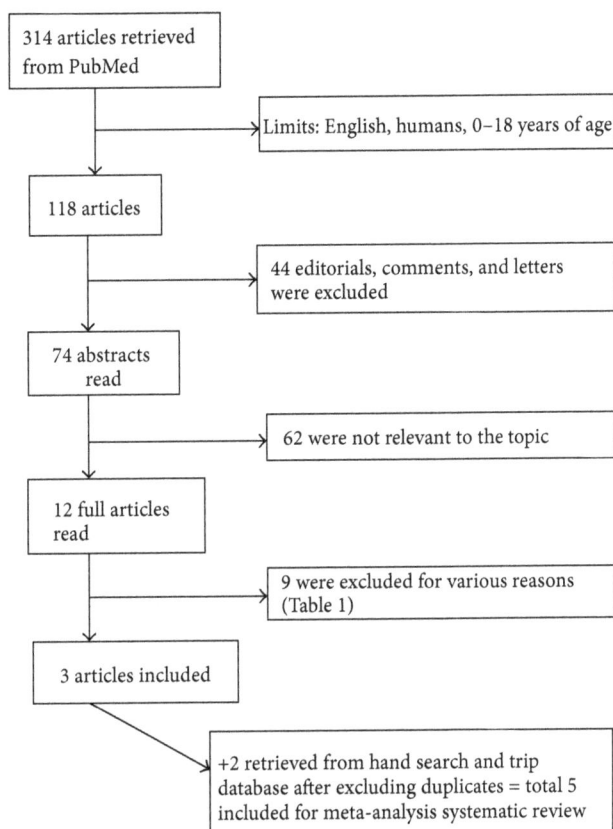

FIGURE 1: Searching details.

Meta analysis

Study name	Odds ratio	Lower limit	Upper limit	Z-value	p value	Odds ratio and 95% CI	Relative weight
Mihrshahi et al. 2003	0.660	0.344	1.266	−1.251	0.211		20.04
Marks et al. 2006	1.160	0.828	1.625	0.863	0.388		31.76
D'Vaz et al. 2012	1.530	0.751	3.117	1.172	0.241		18.26
Birch et al. 2010	0.320	0.108	0.949	−2.054	0.040		10.54
Almqvist et al. 2007	1.310	0.669	2.566	0.787	0.431		19.40
	0.974	0.646	1.469	−0.125	0.900		

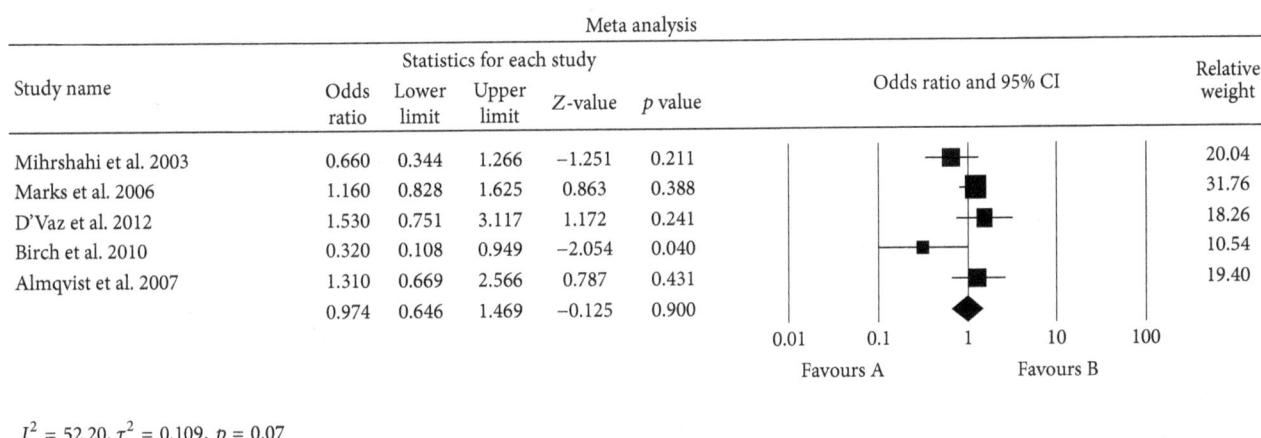

$I^2 = 52.20, \tau^2 = 0.109, p = 0.07$

FIGURE 2: Odds ratio and 95% confidence interval of risk of asthma. The pooled estimates were obtained using a random effects model. The squares represent relative risk in each study, with square size representing the study-specific weight and the 95% CI is represented by horizontal bars. The diamond at the bottom indicates summary risk estimate.

3.5. Sensitivity Analysis. We also did sensitivity analysis to find out whether the pooled result was substantially influenced by one study. On removing one study [31] the heterogeneity reduced substantially to $I^2 = 14.18$, $p = 0.316$, and Tau$^2 = 0.018$. On calculating pooled OR after omitting this study, the pooled result shifted slightly to right (OR 1.122; CI 0.869, 1.448; $p = 0.378$). No other individual studies significantly influenced the results.

4. Discussion

Some clinical trials have shown an increase in levels of omega-3 FA in the offspring with maternal intake of fish oil. They have also reported anti-inflammatory effects of using fish oil supplementation (during pregnancy and lactation) on cytokine production, lipid mediator release, and cellular infiltration [34–38]. A large epidemiological study showed

TABLE 1: Details of excluded studies.

Serial number	Author	Title of paper	Reason for exclusion
1	Hodge et al., 1996 [17]	Consumption of oily fish and childhood asthma risk	Case control study
2	Hodge et al., 1998 [21]	Effect of dietary intake of omega-3 and omega-6 fatty acids on severity of asthma in children	Asthma severity scoring was based on symptoms while, in other study which reported asthma scoring system, it was based on auscultatory findings, hence excluded from meta-analysis
3	Nagakura et al., 2000 [22]	Dietary supplementation with fish oil rich in omega-3 polyunsaturated fatty acids in children with bronchial asthma (asthma severity score)	Asthma severity scoring was based on auscultatory findings while, in other study which reported asthma scoring system, it was based on symptoms, hence excluded from meta-analysis
4	Mihrshahi et al., 2004 [23]	Effect of omega-3 fatty acid concentrations in plasma on symptoms of asthma at 18 months of age	Assessed association of plasma level of omega-3 FA after giving tuna fish and margarine oil with incidence of asthma
5	Chan-Yeung et al., 2005 [24]	Canadian childhood asthma primary prevention study: outcomes at 7 years of age	Did not use omega-3 FA as intervention
6	Almqvist et al., 2007 [25]	Omega-3 and omega-6 fatty acid exposure from early life does not affect atopy and asthma at age 5 years	Observational study
7	Al Biltagi et al., 2009 [26]	Omega-3 fatty acids, vitamin C, and Zn supplementation in asthmatic children: a randomized self-controlled study	Simultaneously used omega-3 FA, vit. C, and Zn supplementation
8	Manley et al., 2011 [27]	High-dose docosahexaenoic acid supplementation of preterm infants: respiratory and allergy outcomes	Supplementation given to mothers and EBM (expressed breast milk) fed to the babies
9	Lang et al., 2013 [28]	Nutrigenetic response to omega-3 fatty acids in obese asthmatics (NOOA): rationale and methods	Results not stated

an inverse association of intake of omega-3 FA with asthma morbidity. Since then, many studies focusing on omega-3 FA intake or supplements have been conducted. Most of them reported a protective effect of omega-3 FA supplementation given to mothers during pregnancy or lactation on the incidence of asthma or wheezing episodes or other allergic outcomes during infancy or childhood [8–12].

There have been some studies which assessed effect of omega-3 supplementation to infants or children. The cohort studies reported a preventive role of fish intake during infancy or childhood on allergic outcomes [11, 13–17]. The clinical intervention studies also showed a decline in prevalence of wheeze and use of bronchodilator at 18 months of age, with fish oil supplementation in infants/children of age group 6 months to 5 years [23, 29]. They also reported reduced allergic sensitization and prevalence of cough at 3 years of age. One out of two studies which examined the effect of fish oil supplements on asthmatic symptoms and lung function in children reported significant reduction in asthma severity [21, 39].

However, in adults, there have been inconsistent reports regarding benefits of fish or fish oil intake on asthmatic episodes [40–45]. Some studies have reported improved lung function and prevention of asthma with high intake of DHA [42, 43]. However, another study showed increased respiratory symptoms with reduced omega-3 FA intake [46]. This pattern was explained previously by the fact that chronic

inflammation may affect the immune system [4] which has been suggested to be "particularly true in children because a child's immune system is under development" [18]. From this, it can be presumed that omega-3 FA are important in the stage of immune system development. In other words, children may be more sensitive to omega-3 FA intake than adults. A recent meta-analysis of observational studies found that "the potential beneficial effect of fish or Omega-3 FA intake was more pronounced in children. It might be explained by the suggestion that children are more sensitive to omega-3 FA." [20].

Some other meta-analyses of RCTs have been done previously, which reported no improvements in asthmatic symptoms with omega-3 fatty acid supplementation [47, 48] both in children and adults. All included RCTs in that meta-analysis [47] had relatively small sample sizes (from 12 to 45) and short follow-up periods (from 8 weeks to 12 months). Also, fish oil was used as supplement which may reflect a different health impact from consuming whole fish, a package of nutrients [48]. Our study is different as we included only RCTs in which omega-3 fatty acids supplementation was given exclusively to children and not to mothers during pregnancy or lactation. All the studies had good sample sizes ranging from 200 to 600; the supplementation was given in the form of fish oil capsules with predetermined contents and quantities and the mean duration of follow-up was 3.5

TABLE 2: Details of included studies.

Serial number	Author	Year	Place	Sample size	Age/sex	Intervention and dose	Comparator and dose	Follow-up (years)	Outcomes studied	Conflict of interests	Funding
1	Mihrshahi et al. [29]	2003	Australia	616/554	6–18 months/ both	o-3–rich tuna fish oil (500 mg) from the age of 6 months.	Sunola oil	1	Number of episodes of wheeze or cough lasting for >1 week not associated with colds	None	Institute of Health
2	Marks et al. [30]	2006	Australia	616/516	6 months to 5 years	Oil capsules with 500 mg tuna fish oil (37% o-3 PUFA + 6% o-6)	Oil capsules with 0.3% o-3 + 7% o-6 PUFA	5	Episodes of wheeze, asthma	None	Institute of Health
3	Birch et al. [31]	2010	USA	147/89	<5 days–12 months/ both	DHA and ARA as 0.32%–0.36% and 0.64%–0.72% of total FA	Enfamil with iron	3	Diagnoses of wheezing, asthma	None	National Institute of Health USA
4	D'Vaz et al. [32]	2012	Australia	420/323	0–6 months/ both	650 mg fish oil capsules (280 mg DHA + 110 mg EPA) daily	650 mg olive oil (66.6% n-9 oleic acid)	0.5	Physician diagnosed IgE-mediated asthma episodes	None	National Health and Medical Research Council (NHMRC)
5	Ng et al. [33]	2010	Australia	616/450	Birth to 5 years/ both	Oil capsules, 500 mg tuna fish oil (37% o-3 PUFA + 6% o-6 PUFA)	500 mg Sunola oil capsules (0.3% o-3 + 7% o-6 PUFA)	8	ARR of wheezing episodes, asthma	None	Institute of Health

DHA: docosahexaenoic acid; EPA: eicosapentaenoic acid; ARA: arachidonic acid; PUFA: polyunsaturated fatty acid; ARR: absolute risk reduction; o-3: omega-3; o-6: omega-6; FA: fatty acids; sample size: number of participants who were given supplements/number of participants who completed the trial.

TABLE 3: Risk of bias amongst the included studies.

Serial number	Author	Randomization	Allocation concealment	Blinding	Incomplete data outcome reporting	Outcome
1	Mihrshahi et al. [29]	Randomized	Yes	Double blind	Not stated	Low
2	Marks et al. [30]	Randomized	Yes	Double blind	Not stated	Low
3	Birch et al. [31]	Randomized	Not clear	Double blind	Not done	Moderate
4	D'Vaz et al. [32]	Randomized	Yes	Double blind	Yes	No
5	Ng et al. [33]	Randomized	Yes	Double blind	Not stated	Low

years. A limitation of our study was that out of the five studies included in meta-analysis, three were parts of the same CAPS (Childhood Asthma Prevention Study); however, we considered them separate studies as the duration of follow-up in those was different and the data were analyzed separately in the three studies. Another peculiar observation was that four out of the five RCTs were carried out in Australia while one was from US. Hence, RCTs from other parts of the world were lacking. We also did not find any significant reduction in incidence of asthma on meta-analysis of these studies. The pooled result did not change much on sensitivity analysis but showed a drift towards right on eliminating one [31] study.

We found two studies assessing change in FEV1 [21, 26] and two studies assessing change in asthma severity scores [21, 22] after supplementation of omega-3 FA in asthmatic children. One of the studies which assessed asthma severity score used symptoms for scoring while the other used auscultatory findings for the same; hence it was not possible to pool the results. Out of those which had FEV1 as outcome measure, one study used omega-3 FA with vitamin C and Zn for supplementation [26], so pooling the results was not logical in this case either. Thus, we excluded all these from meta-analysis. However, it was noted that in these studies also there was inconsistent result regarding improvement in lung function after the supplementation. One [21] of these studies showed no significant improvement while the other two reported improved lung function with the supplementation. Although one study [26] showed improvement, it was only with combined supplementation of omega-3 FA, vitamin C, and Zn; there was no significant improvement on mono supplementation with either of them.

Thus, although many studies have reported significant reduction in incidence of asthma or wheezing episode with omega-3 FA supplementation given to mother during pregnancy or lactation, there are insignificant results with supplementation in adults. In our study, we observed lack of RCTs assessing effect of omega-3 supplementation in infancy or childhood in preventing asthmatic or wheezing episodes. The result in our study also did not show any significant reduction in incidence of asthma or wheezing episode after omega-3 supplementation exclusively in infancy or childhood. There are many theories to explain the anti-inflammatory effect of omega-3 FA but none of them appears to explain this difference, although it can be said that some substance present in maternal tissue or breast milk or some biochemical process during secretion of breast milk might be responsible. So, this study highlights the need of a multicentric RCT to find out the preventive effect of omega-3 supplementation in infancy and childhood on later asthmatic and wheezing episodes. This may answer the query of the best time of supplementation with omega-3 FA to prevent asthmatic or wheezing episodes in children.

5. Conclusion

We did not find any role of omega-3 fatty acid supplementation in children in primary prevention of asthma. However, there are very few RCTs available. As some studies have shown association of maternal supplementation with prevention of asthma in children, a multicentric RCT is required to assess the effect of omega-3 FA supplementation exclusively to infants or children to predict the best time of omega-3 FA supplementation to prevent asthmatic or wheezing episodes later in life.

Conflict of Interests

The authors declare that they have no conflict of interests.

References

[1] S. S. Braman, "The global burden of asthma," *Chest*, vol. 130, no. 1, supplement, 2006.

[2] M. C. Bell and W. W. Busse, "Severe asthma: an expanding and mounting clinical challenge," *Journal of Allergy and Clinical Immunology: In Practice*, vol. 1, no. 2, pp. 110–121, 2013.

[3] P. Saravanan, N. C. Davidson, E. B. Schmidt, and P. C. Calder, "Cardiovascular effects of marine omega-3 fatty acids," *The Lancet*, vol. 376, no. 9740, pp. 540–550, 2010.

[4] A. Muley, P. Muley, and M. Shah, "ALA, fatty fish or marine n-3 fatty acids for preventing DM?: a systematic review and meta-analysis," *Current Diabetes Reviews*, vol. 10, no. 3, pp. 158–165, 2014.

[5] P. C. Calder, "Omega-3 polyunsaturated fatty acids and inflammatory processes: nutrition or pharmacology?" *British Journal of Clinical Pharmacology*, vol. 75, no. 3, pp. 645–662, 2013.

[6] C. M. Yates, P. C. Calder, and G. Ed Rainger, "Pharmacology and therapeutics of omega-3 polyunsaturated fatty acids in chronic inflammatory disease," *Pharmacology & Therapeutics*, vol. 141, no. 3, pp. 272–282, 2014.

[7] J. Miyata and M. Arita, "Role of omega-3 fatty acids and their metabolites in asthma and allergic diseases," *Allergology International*, vol. 64, no. 1, pp. 27–34, 2015.

[8] M. Calvani, C. Alessandri, S. M. Sopo et al., "Consumption of fish, butter and margarine during pregnancy and development of allergic sensitizations in the offspring: role of maternal atopy," *Pediatric Allergy and Immunology*, vol. 17, no. 2, pp. 94–102, 2006.

[9] I. Romieu, M. Torrent, R. Garcia-Esteban et al., "Maternal fish intake during pregnancy and atopy and asthma in infancy," *Clinical and Experimental Allergy*, vol. 37, no. 4, pp. 518–525, 2007.

[10] M. T. Salam, Y.-F. Li, B. Langholz, and F. D. Gilliland, "Maternal fish consumption during pregnancy and risk of early childhood asthma," *Journal of Asthma*, vol. 42, no. 6, pp. 513–518, 2005.

[11] S. Sausenthaler, S. Koletzko, B. Schaaf et al., "Maternal diet during pregnancy in relation to eczema and allergic sensitization in the offspring at 2 y of age," *The American Journal of Clinical Nutrition*, vol. 85, no. 2, pp. 530–537, 2007.

[12] S. M. Willers, G. Devereux, L. C. A. Craig et al., "Maternal food consumption during pregnancy and asthma, respiratory and atopic symptoms in 5-year-old children," *Thorax*, vol. 62, no. 9, pp. 772–779, 2007.

[13] K. Andreasyan, A.-L. Ponsonby, T. Dwyer et al., "A differing pattern of association between dietary fish and allergen-specific subgroups of atopy," *Allergy*, vol. 60, no. 5, pp. 671–677, 2005.

[14] L. Chatzi, M. Torrent, I. Romieu et al., "Diet, wheeze, and atopy in school children in Menorca, Spain," *Pediatric Allergy and Immunology*, vol. 18, no. 6, pp. 480–485, 2007.

[15] T. Dunder, L. Kuikka, J. Turtinen, L. Räsänen, and M. Uhari, "Diet, serum fatty acids, and atopic diseases in childhood," *Allergy: European Journal of Allergy and Clinical Immunology*, vol. 56, no. 5, pp. 425–428, 2001.

[16] T. Antova, S. Pattenden, B. Nikiforov et al., "Nutrition and respiratory health in children in six Central and Eastern European countries," *Thorax*, vol. 58, no. 3, pp. 231–236, 2003.

[17] L. Hodge, C. M. Salome, J. K. Peat, M. M. Haby, W. Xuan, and A. J. Woolcock, "Consumption of oily fish and childhood asthma risk," *Medical Journal of Australia*, vol. 164, no. 3, pp. 137–140, 1996.

[18] I. Kull, A. Bergström, G. Lilja, G. Pershagen, and M. Wickman, "Fish consumption during the first year of life and development of allergic diseases during childhood," *Allergy*, vol. 61, no. 8, pp. 1009–1015, 2006.

[19] P. Nafstad, W. Nystad, P. Magnus, and J. J. K. Jaakkola, "Asthma and allergic rhinitis at 4 years of age in relation to fish consumption in infancy," *Journal of Asthma*, vol. 40, no. 4, pp. 343–348, 2003.

[20] H. Yang, P. Xun, and K. He, "Fish and fish oil intake in relation to risk of asthma: a systematic review and meta-analysis," *PLoS ONE*, vol. 8, no. 11, Article ID e80048, 2013.

[21] L. Hodge, C. M. Salome, J. M. Hughes et al., "Effect of dietary intake of omega-3 and omega-6 fatty acids on severity of asthma in children," *European Respiratory Journal*, vol. 11, no. 2, pp. 361–365, 1998.

[22] T. Nagakura, S. Matsuda, K. Shichijyo, H. Sugimoto, and K. Hata, "Dietary supplementation with fish oil rich in ω-3 polyunsaturated fatty acids in children with bronchial asthma," *European Respiratory Journal*, vol. 16, no. 5, pp. 861–865, 2000.

[23] S. Mihrshahi, J. K. Peat, K. Webb, W. Oddy, G. B. Marks, and C. M. Mellis, "Effect of omega-3 fatty acid concentrations in plasma on symptoms of asthma at 18 months of age," *Pediatric Allergy and Immunology*, vol. 15, no. 6, pp. 517–522, 2004.

[24] M. Chan-Yeung, A. Ferguson, W. Watson et al., "The Canadian childhood asthma primary prevention study: outcomes at 7 years of age," *Journal of Allergy and Clinical Immunology*, vol. 116, no. 1, pp. 49–55, 2005.

[25] C. Almqvist, F. Garden, W. Xuan et al., "Omega-3 and omega-6 fatty acid exposure from early life does not affect atopy and asthma at age 5 years," *Journal of Allergy and Clinical Immunology*, vol. 119, no. 6, pp. 1438–1444, 2007.

[26] M. Al Biltagi, A. Abdul Baset, M. Bassiouny, M. Al Kasrawi, and M. Attia, "Omega-3 fatty acids, vitamin C and Zn supplementation in asthmatic children: a randomized self-controlled study," *Acta Paediatrica*, vol. 98, no. 4, pp. 737–742, 2009.

[27] B. J. Manley, M. Makrides, C. T. Collins et al., "High-dose docosahexaenoic acid supplementation of preterm infants: respiratory and allergy outcomes," *Pediatrics*, vol. 128, no. 1, pp. e71–e77, 2011.

[28] J. E. Lang, E. B. Mougey, H. Allayee et al., "Nutrigenetic response to omega-3 fatty acids in obese asthmatics (NOOA): rationale and methods," *Contemporary Clinical Trials*, vol. 34, no. 2, pp. 326–335, 2013.

[29] S. Mihrshahi, J. K. Peat, G. B. Marks et al., "Eighteen-month outcomes of house dust mite avoidance and dietary fatty acid modification in the Childhood Asthma Prevention Study (CAPS)," *Journal of Allergy and Clinical Immunology*, vol. 111, no. 1, pp. 162–168, 2003.

[30] G. B. Marks, S. Mihrshahi, A. S. Kemp et al., "Prevention of asthma during the first 5 years of life: a randomized controlled trial," *Journal of Allergy and Clinical Immunology*, vol. 118, no. 1, pp. 53–61, 2006.

[31] E. E. Birch, J. C. Khoury, C. L. Berseth et al., "The Impact of early nutrition on incidence of allergic manifestations and common respiratory illnesses in children," *Journal of Pediatrics*, vol. 156, no. 6, pp. 902–906, 2010.

[32] N. D'Vaz, S. J. Meldrum, J. A. Dunstan et al., "Postnatal fish oil supplementation in high-risk infants to prevent allergy: randomized controlled trial," *Pediatrics*, vol. 130, no. 4, pp. 674–682, 2012.

[33] K. K. W. Ng, D. Crisafulli, E. G. Belousova et al., "Eight-year outcomes of the Childhood Asthma Prevention Study," *Journal of Allergy and Clinical Immunology*, vol. 126, no. 2, pp. 388–389.e3, 2010.

[34] A. E. Barden, T. A. Mori, J. A. Dunstan et al., "Fish oil supplementation in pregnancy lowers F2-isoprostanes in neonates at high risk of atopy," *Free Radical Research*, vol. 38, no. 3, pp. 233–239, 2004.

[35] J. A. Dunstan, L. R. Mitoulas, G. Dixon et al., "The effects of fish oil supplementation in pregnancy on breast milk fatty acid composition over the course of lactation: a randomized controlled trial," *Pediatric Research*, vol. 62, no. 6, pp. 689–694, 2007.

[36] J. A. Dunstan, T. A. Mori, A. Barden et al., "Effects of n-3 polyunsaturated fatty acid supplementation in pregnancy on maternal and fetal erythrocyte fatty acid composition," *European Journal of Clinical Nutrition*, vol. 58, no. 3, pp. 429–437, 2004.

[37] S. Krauss-Etschmann, R. Shadid, C. Campoy et al., "Effects of fish-oil and folate supplementation of pregnant women on maternal and fetal plasma concentrations of docosahexaenoic acid and eicosapentaenoic acid: a European randomized multi-center trial," *American Journal of Clinical Nutrition*, vol. 85, no. 5, pp. 1392–1400, 2007.

[38] K. Warstedt, C. Furuhjelm, K. Duchen, K. Fälth-Magnusson, and M. Facerás, "The effects of omega-3 fatty acid supplementation in pregnancy on maternal eicosanoid, cytokine, and chemokine secretion," *Pediatric Research*, vol. 66, no. 2, pp. 212–217, 2009.

[39] T. Nagakura, S. Matsuda, K. Shichijyo, H. Sugimoto, and K. Hata, "Dietary supplementation with fish oil rich in omega-3 polyunsaturated fatty acids in children with bronchial asthma," *European Respiratory Journal*, vol. 16, no. 5, pp. 861–865, 2000.

[40] R. Barros, A. Moreira, J. Fonseca et al., "Dietary intake of alpha-linolenic acid and low ratio of n-6:n-3 PUFA are associated with decreased exhaled NO and improved asthma control," *British Journal of Nutrition*, vol. 106, no. 3, pp. 441–450, 2011.

[41] R. Kitz, M. A. Rose, R. Schubert et al., "Omega-3 polyunsaturated fatty acids and bronchial inflammation in grass pollen allergy after allergen challenge," *Respiratory Medicine*, vol. 104, no. 12, pp. 1793–1798, 2010.

[42] I. Kompauer, H. Demmelmair, B. Koletzko, G. Bolte, J. Linseisen, and J. Heinrich, "Association of fatty acids in serum phospholipids with lung function and bronchial hyperresponsiveness in adults," *European Journal of Epidemiology*, vol. 23, no. 3, pp. 175–190, 2008.

[43] J. Li, P. Xun, D. Zamora et al., "Intakes of long-chain omega-3 (n-3) PUFAs and fish in relation to incidence of asthma among American young adults: the CARDIA study," *American Journal of Clinical Nutrition*, vol. 97, no. 1, pp. 173–178, 2013.

[44] T. M. McKeever, S. A. Lewis, P. A. Cassano et al., "The relation between dietary intake of individual fatty acids, FEV1 and respiratory disease in Dutch adults," *Thorax*, vol. 63, no. 3, pp. 208–214, 2008.

[45] R. K. Woods, J. M. Raven, E. H. Walters, M. J. Abramson, and F. C. K. Thien, "Fatty acid levels and risk of asthma in young adults," *Thorax*, vol. 59, no. 2, pp. 105–110, 2004.

[46] J. S. Burns, D. W. Dockery, L. M. Neas et al., "Low dietary nutrient intakes and respiratory health in adolescents," *Chest*, vol. 132, no. 1, pp. 238–245, 2007.

[47] R. K. Woods, F. C. Thien, and M. J. Abramson, "Dietary marine fatty acids (fish oil) for asthma in adults and children," *Cochrane Database of Systematic Reviews*, no. 3, Article ID CD001283, 2002.

[48] C. Anandan, U. Nurmatov, and A. Sheikh, "Omega 3 and 6 oils for primary prevention of allergic disease: systematic review and meta-analysis," *Allergy*, vol. 64, no. 6, pp. 840–848, 2009.

10

Meta-Analysis of the Efficacy of Ectoine Nasal Spray in Patients with Allergic Rhinoconjunctivitis

Andrea Eichel,[1] Andreas Bilstein,[2] Nina Werkhäuser,[2] and Ralph Mösges[1]

[1] *Institute of Medical Statistics, Informatics and Epidemiology, Faculty of Medicine, University of Cologne, Lindenburger Allee 42, 50931 Cologne, Germany*

[2] *Bitop AG, Stockumer Straße 28, 58453 Witten, Germany*

Correspondence should be addressed to Andrea Eichel; andrea.eichel@uni-koeln.de

Academic Editor: Desiderio Passali

Objectives. The meta-analysis aims to investigate the efficacy of ectoine nasal spray and eye drops in the treatment of allergic rhinitis and rhinoconjunctivitis symptoms. *Design and Methods.* This meta-analysis is based on yet unpublished data of four studies. Both nasal and eye symptoms were documented in patient diary cards. All scales were transformed into a 4-point scale: 0 = no, 1 = mild, 2 = moderate, and 3 = severe symptoms. Each symptom was analysed individually in a meta-analysis of the area under the curve values as well as in a meta-analysis of pre- and posttreatment comparison. *Results.* After seven days of treatment with ectoine nasal spray both nasal and ocular symptoms decreased significantly. A strong reduction of symptom severity was shown for the parameters rhinorrhoea (31.76% reduction) and nasal obstruction (29.94% reduction). Furthermore, the meta-analyses of individual symptoms to investigate the strength of effect after seven days of medication intake showed significant improvement for nasal obstruction, rhinorrhoea, nasal itching, sneezing, itching of eyes, and redness of eyes. The improvement of the symptom nasal obstruction was associated with a strong effect 0.53 (±0.26). *Conclusions.* The ectoine nasal spray and eye drops seem to be equally effective as guideline-recommended medication in the treatment of rhinoconjunctivitis symptoms.

1. Introduction

Allergic rhinitis is clinically defined as an inflammation of the nose with characteristic symptoms such as rhinorrhoea, nasal obstruction, sneezing, and/or itching of the nose. The symptomatic disorder of the nasal mucosa and tissue is associated with an IgE-mediated immune response to allergens and is characterised by two phases: an immediate response after allergen exposure (early phase) and a late phase occurring up to 12 hours later, which predominantly causes nasal congestion [1]. If a concurrent respiratory infection is present, a patient's probability of developing bronchial asthma as comorbidity increases. Likewise, the risk of developing further allergies with more severe symptoms rises over the time of the disease [2].

A variety of causes for rhinitis exist in both children and adults, but 50% of all cases can be ascribed to allergy [3]. Due to its prevalence, impact on quality of life, impairment of work or school performance, reducing effect on productivity, economic burden, and risk of comorbidities, allergic rhinitis is regarded worldwide as a major chronic respiratory disease. Moreover, it can be associated with significant fatigue, mood changes, cognitive impairments, depression, and anxiety [4–8].

The optimal treatment of allergic rhinitis depends on several individual factors. A stepwise therapeutic approach, however, is generally recommended. Current guidelines favour second-generation oral or topical H1 antihistamines for treating allergic rhinitis [1, 9, 10]. Moreover, intranasal glucocorticosteroids and intranasal decongestants are highly recommended as effective treatments for nasal blockage [11].

Ectoine (2-methyl-1,4,5,6-tetrahydropyrimidine-4-carboxyclic acid) is a compatible solute which is naturally produced by bacteria, conferring resistance to external stress factors such as extreme temperatures, high salt concentrations, and ultraviolet radiation. It acts via a mechanism called "preferential exclusion" and "preferential hydration" [12]. Ectoine is expelled from proteins or lipid membranes, resulting in the modulation of the solvent characteristic of surrounding water. Thus, ectoine is able to form a protective and stabilising hydrate capsule around the protein and therefore helps to protect biomolecules and proteins from irreversible structural modifications by inhibiting dehydration. This indirect effect leads to a more compact and more stable folding of proteins and increases the stability of lipid membranes by increasing their fluidity [13]. The effect derives from the mechanism of halophilic bacteria which stabilises the osmotic balance in the microorganic cell, where extremolytes such as ectoine are accumulated in the cytosol to equal out the varying salt concentration in the outer area [14, 15]. Stabilisation of membranes such as those lining the airways or eyes might reduce the potential water loss of such membranes and protect them against invading allergens, thereby limiting the inflammatory cascade induced by stress mediators at the membrane level, as has been shown for lung epithelia and skin cells [16]. *In vitro* experiments have further shown that ectoine inhibits apoptosis, triggered by nanoparticles [17], and likewise blocks the activity of ceramides, which are regarded as central molecules in the sphingolipid metabolism as well as in the induction of apoptosis [18]. Currently, ectoine is used in dermatological products for successfully treating skin diseases such as atopic dermatitis [19]. Still widely unknown is the use of ectoine in nasal sprays or eye drops. In such medical devices, ectoine may strengthen the hydroprotection of the nasal membrane and may alleviate the infection of the inflamed tissue [20].

Toxicological studies and results of human studies reflect the excellent safety profile of products containing ectoine, therewith making them promising candidates for the treatment of allergic rhinoconjunctivitis [14, 20].

With this meta-analysis we aimed to investigate the efficacy of ectoine nasal spray in the treatment of allergic rhinitis and rhinoconjunctivitis symptoms.

2. Material and Methods

2.1. Literature Search. In order to investigate the efficacy of treatment with ectoine, data from published as well as unpublished clinical studies were reviewed.

Bitop AG, a German medical device company, kindly supplied us with detailed results from several clinical and noninterventional studies launched between 2008 and 2011 investigating its allergy nasal spray based on ectoine. Additionally, we conducted a systematic and comprehensive search of scientific and medical databases for further studies and reports published until January 2013. For this purpose, a catalogue of search criteria was generated in due consideration of the question posed by this meta-analysis. Using PubMed's MeSH database, the literature search was based on the following search criteria: "Ectoin," "ectoine", "(S)-2-Methyl-1,4,5,6-tetrahydropyrimidin-4-carbonsäure," "$C_6H_{10}N_2O_2$", "1,4,5,6-tetrahydro-2-methyl-4-pyrimidine-carboxylic acid," "cryoprotective cyclic amino acid," and "rhinitis." Although several electronic databases were searched including *PubMed, Medline, Medpilot, Web of Science, CENTRAL, EMBASE,* and *Google Scholar,* no further

studies on this topic were found. Given the lack of appropriate hits, no additional limits regarding language, participants, publishing date, or study phase were set.

Therefore, this meta-analysis is based on unpublished data provided by Bitop AG. The study data have not been published to date since the number of participants in each trial was too small. Nowadays, large randomised controlled trials with more than 250 patients per treatment group are usually required to be considered for publication [21, 22]. In total four studies were assessed which fulfilled the inclusion criteria described below. The paediatric, randomised controlled study had been formally approved by the respective ethical review committee, whereas no ethical approval was necessary for observational trials in Germany. In all studies, patients had to sign the informed consent form to be eligible for participation.

2.2. Patients and Outcome Parameters. The study population comprised both adults and children with a history of allergic rhinitis or rhinoconjunctivitis, who recorded their daily allergy symptoms for at least 7 days in a patient diary. Each symptom had to be scored numerically on a 4-point scale (0 = no symptoms, 1 = mild symptoms, 2 = moderate symptoms, and 3 = severe symptoms). In case of different scaling schemes applied in a study, scores were adapted to this 4-point scale for comparability reasons.

The primary efficacy parameter was the improvement of each individual symptom (nasal congestion, rhinorrhoea, itching of the nose, sneezing, red/watery eyes, and itching of the eyes) after 7 days of treatment. Generally, patient reported that rhinitis-related symptoms occurred in the nose, eyes, and ears/palate, whereas nasal congestion and rhinorrhoea were frequently reported as most predominant.

2.3. Statistical Methods. For continuous data, we calculated individual and pooled statistics as mean differences with 95% confidence intervals. The efficacy parameters for each study included in the analysis were analysed using the ANOVA model [23]. Scores for each individual symptom after 7 days of medication intake were evaluated in comparison to the baseline values at Day 1. All deviating scaling systems for rating the intensity of rhinitis symptoms were adapted to a 4-point scale. If symptoms were originally rated from 0 to 8 (0 being no symptoms and 8 being very severe symptoms) the scores were transformed according to the following scheme: 0, 1 = no symptoms; 2, 3 = mild symptoms; 4, 5 = moderate symptoms; 6, 7, 8 = severe symptoms. Likewise, 12-point scales were translated into 0, 1, 2 = no symptoms; 3, 4, 5 = mild symptoms; 6, 7, 8 = moderate symptoms; 9, 10, 11, 12 = severe symptoms. In case of missing data the last-value-carried forward method was applied. If data of Day one were not available, we used the score of the following day as baseline value. Additionally, the area under the curve (AUC) from Day 1 to Day 7 was assessed for each symptom. The AUC expresses the cumulative effect of the investigational products over the course of seven days by adding up the baseline adjusted symptom scores of each day. A noninferiority margin δ to ensure a clinically relevant effect was not determined, since

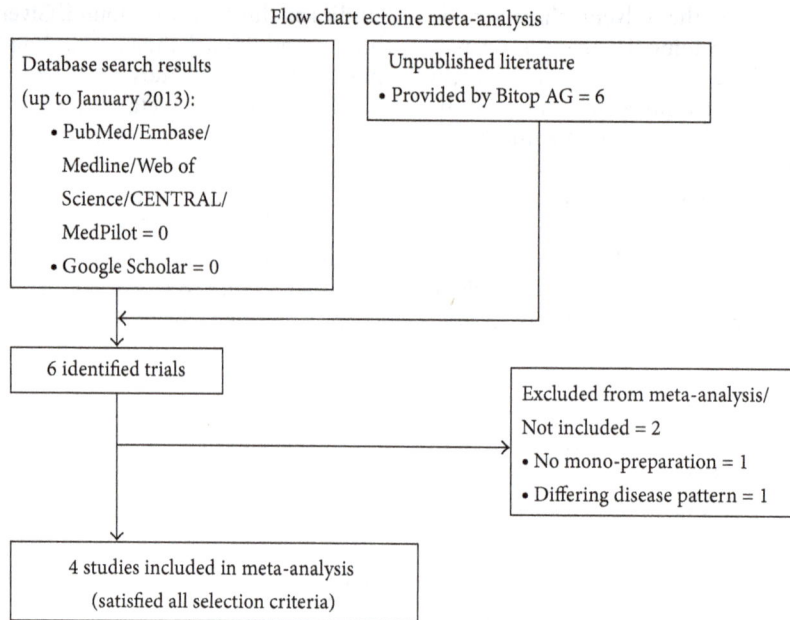

FIGURE 1: Flow chart.

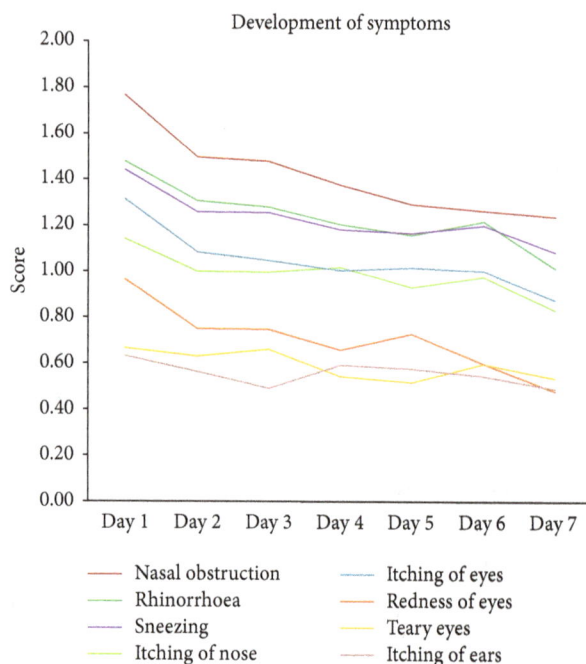

FIGURE 2: Development of symptoms.

was assessed using I^2 statistics and the random-effect model was applied for data synthesis [25].

SPSS version 19 and Review Manager 5 (RevMan 5) were used for statistical analyses and quantitative data synthesis.

3. Results

3.1. Literature Search and Study Population. We identified six studies with unpublished data, provided and conducted by Bitop AG, which matched our inclusion criteria (see Figure 1). One study investigating ectoine in combination with dexpanthenol had to be excluded, since the additional active agent dexpanthenol instead of a mono-preparation would have introduced a severe bias to this meta-analysis. Another study, which investigated patients suffering from Rhinitis Sicca, was rejected because of the differing disease pattern. Thus, the meta-analysis was based on data from four unpublished studies. Of these, three studies included only adults, while one study investigated the efficacy of ectoine in children. Details on the integrated studies are shown in Table 1.

All studies were performed in ENT medical practices in Germany.

In total, 112 patients were included in the analyses comparing the symptom scores on Day 7 and at baseline (Day 1), while the meta-analysis based on the AUC comprised 213 participants. This difference was due to unbalanced numbers of patients in each group of comparison. We performed the meta-analysis in line with a statement proposed by the international MOOSE group [26] about the conduct of meta-analyses of observational studies. Their recommendations concern the entire process of performing a meta-analysis—from describing background, search strategy,

no solid historical data were available. Thus, noninferiority was assumed, when the 95% confidence interval of the overall effect size included the neutral number "0."

Results were displayed graphically as forest plots with associated 95% confidence intervals according to Clopper and Pearson [24]. The area of each square (point estimator for odds ratio) is proportional to the weight of the corresponding study and therefore proportional to the number of patients included as well as to the precision of the effect. Heterogeneity

TABLE 1: Description of included studies.

Study ID	Indication of study	Comparator	Study design	N (Ectoine and control)	Inclusion criteria/exclusion criteria	Duration and dosage	Outcome Parameter	Rating scales
Ectoine versus azelastine, 2010	Allergic rhinitis and conjunctivitis	Azelastine nasal spray and azelastine eye drops	Observational	Ectoine: 21 Control: 21	AR proven by a diagnostic tool or by an allergist Moderate-to-strong nasal symptoms and at least mild eye symptoms at inclusion Signed informed consent Exclusion: allergy to ectoine or azelastine, pregnancy, operation of nose	1 week, ectoine: 4 times daily Azelastine: 2 times daily	Primary: Nasal congestion, rhinorrhoea, sneezing, nasal itching, itching of eyes, itching of palate, teary eyes, conjunctivitis. Secondary: Efficacy, safety.	8-point scale
Ectoine versus cromoglicic acid 2009	Allergic rhinitis	Cromoglicic nasal spray	Observational, cross-over trial	Ectoine: 25 Control: 25	Inclusion: AR proven by skin prick test or by an allergist Moderate-to-strong nasal symptoms at inclusion Signed informed consent Exclusion: allergy to ectoine or cromoglicic acid, pregnancy, operation of nose	1 week, ectoine: 5 times daily Cromoglicic acid: 4 times daily	Primary: Nasal congestion, rhinorrhoea, sneezing. Secondary: Itching of eyes, itching of palate, teary eyes, conjunctivitis, nasal concha hyperplasia, efficacy, safety.	8-point scale
Ectoine versus Livocab, 2011	Seasonal allergic rhinitis	Levocabastine with beclomethasone 0.05% (nasal spray)	Observational	Ectoine: 25 Control: 25	Inclusion: 18–70 years Signed informed consent	2 weeks, intake of medication according to prescribing information	Primary: Total Nasal Symptom Score as sum of nasal congestion, rhinorrhoea, sneezing and nasal itching. Secondary: Itching of palate and ears, efficacy, safety.	4-point scale
Paediatric trial Ectoine versus placebo, 2011	Seasonal allergic rhinitis	Placebo nasal spray and eye drops	RCT	Ectoine: 41 Control: 30	Inclusion: 5–17 years Seasonal AR, general good health status, free of any concomitant conditions that could interfere with conduct of study, sum of TNSS >5, sum of TOSS >3 Signed informed consent (also by parents)	2 weeks Nasal spray: 1 puff per nostril 3 times daily Eye drops: 3 times daily	Primary: Safety Secondary: Efficacy assessment, Total Nasal Symptom Score as sum of runny nose, itchy nose, nasal congestion, sneezing; Total Ocular Symptom Score as sum of itchy eyes, red eyes, watery eyes.	4-point scale

Study or subgroup	Baseline Mean	SD	Total	Day 7 Mean	SD	Total	Weight	Mean difference IV, random, 95% CI	Mean difference IV, random, 95% CI
Ectoine versus Azelastine	1.9	0.94	21	1.48	1.08	21	18.3%	0.42 [−0.19, 1.03]	
Ectoine versus Cromoglycin	1.92	0.91	25	1.2	0.87	25	28.1%	0.72 [0.23, 1.21]	
Ectoine versus Livocab	1.68	0.99	25	1.08	1	25	22.5%	0.60 [0.05, 1.15]	
Pediatric trial	1.56	1.18	41	1.2	0.98	41	31.1%	0.36 [−0.11, 0.83]	
Total (95% CI)			**112**			**112**	**100.0%**	**0.53 [0.26, 0.79]**	

Heterogeneity: $\tau^2 = 0.00$; $\chi^2 = 1.26$, df = 3 ($P = 0.74$); $I^2 = 0\%$
Test for overall effect: $Z = 3.94$ ($P < 0.0001$)

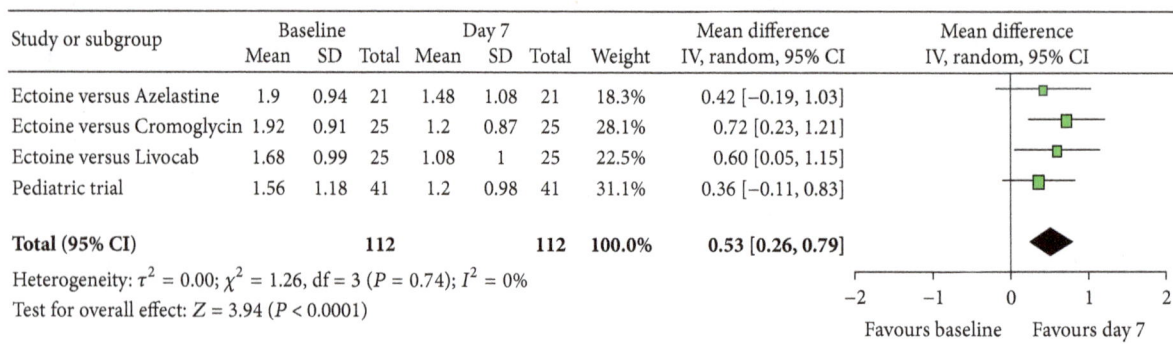

FIGURE 3: Nasal obstruction.

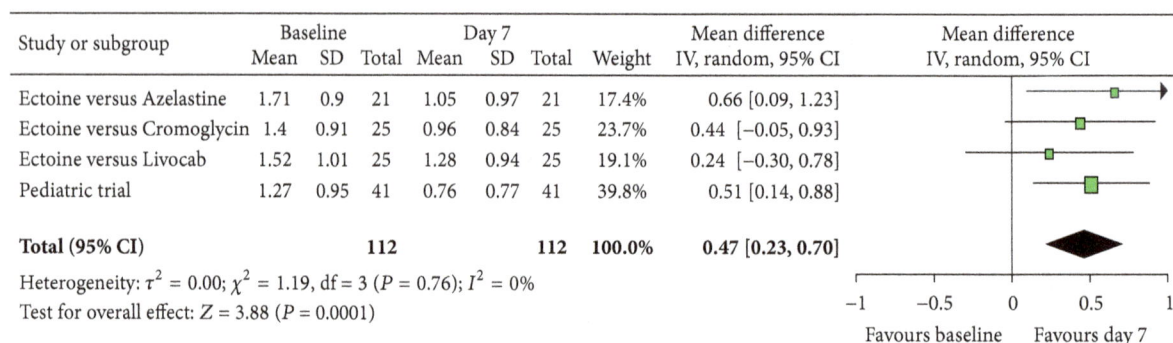

Study or subgroup	Baseline Mean	SD	Total	Day 7 Mean	SD	Total	Weight	Mean difference IV, random, 95% CI	Mean difference IV, random, 95% CI
Ectoine versus Azelastine	1.71	0.9	21	1.05	0.97	21	17.4%	0.66 [0.09, 1.23]	
Ectoine versus Cromoglycin	1.4	0.91	25	0.96	0.84	25	23.7%	0.44 [−0.05, 0.93]	
Ectoine versus Livocab	1.52	1.01	25	1.28	0.94	25	19.1%	0.24 [−0.30, 0.78]	
Pediatric trial	1.27	0.95	41	0.76	0.77	41	39.8%	0.51 [0.14, 0.88]	
Total (95% CI)			**112**			**112**	**100.0%**	**0.47 [0.23, 0.70]**	

Heterogeneity: $\tau^2 = 0.00$; $\chi^2 = 1.19$, df = 3 ($P = 0.76$); $I^2 = 0\%$
Test for overall effect: $Z = 3.88$ ($P = 0.0001$)

FIGURE 4: Rhinorrhoea.

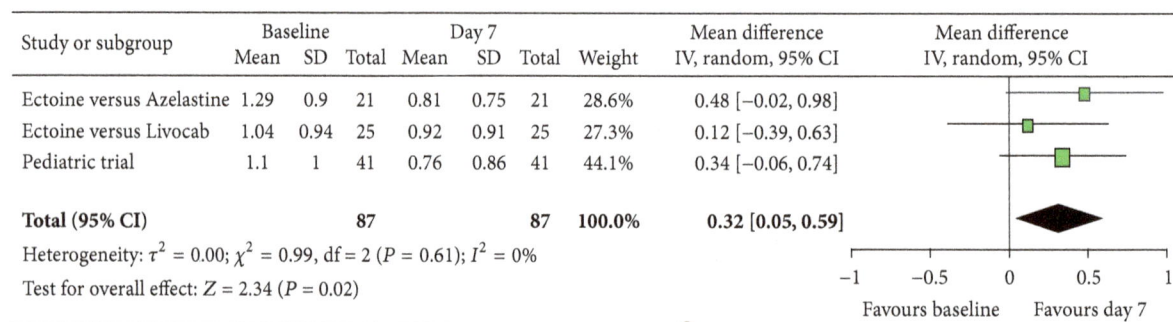

Study or subgroup	Baseline Mean	SD	Total	Day 7 Mean	SD	Total	Weight	Mean difference IV, random, 95% CI	Mean difference IV, random, 95% CI
Ectoine versus Azelastine	1.29	0.9	21	0.81	0.75	21	28.6%	0.48 [−0.02, 0.98]	
Ectoine versus Livocab	1.04	0.94	25	0.92	0.91	25	27.3%	0.12 [−0.39, 0.63]	
Pediatric trial	1.1	1	41	0.76	0.86	41	44.1%	0.34 [−0.06, 0.74]	
Total (95% CI)			**87**			**87**	**100.0%**	**0.32 [0.05, 0.59]**	

Heterogeneity: $\tau^2 = 0.00$; $\chi^2 = 0.99$, df = 2 ($P = 0.61$); $I^2 = 0\%$
Test for overall effect: $Z = 2.34$ ($P = 0.02$)

FIGURE 5: Nasal itching.

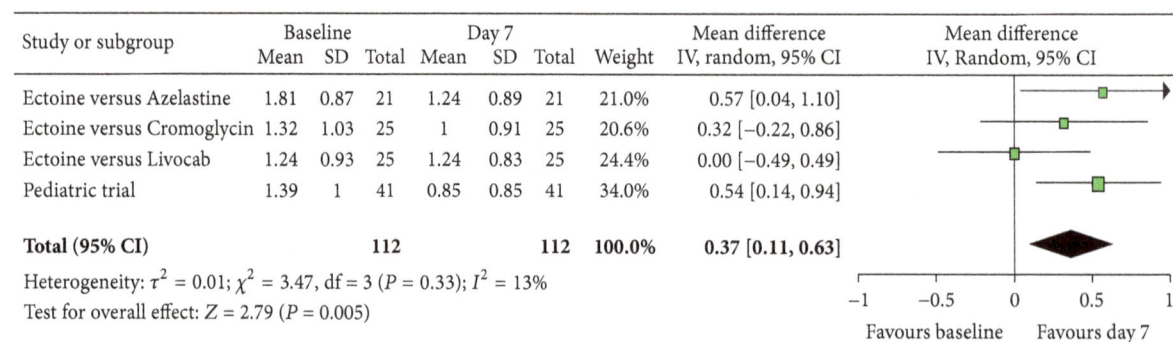

Study or subgroup	Baseline Mean	SD	Total	Day 7 Mean	SD	Total	Weight	Mean difference IV, random, 95% CI	Mean difference IV, Random, 95% CI
Ectoine versus Azelastine	1.81	0.87	21	1.24	0.89	21	21.0%	0.57 [0.04, 1.10]	
Ectoine versus Cromoglycin	1.32	1.03	25	1	0.91	25	20.6%	0.32 [−0.22, 0.86]	
Ectoine versus Livocab	1.24	0.93	25	1.24	0.83	25	24.4%	0.00 [−0.49, 0.49]	
Pediatric trial	1.39	1	41	0.85	0.85	41	34.0%	0.54 [0.14, 0.94]	
Total (95% CI)			**112**			**112**	**100.0%**	**0.37 [0.11, 0.63]**	

Heterogeneity: $\tau^2 = 0.01$; $\chi^2 = 3.47$, df = 3 ($P = 0.33$); $I^2 = 13\%$
Test for overall effect: $Z = 2.79$ ($P = 0.005$)

FIGURE 6: Sneezing.

| Study or subgroup | Baseline | | | Day 7 | | | Weight | Mean difference | Mean difference |
	Mean	SD	Total	Mean	SD	Total		IV, random, 95% CI	IV, random, 95% CI
Ectoine versus Azelastine	1.43	1.03	21	1.19	1	21	27.6%	0.24 [−0.37, 0.85]	
Pediatric trial	1.39	0.97	41	0.83	0.77	41	72.4%	0.56 [0.18, 0.94]	
Total (95% CI)			62			62	100.0%	0.47 [0.15, 0.79]	

Heterogeneity: $\tau^2 = 0.00$; $\chi^2 = 0.76$, df = 1 ($P = 0.38$); $I^2 = 0\%$
Test for overall effect: $Z = 2.87$ ($P = 0.004$)

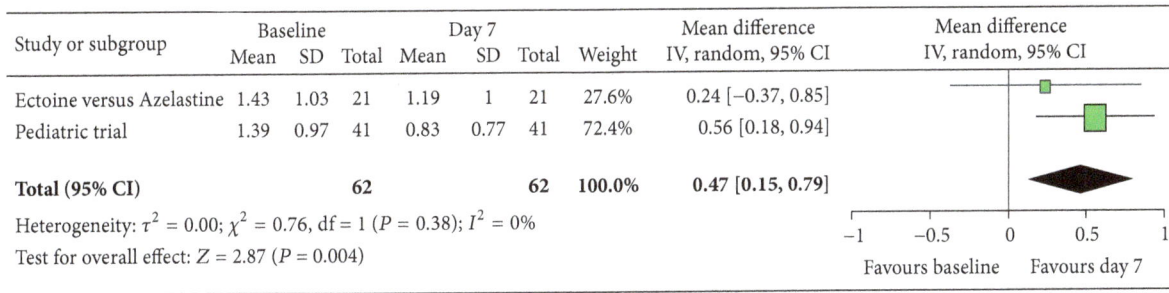

FIGURE 7: Itching of eyes.

and methodology applied to presentation of results and discussion.

All data presented are based on the ITT analysis set of each study.

3.2. Bias. As with any systematic review or meta-analysis, biases may be present and limit the validity of the work. The main concern of this meta-analysis may be the quality of the included studies. In contrast to large systematic reviews, this work was mainly based on observational studies with no blinding of the patients or investigators. Since only one randomised, placebo controlled trial on children has been performed and published on this specific topic, the methodological concepts of the included trials do reach the evidence level IIb but not Ib. We addressed this "garbage in/garbage out" problem [27, 28] in performing a subgroup analysis on observational studies with adults. Apart from that no major conceptional differences between the studies were apparent, which minimises the risk concerning problems with uniformity ("apple-oranges problem") [29]. Endpoints, nasal symptoms, measurements, and the study population were comparable. However, scaling systems in rating the symptom severity differed slightly and had to be transformed into a homogeneous scaling scheme. It is questionable whether this adaption leads to a loss of information or a shift of results. However, the tendency of whether symptoms were released or not is not biased by this approach. Furthermore, the variation of control groups may limit the validity of the meta-analysis. Ectoine was compared to four different control medications, since the major interest was about the efficacy of the active agent ectoine in comparison to general drugs prescribed. As already mentioned before, this meta-analysis was based on only small, unpublished clinical trials. Thus, one can speak of a very untypical publication bias with solely data from yet unpublished studies. Given the small number of included studies, we refrained from performing a funnel plot.

3.3. Development of Symptoms. Figure 2 illustrates the cumulative efficacy of ectoine-based products on both nasal and eye symptoms based on results from the included studies. The descending curve progression affirmed the positive effect of ectoine on rhinitis-related symptoms. At baseline, nasal obstruction presents the most predominant symptom of the allergic disease. After seven days of treatment, each symptom had improved to a mild level of discomfort (see Figure 2).

The strongest decrease in nasal symptom severity was shown for rhinorrhoea and nasal obstruction, both being reduced by approximately 30%. For nasal obstruction, a symptom score of 1.77 at Day 1 decreased to a mean score of 1.24 and the symptom severity of rhinorrhoea eased from 1.48 to 1.01 after seven days of treatment with ectoine nasal spray.

According to the patients' diary entries, however, none of the symptoms was assessed as moderate or severe at baseline, but mild to moderate at the most. The rather mild assessment of symptoms at baseline limited the prospects of significant improvement. However, the apparent decrease in symptom severity suggests the efficacy of ectoine-based treatment.

3.4. Meta-Analyses as Comparison of Baseline (Day 1) to Day 7. The meta-analyses of individual symptoms that were conducted to determine the strength of effect after seven days of medication intake compared to baseline indicated the efficacy of ectoine. All nasal symptoms had significantly improved by Day 7 compared to Day 1.

According to Ferguson the effect size of improvement can be classified in three categories: 0–0.2 reflecting a small effect, 0.2–0.5 indicating a moderate effect, and 0.5–0.8 representing a strong effect [30]. Therefore, the improvement of the main nasal symptom "nasal obstruction" (Figure 3) with a size effect of 0.53 (±0.26) was evaluated as strong. Further nasal symptoms still showed significant moderate effects. The effect size for "rhinorrhoea" (Figure 4) was nearly as high with 0.47 (±0.24), "nasal itching (Figure 5) was calculated as 0.32 (±0.27), and for "sneezing" (Figure 6) the effect size was 0.37 (±0.26). P values of the overall effect (shown underneath each figure) demonstrate significance for all nasal symptoms: both "nasal obstruction" and "rhinorrhoea" were associated with $P < 0.0001$; the symptom "nasal itching" corresponds to $P = 0.02$; the P value for "sneezing" was calculated as $P = 0.005$.

Furthermore, we pooled data from two studies that additionally used ectoine-based eye drops to investigate the effect of ectoine on eye symptoms. After seven days of treatment, "itching of eyes" (Figure 7) and "redness of eyes" (Figure 8) showed significant improvements compared to baseline. Both parameters improved by a moderate-to-strong effect size with 0.47 (±0.32) and 0.54 (±0.30), respectively. Only the reduction of symptom severity in "teary eyes" (Figure 9) was not statistically significant.

Study or subgroup	Baseline			Day 7			Weight	Mean difference IV, random, 95% CI	Mean difference IV, random, 95% CI
	Mean	SD	Total	Mean	SD	Total			
Ectoine versus Azelastine	0.95	0.92	21	0.48	0.68	21	37.6%	0.47 [−0.02, 0.96]	
Pediatric trial	1.15	0.94	41	0.56	0.81	41	62.4%	0.59 [0.21, 0.97]	
Total (95% CI)			62			62	100.0%	**0.54 [0.24, 0.84]**	

Heterogeneity: $\tau^2 = 0.00$; $\chi^2 = 0.14$, df = 1 ($P = 0.70$); $I^2 = 0\%$
Test for overall effect: $Z = 3.56$ ($P = 0.0004$)

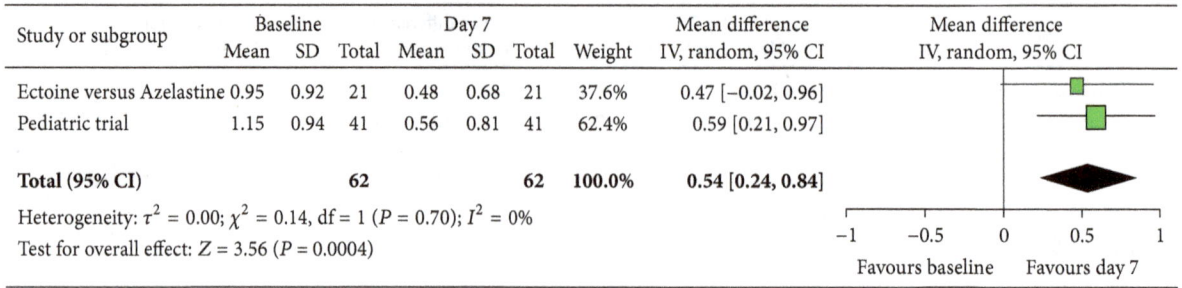

FIGURE 8: Redness of eyes.

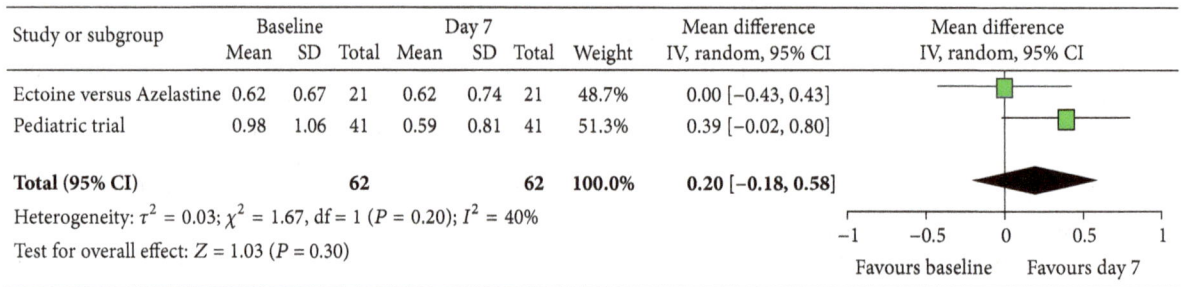

Study or subgroup	Baseline			Day 7			Weight	Mean difference IV, random, 95% CI	Mean difference IV, random, 95% CI
	Mean	SD	Total	Mean	SD	Total			
Ectoine versus Azelastine	0.62	0.67	21	0.62	0.74	21	48.7%	0.00 [−0.43, 0.43]	
Pediatric trial	0.98	1.06	41	0.59	0.81	41	51.3%	0.39 [−0.02, 0.80]	
Total (95% CI)			62			62	100.0%	**0.20 [−0.18, 0.58]**	

Heterogeneity: $\tau^2 = 0.03$; $\chi^2 = 1.67$, df = 1 ($P = 0.20$); $I^2 = 40\%$
Test for overall effect: $Z = 1.03$ ($P = 0.30$)

FIGURE 9: Teary eyes.

Throughout the analyses, the level of heterogeneity was low. As suggested by Higgins et al. [31], values for $I^2 < 25\%$ may express a low level of heterogeneity, although its categorisation and quantification are not that simple in general. Since I^2 was calculated to be in a range of 0% to 13% for most symptoms (apart from the symptom "teary eyes"), the heterogeneity across studies appears to be small.

3.5. Meta-Analyses of the Area under the Curve (AUC) Comparing Ectoine with Control Medication. The meta-analyses of AUC, comprising Day 1 to Day 7, evaluated the efficacy of ectoine treatment in comparison to placebo or to a standard medication (control) for allergic rhinitis. One study used azelastine nasal spray as comparator, in the second study a nasal spray based on cromoglicic acid served as control medication, the third study investigated ectoine nasal spray versus levocabastine (Livocab) with beclomethasone nasal spray, and the paediatric study was set up as a placebo-controlled trial. Although it is principally not recommended to pool data from studies with different control groups, the approach seemed appropriate since we were able to extract original data for each symptom individually. For all symptoms ectoine-containing nasal spray demonstrated similar or better efficacy when compared to controls. Effects were greatest for the symptoms "nasal itching" (−1.97 ± 1.54) (Figure 12) and "sneezing" (−1.69 ± 1.31) (Figure 13) which were associated with significant differences in favour of ectoine. For the remaining nasal symptoms "nasal obstruction" (Figure 10) and "rhinorrhoea" (Figure 11), the meta-analysis revealed that ectoine is similarly effective compared to the control drugs.

Since only two studies investigated the effect of the medication on eye symptoms, we pooled data from these two studies (ectoine versus azelastine and paediatric trial) to evaluate the effect of ectoine on the eyes. The analysis reveals that the symptom "teary eyes" (Figure 16) was significantly improved ($P = 0.02$) by the ectoine-containing nasal spray and eye drops with an effect size of −1.99 (±1.69). The symptoms "itching of eyes" (Figure 14) and "redness of eyes" (Figure 15) both tended slightly towards the ectoine products with effect sizes of −0.54 (±2.75) and −0.40 (±2.24), respectively. However, no statistical significance was reached here.

4. Subgroup Analyses

Subgroup analyses were performed for the two main allergic rhinitis symptoms of nasal obstruction and rhinorrhoea in order to evaluate the effect of ectoine in the specific group of adults with allergic rhinitis. Three studies with a total of 71 patients were included, whereby the level of heterogeneity decreased to 0%. Again, the three control groups of the integrated studies (azelastine, levocabastine/beclomethasone, and cromoglicic acid) were pooled into one control group versus ectoine nasal spray.

The subgroup analyses clearly emphasised the positive effect of ectoine nasal spray after seven days of treatment. Since each individual study consistently expressed the efficacy of ectoine, the overall pooled result for both nasal obstruction and rhinorrhoea was significant in favour of a seven-day medication intake. The corresponding P values were $P = 0.0002$ for the effect on nasal obstruction and $P = 0.005$ for rhinorrhoea. With a total effect of 0.6 (±0.31) for nasal obstruction (Figure 17), the efficacy of the ectoine-based nasal spray after seven days was associated with a strong

Study or subgroup	Ectoine Mean	SD	Total	Control Mean	SD	Total	Weight	Mean difference IV, random, 95% CI
Ectoine versus Azelastine	1.38	4.38	21	2.1	3.13	21	27.0%	−0.72 [−3.02, 1.58]
Ectoine versus Cromoglycin	3.52	3.82	25	0.8	4.52	25	26.9%	2.72 [0.40, 5.04]
Ectoine versus Livocab	2.32	4.16	25	2.12	5.26	25	24.7%	0.20 [−2.43, 2.83]
Pediatric trial	−2.63	7.415	41	0.1	6.07	30	21.4%	−2.73 [−5.87, 0.41]
Total (95% CI)			**112**			**101**	**100.0%**	**0.00 [−2.16, 2.17]**

Heterogeneity: $\tau^2 = 3.12$; $\chi^2 = 8.49$, df = 3 ($P = 0.04$); $I^2 = 65\%$

Test for overall effect: $Z = 0.00$ ($P = 1.00$)

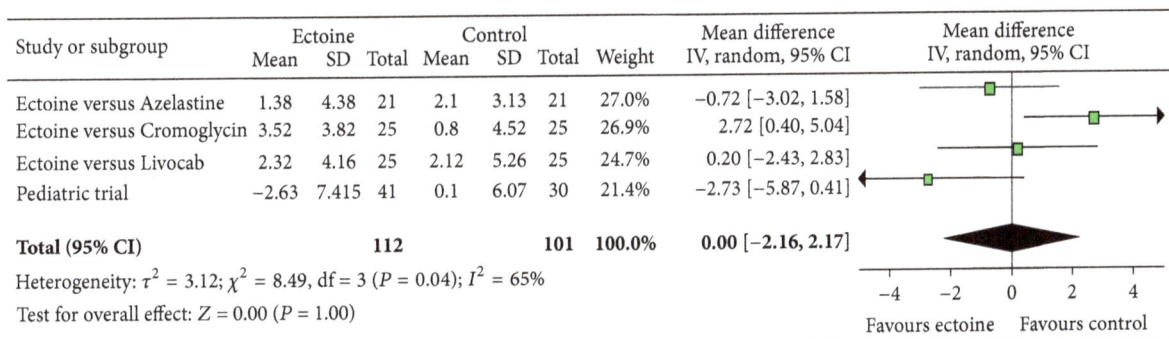

FIGURE 10: AUC nasal obstruction.

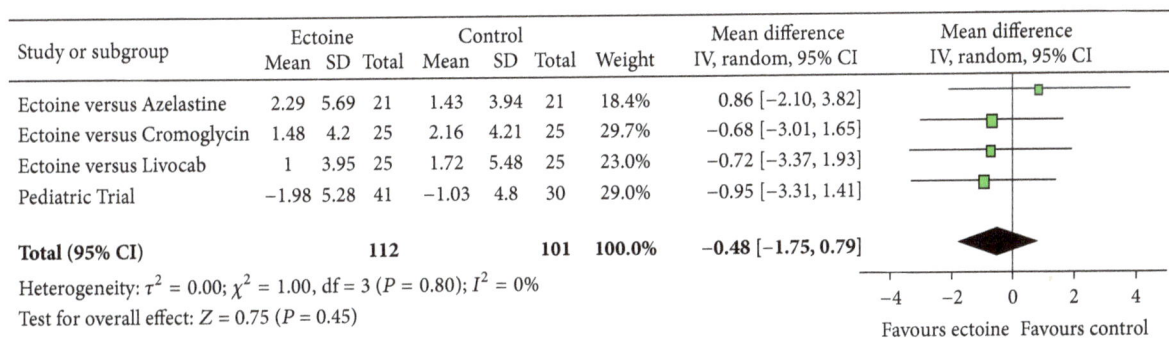

Study or subgroup	Ectoine Mean	SD	Total	Control Mean	SD	Total	Weight	Mean difference IV, random, 95% CI
Ectoine versus Azelastine	2.29	5.69	21	1.43	3.94	21	18.4%	0.86 [−2.10, 3.82]
Ectoine versus Cromoglycin	1.48	4.2	25	2.16	4.21	25	29.7%	−0.68 [−3.01, 1.65]
Ectoine versus Livocab	1	3.95	25	1.72	5.48	25	23.0%	−0.72 [−3.37, 1.93]
Pediatric Trial	−1.98	5.28	41	−1.03	4.8	30	29.0%	−0.95 [−3.31, 1.41]
Total (95% CI)			**112**			**101**	**100.0%**	**−0.48 [−1.75, 0.79]**

Heterogeneity: $\tau^2 = 0.00$; $\chi^2 = 1.00$, df = 3 ($P = 0.80$); $I^2 = 0\%$

Test for overall effect: $Z = 0.75$ ($P = 0.45$)

FIGURE 11: AUC rhinorrhoea.

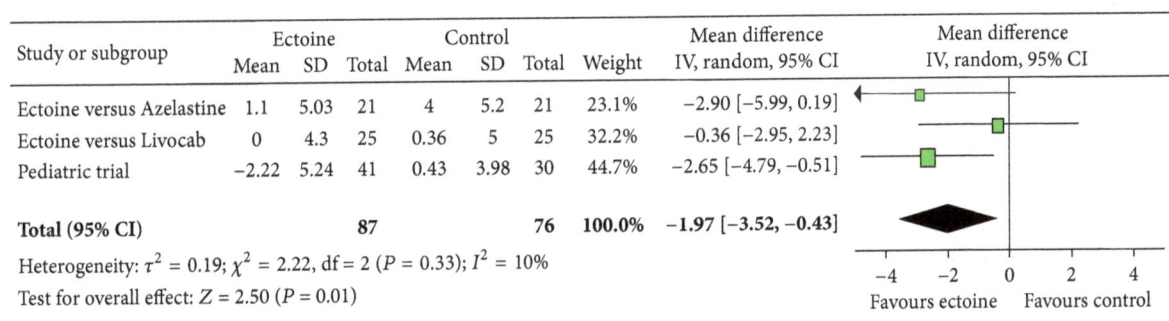

Study or subgroup	Ectoine Mean	SD	Total	Control Mean	SD	Total	Weight	Mean difference IV, random, 95% CI
Ectoine versus Azelastine	1.1	5.03	21	4	5.2	21	23.1%	−2.90 [−5.99, 0.19]
Ectoine versus Livocab	0	4.3	25	0.36	5	25	32.2%	−0.36 [−2.95, 2.23]
Pediatric trial	−2.22	5.24	41	0.43	3.98	30	44.7%	−2.65 [−4.79, −0.51]
Total (95% CI)			**87**			**76**	**100.0%**	**−1.97 [−3.52, −0.43]**

Heterogeneity: $\tau^2 = 0.19$; $\chi^2 = 2.22$, df = 2 ($P = 0.33$); $I^2 = 10\%$

Test for overall effect: $Z = 2.50$ ($P = 0.01$)

FIGURE 12: AUC nasal itching.

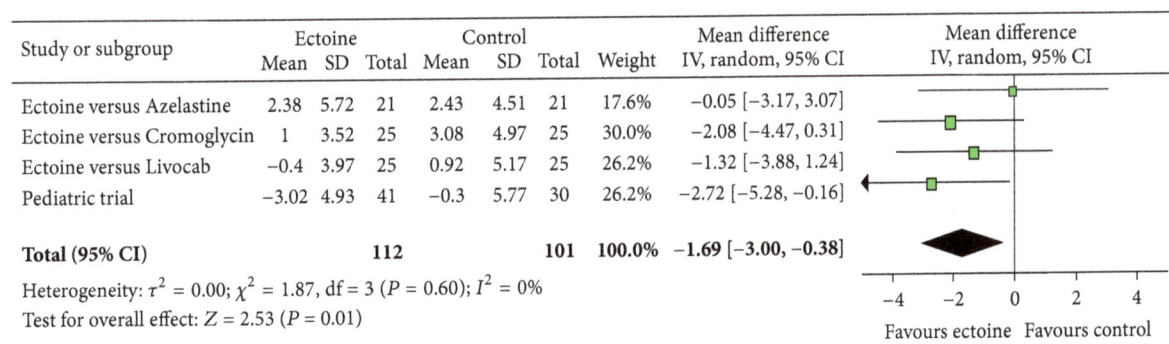

Study or subgroup	Ectoine Mean	SD	Total	Control Mean	SD	Total	Weight	Mean difference IV, random, 95% CI
Ectoine versus Azelastine	2.38	5.72	21	2.43	4.51	21	17.6%	−0.05 [−3.17, 3.07]
Ectoine versus Cromoglycin	1	3.52	25	3.08	4.97	25	30.0%	−2.08 [−4.47, 0.31]
Ectoine versus Livocab	−0.4	3.97	25	0.92	5.17	25	26.2%	−1.32 [−3.88, 1.24]
Pediatric trial	−3.02	4.93	41	−0.3	5.77	30	26.2%	−2.72 [−5.28, −0.16]
Total (95% CI)			**112**			**101**	**100.0%**	**−1.69 [−3.00, −0.38]**

Heterogeneity: $\tau^2 = 0.00$; $\chi^2 = 1.87$, df = 3 ($P = 0.60$); $I^2 = 0\%$

Test for overall effect: $Z = 2.53$ ($P = 0.01$)

FIGURE 13: AUC sneezing.

Study or subgroup	Ectoine Mean	SD	Total	Control Mean	SD	Total	Weight	Mean difference IV, random, 95% CI	Mean difference IV, random, 95% CI
Ectoine versus Azelastine	1.52	5.46	21	0.48	5.46	21	44.0%	1.04 [−2.26, 4.34]	
Pediatric trial	−2.68	5.22	41	−0.9	6.07	30	56.0%	−1.78 [−4.48, 0.92]	
Total (95% CI)			**62**			**51**	**100.0%**	**−0.54 [−3.28, 2.21]**	

Heterogeneity: $\tau^2 = 1.61$; $\chi^2 = 1.68$, df = 1 ($P = 0.19$); $I^2 = 40\%$
Test for overall effect: $Z = 0.38$ ($P = 0.70$)

Favours ectoine   Favours control

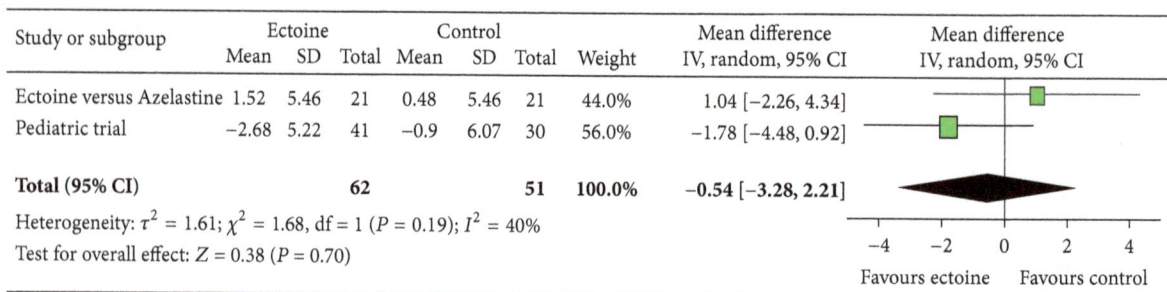

FIGURE 14: AUC itching of eyes.

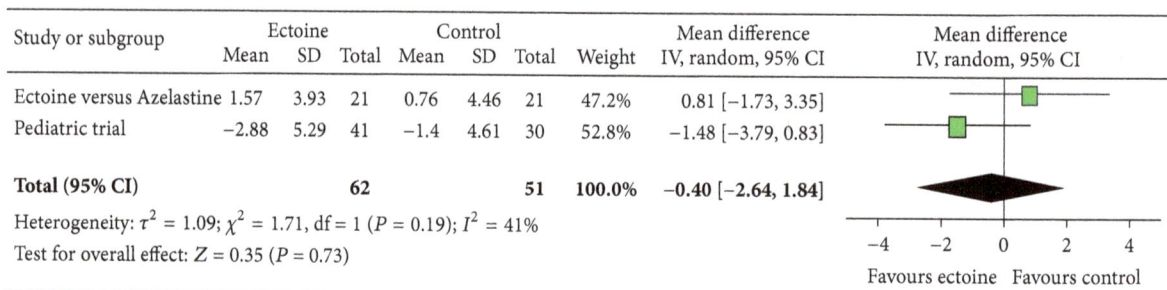

Study or subgroup	Ectoine Mean	SD	Total	Control Mean	SD	Total	Weight	Mean difference IV, random, 95% CI	Mean difference IV, random, 95% CI
Ectoine versus Azelastine	1.57	3.93	21	0.76	4.46	21	47.2%	0.81 [−1.73, 3.35]	
Pediatric trial	−2.88	5.29	41	−1.4	4.61	30	52.8%	−1.48 [−3.79, 0.83]	
Total (95% CI)			**62**			**51**	**100.0%**	**−0.40 [−2.64, 1.84]**	

Heterogeneity: $\tau^2 = 1.09$; $\chi^2 = 1.71$, df = 1 ($P = 0.19$); $I^2 = 41\%$
Test for overall effect: $Z = 0.35$ ($P = 0.73$)

Favours ectoine   Favours control

FIGURE 15: AUC redness of eyes.

effect size. Similarly, the total effect size of 0.44 (±0.31) for rhinorrhoea (Figure 18) signified a moderate effect of ectoine nasal spray. Therefore, the subgroup analyses confirmed the positive effect of ectoine nasal spray in alleviating the predominant symptoms of nasal obstruction and rhinorrhoea in adult patients with allergic rhinitis.

5. Discussion

This meta-analysis served to compare the treatment of allergic rhinitis with ectoine-containing nasal spray and eye drops to traditional treatment agents (antihistamine, glucocorticoid, and cromoglicic acid) or placebo treatment.

The meta-analysis involving ectoine nasal spray in the categories of baseline comparison and AUC determined a reduction in symptom severity for all relevant rhinitis symptoms. An especially strong effect was shown for the symptom of nasal congestion, which dropped significantly by 29.94% after seven days of treatment. According to the classification scheme developed by Ferguson [30], the improvement of nasal obstruction was categorised as strong, while further nasal symptoms such as rhinorrhoea, nasal itching, and sneezing were still associated with a significant improvement of moderate effect size. Likewise, significant improvements with a strong and moderate effect size were also demonstrated for nasal obstruction and rhinorrhoea in the subgroup analysis of adult SAR patients.

While ectoine-based products were shown to act significantly more effective than the control medications in easing the symptom severity of nasal itching, sneezing, and teary eyes, results for the remaining symptoms still confirmed

a similar potency of ectoine nasal spray compared to standard medication.

Two studies during which ectoine-containing eye drops were used additionally to the application of ectoine nasal spray demonstrated improvement of ocular symptoms. Here, a strong size effect was shown in reducing red eyes and moderate size effect in reduction of itching eyes. Likewise, the analysis of accumulated effects revealed a significant improvement for the symptom "teary eyes" in the ectoine group. These results indicate a positive influence of ectoine eye drops on ocular symptoms in seasonal allergic rhinitis. However, further studies are needed to confirm these findings as the possibility that the effect may be explained by the inhibition of the naso-ocular reflex, as it has been suggested in studies with intranasal steroids [32], cannot be excluded based on the current results.

In this meta-analysis, we compared the efficacy of ectoine to three effective, currently guideline-recommended medications, such as the second-generation antihistamine azelastine, the glucocorticoid combination levocabastine/beclomethasone, and the classical cromoglicic acid. The comparison attested the equivalence of ectoine nasal spray to these products. Thus, the ectoine-based products can be regarded as noninferior to topical antihis-tamines, the intranasal glucocorticosteroid combination levocabastine/beclomethasone, or nasal mast cell stabilisers for the treatment of rhinitis symptoms.

The results of this meta-analysis are promising and further supported by the safety profile of products containing ectoine [20, 33]. Clinical studies have shown that treatment with ectoine results in very few adverse events (frequency comparable to placebo) and virtually no safety

Study or subgroup	Ectoine Mean	SD	Total	Control Mean	SD	Total	Weight	Mean difference IV, random, 95% CI	Mean difference IV, random, 95% CI
Ectoine versus Azelastine	−0.52	3.89	21	0.43	4.98	21	39.1%	−0.95 [−3.65, 1.75]	
Pediatric trial	−2.59	5.97	41	0.07	3.24	30	60.9%	−2.66 [−4.82, −0.50]	
Total (95% CI)			62			51	100.0%	**−1.99 [−3.68, −0.30]**	

Heterogeneity: $\tau^2 = 0.00$; $\chi^2 = 0.94$, df = 1 ($P = 0.33$); $I^2 = 0\%$
Test for overall effect: $Z = 2.31$ ($P = 0.02$)

−4 −2 0 2 4
Favours ectoine   Favours control

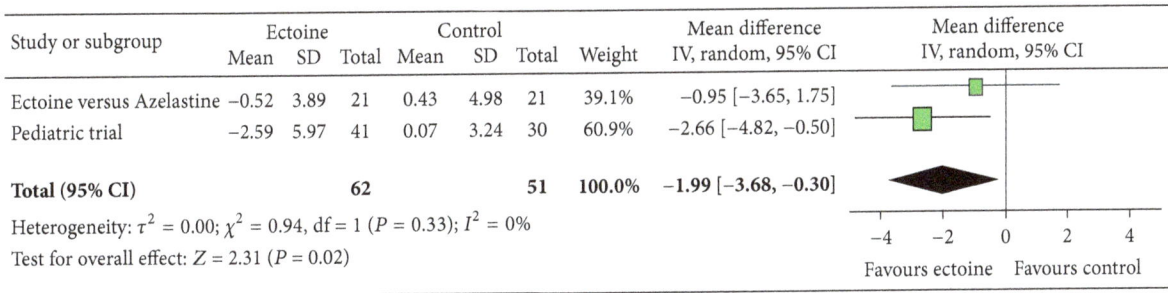

FIGURE 16: AUC teary eyes.

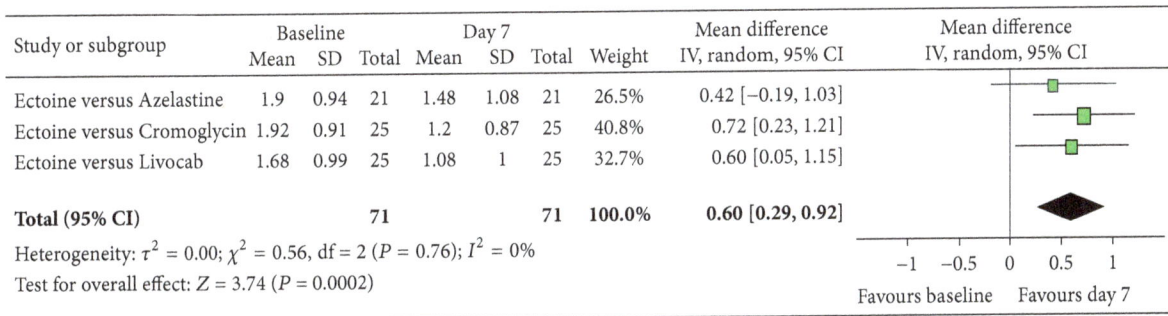

Study or subgroup	Baseline Mean	SD	Total	Day 7 Mean	SD	Total	Weight	Mean difference IV, random, 95% CI	Mean difference IV, random, 95% CI
Ectoine versus Azelastine	1.9	0.94	21	1.48	1.08	21	26.5%	0.42 [−0.19, 1.03]	
Ectoine versus Cromoglycin	1.92	0.91	25	1.2	0.87	25	40.8%	0.72 [0.23, 1.21]	
Ectoine versus Livocab	1.68	0.99	25	1.08	1	25	32.7%	0.60 [0.05, 1.15]	
Total (95% CI)			71			71	100.0%	**0.60 [0.29, 0.92]**	

Heterogeneity: $\tau^2 = 0.00$; $\chi^2 = 0.56$, df = 2 ($P = 0.76$); $I^2 = 0\%$
Test for overall effect: $Z = 3.74$ ($P = 0.0002$)

−1 −0.5 0 0.5 1
Favours baseline   Favours day 7

FIGURE 17: Subgroup nasal obstruction.

concerns [20, 33, 34]. In contrast, the traditional drugs are still associated with side effects, warranting the search for alternative treatments. Thus, particularly antihistamines, such as azelastine, even in nasal spray form, continue to cause sedation/somnolence and nasal burning occasionally (Astelin patient information). Moreover, nasal steroids can also have various adverse effects. For example, the patient information for glucocorticoid nasal spray, for example, fluticasone furoate (Veramyst), warns about possible ocular side effects including glaucoma, cataracts, and increased intraocular pressure. While—in isolated cases—growth retardation has been associated with beclomethasone treatment [35], nasal spray, and eye drops containing ectoine offer adequate relief from allergy symptoms without these added risks. However, those infrequent side effects should not be overestimated, and newer drug formulations show fewer adverse reactions than the earlier agents. Still, the absence of safety concerns makes ectoine-based products particularly interesting candidates for the treatment of allergic rhinitis in children. Since the application of corticosteroids in children has raised some concerns regarding impaired growth and abnormal development, ectoine may provide a safe and convenient alternative for physicians and parents worried about treating their allergic children with pharmaceutical products that have potential harmful side effects. However, the safety of ectoine nasal spray needs to be further investigated in future studies to confirm the safety profile of the product.

The mode of action of ectoine-based products in preventing and relieving allergic symptoms is based on the physical interaction of ectoine with water and the resulting effects on the membrane of the tissue treated. Stabilisation of cell membranes with consequent enhancement of the tissues' barrier function may reduce the allergen-membrane interactions and inflammation which usually cause ocular, nasal, and nonnasal symptoms in patients with allergic rhinitis.

There is one constraint to this meta-analysis: upon inclusion, patients had mostly mild symptoms. Hence, no large improvements could be expected from a one- to two-week course of treatment. Considering these baseline values, the verified improvement can indeed be interpreted as convincing. Future studies including patients with more severe baseline symptoms would be needed to further investigate the effectiveness of ectoine treatment in rhinitis patients. A further limitation concerns the methodology, since only data from unpublished studies are included in this meta-analysis. The included study data have not been published to date, since the number of participants in each trial was too small to show interesting results. Nowadays, large randomised controlled trials with more than 250 patients per treatment group are commonly required to be considered for publication [21, 22]. Likewise, published noninterventional studies are usually performed with numbers larger than 1000 patients to be powered adequately [36, 37]. To date, no publications investigating ectoine as a nasal spray ingredient exist.

6. Conclusion

Taken together, this meta-analysis demonstrated that the application of ectoine-based nasal spray and eye drops improves symptoms of allergic rhinitis and rhinoconjunctivitis. This easy-to-apply, well-tolerated, naturally-based nasal and ocular treatment, which has no unpleasant taste and

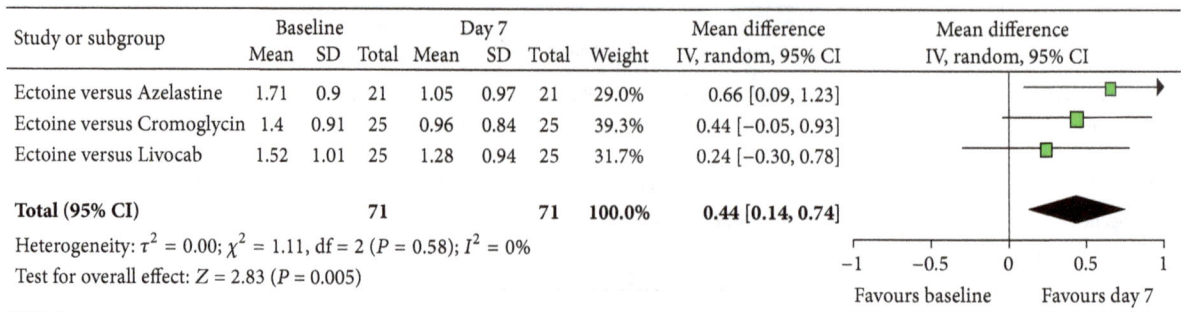

Study or subgroup	Baseline			Day 7			Weight	Mean difference IV, random, 95% CI	Mean difference IV, random, 95% CI
	Mean	SD	Total	Mean	SD	Total			
Ectoine versus Azelastine	1.71	0.9	21	1.05	0.97	21	29.0%	0.66 [0.09, 1.23]	
Ectoine versus Cromoglycin	1.4	0.91	25	0.96	0.84	25	39.3%	0.44 [−0.05, 0.93]	
Ectoine versus Livocab	1.52	1.01	25	1.28	0.94	25	31.7%	0.24 [−0.30, 0.78]	
Total (95% CI)			71			71	100.0%	**0.44 [0.14, 0.74]**	

Heterogeneity: $\tau^2 = 0.00$; $\chi^2 = 1.11$, df = 2 ($P = 0.58$); $I^2 = 0\%$
Test for overall effect: $Z = 2.83$ ($P = 0.005$)

Favours baseline   Favours day 7

FIGURE 18: Subgroup rhinorrhoea.

virtually no side effects, effectively reduces allergic rhinitis symptoms and represents an exciting alternative for rhinoconjunctivitis sufferers.

Conflict of Interests

The authors declare that there is no conflict of interests regarding the publication of this paper.

Acknowledgments

The authors thank Bitop AG, Witten, Germany, for providing the original patient data and for financial support in publishing this paper. Dr. rer. nat. Kijawasch Shah-Hosseini offered valuable advice for the statistical analysis of the original data. Editorial assistance in preparing the paper for publication was provided by Gena Kittel, IMSIE, Faculty of Medicine, University of Cologne, Germany. This work has been supported by an unrestricted research grant from bitop AG.

References

[1] J. Bousquet, N. Khaltaev, A. A. Cruz et al., "Allergic Rhinitis and its Impact on Asthma (ARIA) 2008 update (in collaboration with the World Health Organization, GA2LEN and AllerGen)," *Allergy*, vol. 63, no. 86, pp. 8–160, 2008.

[2] C. Böcking, H. Renz, and P. I. Pfefferle, "Prävalenz und sozioökonomische Bedeutung von Allergien in Deutschland," *Bundesgesundheitsblatt—Gesundheitsforschung—Gesundheitsschutz*, vol. 55, no. 3, pp. 303–307, 2012.

[3] D. P. Skoner, "Allergic rhinitis: definition, epidemiology, pathophysiology, detection, and diagnosis," *Journal of Allergy and Clinical Immunology*, vol. 108, no. 1, supplement, pp. S2–S8, 2001.

[4] C. Kirmaz, O. Aydemir, P. Bayrak, H. Yuksel, O. Ozenturk, and S. Degirmenci, "Sexual dysfunction in patients with allergic rhinoconjunctivitis," *Annals of Allergy, Asthma and Immunology*, vol. 95, no. 6, pp. 525–529, 2005.

[5] P. S. Marshall, C. O'Hara, and P. Steinberg, "Effects of seasonal allergic rhinitis on fatigue levels and mood," *Psychosomatic Medicine*, vol. 64, no. 4, pp. 684–691, 2002.

[6] B. Kremer, H. M. Den Hartog, and J. Jolles, "Relationship between allergic rhinitis, disturbed cognitive functions and psychological well-being," *Clinical and Experimental Allergy*, vol. 32, no. 9, pp. 1310–1315, 2002.

[7] B. Cuffel, M. Wamboldt, L. Borish, S. Kennedy, and J. Crystal-Peters, "Economic consequences of comorbid depression, anxiety, and allergic rhinitis," *Psychosomatics*, vol. 40, no. 6, pp. 491–496, 1999.

[8] X. Lv, L. Xi, D. Han, and L. Zhang, "Evaluation of the psychological status in seasonal allergic rhinitis patients," *ORL*, vol. 72, no. 2, pp. 84–90, 2010.

[9] E. Angier, J. Willington, G. Scadding, S. Holmes, and S. Walker, "Management of allergic and non-allergic rhinitis: a primary care summary of the BSACI guideline," *Primary Care Respiratory Journal*, vol. 19, no. 3, pp. 217–222, 2010.

[10] DEGAM, *Rhinosinusitis DEGAM—Leitlinie Nr.10*, vol. 053/012, Omikron, Düsseldorf, Germany, 2008.

[11] A. Calderon Moises, P. Rodriguez del Rio, and P. Demoly, "Topical nasal corticosteroids versus oral antihistamines for allergic rhinitis," *Cochrane Database of Systematic Reviews*, Article ID CD008232, 2010.

[12] J. Smiatek, R. K. Harishchandra, O. Rubner, H.-J. Galla, and A. Heuer, "Properties of compatible solutes in aqueous solution," *Biophysical Chemistry*, vol. 160, no. 1, pp. 62–68, 2012.

[13] R. K. Harishchandra, A. K. Sachan, A. Kerth, G. Lentzen, T. Neuhaus, and H.-J. Galla, "Compatible solutes: ectoine and hydroxyectoine improve functional nanostructures in artificial lung surfactants," *Biochimica et Biophysica Acta*, vol. 1808, no. 12, pp. 2830–2840, 2011.

[14] T. Dirschka, "Ectoin—Anwendung und Perspektiven für die Dermatologie," *Aktuelle Dermatologie*, vol. 34, no. 4, pp. 115–118, 2008.

[15] G. Lentzen and T. Schwarz, "Extremolytes: natural compounds from extremophiles for versatile applications," *Applied Microbiology and Biotechnology*, vol. 72, no. 4, pp. 623–634, 2006.

[16] A. Bilstein, "Immuno-protective effects of the extremolyte ectoine in animal models and humans," in *Proceedings of the 28 Congress of the European Academy of Allergy and Clinical Immunology*, Warsaw, Poland, 2009.

[17] U. Sydlik, I. Gallitz, C. Albrecht, J. Abel, J. Krutmann, and K. Unfried, "The compatible solute ectoine protects against nanoparticle-induced neutrophilic lung inflammation," *The American Journal of Respiratory and Critical Care Medicine*, vol. 180, no. 1, pp. 29–35, 2009.

[18] U. Sydlik, H. Peuschel, A. Paunel-Gorgulu et al., "Recovery of neutrophil apoptosis by ectoine: a new strategy against lung inflammation," *European Respiratory Journal*, vol. 41, no. 2, pp. 433–442, 2013.

[19] A. M. Vestweber, "Das Stressschutzmolekül MedEctoin zeigt positive Ergebnisse bei der Psoriasis und in der topischen Applikation bei Patienten mit trockener, schuppiger Haut," *Naturheilpraxis mit Naturmedizin*, pp. 2–7, 2009.

[20] Bitop, *Ectoin—The Natural Stress-Protection Molecule*, Scientific Information, Witten, Germany.

[21] W. Carr, J. Bernstein, P. Lieberman et al., "A novel intranasal therapy of azelastine with fluticasone for the treatment of allergic rhinitis," *The Journal of Allergy and Clinical Immunology*, vol. 129, no. 5, pp. 1282.e10–1289.e10, 2012.

[22] E. O. Meltzer, T. Shekar, and A. A. Teper, "Mometasone furoate nasal spray for moderate-to-severe nasal congestion in subjects with seasonal allergic rhinitis," *Allergy and Asthma Proceedings*, vol. 32, no. 2, pp. 159–167, 2011.

[23] B. J. Winer, D. R. Brown, and K. M. Michels, *Statistical Principles in Experimental Design*, vol. 3, McGraw-Hill, New York, NY, USA, 1991.

[24] C. Clopper and E. Pearson, "The use of confidence or fiducial limits illustrated in the case of the binomial," *Biometrika*, vol. 48, no. 3-4, pp. 433–440, 1934.

[25] J. Higgins and S. Green, "Cochrane Handbook for Systematic Reviews of Interventions Version 5.1.0," The Cochrane Collaboration, 2011, http://handbook.cochrane.org.

[26] D. F. Stroup, J. A. Berlin, S. C. Morton et al., "Meta-analysis of observational studies in epidemiology: a proposal for reporting," *Journal of the American Medical Association*, vol. 283, no. 15, pp. 2008–2012, 2000.

[27] H. M. Cooper, L. V. Hedges, and J. C. Valentine, *The Handbook of Research Synthesis and Meta-Analysis*, Russell Sage Foundation, 2009.

[28] M. Egger, K. Dickersin, and G. D. Smith, "Problems and limitations in conducting systematic reviews," in *Systematic Reviews in Health Care*, pp. 43–68, BMJ Publishing Group, 2008.

[29] D. Sharpe, "Of apples and oranges, file drawers and garbage: why validity issues in meta-analysis will not go away," *Clinical Psychology Review*, vol. 17, no. 8, pp. 881–901, 1997.

[30] C. J. Ferguson, "An effect size primer: a guide for clinicians and researchers," *Professional Psychology: Research and Practice*, vol. 40, no. 5, pp. 532–538, 2009.

[31] J. P. T. Higgins, S. G. Thompson, J. J. Deeks, and D. G. Altman, "Measuring inconsistency in meta-analyses," *British Medical Journal*, vol. 327, no. 7414, pp. 557–560, 2003.

[32] F. M. Baroody, K. A. Foster, A. Markaryan, M. DeTineo, and R. M. Naclerio, "Nasal ocular reflexes and eye symptoms in patients with allergic rhinitis," *Annals of Allergy, Asthma and Immunology*, vol. 100, no. 3, pp. 194–199, 2008.

[33] A. Eichel, J. Wittig, K. Shah-Hosseini et al., "A prospective, controlled study of SNS01 (ectoine nasal spray) compared to BNO-101 (phytotherapeutic dragees) in patients with acute rhinosinusitis," *Current Medical Research and Opinion*, vol. 29, no. 7, pp. 739–746, 2013.

[34] A. Marini, K. Reinelt, J. Krutmann et al., "Ectoine-containing cream in the treatment of mild to moderate atopic dermatitis: a randomised, comparator-controlled, intra-individual double-blind, multi-center trial," *Skin Pharmacology and Physiology*, vol. 27, no. 2, pp. 57–65, 2014.

[35] D. P. Skoner, G. S. Rachelefsky, E. O. Meltzer et al., "Detection of growth suppression in children during treatment with intranasal beclomethasone dipropionate," *Pediatrics*, vol. 105, no. 2, p. E23, 2000.

[36] E. Johnson, A. Brookhart, and J. Myers, "Study size planning," in *Developing a Protocol for Observational Comparative Effectiveness Research: A User's Guide*, P. Velentgas, N. A. Dreyer, P. Nourjah et al., Eds., Agency for Healthcare Research and Quality, AHRQ, Rockville, Md, USA, 2013.

[37] M. D. A. Carlson and R. S. Morrison, "Study design, precision, and validity in observational studies," *Journal of Palliative Medicine*, vol. 12, no. 1, pp. 77–82, 2009.

11

Treatment of Allergic Rhinitis with Ectoine Containing Nasal Spray and Eye Drops in Comparison with Azelastine Containing Nasal Spray and Eye Drops or with Cromoglycic Acid Containing Nasal Spray

Nina Werkhäuser,[1] Andreas Bilstein,[1] and Uwe Sonnemann[2]

[1] Bitop AG, Stockumer Straße 28, 58453 Witten, Germany
[2] Private Health Centre, Institute for ENT Elmshorn, Hermann-Ehlers-Weg 4, 25337 Elmshorn, Germany

Correspondence should be addressed to Nina Werkhäuser; werkhaeuser@bitop.de

Academic Editor: Ralph Mösges

Objectives. Allergic rhinitis is a common disease with increasing prevalence and high impact on economic burden and comorbidities. As treatment with pharmacological drugs is not always satisfactory due to side effects and incomplete efficacy, alternative treatment strategies are needed. Ectoine is an osmolyte with membrane stabilizing and inflammation reducing capacities. Nasal spray and eye drops containing ectoine are promising new treatment regimens for allergic rhinitis sufferers. *Design and Methods.* The current two noninterventional trials evaluated the efficacy and safety of ectoine containing nasal spray and eye drops for treating allergic rhinitis in comparison with either azelastine or cromoglycic acid containing products. Nasal and ocular symptom developments as well as judgment of tolerability and efficacy were assessed both by investigators and patients over a time period of one to two weeks. *Results.* Both trials confirmed that ectoine containing products reduced nasal and ocular symptoms in allergic rhinitis patients. Results clearly demonstrated good safety profiles of the ectoine products comparable to those of azelastine and even better to those of cromoglycate products. *Conclusion.* Ectoine containing nasal spray and eye drops are interesting new treatment strategies for sufferers of allergic rhinitis, combining both good efficacy and absence of side effects.

1. Introduction

Allergic rhinitis is a common disease affecting 10–20% of the population [1]. Since it has great impact on patients' quality of life, school performance, work productivity, and comorbid conditions such as asthma, it is considered as an important health problem. Allergic rhinitis is defined as an allergic reaction (most often IgE-dependent) to offending allergens such as dust mites, insects, animal dander, and pollens. Symptoms include rhinorrhea, nasal obstruction, nasal and nasopharyngeal itching, sneezing, and postnasal drip. Often, allergic rhinitis is accompanied by allergic conjunctivitis with ocular symptoms such as itchy and watery eyes, resulting in the term allergic rhinoconjunctivitis. According to its length of duration, allergic rhinitis is classified into intermittent (symptoms present <4 days a week of <4 weeks) and persistent (symptoms present ≥ 4 days a week and for at least 4 weeks) forms. Symptom severity is used to classify allergic rhinitis into mild or moderate-severe forms.

A number of pharmacological treatments of allergic rhinitis exist, such as, for example, oral and topical antihistamines, leukotriene receptor antagonists, intranasal glucocorticoids, and cromoglycic acid (mast cell stabilizers) [2].

Azelastine is a new-generation antihistamine applied topically as nasal spray or eye drops. It is used as treatment of allergic rhinitis, hay fever, and allergic conjunctivitis. Although azelastine is regarded as effective possible first-line treatment for allergic rhinitis, common side effects, such as bitter taste of the drug and local irritation reactions and rare side effects such as fatigue or headache, can occur [3].

Cromoglycic acid is an antiallergic drug which inhibits the degranulation of mast cells, thereby blocking the release of inflammatory mediators [4]. Thus, cromoglycic acid prevents the development of allergic reactions rather than reducing acute symptoms and its onset of action is about four to seven days. Due to its short half-life, cromoglycic acid has to be applied at least 4 times a day. Cromoglycic acid is thought to be a safe medication, and adverse events which might occur are usually mild, such as sneezing and sensation of burning. Due to its good safety profile, cromoglycic acid can be prescribed for treating rhinitis in children and pregnant women.

In general, many allergic rhinitis patients are still unsatisfied with the control of symptoms, complain about incomplete relief of symptoms, and suffer from unwanted side effects [5, 6]. Therefore, it is not surprising that increasing interest in the use of alternative and complementary medicine (CAM) for treating rhinitis exists. Thus, it was demonstrated that 40% of the American population uses CAM, 17% of which uses it for treating otorhinolaryngologic diseases [7]. However, so far no general recommendation for the use of CAM can be given by ARIA guidelines as ambiguous study results are available [8].

The present two individual studies compared treatment of allergic rhinitis with ectoine containing nasal spray and eye drops with azelastine containing products (study 1) or treatment with ectoine containing nasal spray with that of cromoglycic acid containing nasal spray (study 2).

Ectoine is a natural amino acid derivate which is produced by bacteria living under extreme harsh environmental conditions where it serves as osmoregulatory compatible solute [9, 10]. Ectoine works via a mechanism called "preferential exclusion" [11, 12]. If it is present together with proteins or lipids, ectoine is expelled from their surfaces, thereby increasing the hydration of the surface and stabilizing lipid layers [13]. Its membrane stabilizing as well as inflammation reducing capacities makes ectoine an interesting candidate for the treatment of allergic rhinitis. These studies served to investigate the efficacy and safety of ectoine containing nasal spray and eye drops in patients with allergic rhinitis.

2. Materials and Methods

The current paper describes two noninterventional studies carried out with ectoine containing nasal spray and eye drops assessing their efficacy in comparison with azelastine nasal spray and eye drops (study 1, NCT02131051) or cromoglycic acid nasal spray (study 2, NCT02131038).

2.1. Medication. The ectoine eye drops contain an iso-osmotic solution with 2% ectoine and 0.35% hydroxyethyl cellulose; the ectoine nasal spray is a hypertonic solution with 2% ectoine. Additional ingredients of the eye drops were sodium chloride, sodium dihydrogen phosphate dihydrate, sodium monohydrogen phosphate dihydrate, and water. Additional ingredients of the nasal spray were sodium chloride and water. In study 1, both nasal spray and eye drops were used, whereas only the nasal spray was used in study 2.

Azelastine containing products were used as comparator in study 1. The azelastine eye drops contain 0.5 mg/mL azelastine hydrochloride with one drop administering 0.015 mg azelastine hydrochloride, and the azelastine nasal spray contains 1 mg/mL azelastine hydrochloride with one puff administering 0.14 mg azelastine hydrochloride. Additional ingredients of the eye drops were benzalkonium chloride (preservative), sodium edetate, hypromellose, sorbitol, sodium hydroxide, and water. Additional ingredients of the nasal spray were sodium edetate, hypromellose, citric acid, sodium chloride, sodium hydrogen phosphate, and water.

During study 2, a cromoglycic acid containing nasal spray was used as comparator. The spray contained 20 mg/ml cromoglycic acid corresponding to 2.8 mg sodium cromoglycic acid per puff. In addition, the following ingredients were present in the formulation: benzalkonium chloride (preservative 0.014 mg/puff), sodium edetate, sodium chloride, sodium dihydrogen phosphate, sodium monohydrogen phosphate, sorbitol, and water.

2.2. Treatment and Study Design

2.2.1. Study 1. On day 0 (Visit 1) patients were asked to participate in the study, and upon signing the informed consent form and patient information, they were allocated to one of the study groups, without any washout period. Antiallergic medications used the last two days prior to inclusion were recorded by the physician. Patients were treated either with ectoine containing nasal spray and eye drops or with azelastine containing nasal spray and eye drops. Patients of the ectoine group had to apply one eye drop per eye and one puff of the nasal spray per nostril four times per day. Patients of the azelastine group had to apply one eye drop per eye and one puff of the nasal spray per nostril twice per day. The treatment period was 7 days, and patients were asked to document their symptoms, together with possible comedication and adverse effects daily in patient diaries at the evening. Therefore the patients' assessments started after the products had been applied already. Following treatment, patients came back for Visit 2 (day 7), during which symptom scores were evaluated and tolerability, efficacy and compliance, and possibly comedications, antiallergic and others, were assessed.

In- and Exclusion Criteria. Male or female patients aged 18–70 with proven allergy and acute symptoms in nose and eye (sum nasal score $\geq$ 15 and sum oral score $\geq$ 6) were allowed to take part in the study. Allergy diagnosis was based on positive prick test. Exclusion criteria were pregnant and nursing women, drug addicts and persons unable to give consent to study participation, patients with intolerance against ingredients of any of the study treatments, previous eye or nose surgery, concomitant treatment with antiallergic drugs, and diseases which might influence the output of the study according to the physicians' judgment.

Scoring of Nasal and Ocular Symptoms. Single nasal (nasal obstruction, rhinorrhea, and sneezing) and ocular symptoms (eye itching, tearing, and conjunctivitis) were scored with an 8 point scale ranging from no symptoms (0) to very severe symptoms (8).

Scoring of Efficacy, Tolerability, and Compliance. Efficacy, tolerability, and compliance were judged by using a scale ranging from 0 (very good) to 8 (bad). Thus, a general judgment, of either how well to tolerate or how efficient the products were, had to be given by the patients and documented in the patient diaries. Both scoring values were based on the patients' personal opinion/feeling with the products. Whereas efficacy and tolerability were assessed both by patients and by physicians, compliance was solely judged by physicians.

Statistics. The statistical analysis was carried out with SPSS version 18 and SigmaPlot version 12. Both efficacy and safety analyses were performed on the entire study population. Descriptive statistics were used for a quantitative report of the main study population features. Continuous variables were tested for normal distribution via Kolmogorov-Smirnov test. Further analysis was carried out with the Mann-Whitney U test, Wilcoxon test, or Friedman test. The level of significance was set to $P < 0.05$ in all tests. Unavailable data were treated as "missing values" or substituted by the "last value carried forward" method.

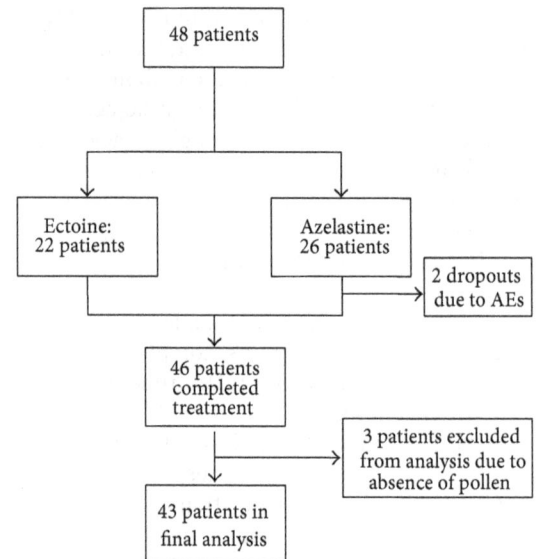

FIGURE 1: Patient flow during study 1.

2.2.2. Study 2. This study was designed as a crossover study, without any washout period within the first week. Half of the patients received ectoine nasal spray whereas the other half received cromoglycic acid containing nasal spray. After 7 days, patients swapped to the other treatment. Thus, patients who started with one week treatment with ectoine nasal spray received cromoglycic acid containing nasal spray within the second week and vice versa. For simplification reasons, patients starting their treatment with ectoine are termed group A, and patients starting their treatment with cromoglycic acid are termed group B in this paper.

The ectoine nasal spray had to be applied at least 5 times per day, whereas the cromoglycic acid spray had to be applied 4 times a day. Thus, patients had to take the ectoine product at least 5 times a day but could upgrade dosing if they felt that medication was not sufficient. The cromoglycic acid product had to be used according to the instruction for use.

Patients had to attend visits to the investigator on day 0 (V1), day 7 (+2 days) (V2), and day 14 (+2 days) (V3). During those visits, the investigator assessed nasal (nasal obstruction, sneezing, and rhinorrhea) and ocular symptoms (eye itching, tearing, and conjunctivitis) as well as palate itching and turbinate hyperplasia. At the end of the study (V3), efficacy, tolerability, and compliance were determined.

In addition to the investigator's assessment, patients had to document daily their ocular and nasal symptoms as well as their judgment of tolerability and efficacy in a patient diary at the evening. Based on the design the patients scoring started after the study medication had been applied.

In- and Exclusion Criteria. Male or female patients with diagnosed allergy and moderate to severe acute symptoms of nasal obstruction, sneezing, and rhinorrhea were allowed to take part in the study. The diagnosis of the allergy was based on a positive prick test. Exclusion criteria were intolerance against ectoine or cromoglycic acid, pregnancy, previous nose

surgeries, or ongoing treatment with additional antiallergic drugs.

Scoring of Nasal, Ocular, and Other Symptoms. Single nasal symptoms (nasal obstruction, rhinorrhea, and sneezing) and ocular symptoms (eye itching, tearing, and conjunctivitis) as well as the symptoms palate itching and turbinate hyperplasia were scored with an 8 point scale ranging from no symptoms (0) to very severe symptoms (8).

Scoring of Efficacy, Tolerability, and Compliance. Efficacy, tolerability, and compliance were judged by using a scale ranging from 0 (very good) to 8 (bad). Thus, a general broad judgment, of how well to tolerate and how efficient the products were, had to be given by the patients and to be documented in the patient diaries. Both scoring values were based on the patients' personal opinion/feeling with the products. Whereas efficacy and tolerability were assessed both by patients and by physicians, compliance was solely judged by physicians.

Pollen Score. In order to reflect the current pollen exposure, data from the online HEXAL pollen calendar were used to grade pollen exposure into mild, moderate, or severe (1, 2, or 3) scores during the course of the study.

Statistics. The statistical analysis was carried out with SPSS version 17 and SigmaPlot version 12. Safety analyses were performed on the entire study population whereas efficacy analysis was performed on all patients who completed the treatment. Continuous variables were tested for normal distribution via Kolmogorov-Smirnov test. Further analysis was carried out with the Mann-Whitney U test, Wilcoxon test, or Friedman test. The level of significance was set to $P < 0.05$ in all tests. Unavailable data were treated as "missing values" or substituted by the "last value carried forward" method.

TABLE 1: Development of single nasal scores (mean ± SD) during study 1 according to patients' and investigators' assessments.

Symptom	Group	Score d1 (patient)	Score d7 (patient)	P value	Score V1 (investigator)	Score V2 (investigator)	P value
Nasal obstruction	Ectoine	4.14 ± 1.93	3.38 ± 2.20	P = 0.003	5.29 ± 1.15	2.86 ± 1.49	P < 0.001
	Azelastine	4.38 ± 2.38	3.60 ± 2.37	P = 0.044	5.91 ± 1.23	3.0 ± 2.13	P < 0.001
Rhinorrhea	Ectoine	3.81 ± 1.86	2.71 ± 1.87	P = 0.054	5.19 ± 1.03	2.24 ± 1.58	P < 0.001
	Azelastine	3.48 ± 2.11	2.8 ± 2.02	P = 0.133	5.45 ± 1.01	2.59 ± 1.89	P < 0.001
Sneezing	Ectoine	3.9 ± 1.92	2.9 ± 1.73	P = 0.475	6.0 ± 1.48	2.43 ± 1.58	P < 0.001
	Azelastine	4.05 ± 1.43	2.45 ± 1.7	P < 0.001	5.77 ± 0.92	2.32 ± 2.10	P < 0.001
Nasal itching	Ectoine	2.81 ± 1.83	2.05 ± 1.56	P = 0.068	4.24 ± 2.32	1.00 ± 1.41	P = 0.001
	Azelastine	3.90 ± 1.70	2.25 ± 1.92	P = 0.002	4.59 ± 1.99	1.41 ± 1.05	P < 0.001

3. Results

Both studies were conducted in accordance with the Declaration of Helsinki. All investigations were carried out with the understanding and consent of all participants.

3.1. Results Study 1. This was a noninterventional trial taking place at two German ear nose throat (ENT) practices starting in June 2010 and being completed in September 2010. Distribution of patients is shown in Figure 1. In total, 48 patients took part in the study, of which 43 were included in the final analysis (31 females and 12 males). Mean age of patients was 35 years, and both groups were comparable in regard to clinical aspects.

3.1.1. Nasal Symptoms. Nasal symptom scores were assessed both as single symptoms and as sum of all nasal symptoms (TNSS). Details of the development of single scores are given in Table 1.

Nasal Obstruction. The mean symptom score of nasal obstruction decreased significantly by 45.95% in the ectoine group and by 49.23% in the azelastine group (V1 to V2, $P <$ 0.001 for both groups). The documentation of the patient diaries also reflected a significant decrease by 18.39% in the ectoine group (P = 0.003) and by 17.83% in the azelastine group (P = 0.044).

Rhinorrhea. A significant decrease in the symptom score was also observed for rhinorrhea from V1 to V2. Mean values decreased by 56.88% in the ectoine group and by 52.50% in the azelastine group ($P <$ 0.001 for both groups). The patient documentation showed a clear decrease of the symptom rhinorrhea which, however, was not significant. Values decreased by 28.75% in the ectoine group (P = 0.054) and by 19.45% in the azelastine group (P = 0.133).

Sneezing. The symptom sneezing decreased significantly from V1 to V2: values decreased by 59.52% in the ectoine group and by 59.84% in the azelastine group ($P <$ 0.001 for both groups). The patient documentation also reflected the symptom decrease which was not significant in the ectoine group (25.61%, P = 0.475) but significant in the azelastine group (39.47%, $P <$ 0.001).

Nasal Itching. Nasal itching decreased significantly from V1 to V2: values decreased by 76.40% in the ectoine group (P =

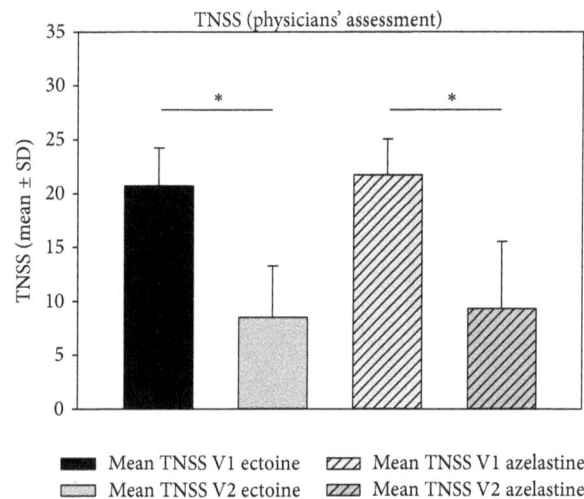

FIGURE 2: Decrease (mean ± SD) of TNSS from V1 to V2 according to the physicians' assessment. $^*P < 0.001$.

0.001) and by 69.31% in the azelastine group ($P <$ 0.001). According to the patient documentation, nasal itching scores decreased by 27.12% in the ectoine group (P = 0.068) and by 42.38% (P = 0.002) in the azelastine group.

3.1.2. Total Nasal Symptom Score (TNSS). The sum of nasal symptom scores (nasal obstruction, rhinorrhea, sneezing, and nasal itching) showed a significant decrease from V1 to V2 (as assessed by physicians): sum scores in the ectoine group decreased from 20.71 ± 3.52 to 8.52 ± 4.74 (decrease of 58.85%; $P <$ 0.001) and sum scores in the azelastine group decreased from 21.73 ± 3.34 to 9.32 ± 6.24 (decrease of 57.11%; $P <$ 0.001). Data are depicted in Figure 2. According to the patients' assessment (see Figure 3), values decreased by 23.05% in the ectoine group (P = 0.076) and by 33.14% in the azelastine group (P = 0.02).

3.1.3. Ocular Symptoms. Ocular symptom scores were also assessed as single symptoms and as sum of all ocular symptoms (TOSS). Details of the development of single scores are given in Table 2.

Conjunctivitis. The symptom conjunctivitis clearly decreased from V1 to V2, as reflected by decline of 48.15% in the

TABLE 2: Development of single ocular symptom scores during study 1 according to patients and investigators' assessments.

Symptom	Group	Score d1 (patient)	Score d7 (patient)	P value	Score V1 (investigator)	Score V2 (investigator)	P value
Conjunctivitis	Ectoine	2.1 ± 1.84	1.38 ± 1.56	P = 0.218	2.67 ± 0.97	1.71 ± 1.62	P = 0.058
	Azelastine	2.05 ± 1.77	2.35 ± 2.32	P = 0.885	3.32 ± 1.73	1.77 ± 1.66	P = 0.013
Eye itching	Ectoine	3.24 ± 1.89	2.67 ± 1.91	P = 0.604	3.86 ± 1.93	2.0 ± 1.79	P = 0.008
	Azelastine	2.9 ± 1.81	2.75 ± 2.1	P = 0.14	4.05 ± 1.89	2.18 ± 2.17	P = 0.002
Tearing	Ectoine	1.71 ± 1.35	1.62 ± 1.63	P = 0.886	2.90 ± 1.3	1.38 ± 1.69	P = 0.003
	Azelastine	1.9 ± 1.84	1.55 ± 1.67	P = 0.357	2.14 ± 1.67	1.27 ± 1.67	P = 0.039

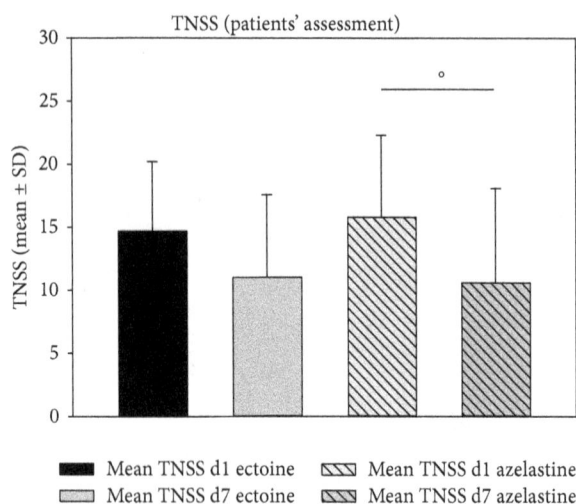

Mean TNSS d1 ectoine Mean TNSS d1 azelastine
Mean TNSS d7 ectoine Mean TNSS d7 azelastine

FIGURE 3: Decrease (mean ± SD) of TNSS from day 1 (d1) to day 7 (d7) according to the patients' assessment. $^{\circ}P = 0.02$.

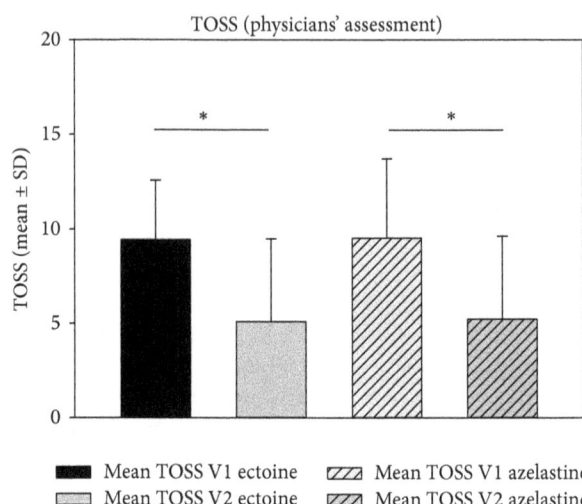

Mean TOSS V1 ectoine Mean TOSS V1 azelastine
Mean TOSS V2 ectoine Mean TOSS V2 azelastine

FIGURE 4: Decrease (mean ± SD) of TOSS from V1 to V2 as assessed by physicians in study 1. $^{*}P < 0.001$.

ectoine group ($P = 0.058$) and of 46.07% in the azelastine group ($P = 0.013$). In the patients documentation, scores of conjunctivitis decreased by 34.09% in the ectoine group ($P = 0.218$) whereas an increase by 14.77% was observed in the azelastine group ($P = 0.885$).

Eye Itching. There was a significant decrease in the symptom scores of eye itching: in the ectoine group, the mean decreased by 48.15% ($P = 0.008$) whereas values of the azelastine group decreased by 46.07% ($P = 0.002$). Corresponding decreases as assessed by the patients were 17.65% in the ectoine group ($P = 0.604$) and 5.33% in the azelastine group ($P = 0.14$).

Tearing. A statistical decrease in the scoring of the symptom tearing was also observed from V1 to V2: in the ectoine group, values decreased by 52.46% ($P = 0.003$) whereas values in the azelastine group decreased by 40.43% ($P = 0.039$). The patient documentation of the symptom tearing also showed a clear decrease of values (5.56% with $P = 0.886$ in the ectoine group and 18.63% with $P = 0.357$ in the azelastine group).

3.1.4. Total Ocular Symptom Score (TOSS). The TOSS (sum of conjunctivitis, eye itching, and tearing) decreased significantly from V1 to V2 in both groups ($P < 0.001$ for ectoine, $P = 0.009$ for azelastine). Starting mean values at V1 were 9.43±3.14 in the ectoine group and 9.5±4.22 in the azelastine group which decreased by 45.96% to 5.10±4.38 in the ectoine

group and by 44.98% to 5.23 ± 4.36 in the azelastine group. Decreases of TOSS values as assessed by patients were not significant (Figure 4) (data not shown).

Palate Itching. As for nasal and ocular symptoms, a clear decrease of the symptom palate itching was observed from V1 to V2: in the ectoine group, values decreased from 2.52 ± 2.71 to 1.19 ± 1.72 ($P = 0.024$), and in the azelastine group, values decreased from 3.36 ± 2.68 to 1.5 ± 1.92 ($P = 0.018$). Values of the patients' documentation did only reach statistical significance in the azelastine group: here, the scoring decreased from 3.81 ± 2.5 to 2.15 ± 2.13 ($P < 0.001$). In the ectoine group, values decreased from 1.76 ± 2.1 to 1.67 ± 2.15 ($P = 0.854$).

Correlation of Pollen Count and Nasal Symptoms. In order to normalize the nasal symptoms (nasal constriction, rhinorrhea, and sneezing) to the pollen burden, a quotient from sum score and pollen counts was determined. Values of quotients decreased significantly from 8.97 ± 3.98 to 5.23 ± 3.59 in the ectoine group ($P = 0.002$) and from 9.73 ± 3.59 to 5.76 ± 5.26 in the azelastine group ($P = 0.011$), thus confirming the decrease of nasal symptoms during the pollen season upon treatment.

Efficacy, Tolerability, and Compliance. The physicians' assessment of efficacy of both products was similar at V2, and

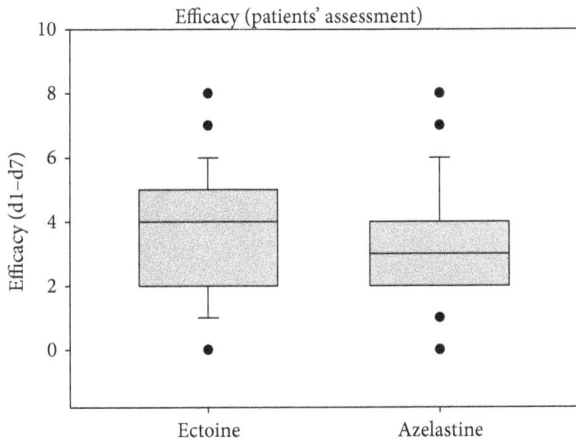

FIGURE 5: Patients' assessment of efficacy during study 1 from day 1 to day 7. Lines within the box mark the median; the upper and lower ends of the box indicate the 75th and 25th percentiles, respectively. Whiskers above and below the box indicate the 90th and 10th percentiles. Dots (•) represent outlying points.

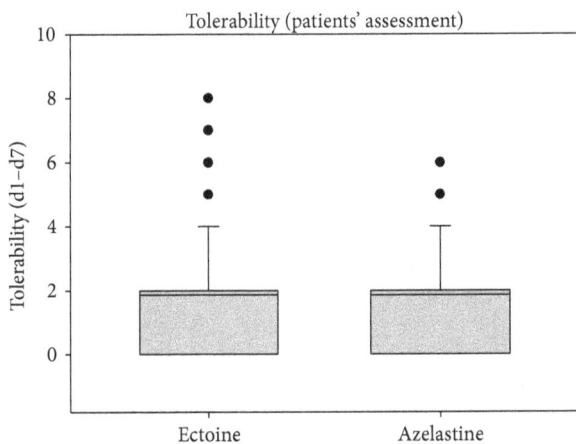

FIGURE 6: Patients' assessment of tolerability during study 1 from day 1 to day 7. Lines within the box mark the median; the upper and lower ends of the box indicate the 75th and 25th percentiles, respectively. Whiskers above the box indicate the 90th percentile. Dots (•) represent outlying points.

with values of 2.48 (good) in the ectoine group and 2.64 (good-satisfactory) in the azelastine group, there was no significant difference between groups. The general tolerability was assessed as very good to good in both groups (1.33 in the ectoine group and 1.45 in the azelastine group), and the compliance was comparably good (values <1) in both groups.

Values of the patients' assessments of efficacy and tolerability are shown in Figures 5 and 6. The patients' evaluations resulted in comparable values of efficacy and tolerability without statistical differences between treatment groups.

Comparison of Reduction of Symptoms between Groups. In order to calculate if reduction of symptoms from V1 to V2 was different between the treatment groups, differences of mean V1 and V2 values were compared via Mann-Whitney U

TABLE 3: Correlation of differences of single symptoms (mean values) between V1 and V2 (based on physicians' evaluations) in study 1.

Symptom	Difference means V1-V2 ectoine	Difference means V1-V2 azelastine	P value
Nasal obstruction	2.43	2.91	0.546
Rhinorrhea	2.95	2.86	0.882
Sneezing	3.57	3.45	0.787
Nasal itching	3.24	3.18	0.768
Conjunctivitis	0.96	1.55	0.409
Eye itching	1.86	1.87	0.863
Tearing	1.52	0.87	0.254
Palate itching	1.33	1.86	0.426

TABLE 4: Correlation of differences of single symptoms (mean values) between d1 and d7 (based on patients' evaluations) in study 1.

Symptom	Difference means d1–d7 ectoine	Difference means d1–d7 azelastine	P value
Nasal obstruction	0.76	0.78	0.814
Rhinorrhea	1.1	0.68	0.446
Sneezing	1.0	1.6	0.54
Nasal itching	0.76	1.65	0.184
Conjunctivitis	0.72	−0.3	0.42
Eye itching	0.57	0.15	0.73
Tearing	0.09	0.35	0.826
Palate itching	0.09	1.66	0.034

test. As shown in Table 3, there were no statistical differences between the ectoine and the azelastine group, thus confirming that both substances worked comparably well. The same calculation was performed for the patient data. Here, no statistical difference was shown except for the symptom palate itching. Details are shown in Table 4.

Adverse Events (AEs). In total, 8 AEs occurred during the study (see Table 5). 2 AEs occurred in the ectoine group, whereas 6 AEs occurred in the azelastine group. 2 AEs in the azelastine group led to dropout of the study. No serious adverse event (SAE) occurred during the study.

3.2. *Results Study 2.* This was a noninterventional trial taking place at a German ear nose throat (ENT) practice starting in May 2009 and being completed in September 2009. Distribution of patients is shown in Figure 7. In total, 50 patients (33 females and 17 males) with an average age of 34 years took part in the study. Both treatment groups were homogeneous from a clinical point of view.

3.2.1. *Nasal Symptoms*

Nasal Obstruction. Both patient groups started with a comparable mean nasal obstruction score of 5.80 in group A and 5.64 in group B (physician's assessment). The symptom scores

TABLE 5: Adverse events during study 1.

	N	Description	Outcome
Ectoine group	2	#1: burning of eyes #2: itching of throat during application of products	Recovered
Azelastine group	6	#1–4: burning of eyes ($n = 4$) #5: nausea #6 headache ($n = 1$)	1 premature determination of study due to AE 1 premature determination of study due to AE

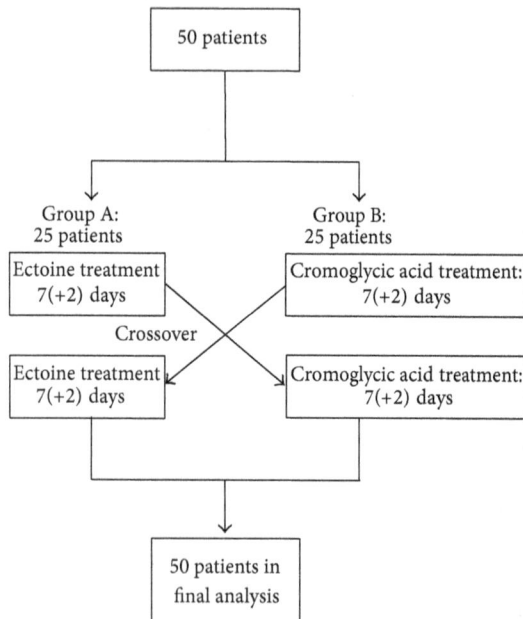

FIGURE 7: Patient flow during study 2.

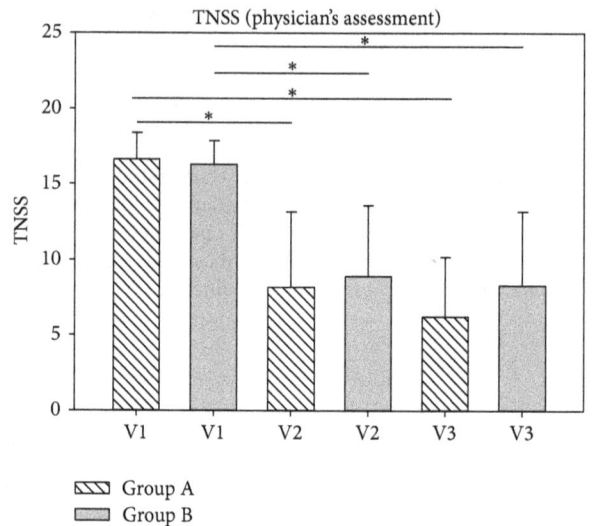

FIGURE 8: TNSS development according to the physician's assessment. TNSS scores decreased from 16.64 (V1, group A) to 8.16 (V2, group A) and further to 6.20 (V3, group A). In group B, values decreased from 16.28 (V1) to 8.92 (V2) and to 8.28 (V3). $^*P < 0.001$.

decreased to 3.2 (group A) and 3.44 (group B) after a week, and a further decrease to 2.52 (group A) and 2.92 (group B) was observed after 2 weeks. Decreases were significant in both groups with P values both for 1 week and for 2 weeks of $P < 0.001$.

Similarly, patient scores of the symptom nasal obstruction decreased from 4.08 (group A) and 3.60 (group B) on day 0 to 2.84 (group A, $P = 0.009$) and 3.24 (group B, $P = 0.464$) on day 7 and further to 2.52 (group A, $P = 0.004$) and 2.56 (group B, $P = 0.041$) on day 14.

Rhinorrhea. The symptom rhinorrhea decreased significantly ($P < 0.001$) for both groups both from V1 to V2 and from V1 to V3 according to the physician's assessment. Values decreased from 5.12 to 2.40 (V2) and further to 1.88 (V3) in group A and from 4.96 to 2.68 (V2) and to 2.76 (V3) in group B.

According to the patients' evaluation, scoring of rhinorrhea decreased from 3.12 to 2.32 (d7, $P = 0.104$) and further to 2.04 (d14, $P = 0.010$) in group A. In group B, values decrease from 3.80 to 3.08 (d7, $P = 0.115$) and further to 2.28 (d14, $P < 0.001$).

Sneezing. The symptom sneezing also decreased significantly ($P < 0.001$) from V1 to V2 and from V1 to V3 in both groups. Baseline scores from group A were 5.72 and decreased to

2.56 (V2) and further to 1.80 (V3), whereas values in group B decreased from 5.68 to 2.80 (V2) and to 2.6 (V3).

According to the patients' evaluation, scoring of the symptom sneezing decreased from 3.16 to 2.44 ($P = 0.20$) on day 7 to 2.12 ($P = 0.265$) on day 14 in group A, whereas values decreased from 4.04 to 2.64 ($P = 0.018$) on day 7 to 2.40 ($P < 0.001$) on day 14 in group B.

3.2.2. Total Nasal Symptom Score (TNSS). To reflect the development of the sum of nasal symptoms, the total nasal score (nasal obstruction, rhinorrhea, and sneezing) was calculated. Results are depicted in Figures 8 and 9. According to the physician's assessment, TNSS scores decreased significantly for both groups both from V1 to V2 ($P < 0.001$) and from V1 to V3 ($P < 0.001$). Scores assessed by patients showed that decreases in TNSS from d1 to d7 were not significant whereas significant decreases in TNSS scores from d1 to d14 were shown both for group A ($P < 0.001$) and group B ($P < 0.001$).

3.2.3. Ocular Symptoms. To investigate the development of ocular symptoms during the treatment period, the single symptoms eye itching, tearing, and conjunctivitis/redness of eyes were assessed both by the investigator and by

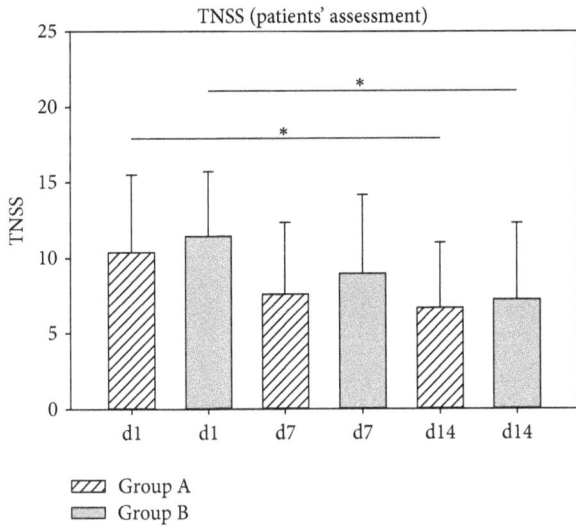

FIGURE 9: TNSS development according to the patients' assessment. TNSS scores decreased from 10.36 (d1, group A) to 7.60 (d7, group A) and further to 6.68 (d14, group A). In group B, values decreased from 11.44 (d1) to 8.96 (d7) and to 7.24 (d14). $^{*}P < 0.001$.

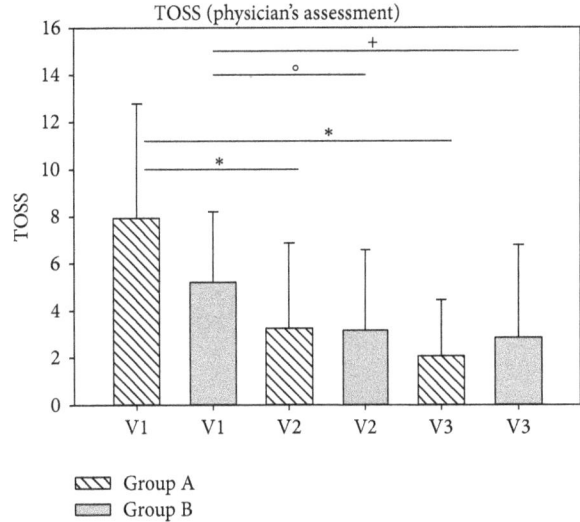

FIGURE 10: Assessment of sum of ocular symptoms (TOSS) according to physician's assessments in study 2. $^{*}P < 0.001$, $^{\circ}P = 0.008$, and $^{+}P = 0.003$.

the patients. Details of scores are listed in Tables 6 and 7. According to the investigator's assessment, all observed ocular symptoms improved significantly from V1 to V3 in group A, whereas only the symptoms eye itching and tearing improved significantly in group B. The patients' assessment of ocular symptoms showed that the symptoms eye itching and eye redness improved significantly in group A, whereas decreases in symptom scores from day 1 to day 14 were not significant in group B.

3.2.4. Total Ocular Symptom Score (TOSS). The development of the sum of ocular symptoms (eye itching, conjunctivitis, and tearing) as assessed by the investigator is depicted in Figure 10. It could be confirmed that ocular symptoms decreased significantly from V1 to V2 ($P < 0.001$ for group 1; $P = 0.008$ for group B) as well as from V1 to V3 ($P < 0.001$ for group 1; $P = 0.003$ for group B).

The development of total ocular symptom score as assessed by patients is shown in Figure 11. Here, a significant decrease of symptom score was only observed in group A from day 1 to day 14 ($P = 0.026$).

Palate Itching and Turbinate Hyperplasia. In addition to nasal and ocular symptoms, the development of the symptom palate itching was determined both by the investigator and the patients. As shown in Table 8, significant decreases in the symptom palate itching were observed by the investigator from V1 to V3. In contrast, patients' assessment of this symptom showed only small decreases in this symptom which were not significant.

Additionally, the development of turbinate hyperplasia was determined by the investigator. As shown in Table 8, treatment resulted in a significant improvement of this symptom within the first week of treatment which was still significantly improved after two weeks of treatment. No

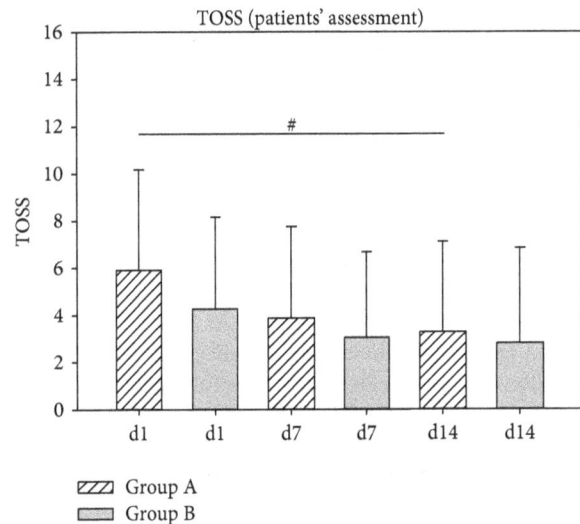

FIGURE 11: Assessment of sum of ocular symptoms TOSS development according to the patients' assessment during study 2. $^{\#}P = 0.026$.

differences between groups could be determined for this symptom (Table 9).

Correlation of Pollen Count and Nasal Symptoms. In order to rule out that results might be influenced by the existence of pollens, data reflecting the current pollen count were included in the analysis. The quotient of TNSS values and pollen count scores confirmed a significant decrease of TNSS values both from V1 to V2 ($P < 0.001$) and from V1 to V3 ($P < 0.001$) (data not shown).

Efficacy, Tolerability, and Compliance. According to the physicians' judgment, the efficacy of treatment was rated "good to satisfactory" with a score of 2.68 ± 1.89 (group A) and

TABLE 6: Development of ocular rhinitis symptoms (mean values) during study 2 (physician's assessment).

Symptom	Group	Mean V1	Mean V2	Mean V3	P value V1 versus V2	P value V2 versus V3
Eye itching	A	3.80 ± 2.29	1.68 ± 1.84	1.00 ± 1.38	P < 0.001	P < 0.001
	B	2.72 ± 2.05	1.60 ± 1.63	1.48 ± 1.78	0.046	0.003
Tearing	A	2.32 ± 1.95	0.76 ± 1.13	0.68 ± 0.95	0.002	P < 0.001
	B	1.32 ± 1.35	0.84 ± 1.37	0.64 ± 1.35	0.107	0.006
Conjunctivitis	A	1.80 ± 2.06	0.80 ± 1.19	0.40 ± 0.58	0.086	0.011
	B	1.12 ± 1.13	0.75 ± 1.22	0.72 ± 1.21	0.094	0.383

TABLE 7: Development of ocular rhinitis symptoms (mean values) during study 2 (patients' assessment).

Symptom	Group	Mean d1	Mean d7	Mean d14	P value d1 versus d7	P value d1 versus d14
Eye itching	A	2.68 ± 1.99	1.56 ± 1.58	1.48 ± 1.81	0.044	0.019
	B	2.04 ± 1.93	1.48 ± 1.61	1.28 ± 1.74	0.250	0.014
Tearing	A	1.24 ± 1.36	1.20 ± 1.26	0.92 ± 1.08	0.992	0.382
	B	1.12 ± 1.36	1.30 ± 1.24	0.68 ± 1.41	0.271	0.297
Eye redness	A	2.00 ± 2.02	1.12 ± 1.24	0.88 ± 1.20	0.150	0.003
	B	1.12 ± 1.42	0.80 ± 1.32	0.84 ± 1.31	0.337	0.292

2.96 ± 1.72 (group B) at V2 and a score of 3.12 ± 2.11 (group A) and 2.80 ± 2.06 (group B) at V3. There were no significant differences between both groups.

Similarly, the patients' assessment of efficacy was "good to satisfactory" both on day 7 (group A: 2.76 ± 1.89; group B: 2.96 ± 1.81) and on day 14 (group A: 2.56 ± 2.00; group B: 2.44 ± 2.16) without statistical differences between groups.

Following 1 week of treatment, the tolerability was judged as "very good" in group A (1.24 ± 1.30) and as "good" (2.40 ± 1.53) in group B. Following crossover of groups, tolerability of the treatment was judged as "satisfactory" (3.0 ± 2.16) in group A and as "very good" (0.88 ± 1.05) in group B. The changes of tolerability between both groups were highly significant (P < 0.001), thus indicating that tolerability was significantly better following a 7-day treatment with ectoine containing nasal spray in comparison to 7-day treatment with cromoglycic acid nasal spray.

Those differences in tolerability scoring were also clearly visible in the patients' assessment of tolerability. Whereas tolerability was judged as "very good" (1.30 ± 1.48) within the first days of treatment in group A, scoring for the second week decreased to a mean score of 2.65 ± 1.89 corresponding to "good to satisfactory." Group B showed the opposite development with a tolerability scoring of 2.35 ± 1.68 ("good") within the first 7 days which improved to a mean score of 0.97 ± 1.24 ("very good") within the second half of the treatment. Details of the patients' tolerability assessment are depicted in Figure 12. In summary, patients judged the tolerability significantly better under treatment with ectoine containing nasal spray compared to treatment with cromoglycic acid nasal spray (P < 0.001).

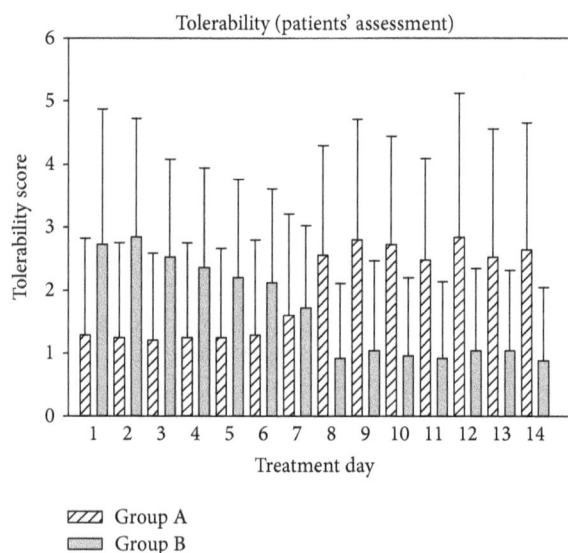

FIGURE 12: Patients' assessment of tolerability of treatments during study 2.

The compliance was assessed as very good by the physician, and values were not statistically different between groups (see Table 10).

Adverse Events (AEs). During the study, no serious adverse events (SAEs) occurred. No adverse events were observed during treatment with ectoine containing nasal spray. In contrast, 13 patients complained about a burning sensation during treatment with cromoglycic acid nasal spray. One

TABLE 8: Physician's assessment of palate itching and turbinate hyperplasia during study 2.

Symptom	Group	Mean V1	Mean V2	Mean V3	P value V1 versus V2	P value V1 versus V3
Palate itching	A	2.32 ± 2.54	1.12 ± 2.05	0.84 ± 1.52	0.054	0.003
	B	2.20 ± 2.36	1.24 ± 2.13	0.92 ± 1.80	0.048	0.002
Turbinate hyperplasia	A	4.68 ± 1.25	3.56 ± 1.08	3.76 ± 1.69	<0.001	0.007
	B	4.80 ± 1.15	3.84 ± 1.25	3.56 ± 1.19	0.005	0.001

TABLE 9: Patients' assessment of palate itching during study 2.

Symptom	Group	Mean d1	Mean d7	Mean d14	P value d1 versus d7	P value d1 versus d14
Palate itching	A	1.80 ± 2.35	1.56 ± 1.87	1.12 ± 1.62	0.962	0.425
	B	1.56 ± 1.89	1.24 ± 2.09	0.92 ± 1.78	0.053	0.035

TABLE 10: Compliance scores (assessed by the investigator) following 1 week (V2) and 2 weeks (V3) of treatment during study 2.

Group	Mean V2	Mean V3
A	1.28 ± 1.24	1.12 ± 0.97
B	0.88 ± 0.93	1.16 ± 1.03

patient complained about displeasing smell, and another patient complained about dehydration effect. The correlation between the observed AEs (burning sensation, displeasing smell, and dehydration effect) was judged as probable.

4. Conclusions

The current studies investigated the efficacy and safety of ectoine containing nasal spray and eye drops in comparison with commonly applied pharmacological treatments of allergic rhinitis. In two noninterventional trials, ectoine products were compared with either azelastine or cromoglycic acid containing products. Although this paper covers results of two separate studies, they were summarized in one document as the indication was very similar and both studies aimed to compare ectoine containing products with other topical medications. As the study with cromoglycic acid was one of the first studies with ectoine products, dosage was slightly higher than in the study comparing ectoine and azelastine products. As a placebo-controlled, randomized trial with ectoine nasal spray and eye drops which was conducted after the study 2 had confirmed that the dose of 4 uses per day was sufficient to show significant superiority over placebo treatment, this dosage was chosen in study 1 [14]. Both studies demonstrated that allergic rhinitis can be successfully and safely treated with ectoine containing products, thus offering a potential new treatment strategy for allergic rhinitis sufferers.

Both studies were intentionally designed as noninterventional studies based on German law. Although this study design forbids randomization of patients, use of placebo, and blinding of study medication, it still reflects the most realistic standard clinical practice. Thus, patients were included independently on their prior medication and no washout period had to be kept. In order to ensure homogeneity of patients, all had to show a certain degree of symptoms at inclusion reflected by a minimum of TNSS values. Additionally, symptom scores were correlated with pollen count scores in order to include objective measures into the analysis. Importantly, sites specialized in the area of ear nose throat practice were chosen to warrant a very precise assessment of symptoms by specialized physicians and to have a homogeneous patient population. Although we believe that valuable results can be drawn from noninterventional trials, one drawback of this study design is the fact that one cannot include a placebo group into the study population. On the other hand, it has been demonstrated that double-blind randomized placebo-controlled trials clearly have their limitations and disadvantages and that particularly patients' awareness of a placebo arm can lead to modifications of results due to patients' expectations and interpretations [15]. This was confirmed by a comparison of open and controlled study designs in neuroleptic studies, indicating that results of well performed open studies earn more attention [16].

In study 1, it was shown that both the ectoine and the azelastine products resulted in a clear decrease of symptoms of allergic rhinitis over the study period of 7 days. According to the physicians' evaluation, the symptoms nasal obstruction, rhinorrhea, sneezing, nose itching, conjunctivitis (azelastine group only), eye itching, and tearing were significantly reduced. The mean decrease of TNSS was −58.85% in the ectoine group and −57.11% in the azelastine group, thus demonstrating a strong clinical relevance. Similarly, mean decreases in TOSS were −45.96% in the ectoine group and −44.98% in the azelastine group and therewith reflect strong clinical relevance, too.

Study 2 also demonstrated a significant decrease of symptom scores upon treatment: within the first week of the study, TNSS values decreased by −50.96% (group A) and by −45.21% (group B), and decreases within the entire study period of 2 weeks were −62.74% (group A) and −49.14% (group B) according to the physician's assessment. Nasal obstruction is often caused by an enlargement of the nasal turbinates which are located on the lateral walls on each side of the nose.

Thus, the significant improvement of turbinate hyperplasia as assessed by the physician underlined the efficacy of both treatments in reducing nasal obstruction.

In comparison to the physicians' assessment of symptoms, generally less strong symptom decreases were observed by patients. This might be most likely due to the fact that starting symptom values as assessed by patients themselves were lower than the physicians' values. This in turn is at least partly accredited to the fact that patients' first assessments of symptoms were documented at the end of the first treatment days whereas physicians documented baseline symptoms during the first site visit prior to the start of treatment. A recent placebo-controlled study in an environmental challenge chamber showed that 3 hours after application of the ectoine nasal spray and eye drops the symptoms were decreased by ~20%. This decrease reflects roughly the difference between the first assessment by the physicians and the first patient diary entry [14]. In addition, physicians are able to carry out ranking of symptoms based on their experience with many patients; thus, their judgment might be considered more objectively. On the other hand, symptoms such as itching of eyes, nose, and palate cannot be measured with a scientifically valid method and are thus prone to personal perception and difficult to be assessed by physicians together with patients. Taken together, an overestimation by the physician or an underestimation by the patients is not likely.

In study 1, the patients' assessment showed that for the azelastine group, decreases were significant for the symptoms nasal obstruction, sneezing, and nasal itching. For the ectoine group, values decreased significantly in the symptom nasal obstruction, whereas a clear but not significant decrease in the symptoms nasal itching, sneezing, and rhinorrhea was observed. In total, decreases of TNSS were −24.68% in the ectoine group and −35.26% in the azelastine group, thus confirming a clinical relevance of the treatment. Clear decreases in the ocular symptoms tearing and eye itching were assessed by patients of both groups; however, values did not reach significance. The symptom conjunctivitis was clearly (but not significantly) decreased in the ectoine group, whereas it became slightly worse in the azelastine group. In total, TOSS as assessed by patients decreased by −19.57% in the ectoine group and by −11.81% in the azelastine group.

Although no ocular treatment was applied in study 2, ocular symptoms of allergic rhinitis clearly improved upon treatment with ectoine or cromoglycic acid nasal spray. According to the physicians' assessment, TOSS values decreased by −59.09% in group A and by −39.32% in group B after 1 week of treatment and by −73.74% in group A and by −45.47% in group B after 2 weeks of treatment. It is not surprising that local and nonpharmaceutical nasal treatment might also influence ocular symptoms as recent studies suggest a crosstalk between the nose and eyes. The mechanism of the influence of symptoms via the nasolacrimal duct is not fully understood but thought to be via a mucosal connection, possibly via a nose-eye reflex.

The patients' assessment of ocular symptom development in study 2 confirmed a significant decrease in the symptom eye itching after two weeks' treatment in both groups.

A significant reduction of the symptom eye redness was observed in group A but not in group B. However, as ocular symptom scores were generally rather small in this study and treatment aimed mainly to reduce nasal symptoms, further studies will be needed to evaluate the efficacy of treatments on ocular symptoms. Interestingly, another published study with azelastine eye drops, cromoglycate eye drops, or placebo eye drops showed superiority of both active treatments versus placebo without significant differences between the two active treatments [17], and a future study comparing treatment with ectoine eye drops only with other pharmacological eye drop formulations would be desirable.

The current studies both showed that ectoine nasal spray and eye drops can safely be applied in patients with allergic rhinitis. Patients judged the tolerability of the products as similarly good as the azelastine products and significantly better than cromoglycic acid nasal spray, and the very low numbers of AEs reflected a very good safety profile of the used treatments.

The crossover design of study 2 bears difficulties as no washout period between the crossover was carried out. However, as symptoms were assessed on a daily basis, effects following one treatment only (after one week) can be analyzed separately from the results following two treatments. As clear improvements of symptoms were already observed after one week of treatment, this time span seems sufficient to evaluate effects of either treatment A or B.

As the efficacy and safety of azelastine has been studied in a huge range of clinical trials during the last decades, one can use historical data to bring the results of the current study into a broader context (for results from comparator studies see Table 11). In addition, results from placebo groups of comparator studies can be used in order to rank the current results. Thus, comparable data confirmed a superiority of azelastine versus placebo treatment, and values indicate that effects of azelastine are usually about 2-3-fold higher than placebo. However, comparing the actual values of the current study with other studies is rather difficult as design (e.g., randomized versus nonrandomized, placebo-controlled versus not placebo-controlled, differences in length of treatment, and differences in scaling of symptoms) and dose (azelastine concentration and number of daily applications) of available studies differs enormously. In addition, most studies used nasal spray only and assessed solely nasal symptoms, whereas the current study is one of few studies acknowledging also ocular symptoms of allergic rhinitis. Taken together, results of the current study 1 showed that effects of ectoine containing products are almost comparable with those of azelastine, a well-studied drug, which has a proven superiority to placebo treatment and is commonly prescribed against allergic rhinitis.

Cromoglycic acid has been a common drug in treating allergic rhinitis, and although it is thought not to be as effective as intranasal steroids or antihistamines, it has been shown to reduce both nasal and ocular symptoms and it is therefore a reasonable therapy option. In particular, its good safety profile makes it an interesting treatment option both for children and pregnant women. As no published studies were identical with the current study design (study

TABLE 11: Comparison of the current study 1 with other azelastine studies.

Study	Treatment	% improvement from baseline to end of treatment	
		TNSS	TOSS
Current study 1[1]	Ectoine	58.85	45.96
	Azelastine	57.11	44.98
Current study 1[2]	Ectoine	24.68	19.57
	Azelastine	35.26	11.81
Lumry et al. 2007 (study 1)[3] [18]	Azelastine	14.1	n.d.
	Placebo	4.5	n.d.
Lumry et al. 2007 (study 2)[3] [18]	Azelastine	22.1	n.d.
	Placebo	12.0	n.d.
Shah et al.[4] [19]	Azelastine 0.1%	24.4	n.d.
	Azelastine 0.15%	29.7	n.d.
	Placebo	12.0	n.d.
Howland et al.[5] [20]	Azelastine 0.15%	19.3	16.7
	Placebo	11.4	6.0
Van Bavel et al.[6] [21]	Azelastine 0.15%	18.7	n.d.
	Placebo	10.5	n.d.
Falser et al.[7] [22]	Azelastine	83.56*	n.d.
	Levocabastine	70.42*	n.d.
Charpin et al.[8] [23]	Azelastine	60.2	65.0
	Cetirizine (tablet)	63.3	60.8

[1]Physicians assessment; [2]patients' assessment; [3]one spray of 0.1% azelastine nasal spray per nostril twice daily for 14 days; [4]two sprays of 0.1% or 0.15% azelastine nasal spray per nostril twice daily for 14 days; [5]two sprays of 0.15% azelastine nasal spray per nostril once daily for 14 days; [6]two sprays of 0.15% azelastine nasal spray per nostril once daily for 2 weeks; [7]azelastine 1.12 mg/day and levocabastine 0.4 mg/day nasal spray administered twice daily for 4 weeks, *TNSS: sneezing, nasal itching, and rhinorrhoea; [8]one spray of 0.1% azelastine nasal spray per nostril twice daily for 14 days. n.d.: not determined.

2) in terms of treatment duration and analysis of end points, only general comparisons to cromoglycic acid studies can be drawn. Several studies have confirmed that cromoglycic acid is superior to placebo in patients with allergic rhinitis [24]. Thus, Schuller and colleagues [25] investigated the efficacy of Cromolyn sodium in comparison to nedocromil sodium and placebo. Over a treatment period of 8 weeks, it was demonstrated that Cromolyn resulted in a clear improvement of nasal symptoms, particularly in the symptom "stuffy nose." A further placebo-controlled study confirmed that cromoglycate acid nasal spray provided significant relief of nasal symptoms within 2 weeks of treatments which were significant for the symptoms sneezing and nasal congestion and clearly visible but not significant for the symptoms rhinorrhea and nasal pruritus [26].

Taken together, ectoine containing nasal spray and eye drops have been demonstrated to be promising alternatives to pharmacological drugs with both good efficacy and a very good safety profile. As the ectoine nasal spray and eye drops act purely physically on the nasal and ocular mucosa,

it makes those products particularly interesting for patients with reservations about pharmacological therapy. An additional study in children and adolescents with seasonal allergic rhinitis (data not yet published) has confirmed the safety of ectoine containing nasal spray and eye drops in the pediatric population. Further studies should be undertaken to further investigate the onset of action and compare it to commonly applied pharmacological drugs. Quick relief of symptoms is crucial for patients and understood to be advantageous when comparing, for example, azelastine with intranasal corticosteroids [27] and should therefore be assessed for the ectoine products. A controlled, ramdomised study which was carried out using a controlled environmental exposure chamber showed a quick onset of action of ectoine nasal spray and eye drops and confirmed the efficacy in reducing both nasal and ocular symptoms [14]. Additional studies applying the ectoine eye drops only are needed to further elucidate their impact on ocular symptoms during allergic rhinitis.

Conflict of Interests

Dr. Nina Werkhäuser and Dr. Andreas Bilstein are employees of bitop AG, a company where medical devices, including the ectoine nasal spray and eye drops, are developed and registered. bitop AG sponsored the trials discussed in this paper. Dr. Uwe Sonnemann received sponsorship by bitop AG to conduct the studies.

Acknowledgment

The authors thank Dr. T. Kottmann for statistical analysis of data.

References

[1] J. L. Broek, J. Bousquet, C. E. Baena-Cagnani et al., "Allergic rhinitis and its impact on asthma (ARIA) guidelines: 2010 revision," *Journal of Allergy and Clinical Immunology*, vol. 126, no. 3, pp. 466–476, 2010.

[2] D. K. Sur and S. Scandale, "Treatment of allergic rhinitis," *American Family Physician*, vol. 81, no. 12, pp. 1440–1446, 2010.

[3] F. Horak and U. P. Zieglmayer, "Azelastine nasal spray for the treatment of allergic and nonallergic rhinitis," *Expert Review of Clinical Immunology*, vol. 5, no. 6, pp. 659–669, 2009.

[4] "Disodium cromoglycate in allergic respiratory disease," *British Medical Journal*, vol. 2, no. 5806, pp. 159–161, 1972.

[5] T. A. Mahr, "Therapy in allergic rhinoconjunctivitis: new horizons," *Allergy and Asthma Proceedings*, vol. 28, no. 4, pp. 404–409, 2007.

[6] HealthSTAR Communications and Schulman Ronca & Bucuvales, *Allergies in America: A Landmark Survey of Nasal Allergy Sufferers: Adult*, 2006.

[7] C. E. Roehm, B. Tessema, and S. M. Brown, "The role of alternative medicine in rhinology," *Facial Plastic Surgery Clinics of North America*, vol. 20, no. 1, pp. 73–81, 2012.

[8] G. Passalacqua, P. J. Bousquet, K.-H. Carlsen et al., "ARIA update: I—systematic review of complementary and alternative medicine for rhinitis and asthma," *Journal of Allergy and Clinical Immunology*, vol. 117, no. 5, pp. 1054–1062, 2006.

[9] E. A. Galinski, H.-P. Pfeiffer, and H. G. Truper, "1,4,5,6-Tetrahydro-2-methyl-4-pyrimidinecarboxylic acid. A novel cyclic amino acid from halophilic phototropic bacteria of the genus Ectothiorhodospira," *European Journal of Biochemistry*, vol. 149, no. 1, pp. 135–139, 1985.

[10] E. Bremer and R. Krämer, "Coping with osmotic challenges: osmoregulation through accumulation and release of compatible solutes in bacteria," in *Bacterial Stress Responses*, pp. 79–97, 2000.

[11] T. Arakawa and S. N. Timasheff, "The stabilization of proteins by osmolytes," *Biophysical Journal*, vol. 47, no. 3, pp. 411–414, 1985.

[12] Y. Oberdörfer, S. Schrot, H. Fuchs, E. Galinski, and A. Janshoff, "Impact of compatible solutes on the mechanical properties of fibronectin: a single molecule analysis," *Physical Chemistry Chemical Physics*, vol. 5, no. 9, pp. 1876–1881, 2003.

[13] R. K. Harishchandra, S. Wulff, G. Lentzen, T. Neuhaus, and H.-J. Galla, "The effect of compatible solute ectoines on the structural organization of lipid monolayer and bilayer membranes," *Biophysical Chemistry*, vol. 150, no. 1–3, pp. 37–46, 2010.

[14] A. Bilstein, A. Salapatek, P. Patel, and G. Lentzen, "Topical treatments based on ectoine, a novel, non-drug, extremophile-based substance, relieves allergic rhinoconjunctivitis symptoms in patients in an environmental eexposure chamber model," in *Proceedings of the 30th Congress of the European Academy of Allergy and Clinical Immunology (EAACI '11)*, June 2011.

[15] B. Colagiuri, "Participant expectancies in double-blind randomized placebo-controlled trials: potential limitations to trial validity," *Clinical Trials*, vol. 7, no. 3, pp. 246–255, 2010.

[16] F.-G. Pajonk, R. Holzbach, and D. Naber, "Evaluation of efficacy of neuroleptics in open versus double-blind trials," *Fortschritte der Neurologie Psychiatrie*, vol. 68, no. 7, pp. 313–320, 2000.

[17] I. G. V. James, L. M. Campbell, J. M. Harrison, P. J. Fell, B. Ellers-Lenz, and U. Petzold, "Comparison of the efficacy and tolerability of topically administered azelastine, sodium cromoglycate and placebo in the treatment of seasonal allergic conjunctivitis and rhinoconjunctivitis," *Current Medical Research and Opinion*, vol. 19, no. 4, pp. 313–320, 2003.

[18] W. Lumry, B. Prenner, J. Corren, and W. Wheeler, "Efficacy and safety of azelastine nasal spray at a dose of 1 spray per nostril twice daily," *Annals of Allergy, Asthma and Immunology*, vol. 99, no. 3, pp. 267–272, 2007.

[19] S. Shah, W. Berger, W. Lumry, C. la Force, W. Wheeler, and H. Sacks, "Efficacy and safety of azelastine 0.15% nasal spray and azelastine 0.10% nasal spray in patients with seasonal allergic rhinitis," *Allergy and Asthma Proceedings*, vol. 30, no. 6, pp. 628–633, 2009.

[20] W. C. Howland, N. J. Amar, W. Wheeler, and H. Sacks, "Efficacy and safety of azelastine 0.15% nasal spray administered once daily in patients with allergy to Texas mountain cedar pollen," *International Forum of Allergy & Rhinology*, vol. 1, no. 4, pp. 275–279, 2011.

[21] J. van Bavel, W. C. Howland, N. J. Amar, W. Wheeler, and H. Sacks, "Efficacy and safety of azelastine 0.15% nasal spray administered once daily in subjects with seasonal allergic rhinitis," *Allergy and Asthma Proceedings*, vol. 30, no. 5, pp. 512–518, 2009.

[22] N. Falser, W. Wober, V. W. Rahlfs, and M. Baehre, "Comparative efficacy and safety of azelastine and levocabastine nasal sprays in patients with seasonal allergic rhinitis," *Arzneimittel-Forschung*, vol. 51, no. 5, pp. 387–393, 2001.

[23] D. Charpin, P. Godard, R. P. Garay, M. Baehre, D. Herman, and F. B. Michel, "A multicenter clinical study of the efficacy and tolerability of azelastine nasal spray in the treatment of seasonal allergic rhinitis: a comparison with oral cetirizine," *European Archives of Oto-Rhino-Laryngology*, vol. 252, no. 8, pp. 455–458, 1995.

[24] P. H. Ratner, P. M. Ehrlich, S. M. Fineman, E. O. Meltzer, and D. P. Skoner, "Use of intranasal cromolyn sodium for allergic rhinitis," *Mayo Clinic Proceedings*, vol. 77, no. 4, pp. 350–354, 2002.

[25] D. E. Schuller, J. E. Selcow, T. H. Joos et al., "A multicenter trial of nedocromil sodium, 1% nasal solution, compared with cromolyn sodium and placebo in ragweed seasonal allergic rhinitis," *Journal of Allergy and Clinical Immunology*, vol. 86, no. 4, pp. 554–561, 1990.

[26] E. O. Meltzer, "Efficacy and patient satisfaction with cromolyn sodium nasal solution in the treatment of seasonal allergic rhinitis: a placebo-controlled study," *Clinical Therapeutics*, vol. 24, no. 6, pp. 942–952, 2002.

[27] P. Patel, C. D'Andrea, and H. J. Sacks, "Onset of action of azelastine nasal spray compared with mometasone nasal spray and placebo in subjects with seasonal allergic rhinitis evaluated in an environmental exposure chamber," *American Journal of Rhinology*, vol. 21, no. 4, pp. 499–503, 2007.

12

Clinical Efficacy of a Spray Containing Hyaluronic Acid and Dexpanthenol after Surgery in the Nasal Cavity (Septoplasty, Simple Ethmoid Sinus Surgery, and Turbinate Surgery)

Ina Gouteva,[1] Kija Shah-Hosseini,[1] and Peter Meiser[2]

[1] Institute of Medical Statistics, Informatics and Epidemiology, University Hospital of Cologne, Lindenburger Allee 42, 50931 Cologne, Germany

[2] Ursapharm Arzneimittel GmbH, Industriestraße 35, 66129 Saarbrücken, Germany

Correspondence should be addressed to Ina Gouteva; inagouteva@yahoo.com

Academic Editor: Carlos E. Baena-Cagnani

Background. This prospective, controlled, parallel-group observational study investigated the efficacy of a spray containing hyaluronic acid and dexpanthenol to optimise regular treatment after nasal cavity surgery in 49 patients with chronic rhinosinusitis. *Methods.* The control group received standard therapy. Mucosal regeneration was determined using rhinoscopy sum score (RSS). Pre- and postoperative nasal patency was tested using anterior rhinomanometry. The participants were questioned about their symptoms. *Results.* Regarding all RSS parameters (dryness, dried nasal mucus, fibrin deposition, and obstruction), mucosal regeneration achieved good final results in both groups, tending to a better improvement through the spray application, without statistically significant differences during the whole assessment period, the mean values being 7.04, 5.00, 3.66, and 3.00 (intervention group) and 7.09, 5.14, 4.36, and 3.33 (control group). No statistically significant benefit was identified for nasal breathing, foreign body sensation, and average rhinomanometric volume flow, which improved by 12.31% (control group) and 11.24% (nasal spray group). *Conclusion.* The investigational product may have additional benefit on postoperative mucosal regeneration compared to standard cleaning procedures alone. However, no statistically significant advantage could be observed in this observational study. Double-blind, controlled studies with larger populations will be necessary to evaluate the efficacy of this treatment modality.

1. Introduction

Ventilation, mucociliary transport, and the epithelial barrier are considerably impaired initially following surgical procedures of the nasal cavity.

Injury of the nasal mucosa involved not only with the procedure but also prior to surgery caused by various pathologies usually results in the reduction of the protective secretion film and damage to the highly sensitive cilia [1]. Rapid wound healing from rhinosurgical procedures therefore reduces the risk of new infections considerably.

Although minimally invasive endoscopic technology and instruments enable functional endoscopic paranasal surgery that is gentle to the mucosa, the final results remain dependent upon proper wound healing of the nasal or paranasal mucosa without extreme scarring. Large-scale crusting, mucosal changes, ventilation disorders due to excessive secretion and edema, secondary hemorrhaging, or the development of synechia with possible reobstruction are critical factors that can lead to postoperative complications.

Besides frequent check-ups and wound debridement on the part of the treating physician, meticulous postoperative care of the mucosa using nasal irrigation, inhalation, sprays, and ointments on the part of the patient complements local treatment approaches and the measures taken to prevent adhesion up to the full and proper healing of the wound. In this connection, no established gold standard exists.

At present, investigations are available on a broad spectrum of topical nasal preparations for the postoperative care of the mucosa. To date, however, studies on the combination of hyaluronic acid (HA) and dexpanthenol as the main components of a nasal spray have not yet been carried out.

Hyaluronic acid belongs to the group of glycosaminoglycans and is an omnipresent macromolecule in the interstitium of vertebrates. It is involved in the modulation of various physiological processes (including morphogenesis, regeneration, wound healing, and tumor invasion [2]) and also controls signaling pathways, ergo cell behavior and interactions [2–4].

If tissue continuity is disrupted because of injury, a relatively uniform inflammatory response is induced in the body to break down necrotic tissue, eliminate pathogenic microorganisms, and restore initial integrity through tissue proliferation and repair [5, 6]. As a fundamental component of the extracellular space, hyaluronic acid functions as a framework for wound healing. In addition, it performs other various functions during the regeneration process. Its involvement and specific interaction in subprocesses are complex and to some extent still unknown for the individual steps to be attributed to a specific property.

As a response to tissue injury in the skin, the unusually high hyaluronic acid level influences tissue hydration during the subsequent inflammatory process. This is relevant with regard to cell proliferation and migration, as the pronounced hygroscopy of the polymer increases the moisture content of the tissue locally, which weakens cell adhesion mechanisms in the extracellular matrix and permits temporary separation for the purpose of cell migration and proliferation [7].

Scarless regeneration in human fetal wounds is attributed to unusual hyaluronic acid abundance in the matrix during embryonic development [8, 9].

Diverse biological effects of hyaluronic acid are related to its molecular size. High molecular sized polymers have antiangiogenic and immunosuppressive functions, thereby reflecting intact tissue, while smaller units are distress signals and potent inducers of inflammation, angiogenesis, and mobilization of immune cells [10–12]. Hyaluronic acid and its degradation products originating from the wound healing process are able to regulate tissue or cellular reactions, most notably the promotion of fibroblast proliferation and angiogenesis [2, 13].

The unique viscoelasticity and mucoadhesive capability of hyaluronic acid [14, 15] together with its high immunological and toxicological product safety have led to its versatile use in a number of application forms for various dermatological [16–22], pharmaceutical [3, 14, 23–32], and tissue engineering [33, 34] purposes, or during surgical procedures as well as for postoperative treatment [35–56].

In support of the therapeutic potential of sodium hyaluronate, hysan *Pflegespray* also contains dexpanthenol, which is a long-established active substance having excellent skin tolerance and penetration capacity [57] and a particularly positive impact on the mucociliary clearance of the respiratory epithelium [58, 59].

In the skin, dexpanthenol (provitamin B5) metabolizes to pantothenic acid (vitamin B5), which is essential for the normal function of the epithelial cells, especially during the energy-intensive early phase of epithelial regeneration (within the first 4 days) [60].

Particularly as a topical dermatological preparation for treating wound healing disorders, dermatoses, scars, extensive burn wounds, or skin transplantations [57, 60–62] as well as for treating wounds following nose surgery, the long-established anti-inflammatory and epithelium-protective effect [63] of dexpanthenol has been used for decades in clinical routine [63–66]. Various studies have scientifically confirmed the effectiveness of its preservative-free nasal ointment (predominantly) or spray application forms in treating rhinitis sicca anterior or after nasal and paranasal surgery [63–69]. It also improves the tolerability of rhinological preparations containing preservatives [1, 66, 69]. The local application of dexpanthenol in acute and chronic rhinitis is a part of routine standard therapy [66].

Corresponding to clinical experience, external therapy with dexpanthenol preparations is normally considered very well tolerated, having a minimum risk of skin irritations or sensitization [70].

Even though hyaluronic acid and dexpanthenol have long been clinically proven to be antiadhesive and mucosal conditioning substances separately, no study has yet investigated the possibility of a more intensive, wound-healing promotive effect based on the synergy of their set combination in a nasal spray. This was the reason that this dual-center, clinical trial examined a CE-labelled medical device (nasal spray) which was used for its intended purpose of regenerating damaged nasal mucosa; the study was carried out in strict accordance with the definition of nonintervention [71].

2. Patients and Methods

2.1. Patients. Included in the study were patients who suffered from chronic rhinosinusitis and who had undergone the following surgical procedures of the nasal cavity: septoplasty, simple ethmoid surgery, turbinate surgery, pansinus surgery, and maxillary sinus surgery.

The total population consisted of 49 patients. Of these, 27 patients were assigned to the intervention group. The other 22 patients comprised the control group which received customary conditioning preparations that were not documented.

2.2. Design. This trial was carried out as a prospective, open-label, observational study in two doctor's offices from 11 September 2008 to 13 September 2011. Investigators collected test results and the patients' subjective assessments at a minimum of five check-up visits, the initial examination, three intermediate examinations, and one final examination, and documented the data in the observation form.

At the initial examination, the patient was thoroughly informed about the planned noninterventional study, indications for surgery, and preoperative rhinomanometry. Patients were not randomised to receive the study medication. The choice of the appropriate postsurgical care was based on the investigator's judgement of the patients' clinical condition after surgery and the patients' willingness to apply the spray regularly instead of using the alternative nasal pipetting or ointments.

All participating patients signed a data privacy declaration form, giving their consent to allow their data in pseudonymous form to be recorded and forwarded to the sponsor or competent authorities.

This observational study examines how wound healing is influenced after the first check-up and after removal of packing material, if inserted. This was not documented in the observation form and was not considered in the results.

Furthermore, the adjuvant postoperative administration of antibiotics, antiphlogistics, or analgesics as concomitant medication, if necessary, was recorded.

A repeated anterior rhinomanometry (at visit 1 in the 1st postoperative week) and anterior rhinoscopy (optional endoscopy) (at all other visits in accordance with the observation schedule) were conducted for documentation purposes, for monitoring the final results of surgical treatment with respect to nasal patency, and for the visual assessment of nasal mucosa conditions. In addition, the patients were questioned about their subjective perceptions with respect to nasal breathing and foreign body sensation, tolerability of the nasal spray, and any noticeable problems or complaints in connection with the preparation used.

This paper was compiled in accordance with the STROBE (strengthening the reporting of observational studies in epidemiology) statement.

2.3. Ethical Aspects and Professional Regulations.

The investigational preparation and the control medication were both CE-certified. According to the Medical Devices Act, this investigation was therefore exempted from requiring approval from the competent federal authority and the competent ethics committee. Investigators in charge of the study received consultation with respect to professional regulations before the study commenced.

2.4. Study Medication.

The object of the investigation was the nonprescription "hysan Pflegespray" manufactured by Ursapharm Arzneimittel GmbH, Saarbrücken, Germany. At the beginning of the study (2008), the product was called "Hylocare-Nasenspray." It was renamed "hysan Pflegespray" in 2011. It is a liquid pharmaceutical preparation with a dosing spray applicator for the prophylactic or curative topical treatment of inflammatory conditions. It can be applied as monotherapy as well as a concomitant adjuvant to therapy with decongestant nasal sprays (or drops) for rhinosinusitis.

Hysan Pflegespray is a sterile, preservative-free solution containing 0.25 mg/mL sodium hyaluronate, 2% dexpanthenol, as well as sodium dihydrogen phosphate × $2H_2O$, sodium monohydrogen phosphate × $2H_2O$, sorbitol, and water. One bottle contains 10 mL of solution, which corresponds to approximately 70 sprays [72].

2.5. Dosage of Study Medication.

One to two puffs of nasal spray to each nostril were to be administered three times, distributed evenly throughout the day. If additional therapy with other nasal sprays was applied, nasal spray was always to be used last, allowing at least 30 minutes to elapse between nasal sprays.

2.6. Conventional Care Preparations.

Treating otolaryngologist Nr. 1 administered a proprietary composed solution for pipetting by the patients 3-4 throughout the day in both nasal cavities, with the following ingredients: glucose-monohydrate: 5.0 g, menthol: 0,025 g, Olynth 0.1% nasal drops (active agent: xylometazoline hydrochloride): 5.0 g, eucerinum anhydricum: 7.0 g, and peanut oil: ad. 50.0 g.

Treating otolaryngologist Nr. 2 prescribed a proprietary composed ointment as a standard local postoperative care formulation which was to be applied twice a day. The ingredients of the mixture were hydrocortisone: 0.01 g, vitamin A (retinoic acid): 0.4 g, Bepanthen ointment (active agent 5% Dexpanthenol): 16.0 g, and Otrivin nasal drops 0.1% (active agent: xylometazoline hydrochloride): 1 g.

Both preparations were individually compounded by a pharmacist.

2.7. Recording of Efficacy.

The primary variable was changed in the sum score (RSS: rhinoscopy sum score), which was attained from the clinical, objectively recorded endoscopy findings: nasal dryness, dried nasal mucus, fibrin deposition, and nasal obstruction. All variables pertaining to rhinoscopic mucosal findings were evaluated using a 4-point scale as follows: absent = 0, mild = 1, moderate = 2, and severe = 3.

For the secondary variable, the patient's subjective perception of unobstructed nasal breathing and foreign body sensation was rated on a scale from 1 to 3 (1 = good, 2 = average, and 3 = poor).

In order to categorize the initial symptom situation and objectivization of patients' statements on symptoms of nasal obstruction and to record the effectiveness of surgery and the monitoring of the final results of surgery, pre- and postoperative active anterior rhinomanometry were carried out at the initial examination.

The treating physician recorded general efficacy and tolerability in free-text format at the end of the observation period.

2.8. Recording of Safety.

In spite of the broad clinical experience with both active ingredients contained in nasal spray, special importance was attached to the documentation of adverse events when collecting data in the present study.

The holder of the marketing authorization for the medical device investigated here was obliged to report the severity or intensity of adverse events to the Bundesinstitut für Arzneimittel und Medizinprodukte (The Federal Institute for Drugs and Medical Devices, Pharmacovigilance Division). The treating physician was also able to document his/her own or the others comments or noticeable signs relating to the patient's general condition, product use, or general remarks about the course of treatment in free-text format on the observation forms under "Other notes."

3. Analysis

3.1. Handling of Documentation Errors and Analysis Problems.

Missing entries resulted in incomplete data sets, so individual parameters could not be evaluated. These missing data were

TABLE 1: Rhinoscopy sum score (RSS), postoperative. Confidence interval 95%.

		RSS week 1	RSS week 2	RSS week 4	RSS week 6
Control group	N (valid)	22	21	19	18
	Mean	**7.09**	**5.14**	**4.36**	**3.33**
	Standard deviation	1.77037	1.98206	1.77045	1.97037
Nasal spray group	N (valid)	24	24	21	19
	Mean	**7.04**	**5.00**	**3.66**	**3.00**
	Standard deviation	2.23566	1.41421	1.49443	1.63299

generally treated as "missing values" and not taken into consideration in the analysis.

3.2. Statistics. The detailed analysis of the parameters was carried out using SPSS 19 statistics software manufactured by SPSS Inc. Frequencies, mean values, standard deviations, medians, and minimum and maximum values within the treatment groups were given for the various variable forms.

To this purpose, patient data were first entered into separate SPSS databases by two people independent of each other. The monitoring person in charge recognized all occurring discrepancies and illogical values. The merged database underwent a plausibility test. Data were then synchronized and subsequently analyzed in SPSS. A significance level of $\alpha = 0.05$ was defined for all statistical tests.

3.3. Data Analysis. Descriptive statistical methods were applied. The statistical values (number, mean value, minimum, maximum, and standard deviation) for continuous variables such as height, age, and time periods were listed in a table. Discrete variables were categorized in the form of frequency distributions with their percentage-wise relationships to the total sample. Free-text answers were transferred post hoc in the appropriate coding schemes and analyzed as frequency distributions. Clinical parameters of disease progression were evaluated and illustrated in the form of intraindividual differential analyses (first versus last examination). Categorically recorded clinical data were analyzed in the form of contingency analyses (before/after). Subgroup analyses were not defined a priori. Any results yielded using comparative statistical methods were of purely explorative character.

4. Results

4.1. Patients: Demographic Data. Overall, 49 patients participated in the study, 8 of whom were female and 41 male. Patients were aged 15 to 58 years (mean age of the total population was 33.12 years, SD: ±11.04 years).

4.2. Rhino-/Endoscopic Mucosal Findings. A scale from 0 to 3 (0 = none, 1 = mild, 2 = moderate, and 3 = severe) was used to assess all parameters (nasal dryness, dried nasal mucus, fibrin deposition, and development of obstructions). The treating physician thereby documented, added, and averaged the mucosal findings obtained via rhinoscopy/endoscopy during the weeklong application of the nasal spray. The resulting

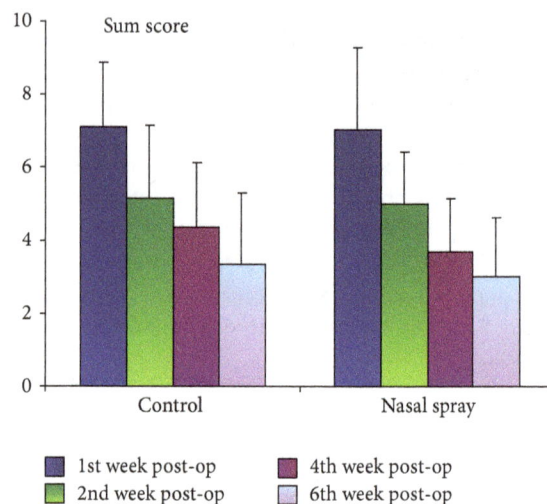

FIGURE 1: Rhinoscopy sum score (RSS) of the individual groups.

rhinoscopy sum score (RSS) is shown in Table 1 and illustrated in Figure 1. Details for each individual parameter can be found in Table 2.

4.3. Patient Evaluation of Nasal Breathing and Foreign Body Sensation. A scale from 1 to 3 (1 = good, 2 = moderate, and 3 = poor) was used for the patients' self-assessment of nasal breathing. The patients rated their subjective perception of a foreign body during the entire postoperative follow-up interval on a scale from 0 to 2 (0 = absent, 1 = moderate, and 2 = severe).

4.4. Pre- and Postoperative Rhinomanometry (8th–10th Postoperative Day). The comparison between pre- and postoperative rhinomanometry shows a similar percentage increase for the mean volume flow in both comparison groups: hysan group 11.24% and control 12.31% (Table 4, Figure 2). Here, the mean preoperative volume flow of 688.13 mL/s (±209.524 mL/s) in the hysan group was slightly above the initial value for the control group at 643.16 mL/s (±188.253 mL/s).

5. Discussion

In spite of gender inhomogeneity, both patient populations were comparable.

TABLE 2: Individual rhinoscopy findings during the examination period (1st–6th postoperative week).

Post-op week		"Dryness"				"Dried nasal mucus"				"Fibrin deposition"				"Obstruction"			
		1.	2.	4.	6.	1.	2.	4.	6.	1.	2.	4.	6.	1.	2.	4.	6.
Control group	N (valid)	22	21	19	18	22	21	19	18	22	21	19	18	22	21	19	18
	MV	1.64	1.24	1.21	0.83	1.95	1.33	1.16	0.89	1.86	1.33	1.11	0.89	1.64	1.24	0.89	0.72
	SD	0.581	0.539	0.535	0.514	0.653	0.658	0.501	0.583	0.468	0.483	0.567	0.583	0.581	0.539	0.459	0.575
Nasal spray group	N (valid)	24	24	21	19	24	24	21	19	24	24	21	19	24	24	21	19
	MV	1.67	1.25	1.00	0.84	1.92	1.29	0.95	0.74	1.83	1.42	0.90	0.74	1.63	1.04	0.81	0.68
	SD	0.702	0.442	0.316	0.375	0.717	0.464	0.384	0.452	0.702	0.504	0.436	0.452	0.576	0.359	0.602	0.478

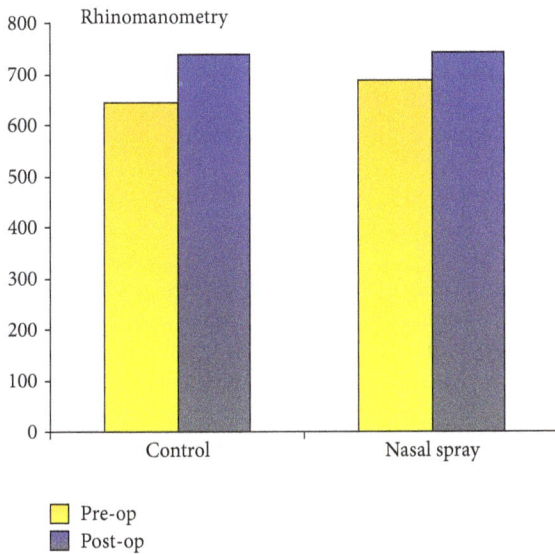

FIGURE 2: Values for pre- and postoperative rhinomanometry in [mL/s] at 150 Pa, sum left and right nasal cavity. Bar graph.

It was up to the treating physician to decide whether the patient required concomitant medication in the postoperative healing period. No valid conclusion could be made with regard to the possible influence of antibiotics, antiphlogistics, or analgesics on the effect of hysan nasal spray.

In both patient populations, the condition of the endonasal mucosa improved continuously during the follow-up period with respect to the defined objective parameters (nasal dryness, dried nasal mucus, fibrin deposition, and obstruction). The mean RSS values, however, exhibited no significant differences between both populations (see Table 1). Nevertheless, the hysan group showed lower values in the 4th and 6th week (3.66 pts. and 3.00 pts., resp.) compared to the control group (4.36 pts. and 3.33 pts., resp.). A clinical comparison of an isotonic saline spray containing dexpanthenol with a simple saline spray for postoperative treatment over 6 weeks showed comparable efficacy regarding all objective parameters of the endoscopic mucosal analysis and the majority of subjective symptoms as well [59]. Another similarly designed study compared an ointment containing hyaluronic acid (Rhinogen) with a plant-based ointment (H.E.C.). Both preparations, yet again, did not differ significantly with respect to the objective parameters of

mucosal dehydration, formation of blood clots, and mucosal lesions [73].

Furthermore, the application of the control substances might have led to falsified results in the control group, because of the potentially positive effects of their active agents on the wound healing process. An enhancing effect on morphological and functional cilia regeneration has been ascribed to retinoic acid [74–77]. Systemic prednisolone administration together with local application of 5% of dexpanthenol ointment had a beneficial effect especially on the late spontaneous wound closure in a standardized animal model [68]. On the other hand, the addition of dexpanthenol (5%) resulted in a statistically significant reduction of the toxicity of α-sympathomimetic decongestants like xylomethazoline [63].

Mean values for the rhinoscopic parameter of nasal dryness were almost identical in both groups of this observational study except in the 4th postoperative week (Table 2). In the control group, the mean value at visit 2 (1.24 pt.) dropped only slightly by visit 3 (1.21 pt.), while it decreased more in the intervention group (from 1.25 to 1.00 pt.: no statistical significance). This fact could be attributed to the intense hydration effect of hyaluronic acid. This explanation was based on the important clinical observations made by Soldati et al. that the application of the hyaluronic acid containing ointment prevented large-scale crusting in the first postoperative week compared to the control substance [73].

The mean values for the parameter dried nasal mucus exhibited almost analogous dynamics (Table 2). Although a greater decrease in the mean value for the degree of dried nasal mucus was observed among hysan users in the 4th and 6th weeks, it did not reach a level of significance. This was probably ascribed to the increased local hydration due to hyaluronic acid, which formed an even, stable, and long-lasting moisture film on the nasal mucosa, thereby serving as a lubricant during the vulnerable regeneration process and as a vehicle for dexpanthenol in the late phase of wound healing phase, allowing its full cilia-protective effect to unfold. Consequently, the improved mucociliary clearance helped gently loosen dried nasal mucus.

The significantly decreased crusting during the 1st and 2nd postoperative weeks after applying a combination solution for mucosal care (that contained isotonic saline, algae extract, hyaluronic acid, panthenol, and Tonimer Gel Spray) may also support this assumption [78]. Another clinical

TABLE 3: Patient evaluation of nasal breathing and foreign body sensation.

Postoperative week		Nasal breathing				Foreign body sensation
		1.	2.	4.	6.	1–6.
Control group	N (valid)	21	21	19	18	21
	Mean value	**1.90**	**1.48**	**1.11**	**1.00**	**0.52**
	SD	0.625	0.512	0.315	0.000	0.512
Nasal spray group	N (valid)	24	24	20	19	24
	Mean value	**1.58**	**1.25**	**1.10**	**0.95**	**0.71**
	SD	0.584	0.442	0.447	0.229	0.464

comparison between dexpanthenol seawater spray (Mar plus) and normal saline irrigation resulted in less crusting at the 2nd check-up visit and better mucociliary clearance at the 4th check-up in the intervention group [79].

A clinical reduction in the formation of dried nasal mucus was observed after an 8-week treatment with dexpanthenol in a spray application form in patients with chronic rhinitis sicca as well [65]. Analogous results were shown by Hahn et al. after the four-week application of a dexpanthenol ointment [80].

The mean values for fibrin deposition in the hysan group were somewhat lower in the late phase of wound healing between the 4th and 6th postoperative weeks compared to the prior weeks (Table 2).

The last mucosal findings collected by the treating physician concerned nasal obstruction as observed via rhinoscopy. At all scheduled examinations, the results of both groups were of similar magnitude and without statistically significant differences (Table 2). Notable were the initially rapid drop of the mean value in the hysan group in the 2nd week and the consistent small decline over the remaining three visits. This tendency gave rise to the presumption that the use of the nasal spray greatly reduced nasal mucosal obstruction in the early phase of wound healing and was responsible for lower mean values in general over the entire period of application. In the end, however, no considerably better results were obtained than in the control group.

This correlation could lead one to assume that, due to hyaluronic acid, increased tissue hydration, which according to Kühnel et al. enables the early reduction of dried nasal mucus [81], and the reduced formation of hyperplastic granulation tissue [68, 82], as well as the accelerated reepithelialization due to dexpanthenol [82], resulted synergistically in diminished postoperative nasal obstruction symptoms. Our study, however, could not clearly verify this theory.

The subjects were asked to categorize their subjective perceptions of free nasal breathing and foreign body sensation on the observation form, since according to definition an observational study is to consider the individual assessments of the product users as an important influencing factor. The results are summarized in Table 3.

The responses from the nasal spray patients at the first two examinations are striking with their low mean values for free nasal breathing, again without significant differences to the control group. The results were almost identical for the last visits in both groups (Table 3). This fact suggests

that patients tended to perceive nasal breathing as freer while using hysan spray during early postoperative tissue regeneration. A possible explanation for this could be the film formed by the aerosol of the nasal spray that temporarily covered the mucosal areas and which the patient mistakenly interpreted as mildly impaired nasal breathing in the last two weeks.

Similar results of positive influence of an isotonic seawater spray containing dexpanthenol on the total nasal subjective symptom score and on patient satisfaction, although again without significance, were confirmed by Fooanant et al. [79].

In this connection, conflicting results have been mostly published in the literature. A significant improvement of the patient-reported comfort (ease of breathing, nasal tension, and feeling of dryness) has been observed by Ercan et al. [78]. Soldati et al. also confirmed a significant improvement in respiration among subjects who applied ointment containing hyaluronic acid, with nasal patency being highly significant on the 7th postoperative day and significant on the 14th postoperative day [73]. Kehrl and Sonnemann [65] and Hahn [80] verified positive dynamics in the subjective sensory scale in terms of nasal airway obstruction among dexpanthenol spray users with rhinitis sicca. Significant improvement of nasal obstruction showed a saline aerosol containing hyaluronic acid in the phase of functional regeneration during sinonasal remodeling, as described by Macchi et al. [83].

The mean value for patient's self-assessment of foreign body sensation was in general relatively positive (Table 3). Limitations existed with respect to the time at which this symptom appeared (the parameter was not enquired upon at every scheduled examination but instead globally assessed for the entire postoperative interval). Contrary to expectations, at a value of 0.52 points in the control group it tended to fall into the category "not present," and at 0.71 points, the parameter tended slightly to "moderately pronounced" among hysan users. One reason for this could be the protective film on the mucosa as mentioned earlier that compromised the patients' perception of a foreign body.

Rhinomanometry data confirmed volume enlargement of the nasal cavity by 12.31% in the control group and by 11.24% in the intervention group, the difference not being statistically significant (Table 4). The application of the test substance (period: 8th–10th postoperative day) resulted

TABLE 4: Values for pre- and postoperative rhinomanometry in [mL/s] at 150 Pa, sum left and right nasal cavity.

		Preoperative rhinomanometry sum left and right at 150 Pa in [mL/s]	Postoperative rhinomanometry sum left and right at 150 Pa in [mL/s]	Delta rhinomanometry	Improvement in %
Control group	N (valid)	19	18	16	
	Mean value	643.16	737.67	79.19	12.31
	SD	188.253	118.457	179.300	
Nasal spray group	N (valid)	23	19	18	
	Mean value	688.13	743.05	77.33	11.24
	SD	209.524	140.956	206.292	

in no significant, objectively measured reduction in nasal resistance. Volume enlargement of the nasal cavity relies in fact only on structure-reducing measures which successfully eliminated any obstruction to nasal breathing.

The investigator's impressions concerning the good tolerability and efficacy of the preparation agreed to a large extent with those of the patients and with the literature.

Soldati et al. also reported high acceptance, safety, and tolerability of the ointment containing hyaluronic acid. Worth mentioning, besides the positive organoleptic evaluation relating to the smell and the sensation of cooling upon application, was also the absence of adverse reactions [73]. The study conducted by Fooanant et al. yielded similarly good results for the dexpanthenol spray with respect to effectiveness and patient satisfaction [79]. The positive influence of dexpanthenol preparations on the subjective symptoms in patients with rhinitis sicca [65, 80] and their high acceptance were, yet again, able to confirm the clinically relevant and statistically significant superiority of the substance.

Dropouts were the most common subject appearing in the text field "other doctor's comments." Only one mild irritation was noted, probably due to intolerance of one of the ingredients; no entry, however, was made under the item "adverse events" on the observation form.

6. Conclusion

Surgical procedures of the paranasal sinuses leave behind extensive wounds that are left up to the secondary self-healing process [6, 84]. The aim of postoperative treatment is optimum wound healing with minimal morbidity.

The present limited observational study showed that the nasal spray is a safe preparation for care of the mucosa after rhinosurgical procedures. Its use did not negatively affect postoperative mucosal regeneration, yet no significant improvement of mucosal conditions could be observed either.

The results might have been impaired by the two treating physicians, who might have not always assessed the nasal mucosa conditions identically, by the possible positive influence of the active ingredients of the conventional care preparations on the control group, or by the unbalanced concomitant use of antibiotics and anti-inflammatory medication. Furthermore, the conclusions of the study might have somewhat been affected by the limited participants

number, by the lack of randomization and blinding, by the heterogeneity of the initial pathology state among the patients, or by the variety of the surgical procedures that are scarcely comparable.

Additional multicenter, double-blind studies with larger populations, having a comparable degree of pathology and extent of mucosal extirpation in the same surgical procedure along with detailed surveys, are necessary to clarify further aspects of postoperative wound healing processes of the respiratory epithelium and the influence thereof for achieving adequate functional regeneration and better quality of life.

Conflict of Interests

The authors declare that there is no conflict of interests regarding the publication of this paper.

Acknowledgments

The authors would like to thank Gena Kittel for her editorial assistance. Hysan spray was provided by Ursapharm-Arzneimittel GmbH, Saarbrücken, Germany.

References

[1] T. Verse, C. Sikora, P. Rudolph, and N. Klöcker, "Die Verträglichkeit von Nasalia unter besonderer Berücksichtigung des Einflusses von Konservierungsmitteln und physikalisch-chemischen Parametern," Laryngo-Rhino-Otologie, vol. 82, no. 11, pp. 782–789, 2003.

[2] B. P. Toole, "Hyaluronan in morphogenesis," Seminars in Cell and Developmental Biology, vol. 12, no. 2, pp. 79–87, 2001.

[3] Y.-H. Liao, S. A. Jones, B. Forbes, G. P. Martin, and M. B. Brown, "Hyaluronan: pharmaceutical characterization and drug delivery," Drug Delivery, vol. 12, no. 6, pp. 327–342, 2005.

[4] B. P. Toole, "Hyaluronan is not just a goo!," The Journal of Clinical Investigation, vol. 106, no. 3, pp. 335–336, 2000.

[5] R. Weber, R. Keerl, A. Huppmann, B. Schick, and W. Draf, "Der Einfluß der Nachbehandlung auf die Wundheilung nach endonasaler Nasennebenhöhlenoperation," Laryngo-Rhino-Otologie, vol. 75, no. 4, pp. 208–214, 1996.

[6] W. Hosemann, L. Dunker, U. Göde, and M. E. Wigand, "Experimentelle Untersuchungen zur Wundheilung in den Nasennebenhöhlen. III. Endoskopie und Histologie des Operationsgebietes nach einer endonasalen Siebbeinausräumung," HNO, vol. 39, pp. 111–115, 1991.

[7] W. Y. Chen and G. Abatangelo, "Functions of hyaluronan in wound repair," *Wound Repair and Regeneration*, vol. 7, no. 2, pp. 79–89, 1999.

[8] J. A. Iocono, H. P. Ehrlich, K. A. Keefer, and T. M. Krummel, "Hyaluronan induces scarless repair in mouse limb organ culture," *Journal of Pediatric Surgery*, vol. 33, no. 4, pp. 564–567, 1998.

[9] P. Samuels and A. K. Tan, "Fetal scarless wound healing," *The Journal of Otolaryngology*, vol. 28, no. 5, pp. 296–302, 1999.

[10] R. Stern and H. I. Maibach, "Hyaluronan in skin: aspects of aging and its pharmacologic modulation," *Clinics in Dermatology*, vol. 26, no. 2, pp. 106–122, 2008.

[11] P. W. Noble, "Hyaluronan and its catabolic products in tissue injury and repair," *Matrix Biology*, vol. 21, no. 1, pp. 25–29, 2002.

[12] R. Krasinski and H. Tchorzewski, "Hyaluronan-mediated regulation of inflammation," *Postępy Higieny i Medycyny Doświadczalnej*, vol. 61, pp. 683–689, 2007.

[13] M. Prosdocimi and C. Bevilacqua, "Exogenous hyaluronic acid and wound healing: an updated vision," *Panminerva Medica*, vol. 54, no. 2, pp. 129–135, 2012.

[14] A. Ludwig, "The use of mucoadhesive polymers in ocular drug delivery," *Advanced Drug Delivery Reviews*, vol. 57, no. 11, pp. 1595–1639, 2005.

[15] M. F. Saettone, D. Monti, M. T. Torracca, and P. Chetoni, "Mucoadhesive ophthalmic vehicles: evaluation of polymeric low-viscosity formulations," *Journal of Ocular Pharmacology*, vol. 10, no. 1, pp. 83–92, 1994.

[16] R. J. Rohrich, A. Ghavami, and M. A. Crosby, "The role of hyaluronic acid fillers (Restylane) in facial cosmetic surgery: review and technical considerations," *Plastic and Reconstructive Surgery*, vol. 120, no. 6, 2007.

[17] K. L. Beasley, M. A. Weiss, and R. A. Weiss, "Hyaluronic acid fillers: a comprehensive review," *Facial Plastic Surgery*, vol. 25, no. 2, pp. 86–94, 2009.

[18] T. Y. Han, J.W. Lee, J. H. Lee et al., "Subdermal minimal surgery with hyaluronic acid as an effective treatment for neck wrinkles," *Dermatologic Surgery*, vol. 37, no. 9, pp. 1291–1296, 2011.

[19] C. Muhn, N. Rosen, N. Solish et al., "The evolving role of hyaluronic acid fillers for facial volume restoration and contouring: a Canadian overview," *Clinical, Cosmetic and Investigational Dermatology*, vol. 5, pp. 147–158, 2012.

[20] V. S. Lambros, "Hyaluronic acid injections for correction of the tear trough deformity," *Plastic and Reconstructive Surgery*, vol. 120, no. 6, pp. 74S–80S, 2007.

[21] S. Nanda and S. Bansal, "Upper face rejuvenation using botulinum toxin and hyaluronic acid fillers," *Indian Journal of Dermatology, Venereology and Leprology*, vol. 79, no. 1, pp. 32–40, 2013.

[22] A. Redaelli, "Medical rhinoplasty with hyaluronic acid and botulinum toxin A: a very simple and quite effective technique," *Journal of Cosmetic Dermatology*, vol. 7, no. 3, pp. 210–220, 2008.

[23] K. P. Vercruysse and G. D. Prestwich, "Hyaluronate derivatives in drug delivery," *Critical Reviews in Therapeutic Drug Carrier Systems*, vol. 15, no. 5, pp. 513–555, 1998.

[24] K. Morimoto, H. Yamaguchi, Y. Iwakura, K. Morisaka, Y. Ohashi, and Y. Nakai, "Effects of viscous hyaluronate-sodium solutions on the nasal absorption of vasopressin and an analogue," *Pharmaceutical Research*, vol. 8, no. 4, pp. 471–474, 1991.

[25] Türker S., E. Onur, and Y. Ozer, "Nasal route and drug delivery systems," *Pharmacy World and Science*, vol. 26, no. 3, pp. 137–142, 2004.

[26] M. I. Ugwoke, R. U. Agu, N. Verbeke, and R. Kinget, "Nasal mucoadhesive drug delivery: background, applications, trends and future perspectives," *Advanced Drug Delivery Reviews*, vol. 57, no. 11, pp. 1640–1665, 2005.

[27] Y. Huh, H. Cho, I. Yoon et al., "Preparation and evaluation of spray-dried hyaluronic acid microspheres for intranasal delivery of fexofenadine hydrochloride," *European Journal of Pharmaceutical Sciences*, vol. 40, no. 1, pp. 9–15, 2010.

[28] K. Y. Cho, T. W. Chung, B. C. Kim et al., "Release of ciprofloxacin from poloxamer-graft-hyaluronic acid hydrogels in vitro," *International Journal of Pharmaceutics*, vol. 260, no. 1, pp. 83–91, 2003.

[29] S. T. Lim, G. P. Martin, D. J. Berry, and M. B. Brown, "Preparation and evaluation of the in vitro drug release properties and mucoadhesion of novel microspheres of hyaluronic acid and chitosan," *Journal of Controlled Release*, vol. 66, no. 2-3, pp. 281–292, 2000.

[30] H. Wolburg, K. Wolburg-Buchholz, H. Sam, S. Horvát, M. A. Deli, and A. F. Mack, "Epithelial and endothelial barriers in the olfactory region of the nasal cavity of the rat," *Histochemistry and Cell Biology*, vol. 130, no. 1, pp. 127–140, 2008.

[31] C. M. Lehr, "Lectin-mediated drug delivery: the second generation of bioadhesives," *Journal of Controlled Release*, vol. 65, no. 1-2, pp. 19–29, 2000.

[32] S. Horvát, A. Fehér, H. Wolburg et al., "Sodium hyaluronate as a mucoadhesive component in nasal formulation enhances delivery of molecules to brain tissue," *European Journal of Pharmaceutics and Biopharmaceutics*, vol. 72, no. 1, pp. 252–259, 2009.

[33] J. Aigner, J. Tegeler, P. Hutzler et al., "Cartilage tissue engineering with novel nonwoven structured biomaterial based on hyaluronic acid benzyl ester," *Journal of Biomedical Materials Research*, vol. 42, no. 2, pp. 172–181, 1998.

[34] T.-W. Huang, Cheng P. W., Y. H. Chan, T. H. Yeh, Y. H. Young, and T. H. Young, "Regulation of ciliary differentiation of human respiratory epithelial cells by the receptor for hyaluronan-mediated motility on hyaluronan-based biomaterials," *Biomaterials*, vol. 31, no. 26, pp. 6701–6709, 2010.

[35] E. A. Balazs, "Hyaluronan as an ophthalmic viscoelastic device," *Current Pharmaceutical Biotechnology*, vol. 9, no. 4, pp. 236–238, 2008.

[36] C. Schramm, M. S. Spitzer, S. Henke-Fahle et al., "The cross-linked biopolymer hyaluronic acid as an artificial vitreous substitute," *Investigative Ophthalmology and Visual Science*, vol. 53, no. 2, pp. 613–621, 2012.

[37] K. Takeuchi, M. Nakazawa, T. Metoki, H. Yamazaki, Y. Miyagawa, and T. Ito, "Effects of solid hyaluronic acid film on postoperative fibrous scar formation after strabismus surgery in animals," *Journal of Pediatric Ophthalmology and Strabismus*, vol. 48, no. 5, pp. 301–304, 2011.

[38] K. Takeuchi, M. Nakazawa, H. Yamazaki et al., "Solid hyaluronic acid film and the prevention of postoperative fibrous scar formation in experimental animal eyes," *Archives of Ophthalmology*, vol. 127, no. 4, pp. 460–466, 2009.

[39] P. I. Condon, C. G. McEwen, M. Wright, G. Mackintosh, R. J. Prescott, and C. McDonald, "Double blind, randomised, placebo controlled, crossover, multicentre study to determine the efficacy of a 0.1% (w/v) sodium hyaluronate solution (Fermavisc) in the treatment of dry eye syndrome," *The British Journal of Ophthalmology*, vol. 83, no. 10, pp. 1121–1124, 1999.

[40] C. C. McDonald, S. B. Kaye, F. C. Figueiredo, G. Macintosh, and C. Lockett, "A randomised, crossover, multicentre study to

compare the performance of 0.1% (w/v) sodium hyaluronate with 1.4% (w/v) polyvinyl alcohol in the alleviation of symptoms associated with dry eye syndrome," *Eye*, vol. 16, no. 5, pp. 601–607, 2002.

[41] P. Aragona, G. Di Stefano, F. Ferreri, R. Spinella, and A. Stilo, "Sodium hyaluronate eye drops of different osmolarity for the treatment of dry eye in Sjögren's syndrome patients," *British Journal of Ophthalmology*, vol. 86, no. 8, pp. 879–884, 2002.

[42] M. Berlucchi, P. Castelnuovo, A. Vincenzi, B. Morra, and E. Pasquini, "Endoscopic outcomes of resorbable nasal packing after functional endoscopic sinus surgery: a multicenter prospective randomized controlled study," *European Archives of Oto-Rhino-Laryngology*, vol. 266, no. 6, pp. 839–845, 2009.

[43] R. Valentine and P. Wormald, "Nasal dressings after endoscopic sinus surgery: what and why?" *Current Opinion in Otolaryngology & Head and Neck Surgery*, vol. 18, no. 1, pp. 44–48, 2010.

[44] R. K. Weber and U. Hay, "Ist die Nasentamponade noch zeitgemäß?" *Laryngo-Rhino-Otologie*, vol. 82, no. 9, pp. 650–654, 2003.

[45] B. A. Woodworth, R. K. Chandra, M. J. Hoy, F. S. Lee, R. J. Schlosser, and M. B. Gillespie, "Randomized controlled trial of hyaluronic acid/carboxymethylcellulose dressing after endoscopic sinus surgery," *ORL*, vol. 72, no. 2, pp. 101–105, 2010.

[46] K. E. Rodgers, D. B. Johns, W. Girgis, J. Campeau, and G. S. diZerega, "Reduction of adhesion formation with hyaluronic acid after peritoneal surgery in rabbits," *Fertility and Sterility*, vol. 67, no. 3, pp. 553–558, 1997.

[47] D. B. Johns, Rodgers K. E., Donahue W. D., T. C. Kiorpes, and G. S. diZerega, "Reduction of adhesion formation by postoperative administration of ionically cross-linked hyaluronic acid," *Fertility and Sterility*, vol. 68, no. 1, pp. 37–42, 1997.

[48] R. E. Leach, J. W. Burns, E. J. Dawe, M. D. Smithbarbour, and M. P. Diamond, "Reduction of postsurgical adhesion formation in the rabbit uterine horn model with use of hyaluronate/carboxymethylcellulose gel," *Fertility and Sterility*, vol. 69, no. 3, pp. 415–418, 1998.

[49] J. W. Burns, K. Skinner, M. J. Colt, L. Burgess, R. Rose, and M. P. Diamond, "A hyaluronate based gel for the prevention of postsurgical adhesions: evaluation in two animal species," *Fertility and Sterility*, vol. 66, no. 5, pp. 814–821, 1996.

[50] E. P. Goldberg, J. W. Burns, and Y. Yaacobi, "Prevention of postoperative adhesions by precoating tissues with dilute sodium hyaluronate solutions," *Progress in Clinical and Biological Research*, vol. 381, pp. 191–204, 1993.

[51] J. M. Becker, M. T. Dayton, V. W. Fazio et al., "Prevention of postoperative abdominal adhesions by a sodium hyaluronate-based bioresorbable membrane: a prospective, randomized, double-blind multicenter study," *Journal of the American College of Surgeons*, vol. 183, no. 4, pp. 297–306, 1996.

[52] G. T. Fossum, K. M. Silverberg, C. E. Miller, M. P. Diamond, and L. Holmdahl, "Gynecologic use of Sepraspray Adhesion Barrier for reduction of adhesion development after laparoscopic myomectomy: a pilot study," *Fertility and Sterility*, vol. 96, no. 2, pp. 487–491, 2011.

[53] L. S. Lohmander, N. Dalén, G. Englund et al., "Intra-articular hyaluronan injections in the treatment of osteoarthritis of the knee: a randomised, double blind, placebo controlled multicentre trial," *Annals of the Rheumatic Diseases*, vol. 55, no. 7, pp. 424–431, 1996.

[54] R. W. Jubb, S. Piva, L. Beinat, J. Dacre, and P. Gishen, "A one-year, randomised, placebo (saline) controlled clinical trial of 500–730 kDa sodium hyaluronate (Hyalgan) on the radiological change in osteoarthritis of the knee," *International Journal of Clinical Practice*, vol. 57, no. 6, pp. 467–474, 2003.

[55] J. Karlsson, L. S. Sjögren, and L. S. Lohmander, "Comparison of two hyaluronan drugs and placebo in patients with knee osteoarthritis. A controlled, randomized, double-blind, parallel-design multicentre study," *Rheumatology*, vol. 41, no. 11, pp. 1240–1248, 2002.

[56] S. S. Leopold, B. B. Redd, W. J. Warme, P. A. Wehrle, P. D. Pettis, and S. Shott, "Corticosteroid compared with hyaluronic acid injections for the treatment of osteoarthritis of the knee. A prospective, randomized trial," *The Journal of Bone and Joint Surgery A*, vol. 85, no. 7, pp. 1197–1203, 2003.

[57] F. Ebner, A. Heller, F. Rippke, and I. Tausch, "Topical use of dexpanthenol in skin disorders," *American Journal of Clinical Dermatology*, vol. 3, no. 6, pp. 427–433, 2002.

[58] T. Verse, N. Klöcker, F. Riedel, W. Pirsig, and M. Scheithauer, "Dexpanthenol—Nasenspray versus Nasensalbe: Prospektive, randomisierte, offene Cross-over-Studie zur mukoziliaren Clearance," *HNO*, vol. 52, no. 7, pp. 611–615, 2004.

[59] P. Tantilipikorn, P. Tunsuriyawong, P. Jareoncharsri et al., "A randomized, prospective, double-blind study of the efficacy of dexpanthenol nasal spray on the postoperative treatment of patients with chronic rhinosinusitis after endoscopic sinus surgery," *Journal of the Medical Association of Thailand*, vol. 95, no. 1, pp. 58–63, 2012.

[60] S. Presto, A. Wehmeyer, A. Filbry, F. Rippke, and S. Bielfeldt, "Stimulation der epidermalen Regeneration durch 5% Dexpanthenol—Ergebnisse einer Placebo-kontrollierten Doppelblindstudie," *H & G*, vol. 76, no. 2, pp. 114–115, 2001.

[61] H. Eggensperger, *Multiaktive Wirkstoffe für Kosmetika*, 1995.

[62] W. Gehring and M. Gloor, "Effect of topically applied dexpanthenol on epidermal barrier function and stratum corneum hydration. Results of a human in vivo study," *Arzneimittel-Forschung*, vol. 50, no. 7, pp. 659–663, 2000.

[63] N. Klöcker, T. Verse, and P. Rudolph, "Die schleimhautprotektive Wirkung von Dexpanthenol in Nasensprays. Erste Ergebnisse zytotoxischer und zilientoxischer Versuche in vitro," *Laryngo-Rhino-Otologie*, vol. 82, no. 3, pp. 177–182, 2003.

[64] S. Hauptmann, H. Schäfer, A. Fritz, and P. Hauptmann, "Untersuchung der wachstumsbeeinflussenden Wirkung von Wundsalben an der Zellkultur," *Der Hautarzt*, vol. 43, pp. 432–435, 1992.

[65] W. Kehrl and U. Sonnemann, "Dexpanthenol-Nasenspray als wirksames Therapieprinzip zur Behandlung der Rhinitis sicca anterior," *Laryngo-Rhino-Otologie*, vol. 77, no. 9, pp. 506–512, 1998.

[66] W. Kehrl and U. Sonnemann, "Verbesserung der Wundheilung nach Nasenoperationen durch kombinierte Anwendung von Xylometazolin und Dexpanthenol," *Laryngo-Rhino-Otologie*, vol. 79, no. 3, pp. 151–154, 2000.

[67] Monographie des BfArM, "Dexpanthenol/Panthenol und Salze der Pantothensäure zur topischen Anwendung," Bundesanzeiger Nr. 24 v. 05.02.1993, S. 845, 1993.

[68] W. Hosemann, U. Göde, F. Länger, and M. E. Wigand, "Experimentelle Untersuchungen zur Wundheilung in den Nasennebenhöhlen. II. Spontaner Wundschluss und medikamentöse Effekte im standardisierten Wundmodell," *HNO*, vol. 39, pp. 48–54, 1991.

[69] W. Kehrl, U. Sonnemann, and U. Dethlefsen, "Fortschritt in der Therapie der akuten Rhinitis," *Laryngo-Rhino-Otologie*, vol. 82, no. 4, pp. 266–271, 2003.

[70] C. Skudlik, A. Schnuch, W. Uter, and H. J. Schwanitz, "Berufsbedingtes Kontaktekzem nach Anwendung einer Dexpanthenolhaltigen Salbe und Überblick über die IVDK-Daten zu Dexpanthenol," *Aktuelle Dermatologie*, vol. 28, no. 11, pp. 398–401, 2002.

[71] BfArM, "Klinische Prüfungen—Fragen und Antworten zur Klinik—Anwendungsbeobachtungen," 2013, http://www.bfarm.de/DE/Service/FAQ/_functions/Arzneimittelzulassung/klinPr/klinik/3anwendbeob/_node.html.

[72] *Gebrauchsinformation, Stand März 2011*, Ursapharm Arzneimittel GmbH, Saarbrücken, Germany, 2011.

[73] D. Soldati, F. Rahm, and P. Pasche, "Mucosal wound healing after nasal surgery. A controlled clinical trial on the efficacy of hyaluronic acid containing cream," *Drugs under Experimental and Clinical Research*, vol. 25, no. 6, pp. 253–261, 1999.

[74] M. S. Maccabee, D. R. Trune, and P. H. Hwang, "Effects of topically applied biomaterials on paranasal sinus mucosal healing," *American Journal of Rhinology*, vol. 17, no. 4, pp. 203–207, 2003.

[75] M. Leung and P. H. Hwang, "Rehabilitation of surgically traumatized paranasal sinus mucosa using retinoic acid," *American Journal of Rhinology*, vol. 21, no. 3, pp. 271–275, 2007.

[76] M. S. Maccabee, D. R. Trune, and P. H. Hwang, "Paranasal sinus mucosal regeneration: the effect of topical retinoic acid," *American Journal of Rhinology*, vol. 17, no. 3, pp. 133–137, 2003.

[77] V. R. Erickson, M. Antunes, B. Chen, N. A. Cohen, and P. H. Hwang, "The effects of retinoic acid on ciliary function of regenerated sinus mucosa," *American Journal of Rhinology*, vol. 22, no. 3, pp. 334–336, 2008.

[78] I. Ercan, B. O. Cakir, M. Ozcelik, and S. Turgut, "Efficacy of Tonimer gel spray on postoperative nasal care after endonasal surgery," *ORL*, vol. 69, no. 4, pp. 203–206, 2007.

[79] S. Fooanant, S. Chaiyasate, and K. Roongrotwattanasiri, "Comparison on the efficacy of dexpanthenol in sea water and saline in postoperative endoscopic sinus surgery," *Journal of the Medical Association of Thailand*, vol. 91, no. 10, pp. 1558–1563, 2008.

[80] C. Hahn, *Vergleich der Verträglichkeit und der Auswirkungen auf die Lebensqualität der Behandlungsmethode mit einem liposomalen Nasenspray gegenüber der Anwendung Dexpanthenolhaltiger Nasensalbe bzw. isotonem NaCl-Spray bei Patienten mit Rhinitis sicca*, 2013.

[81] T. Kühnel, W. Hosemann, W. Wagner, and K. Fayad, "Wie traumatisierend ist die mechanische Schleimhautpflege nach Eingriffen an den Nasennebenhöhlen?" *Laryngo-Rhino-Otologie*, vol. 75, no. 10, pp. 575–579, 1996.

[82] W. Hosemann, M. E. Wigand, U. Göde, F. Länger, and I. Dunker, "Normal wound healing of the paranasal sinuses: clinical and experimental investigations," *European Archives of Oto-Rhino-Laryngology*, vol. 248, no. 7, pp. 390–394, 1991.

[83] A. Macchi, P. Terranova, E. Digilio, and P. Castelnuovo, "Hyaluronan plus saline nasal washes in the treatment of rhino-sinusal symptoms in patients undergoing functional endoscopic sinus surgery for rhino-sinusal remodeling," *International Journal of Immunopathology and Pharmacology*, vol. 26, no. 1, pp. 137–145, 2013.

[84] A. G. Beule and W. Hosemann, "Wundheilung und postoperative Behandlung nach Nasennebenhöhlenoperationen," *HNO*, vol. 57, no. 8, pp. 763–771, 2009.

13

A Model for the Determination of Pollen Count Using Google Search Queries for Patients Suffering from Allergic Rhinitis

Volker König and Ralph Mösges

Institute of Medical Statistics, Informatics and Epidemiology, University of Cologne, 50924 Cologne, Germany

Correspondence should be addressed to Volker König; volker.koenig@uni-koeln.de

Academic Editor: Carlos E. Baena-Cagnani

Background. The transregional increase in pollen-associated allergies and their diversity have been scientifically proven. However, patchy pollen count measurement in many regions is a worldwide problem with few exceptions. *Methods.* This paper used data gathered from pollen count stations in Germany, Google queries using relevant allergological/biological keywords, and patient data from three German study centres collected in a prospective, double-blind, randomised, placebo-controlled, multicentre immunotherapy study to analyse a possible correlation between these data pools. *Results.* Overall, correlations between the patient-based, combined symptom medication score and Google data were stronger than those with the regionally measured pollen count data. The correlation of the Google data was especially strong in the groups of severe allergy sufferers. The results of the three-centre analyses show moderate to strong correlations with the Google keywords (up to >0.8 cross-correlation coefficient, $P < 0.001$) in 10 out of 11 groups (three averaged patient cohorts and eight subgroups of severe allergy sufferers: high IgE class, high combined symptom medication score, and asthma). *Conclusion.* For countries with a good Internet infrastructure but no dense network of pollen traps, this could represent an alternative for determining pollen levels and, forecasting the pollen count for the next day.

1. Introduction

Allergic rhinitis (AR), together with the comorbidity of asthma, ranks among the most frequent chronic diseases of our time [1, 2]. Its prevalence rates continue to rise and are thereby defining it as a global health problem. In several countries, the prevalence rate of AR in young adults is over 40% [2]. In the therapeutic ranking the avoidance of the allergen exposure comes first. An already established measurement supporting the avoidance of pollen exposure of affected persons suffering from seasonal AR is the measurement of the pollen count on the basis of pollen traps [3, 4]. This is especially drawing attention to the strength of the pollen count. Forecasting and providing the patients suffering from AR with these forecasts allow them to take measures to specifically avoid either strong or any pollen exposure. Possible measures could be an airing according to the time of the day and a postponement of outdoor activities. The warning of a high pollen count furthermore enables the

patients to prepare themselves these days by taking along symptomatic medication especially for asthmatics.

Data from clinical trials on AR must be interpreted in the context of pollen exposure. Only when it is ensured that the patients were in fact exposed to the allergens of their individual pollinosis, can it be assumed that therapy has induced symptom improvement. In placebo-controlled double-blind trials, it has therefore also become standard procedure to determine regional pollen concentrations. Based on such data it is possible to detect a more precise contrast between the symptoms of the placebo group and those of patients receiving active treatment. One requirement for this is a frequent documentation of local pollen concentrations, as is the case in Kuwait [5]. In countries with larger areas, it encounters limits since the number of stations needed can quickly reach magnitudes that are no longer affordable. Furthermore, it must be considered that each type of pollen differs in terms of its travel duration, dispersal distance, and time/period of release. Birch pollen grains, for example, can

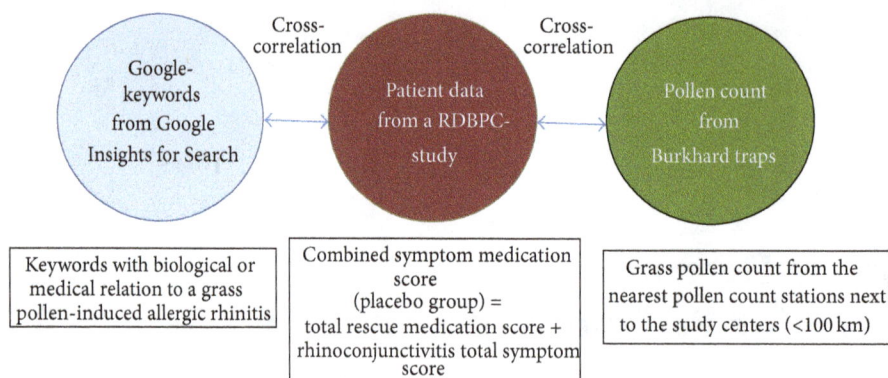

FIGURE 1: The three data pools.

be carried over 1000 km, while grass pollen usually does not travel more than 100 km [6–9]. With few exceptions [5], it is precisely the patchy pollen count coverage in many regions that poses a worldwide problem. Even the highly financed network of German pollen count stations is not complete, with distances of more than 100 km between the counting stations. In the vast expanses of the USA, the method of pollen measurement reaches its limits entirely. Alternatives, such as those in which each participant in a clinical trial is equipped with an individual allergen sampler, have not been able to assert themselves [10].

In 2008, the company Google launched Google Insights for Search, an Internet-based information service that displays all queries (keywords) entered by users in the Google search engine in terms of numbers and regions. The time- and region-stamped queries could help support the previous pollen count measurement and also analytically derive a denser network of pollen count analysis. At the end of September 2012, Google Insights for Search was integrated into Google Trends and continues to be available as an analysis tool.

We have recently found that regionally measured pollen concentrations and Google queries using allergy-typical search terms exhibit a similar time period [11]. Several investigations, although unrelated to AR, have already been published on the use of these modern, Internet-based source data from Google Insights for Search or Google Trends [12–16].

The aim of the analyses described below was therefore to examine whether the frequency of Google searches for allergy-typical terms correlates similarly well with the disease severity of patients with pollen-induced AR, as it has been assumed for regionally measured pollen concentrations and verified in numerous studies [17, 18].

2. Methods

Figure 1 gives a rough overview on the methods for the correlation analysis of the data pool used, which is described in the following section. Besides, the middle circle represents the gold standard for the analysis, defined by the pooled combined symptom and medication score

from patients of a randomized, double-blind, and placebo-controlled (RDBPC) clinical study.

2.1. The Clinical Study. As part of this investigation, a prospective, double-blind, randomised, placebo-controlled, multicentre subcutaneous immunotherapy study was examined with regard to a correlation between the pollen count at the time and the symptom-medication values of the patients (placebo group). This thirteen-month study included patients aged 18 to 75 years who had the clinical picture of AR and/or allergic rhinoconjunctivitis with/without seasonally controlled allergic asthma. These patients had to be sensitised to grasses (positive prick test for grass, wheal diameter > 3 mm), and AR symptoms had to appear primarily during the grass pollen season. Furthermore, the 18-level total symptoms sum score in RRTSS (retrospective rhinoconjunctivitis total symptom score, 0: no symptoms; 18: maximal symptoms) [19] of the respective patient had to be ≥8 in the previous pollen season. An exclusion criterion was the predominance of perennial AR. Moreover, the patients were required to keep a diary in which they were to record their symptoms and possible consumption of concomitant medication on a daily basis. Entries were limited to the months of May, June, and July 2009. These diary data are the basis for this investigation.

Overall, three study centres participated in the study ((1) Aachen/German state of North Rhine-Westphalia (NRW), (2) Hamburg/German state of Hamburg, and (3) Wiesbaden/German state of Hesse). Subsequent analyses were only performed for the placebo group to rule out drug-related biases.

The three cohorts were then examined with respect to the rhinoconjunctivitis total symptom score (RTSS 0–3, symptoms: sneezing, runny nose, itchy nose, nasal congestion, tearing, and itchy eyes) and the total rescue medication score (TRMS: chromones (eyedrops) = 1 point, antihistamine (oral) = 2 points, corticosteroids (nasal) = 3 points, on demand: leukotriene antagonists = 5 points). Afterwards, both scores were added together to a combined symptom medication score (CSMS) to compare the data with the Google data and the pollen count data.

Four subgroups were formed for the three cohorts in order to more exactly interpret the significance of the strengths of the correlations with pollen counts.

Subgroup 1 (Patient Cohort according to Average CSMS). The basis of calculation in this group was the averaged CSMS. The scores of all patients from one centre were added together and the mean was generated.

Subgroup 2 (Determining the IgE Classes). Besides the total IgE value, the specific IgE values were analysed for the single allergen timothy grass in this study. Together with the clinical picture (inclusion criteria in the study: positive history and skin prick test for grasses), this suggests a grass allergy in a patient [20]. Two subgroups were formed according to the grass pollen-specific IgE classes of "IgE low" (0: <0.35/I: 0.35–0.69/II: 0.70–3.49) to "IgE high" (III: 3.50–17.49/IV: 17.5–49.99/V: 50–100/VI: >100).

Subgroup 3 (Comorbidity-Asthma). In this analysis, the patients from all centres were divided into "asthma" and "no asthma" groups.

Subgroup 4 (Grouping according to CSMS). Patients were divided into the two groups "CSMS high" and "CSMS low." The basis for allocating the patients to the respective groups was the calculation of the group-specific mean CSMS of the respective centre. The patients CSMS in the "CSMS low" group were below 50% of the calculated mean of the respective patient population of the individual centres.

2.2. Keyword Analysis.

To find appropriate terms for a suitable correlation, all terms of interest to a pollen allergy sufferer were investigated. In doing so, general terms such as "allergy" or "pollen count" and more specific allergological terms were of interest, such as the names of respective drugs most frequently requested in Germany.

The first step involved entering the search terms in the "Google AdWords" keyword tool (Step 1). This instrument displays search terms according to number and the location (state) chosen. This step investigates whether the keywords were entered in Google using the same or similar syntax. This tool also suggests synonyms, related words, or word combinations, which would be an interesting aspect for further analysis (Step 2).

Another option for identifying suitable keywords is "Google Correlate." This is an analysis tool that outputs queries correlating best with the entered keyword. In this case, the term "hay fever" was investigated, since it constitutes the strongest medical correlation. The strongest 20 terms were included for further analyses.

Step 2 consisted of entering the identified keywords into the tool "Google Insights for Search." In addition to the simple search of the identified keywords, the keywords were also entered in combination. In this step, all terms were excluded for which there was no sufficient frequency and therefore no data in the patient diary. Insufficient data and hence the exclusion for the following analyses are based on the fact that the output of "Google Insights for Search" only includes

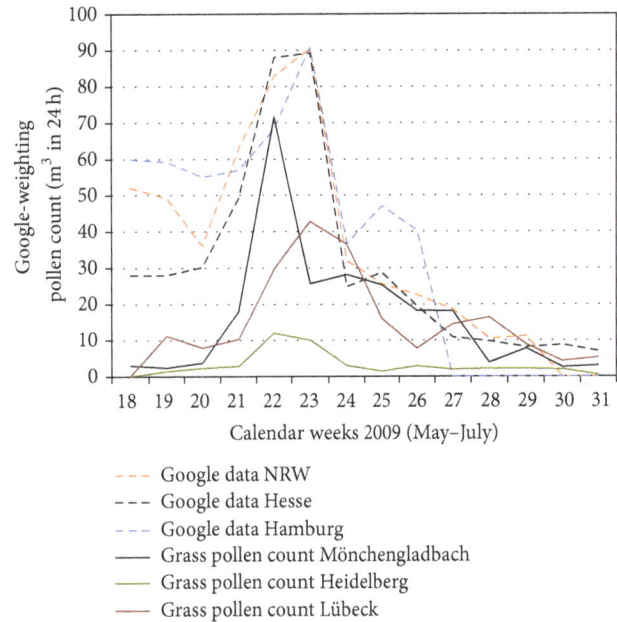

FIGURE 2: Courses of Google data depicted on the exemplary keyword "hay fever" versus grass pollen count from the pollen count stations.

keywords or combinations for popular search terms and does not depict terms with low volume. The absolute number or the limits of the search requests are not mentioned by Google. The data put out by Google for the requested period and region are normalised on a scale from 0 to 100. Repeated queries from a certain user over a short period of time were eliminated.

2.2.1. Overlap of Birch and Grass Pollen Count.

Obviously, other levels of baseline values were recognised in the Google data than in the actual pollen count data (grasses). Real pollen counts begin at zero in May and peak once before subsiding at the end of July. The Google data, on the other hand, start at a weighting of 30–60% and, except for Hamburg, subside similarly after peaking once (Figure 2). The reason for this is the effect of birch pollen up to the beginning/middle of May in connection with keyword searches not specific to the grass pollen allergy (Figure 3). For the subsequent correlation analyses, weighting of the Google data was therefore adjusted in a second step with the pollen counts (birch, travel distance up to 1,000 km) from the separate counting stations, to minimise the influence of the birch pollen count. These values were displayed and analysed as "Google data (2)." The basis of the calculation was the division of the grass pollen count data by the pooled data of the birch and grass pollen counts on the respective day in the observation period. Afterwards, the Google data (1) were adjusted according to the resulting values. The numbers of Google data in the figures reflect how many searches have been done using the identified keyword or the keyword-combination, relative to the total number of searches done on Google over the time period from May to July 2009.

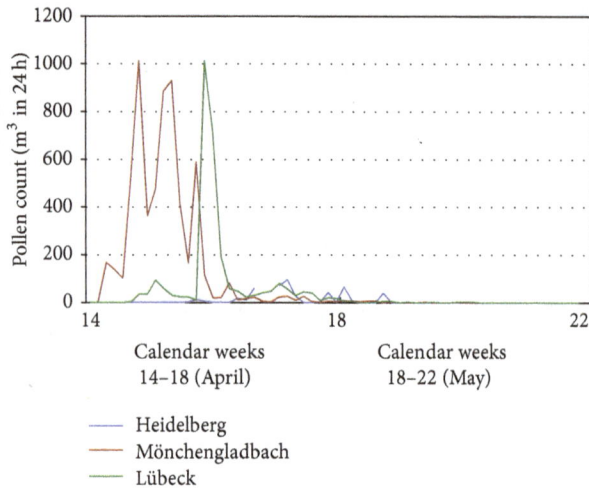

FIGURE 3: Birch pollen count, April-May 2009.

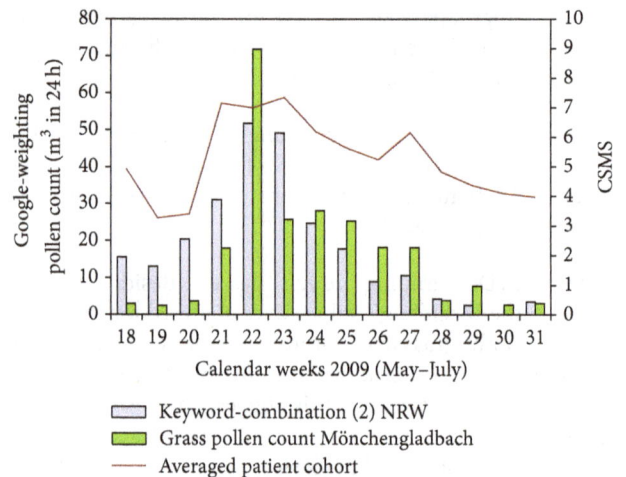

FIGURE 4: Course for Subgroup 1 (Aachen study centre). *Legend*: the averaged weekly values from Google ("Search Volume Index") and the pollen count data (pollen count/m^3 in 24 h) are presented together on the y-axis for the sake of clarity. Scaling of the averaged weekly CSMS of the patients is displayed on the opposite axis.

2.3. Statistics. All analyses were performed using the SPSS statistics software package by IBM (version 20). For data consistency, descriptive analyses were conducted to identify possible duplicates or values outside the norm.

Possible relationships were measured by cross-correlation analysis. This statistical procedure measures the correlation between two time series and has the advantage of calculating such correlations under consideration of a time shift. The term "lag" used here indicates the shift of days on which the respective cross-correlation coefficient (CCF) value was measured. The CCF reflects the strength of the correlation (0 < CCF < 0.5 = weak correlation, 0.5 ≤ CCF < 0.8 = moderate correlation, 0.8 ≤ CCF ≤ 1.0 = strong correlation). Besides the correlation coefficient and the lag, the standard deviation (SE: standard error) was also calculated. Additionally, the correlation strengths were examined with regard to their two-sided significance.

3. Results

After carrying out all investigations in the aforementioned steps, the keywords and combinations of these keywords were analysed for each centre via cross-correlation analysis using the data from Subgroup 1 (patient cohort according to average CSMS). Here, a combination of several keywords proved particularly suitable for further analysis. Hence, only this combination is introduced further in this work, which is also fulfilling the following criteria:

(i) sufficient data available for all three German states,

(ii) a clinical or biological relationship to grass pollen count or pollinosis,

(iii) long-term significance of the keywords.

The long-term significance of the keywords is of special importance with regard to future analyses in this area, irrespective of location and time. In contrast, there are drug names, for example, that can be replaced over time by more modern products (new generation antihistamines).

3.1. Cohort 1 (Aachen). In this centre, 16 patients in total received placebo. The cities of Aachen (study centre), Bonn (pollen count station, 71.49 km from the study centre), and Mönchengladbach (pollen count station, 52.55 km from the study centre) are located in the state of NRW. Therefore, the Google data from NRW using the respective keywords were compared with the patient data from Aachen.

No asthma patient was treated in this patient population. Thus, there are no investigations for Subgroup 3.

In Subgroup 1, the best values were determined for this patient cohort (Table 1). The grass pollen data for Bonn had a CCF of 0.466 (lag = −1, $P < 0.001$) and 0.630 (lag = 0. $P < 0.001$) for the data from Mönchengladbach compared to the CSMS of the patients. The keyword-combination (2) indeed showed stronger correlations; the value here was at a CCF of 0.715 (lag = −1, $P < 0.001$). Figure 4 depicts the corresponding course for this group.

3.2. Cohort 2 (Hamburg). In the Hamburg centre (state of Hamburg), a total number of 14 patients received placebo. Valid data were available for analysis from Lübeck (pollen count station, 57.77 km from the study centre) in the neighbouring German state of Schleswig-Holstein. Google data from the state of Hamburg could be analysed for Cohort 2.

Unlike in the Wiesbaden and Aachen study centres, two peaks were observed for the Hamburg patient cohort at the end of May and June, respectively. The IgE value was missing for one patient who was consequently excluded from Subgroup 2 analysis.

The correlation for the averaged patient cohort with the keyword-combination (1) was a CCF = 0.524. For the grass pollen data from Lübeck, only a weak correlation of 0.389 CCF (lag = 0) was calculated for the averaged cohort.

On the other hand, the "IgE high" (0.536) and "CSMS high" (0.557) groups each showed the strongest correlations

TABLE 1: Results of cross-correlations for the Aachen study centre.

	Subgroup 1 Averaged CSMS (n = 16)				Subgroup 2 IgE ≥ class III (3.5 kU/L) (n = 8)				Subgroup 2 IgE < class III (3.5 kU/L) (n = 8)				Subgroup 4 CSMS ≥ 50% of mean (n = 13)				Subgroup 4 CSMS < 50% of mean (n = 3)			
	CCF	lag	SE	P value	CCF	lag	SE	P value	CCF	lag	SE	P value	CCF	lag	SE	P value	CCF	lag	SE	P value
Grass pollen count Bonn	0.466	−1	0.107	<0.001	0.441	6	0.110	<0.001	0.386	−1	0.107	<0.001	0.461	−1	0.107	<0.001	0.395	7	0.111	<0.001
Grass pollen count Mönchengladbach	0.630	0	0.107	<0.001	0.607	0	0.107	<0.001	0.412	−7	0.111	<0.001	0.622	0	0.107	<0.001	0.339	3	0.108	<0.01
Keyword-combination (1) NRW	0.643	−1	0.106	<0.001	0.517	−1	0.106	<0.001	**0.645**	**−1**	**0.106**	**<0.001**	0.607	−1	0.106	<0.001	**0.486**	**1**	**0.106**	**<0.001**
Keyword-combination (2) NRW	**0.715**	**−1**	**0.106**	**<0.001**	**0.608**	**−1**	**0.106**	**<0.001**	0.622	−1	0.106	<0.001	**0.688**	**−1**	**0.106**	**<0.001**	0.420	1	0.106	<0.001

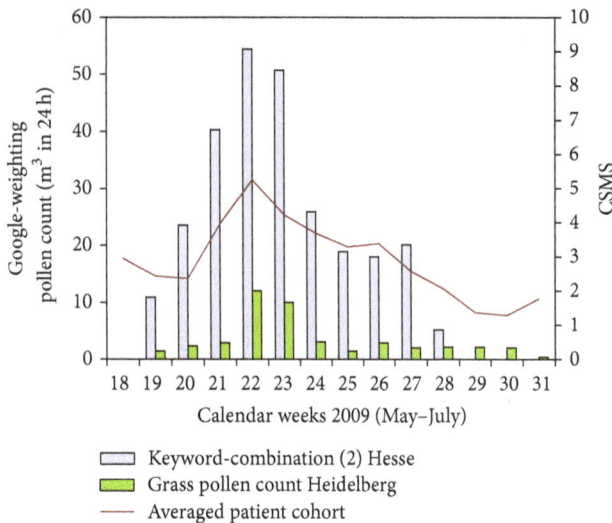

FIGURE 5: Course for Subgroup 1 (Wiesbaden study centre).

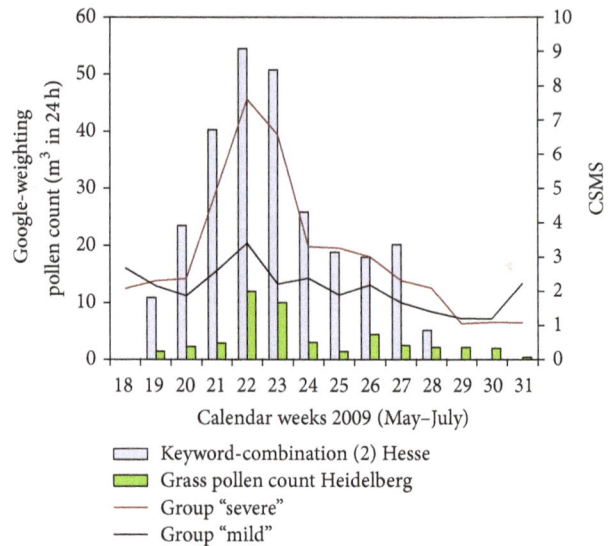

FIGURE 6: Course of the "severe" and "mild" group (Wiesbaden centre).

for the keyword-combination (1). No CCF over 0.5 was observed for the "IgE low" and "CSMS low" groups.

The grass pollen count data from Lübeck did not exceed a CCF of 0.5 in any group. The best value here was a CCF of 0.417 (lag = 0) in the "no asthma" group.

3.3. Cohort 3 (Wiesbaden). The Wiesbaden study centre is located in the state of Hesse. The nearest pollen count station was located in Heidelberg (82.32 km from the study centre) in the neighbouring state. Data directly from the state of Hesse were used for the Google-specific analysis. Overall, 22 patients from this centre received placebo.

The value in the averaged Wiesbaden patient cohort for the keyword-combination (1 and 2) was a CCF of 0.766 (lag = −1, $P < 0.001$) (Table 2, Figure 5). The correlation strength of the grass pollen count data from the nearest pollen count station in Heidelberg was 0.495 (lag = 0, $P < 0.001$). In this population, a correlation strength of 0.752 (lag = −1, SE = 0.106, $P < 0.01$) was ascertained for the keyword-combination (2) in the "CSMS high" subgroup and a strength of 0.753 (lag = −1, SE = 0.106, $P < 0.01$) for the keyword-combination (1) in the "IgE high" subgroup. The comparative values for the pollen count data from Heidelberg for these two subgroups had a CCF of about 0.5.

3.4. Other Subgroup Analyses. Because of the significantly weaker correlation strengths in the subgroups with less allergic patients, additional "severe" (IgE ≥ class III (3.5 kU/L), CSMS ≥ 50% of the mean, asthma) and "mild" (IgE < class III (3.5 kU/L), CSMS < 50% of the mean, no asthma) groups were created. In all comparisons between these two groups at Aachen, Hamburg, and Wiesbaden centres, consistently higher CCF values were identified in the group of severely affected allergy sufferers for the keyword-combination (2). In the Wiesbaden centre, the highest superiority of the keyword-combination (2) could be observed. Figure 6 shows the data evaluated for the averaged "severe" and "mild" group from

the Wiesbaden centre. The keyword-combination (2) had a CCF of 0.808 (lag = −1) for the group "severe" (group "mild," 0.616 CCF (lag = −1)). The corresponding grass pollen count data from Heidelberg showed a CCF of 0.553 (lag = −2).

4. Discussion

The results of the three centre analyses show moderate to strong correlations with the Google keyword-combination (up to >0.8 CCF) in 10 out of 11 groups (three averaged patient cohorts and the eight subgroups of severe allergy sufferers). The "asthma" ($n = 2$) group from Hamburg is the only exception with a CCF under 0.5. Thus, the correlation strengths of the Google data in these groups were invariably better than those of the grass pollen count data from the nearest pollen count stations. Other pooled group analyses with the severe allergy sufferers further strengthened the good results of the Google data.

Adjustment of the Google data (Google data (2)) due to the birch pollen season at the beginning of May showed an even stronger correlation. It is therefore possible to process the data later for certain pollen allergy sufferers.

The Hamburg study site, besides having the aforementioned outlier group of severe allergy sufferers, was the centre with the weakest correlations with the Google data. This centre showed extraordinary, erratic CSMS courses of the patients, which could be due on the one hand to a smaller patient data pool ($n = 14$) and on the other hand—compared to the other centres—to the highest TRMS.

4.1. Estimation of the Forecast. A negative lag of −1 was often observed for the Google data values. This could indicate that possible preventive measures were taken before pollen exposure, since the media often report the start of the pollen season or high pollen counts and allergy sufferers are possibly getting more information on the Internet. In addition, patient

TABLE 2: Results of cross-correlations for the Wiesbaden study centre.

	Subgroup 1 Averaged CSMS (n = 22)				Subgroup 2 IgE ≥ class III (3.5 kU/L) (n = 17)				Subgroup 2 IgE < class III (3.5 kU/L) (n = 5)				Subgroup 3 Asthma (n = 2)				Subgroup 3 No asthma (n = 20)				Subgroup 4 CSMS ≥ 50% of mean (n = 17)				Subgroup 4 CSMS < 50% of mean (n = 5)			
	CCF	lag	SE	P value	CCF	lag	SE	P value	CCF	lag	SE	P value	CCF	lag	SE	P value	CCF	lag	SE	P value	CCF	lag	SE	P value	CCF	lag	SE	P value
Grass pollen count Heidelberg	0.495	0	0.107	<0.001	0.492	−1	0.108	<0.001	0.321	−7	0.112	<0.01	0.574	−2	0.108	<0.001	0.441	0	0.107	<0.001	0.511	0	0.107	<0.001	0.300	−5	0.110	<0.01
Keyword-combination (1) HE	**0.766**	**−1**	**0.106**	**<0.001**	**0.753**	**−1**	**0.106**	**<0.001**	**0.352**	**−4**	**0.108**	**<0.01**	**0.726**	**−1**	0.105	<0.001	**0.685**	**−1**	**0.106**	**<0.001**	0.728	−1	0.106	<0.001	**0.524**	**−1**	**0.106**	**<0.001**
Keyword-combination (2) HE	**0.766**	**−1**	**0.106**	**<0.001**	0.748	−1	0.106	<0.001	0.336	−4	0.108	<0.01	**0.743**	**−1**	**0.106**	<0.001	0.680	−1	0.106	<0.001	**0.752**	**−1**	**0.106**	**<0.001**	0.400	−1	0.106	<0.001

symptoms begin with the start of the pollen season and Internet queries could be made before the symptoms are strongest or before they become even stronger. This influence, known in the statistics as confounding, offers the possibility to determine the pollen count a day in advance. Therefore it offers the possibility to avoid or reduce the allergen exposure for all those who are suffering from pollen allergies and is thus supporting the most important factor in the therapeutic ranking.

4.2. Confounder. Since the patient's exact location was unknown, it was assumed that the patients were from the region surrounding the respective study centre. Based on the long-term design of the study (>1 year, 14 visits), however, this is to be expected. Because the Google data were generated according to state, one can also presume the direct correlation for this analysis.

4.3. Modern Data Analysis. The Google search engine has continued to improve during the past four years in that even more exact search results can be displayed based on the availability of more data. For example, in 2011, an analysis using the keyword-combination could be performed for all 16 states in Germany. In comparison, there were only nine analysable states in 2009. Based thereon and on the growth of worldwide Internet use [21], it is to be expected that an even more exact analysis of the pollen count can be conducted not for Germany alone. Regionally pooled Google data could therefore be used to derive correlations especially for pollen types that do not travel great distances.

4.4. Clinical Studies. The impact of pollen count on studies with pollinosis patients is well known and correlations have already been proven [17, 18]. The costs and expense for recruiting a suitable patient population are very high [22]. For the area of allergology, the results presented here can yield more validity of the study data. In the case of placebo-controlled studies, the data of placebo populations in particular can be examined and interpreted more precisely, especially in the context of the cohort receiving the study drug. Already completed studies as far back as 2004 could also be analysed in retrospect for differences in the symptom and medication scores of the study subjects based on freely available Google data.

The complexity of the pollen flight and the different clinical pictures of a person with pollinosis are of course difficult to be analysed with a general search engine based algorithm, as it is possible for other diseases. In our analysis we performed an algorithm for patients with a grass pollen allergy only.

5. Conclusion

Particularly for countries that do not have a dense network of pollen count stations, this Google-based algorithm would represent an alternative for determining pollen counts and even provide forecasts for the next day. It thus considers and supports the most important factor in the therapeutic

approach to the clinical picture of pollinosis, namely, the avoidance of the allergen exposure. A prerequisite, of course, is the availability of an Internet infrastructure in the respective regions.

The correlations determined here are very clearly connected, but they must be further confirmed using a larger, transregional patient pool.

Abbreviations

AR: Allergic rhinitis
CCF: Cross-correlation coefficient
CSMS: Combined symptom medication score
HE: Hesse
NRW: North Rhine-Westphalia
RDBPC: Randomized, double-blind, placebo-controlled
RRTSS: Retrospective rhinoconjunctivitis total symptom score
RTSS: Rhinoconjunctivitis total symptom score
TRMS: Total rescue medication score.

Conflict of Interests

Volker König and Ralph Mösges report no conflict of interests concerning this paper.

Authors' Contribution

Volker König and Ralph Mösges have contributed to, seen, and approved the paper.

Acknowledgments

The authors thank ROXALL Medizin GmbH for provision of data from the clinical study. The authors would like to acknowledge Gena Kittel, B.A., and Marie-Josefine Joisten, M.A., for proofreading the paper.

References

[1] J. Bousquet, N. Khaltaev, A. A. Cruz et al., "Allergic Rhinitis and its Impact on Asthma (ARIA) 2008 update (in collaboration with the World Health Organization, GA2LEN and AllerGen)," *Allergy*, vol. 63, no. 86, pp. 8–160, 2008.

[2] J. Bousquet, H. J. Schunemann, T. Zuberbier et al., "Development and implementation of guidelines in allergic rhinitis—an ARIA-GA2LEN paper," *Allergy*, vol. 65, no. 10, pp. 1212–1221, 2010.

[3] E. Levetin and P. K. van de Water, "Pollen count forecasting," *Immunology and Allergy Clinics of North America*, vol. 23, no. 3, pp. 423–442, 2003.

[4] H. Moriguchi, M. Matsumoto, Y. Nishimoto, and K. Kuwada, "The development of a pollen information system for the improvement of QOL," *The Journal of Medical Investigation*, vol. 48, no. 3-4, pp. 198–209, 2001.

[5] N. Behbehani, N. Arifhodzic, M. Al-Mousawi et al., "The seasonal variation in allergic rhinitis and its correlation with

outdoor allergens in Kuwait," *International Archives of Allergy and Immunology*, vol. 133, no. 2, pp. 164–167, 2004.

[6] L. Cecchi, M. Morabito, M. P. Domeneghetti, A. Crisci, M. Onorari, and S. Orlandini, "Long distance transport of ragweed pollen as a potential cause of allergy in central Italy," *Annals of Allergy, Asthma and Immunology*, vol. 96, no. 1, pp. 86–91, 2006.

[7] M. Sofiev, P. Siljamo, H. Ranta, and A. Rantio-Lehtimäki, "Towards numerical forecasting of long-range air transport of birch pollen: theoretical considerations and a feasibility study," *International Journal of Biometeorology*, vol. 50, no. 6, pp. 392–402, 2006.

[8] P. K. van de Water, T. Keever, C. E. Main, and E. Levetin, "An assessment of predictive forecasting of Juniperus ashei pollen movement in the Southern Great Plains, USA," *International Journal of Biometeorology*, vol. 48, no. 2, pp. 74–82, 2003.

[9] S. F. Wood, "Review of hay fever. 1. Historical background and mechanisms," *Family Practice*, vol. 3, no. 1, pp. 54–63, 1986.

[10] A. Custovic, S. C. O. Taggart, H. C. Francis, M. D. Chapman, and A. Woodcock, "Exposure to house dust mite allergens and the clinical activity of asthma," *Journal of Allergy and Clinical Immunology*, vol. 98, no. 1, pp. 64–72, 1996.

[11] R. Mosges, M. Adrian, E. El Hassan, and V. Konig, "What Google(R) knows about the pollen season," *Allergy*, vol. 66, no. 5, pp. 707–708, 2011.

[12] N. Askitas and K. F. Zimmermann, "Google econometrics and unemployment forecasting," *Aplied Economics Quarterly*, vol. 55, no. 2, pp. 107–120, 2009.

[13] B. N. Breyer, S. Sen, D. S. Aaronson, M. L. Stoller, B. A. Erickson, and M. L. Eisenberg, "Use of google insights for search to track seasonal and geographic kidney stone incidence in the United States," *Urology*, vol. 78, no. 2, pp. 267–271, 2011.

[14] M. P. Connolly, M. Postma, and S. J. Silber, "What's on the mind of IVF consumers?" *Reproductive BioMedicine Online*, vol. 19, no. 6, pp. 767–769, 2009.

[15] J. Ginsberg, M. H. Mohebbi, R. S. Patel, L. Brammer, M. S. Smolinski, and L. Brilliant, "Detecting influenza epidemics using search engine query data," *Nature*, vol. 457, no. 7232, pp. 1012–1014, 2009.

[16] C. T. Leffler, B. Davenport, and D. Chan, "Frequency and seasonal variation of ophthalmology-related internet searches," *Canadian Journal of Ophthalmology*, vol. 45, no. 3, pp. 274–279, 2010.

[17] J. A. Qasem, H. Nasrallah, B. N. Al-Khalaf et al., "Meteorological factors, aeroallergens and asthma-related visits in Kuwait: a 12-month retrospective study," *Annals of Saudi Medicine*, vol. 28, no. 6, pp. 435–441, 2008.

[18] K. Takasaki, K. Enatsu, H. Kumagami, and H. Takahashi, "Relationship between airborne pollen count and treatment outcome in Japanese cedar pollinosis patients," *European Archives of Oto-Rhino-Laryngology*, vol. 266, no. 5, pp. 673–676, 2009.

[19] E. Röder, M. Y. Berger, W. C. J. Hop, R. M. D. Bernsen, H. de Groot, and R. Gerth van Wijk, "Sublingual immunotherapy with grass pollen is not effective in symptomatic youngsters in primary care," *Journal of Allergy and Clinical Immunology*, vol. 119, no. 4, pp. 892–898, 2007.

[20] AWMF AdWMF, "In-vitro-Allergiediagnostik," AWMF-Leitlinien-Register, 2009.

[21] IDS, "Individuals using the Internet per 100 inhabitants, 2001–2011," International Telecommunication Union, Geneva, Switzerland, 2011, http://www.itu.int/ITU-D/ict/statistics/.

[22] E. L. Eisenstein, R. Collins, B. S. Cracknell et al., "Sensible approaches for reducing clinical trial costs," *Clinical Trials*, vol. 5, no. 1, pp. 75–84, 2008.

14

Impact of Adiponectin Overexpression on Allergic Airways Responses in Mice

Norah G. Verbout,[1] **Leandro Benedito,**[1] **Alison S. Williams,**[1]
David I. Kasahara,[1] **Allison P. Wurmbrand,**[1] **Huiqing Si,**[1] **Andrew J. Halayko,**[2]
Christopher Hug,[3] **and Stephanie A. Shore**[1]

[1] *Department of Environmental Health, Harvard School of Public Health, 665 Huntington Avenue, Boston, MA 02115, USA*
[2] *Departments of Physiology and Internal Medicine, University of Manitoba, Winnipeg, MB, Canada R3A 1R9*
[3] *Children's Hospital, Boston, MA 02115, USA*

Correspondence should be addressed to Stephanie A. Shore; sshore@hsph.harvard.edu

Academic Editor: Akshay Sood

Obesity is an important risk factor for asthma. Obese individuals have decreased circulating adiponectin, an adipose-derived hormone with anti-inflammatory properties. We hypothesized that transgenic overexpression of adiponectin would attenuate allergic airways inflammation and mucous hyperplasia in mice. To test this hypothesis, we used mice overexpressing adiponectin (Adipo Tg). Adipo Tg mice had marked increases in both serum adiponectin and bronchoalveolar lavage (BAL) fluid adiponectin. Both acute and chronic ovalbumin (OVA) sensitization and challenge protocols were used. In both protocols, OVA-induced increases in total BAL cells were attenuated in Adipo Tg versus WT mice. In the acute protocol, OVA-induced increases in several IL-13 dependent genes were attenuated in Adipo Tg versus WT mice, even though IL-13 per se was not affected. With chronic exposure, though OVA-induced increases in goblet cells numbers per millimeter of basement membrane were greater in Adipo Tg versus WT mice, mRNA abundance of mucous genes in lungs was not different. Also, adiponectin overexpression did not induce M2 polarization in alveolar macrophages. Our results indicate that adiponectin protects against allergen-induced inflammatory cell recruitment to the airspaces, but not development of goblet cell hyperplasia.

1. Introduction

Obesity is an important risk factor for asthma. Obesity increases the prevalence, the incidence, and possibly the severity of asthma, while weight loss improves many asthma outcomes in the obese [1, 2]. In addition, standard asthma therapeutic agents are less effective in obese versus lean asthmatics [3, 4].

Adiponectin is an adipocyte-derived hormone that declines in obesity [5]. Loss of adiponectin in obesity appears to have important functional consequences. In animal models, adiponectin deficiency exacerbates several obesity-related conditions, including insulin resistance and atherosclerosis [6, 7]. In obese human subjects, serum adiponectin levels are inversely correlated with the risk of type 2 diabetes,

atherosclerosis, and hypertension [8–10]. Some, but not all, epidemiological studies suggest that obesity-related declines in adiponectin may also contribute to obesity-related asthma. For example, in a cohort of premenopausal women, the risk of asthma was greatest in subjects in the lowest tertile of serum adiponectin [11]. Similarly, in C57BL/6 mice, adiponectin deficiency worsens airway eosinophilia and macrophage recruitment induced by chronic allergen challenge [12]. In addition, we have shown that in lean Balb/C mice, continuous infusion of adiponectin via mini-Alzet pumps suppresses acute allergen-induced airway hyperresponsiveness, airway inflammation, and Th2 cytokine production [13]. Similarly, Ionescu et al. reported a reduction in allergic airway inflammation in allergen challenged mice treated intranasally with recombinant adiponectin [14]. These data suggest that manipulating adiponectin levels might have beneficial effects for asthma. However, none of these studies examined goblet cell metaplasia, a common feature of asthma (reviewed in [15]) and of animal models of asthma. Adiponectin receptors are expressed on airway epithelial cells [16], and we have previously reported that compared to wildtype (WT) mice, acute allergen sensitization and challenge results in reduced mucous cell staining in the airways of T-cadherin deficient mice, which have increased circulating adiponectin [17]. These data suggest that adiponectin may have the capacity to impact goblet cell metaplasia.

Some of the observed beneficial effects of adiponectin in the airways [13, 14] may be related to its anti-inflammatory effects, particularly its effects on macrophages, although adiponectin also has proinflammatory effects [18–20]. Adiponectin decreases the ability of LPS or Toll-like receptor activation to elicit TNFα and IL-6 production from macrophages [21–24] and reduces eotaxin expression in bone marrow derived macrophages stimulated with TNFα and IL-4 [12]. Adiponectin also inhibits the transformation of macrophages to foam cells [25], which may explain the antiatherosclerotic effects of adiponectin. Cultured alveolar macrophages from adiponectin deficient mice demonstrate increased production of TNFα, both innately and upon stimulation with LPS [26]. Adiponectin has also been shown to promote an anti-inflammatory, M2 phenotype in macrophages of various origins [27–29]. Such effects may be magnified in the setting of allergic lung disease which is associated with induction of Th2 cytokines that also promote M2 polarization.

The purpose of this study was to determine whether transgenic overexpression of adiponectin could affect allergic airways responses, including goblet cell hyperplasia. To do so, we used mice overexpressing adiponectin from a chicken beta-actin promoter/cytomegalovirus enhancer. We have previously reported that these mice have marked increases in serum adiponectin [30]. Two allergen sensitization and challenge protocols were employed. The first, an acute challenge protocol, was similar to that used in a previous study in which we examined the effects of adiponectin administered by mini-Alzet pumps [13] and was used as a proof of concept that adiponectin overexpressed in this manner would be effective. The second protocol, a chronic challenge protocol, results in allergic airways inflammation and goblet cell metaplasia, that is dependent on mast cells [31], as is allergic asthma in humans, whereas the acute protocol requires T cells but not mast cells [32]. The transgenic expression of adiponectin allowed increased levels of this adipokine to be present throughout the extended challenge period needed for this protocol.

2. Materials and Methods

2.1. Animals. This study was approved by the Harvard Medical Area Standing Committee on Animals. Transgenic mice overexpressing adiponectin (Adipo Tg) driven by a chicken beta-actin promoter with a cytomegalovirus enhancer and backcrossed onto a C57BL/6J background were generated as previously described [33]. Adipo Tg mice (which were ±

for the transgene) were mated with WT littermates, and the Adipo Tg and littermate WT offspring of these matings were used in experiments described below. Primers used for genotyping were 5′-GCT TAT ATG TAT CGC TCA GCG TTC AG-3′ and 5′-CTT GTC GTC GTC GTC CTT GTA GTC-3′. Using these primers, a 438 bp product was observed in the Adipo Tg but not the WT mice.

2.2. Allergen Sensitization and Challenge

2.2.1. Acute Protocol. Four-week-old male mice were sensitized to chicken egg albumin (ovalbumin (OVA), Grade V, Sigma-Aldrich Co., St. Louis, MO) on *day 1* by intraperitoneal injection of 20 μg of OVA and adjuvant, 2 mg of aluminum hydroxide (Al(OH)$_3$; J. T. Baker, Phillipsburg, NJ) dispersed in 0.2 mL of PBS. Mice were given a second injection of identical reagents on *day 14*. On *days 28* through *30*, mice were challenged for 30 min with an aerosol of either PBS containing 1% OVA or PBS alone, as previously described [34]. Mice were studied 24 h after the last OVA challenge.

2.2.2. Chronic Protocol. Four-week-old male mice were sensitized to OVA on *days 1, 4, and 7* by intraperitoneal injection of 50 μg OVA dispersed in 0.1 mL of PBS without alum. Beginning on *day 12*, mice were intranasally challenged once a week for 4 weeks with either sterile PBS or OVA (20 μg in 30 μL PBS) as described by others [31]. Mice were studied 24 h after the last OVA challenge.

2.3. Bronchoalveolar Lavage (BAL). Mice were euthanized with an overdose of sodium pentobarbital, blood was drawn by cardiac puncture, and serum stored at −20°C for subsequent measurement of total serum adiponectin and IgE by ELISA. BAL was performed and the BAL cells and differentials counted as described previously [13, 34]. BAL supernatant was stored at −80°C and subsequently analyzed by ELISA for adiponectin, eotaxin, and IL-13 (R&D Systems Inc.). OVA specific IgE in serum was analyzed by ELISA (Cayman Chemical).

2.4. Histology and Morphometry. For mice in the chronic OVA protocol, twenty-four hours after the last exposure to OVA or PBS, mice were euthanized and lungs processed for histology as previously described [35]. Briefly, the lungs were inflated in situ at 20 cm of water with 4% paraformaldehyde and then removed en bloc. The left lung was cut, embedded in paraffin, and sections stained with periodic acid Schiff (PAS) to assess mucous-containing goblet cells. Sections were viewed using an upright light microscope equipped with SPOT CCD camera and Image Pro software (Olympus Canada, Mississauga, ON). Airways were selected for analysis that exhibited a maximum diameter: minimum diameter ratio that was less than ≤2 to avoid artifacts from airways cut obliquely. Basement membrane (BM) length was measured for all airways. For measurement of goblet cell abundance, a band-shaped region of interest extending from the BM to the edge of the epithelium was drawn, using a maximum length that avoided sectioning artifacts. Using Image Pro (Olympus)

TABLE 1: Primers used for qRT-PCR.

Gene	Forward primer (5′ → 3′)	Reverse primer (5′ → 3′)
Alox15	ATGGTGCTGAAGCGGTCTAC	ATCCGCTTCAAACAGAGTGC
Cxcl9	TCCTCTTGGGCATCATCTTC	TGAGGGATTTGTAGTGGATCG
Il13	CAGCATGGTATGGAGTGTGG	AGGCCATGCAATATCCTCTG
Il17a	CTCCAGAAGGCCCTCAGACTA	AGCTTTCCCTCCGCATTGACACAG
Itln1	AGAACCTGGACACCAACAGG	GTGCGCAGGAAATAGAGACC
Clec10a	CAGTGGAGAAGAGGGAGCAG	AGCCGTTGTTCTTGAGGTTG
Muc5ac	ACCCAGAGGGTCAGTGTGAG	TTGGGATAGCATCCTTCCAG
Retnla	TCGTGGAGAATAAGGTCAAGG	GGAGGCCCATCTGTTCATAG
Chi3l3	GAAGGAGCCACTGAGGTCTG	TTGTTGTCCTTGAGCCACTG
Clca3	GATTCCCGAGAGCTGGAAG	TGTTCGGTGTAGGGCTCATC
Agr2	GCGATCAGCTCATCTGGACT	GCTTGACTGTGTGGGCATT
18S ribosomal RNA	GTAACCCGTTGAACCCCATT	CCATCCAATCGGTAGTAGCG

software, thresholds for detecting goblet cells were set to enable discrimination between individual mucous-positive cells, so that the numbers of cells per mm of BM could be determined. Images of at least 3 different airways were captured for each animal. Other sections were stained with hematoxylin and eosin to determine the inflammation index, a product of the severity and prevalence of inflammation, as described by Hamada et al. [36]. Severity was assigned a numerical value based upon the number of inflammatory cell infiltrate layers surrounding the airways or blood vessels (0, no cells; 1, ≤3 cell layers; 2, 4–9 cell layers; 3, 10 cell layers). Prevalence of inflammation was assigned a numerical value according to the percentage of airways or blood vessels in each section encompassed by inflammatory cells (0, none; 1, ≤25%; 2, 25–50%; 3, >50%). Medium to large sized airways were analyzed, and in each mouse, a minimum of 8 airways were examined. For both goblet cell hyperplasia and inflammation, a mean value for each mouse was computed and used for statistical analyses.

2.5. RNA Extraction and Real-Time PCR. Lungs were harvested, frozen at −80°C, and subsequently homogenized for RNA extraction with RNeasy (Qiagen). Total RNA (1 μg) was reverse transcribed using random hexamer primers and Superscript III (Invitrogen). Quantitative mRNA expression for each gene was performed using real-time PCR and SYBR Green (Applied Biosystems). Primers are described in Table 1. Values were calculated based on the ΔΔCT method, and 18S was used to control for total mRNA. For each set of primers, melting curve analysis yielded a single peak consistent with one PCR product.

2.6. Statistical Analysis of Results. Data were analyzed by factorial ANOVA (BAL and serum moieties, histological analyses, and lung mRNA expression) using STATISTICA software (StatSoft, Tulsa, OK). BAL cells were log transformed in order to conform to a normal distribution. Fisher's LSD test was used for post hoc comparisons. A P value < 0.05 was considered statistically significant.

3. Results

3.1. Acute Allergen Challenge Protocol

3.1.1. Adiponectin Expression and Body Weight. Compared to WT littermates, Adipo Tg mice had marked increases in both serum and BAL fluid adiponectin (Figure 1). Adiponectin levels in the serum were not significantly altered by exposure to OVA, though there was a trend towards increased BAL adiponectin in OVA versus PBS treated mice ($P = 0.076$). Neither adiponectin genotype nor OVA had any effect on body mass. Body mass averaged 26.9±0.5, 26.7±0.6, 26.5±1.0, and 27.0±0.7 g in WT mice challenged with PBS or OVA, and Adipo Tg mice challenged with PBS or OVA respectively.

3.1.2. Pulmonary Inflammation. Factorial ANOVA indicated a significant effect of OVA versus PBS exposure on total BAL cells. Follow-up analysis indicated that the effect occurred in the WT mice. Total BAL cells increased from 2.7 ± 0.5 to $9.1 \pm 4.2 \times 10^4$ cells/mL in WT mice ($P < 0.05$), whereas there was no significant effect of OVA versus PBS exposure in Adipo Tg mice (2.1 ± 0.2 versus $3.9 \pm 0.5 \times 10^4$ cells/mL). OVA induced a significant increase in neutrophils, eosinophils, and lymphocytes (Figure 2(a)) in WT mice. Compared to WT mice, OVA-induced increases in lymphocytes were significantly reduced in adiponectin transgenic mice. A similar trend was observed for neutrophils and eosinophils but did not reach statistical significance. There was no effect of either OVA exposure or genotype on BAL epithelial cells (data not shown). In contrast, circulating leukocytes were not different between wildtype and adiponectin transgenic mice, except for a reduction in circulating neutrophils in WT OVA versus PBS treated mice (Figure 2(b)). These observations suggest that genotype-related reductions in infiltration of airspaces by inflammatory cells were not the result of a deficiency in the availability of these cells in the blood.

Compared to PBS, OVA challenge increased BAL IL-13 (Figure 2(c)). There was no significant genotype-related difference, although there was a trend for reduced BAL IL-13

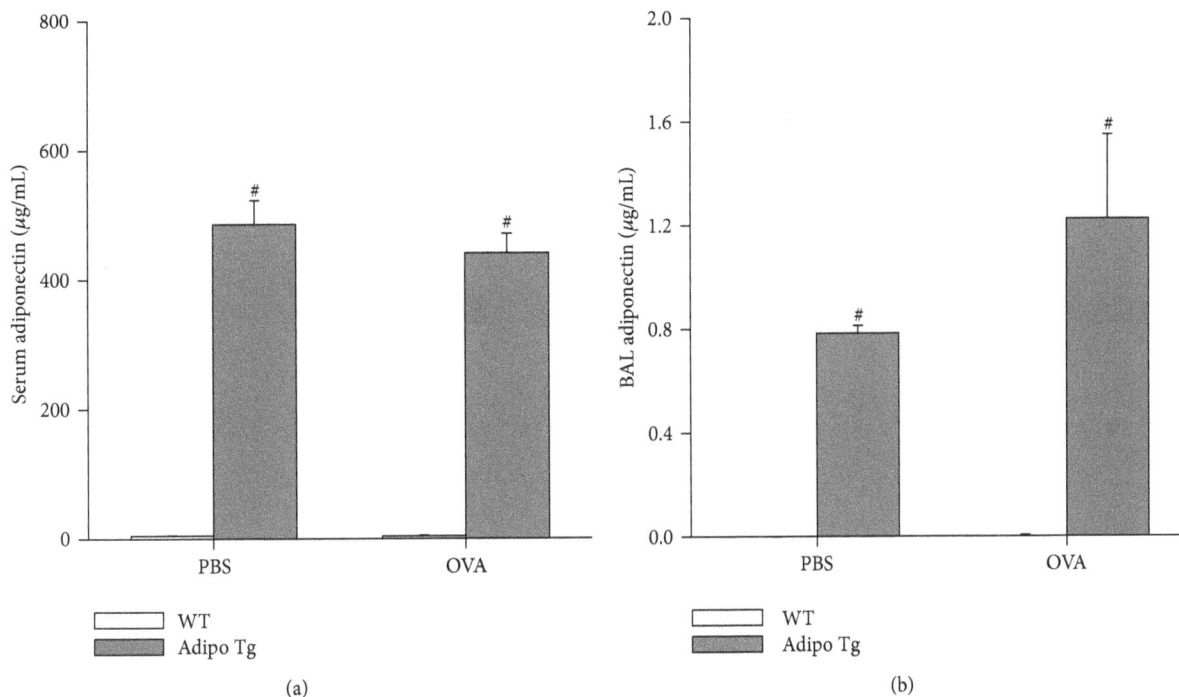

FIGURE 1: Serum (a) and bronchoalveolar lavage (BAL) fluid (b) adiponectin concentrations in wildtype (WT) and adiponectin transgenic (Adipo Tg) mice sensitized to ovalbumin (OVA) and challenged with aerosols of OVA or PBS every day for 3 days. Data shown are mean ± SEM of 5–7 mice per group. $^{#}P < 0.05$ versus WT mice with the same exposure.

in Adipo Tg mice. OVA induced a significant increase in BAL eotaxin in WT but not Adipo Tg mice (Figure 2(d)). Similarly, OVA exposure increased OVA-specific serum IgE (Figure 2(e)) in WT mice, but not in Adipo Tg mice.

3.1.3. Pulmonary Gene Expression.

Real-time PCR was used to measure changes in mRNA abundance of genes known to be strongly induced in the lungs by OVA challenge in this protocol [37–44]. In WT mice, inhalation of OVA significantly increased pulmonary expression of *Retnla*, *Itln1*, *Alox15*, *Muc5ac*, *Cxcl9*, *Clca3*, *Agr2*, and *Il17a* mRNA (Figure 3). OVA-induced *Retnla*, *Itln1*, *Alox15*, *Clca3*, and *Agr2* mRNA abundance was significantly lower in Adipo Tg than WT mice. A similar trend was observed for *Muc5ac* and *Cxcl9*, but the effect did not reach statistical significance. *Il17a* mRNA abundance was not different in Adipo Tg and WT mice.

3.2. Chronic Allergen Challenge Protocol

3.2.1. Pulmonary Inflammation.

Compared to PBS challenge, repeated intranasal OVA challenge caused significant increases in BAL neutrophils, eosinophils, and lymphocytes (Figure 4(a)), although eosinophils were lower than those induced with the acute challenge protocol (Figure 2(a)). Importantly, OVA-induced increases in BAL neutrophils and eosinophils were significantly attenuated in Adipo Tg versus WT mice. There was no effect of either OVA challenge or adiponectin genotype on circulating leukocytes (Figure 4(b)). Compared to PBS, OVA challenge increased BAL IL-13 in WT mice (Figure 4(c)). BAL IL-13 was

significantly reduced in Adipo Tg versus WT OVA exposed mice. BAL eotaxin was also significantly lower in Adipo Tg versus WT OVA exposed mice (Figure 4(d)). Compared to PBS, OVA challenge caused a significant increase in serum OVA-specific IgE, but there was no effect of genotype (Figure 4(e)).

OVA challenge resulted in accumulation of inflammatory cells around airways (Figure 5), but there was no significant difference in the extent of these cell infiltrates in WT versus Adipo Tg mice (Figure 6(a)). We also examined goblet cell hyperplasia in these mice. Compared to PBS, chronic OVA i.n. challenge significantly increased the number of goblet cells per mm of BM in the airways in both WT and Adipo Tg mice (Figures 5 and 6(b)). However, there was a small but significant *increase* in goblet cell hyperplasia in the OVA challenged Adipo Tg versus WT mice.

3.2.2. Gene Expression.

Similar to the results obtained with the acute OVA exposure protocol, chronic intranasal instillation of OVA significantly increased pulmonary expression of *Retnla*, *Itln1*, *Alox15*, *Clca3*, *Agr2*, *Muc5ac*, and *Cxcl9* (Figure 7), although the magnitude of these changes was substantially reduced compared to the acute OVA protocol (Figure 3). However, in contrast to the acute OVA exposure protocol, OVA-induced increases in the expression of these genes were not significantly affected by transgenic status. *Il17a* mRNA expression was not induced by i.n. OVA (Figure 7(h)).

Since others have reported effects of adiponectin on macrophage phenotype [27, 29], we also measured additional markers of M2 phenotype in the lungs of these

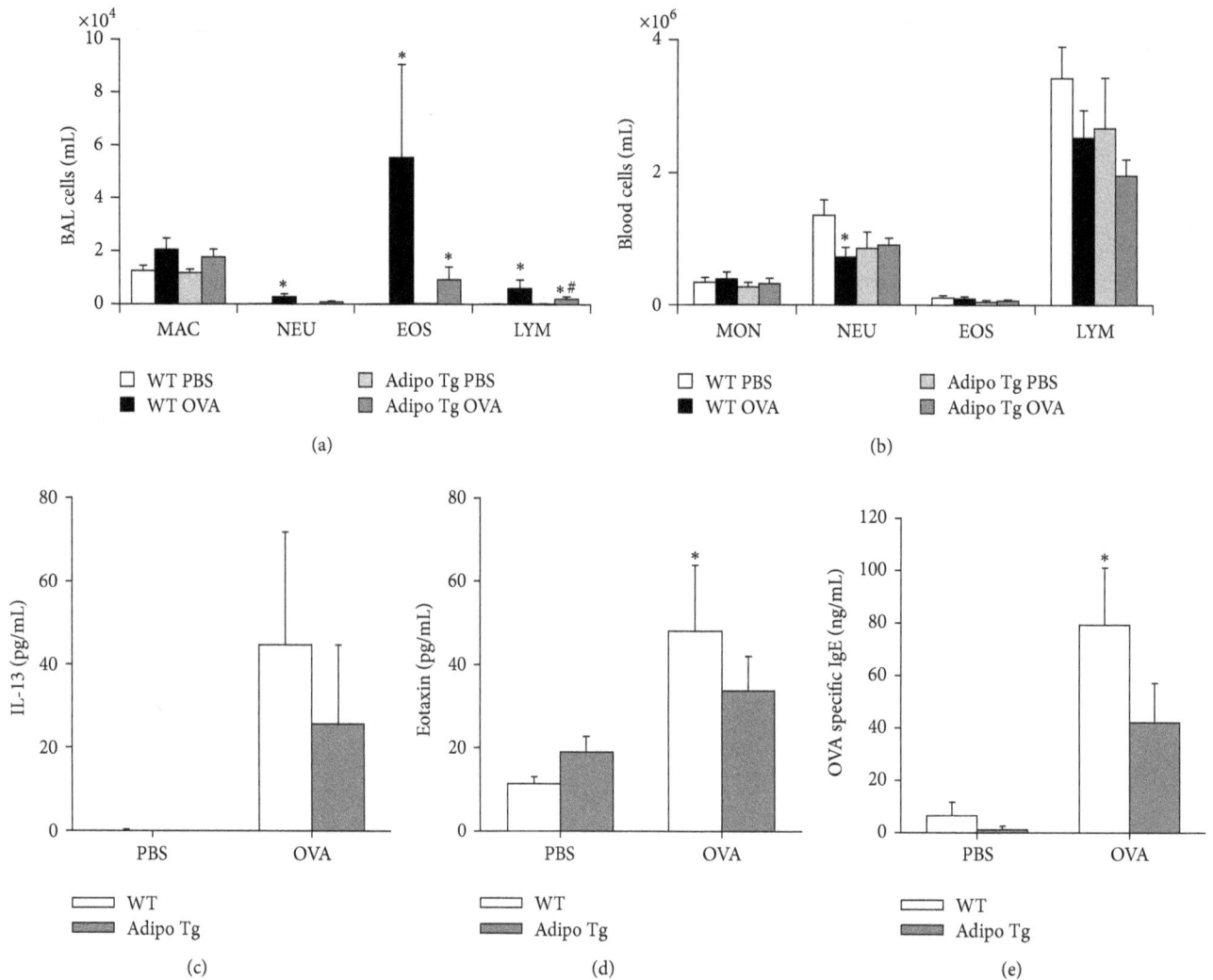

FIGURE 2: Leukocytes in BAL fluid (a) and blood (b) and BAL IL-13 (c), BAL eotaxin (d), and serum OVA-specific IgE (e) of wildtype (WT) and adiponectin transgenic (Adipo Tg) mice sensitized with ovalbumin (OVA) and exposed to aerosols of OVA or PBS. Data shown are mean ± SEM of 5-6 PBS and 9-10 OVA treated mice per group except for OVA-specific IgE (n = 5-6 for PBS and 12-13 for OVA). $^{*}P < 0.05$ versus PBS challenged mice of the same genotype; $^{#}P < 0.05$ versus WT mice with the same exposure. MAC: macrophages; NEU: neutrophils; EOS: eosinophils; LYM: lymphocytes; MON: mononuclear cells.

mice. Compared to PBS, chronic OVA challenge caused a significant increase in both *Chi3l3* and *Clec10a* (Mgl1), but there was no genotype-related difference in the induction of these genes by OVA (Figures 8(a) and 8(b)). We also evaluated expression of M2 associated genes in alveolar macrophages isolated from *naïve* WT and Adipo Tg mice (Figure 8(c)). *Chi3l3, Clec10a,* and *Retnla* mRNA levels were not different in macrophages isolated from WT and Adipo Tg mice.

4. Discussion

Our data indicate that adiponectin overexpression results in a significant reduction in inflammatory cell recruitment to the airspaces (Figure 2) and in the induction of genes known to drive airway inflammation (Figure 3) after acute OVA challenge. A similar reduction in BAL inflammatory cells as well as reductions in BAL eotaxin and IL-13 with

adiponectin overexpression was observed (Figure 4) when we used a chronic OVA challenge protocol in which inflammation is dependent on mast cells [31], a feature relevant to human allergic asthma. Importantly, others have previously reported that adiponectin deficiency results in increased allergic airways inflammation in this chronic challenge protocol, likely as a result of effects on chemokine expression, especially eotaxin [12]. Since mucous hypersecretion is largely refractory to current therapies, we also used the chronic protocol to determine whether adiponectin overexpression might also be effective against this aspect of the allergic airways phenotype. Interestingly, despite having no effect on Muc5ac mRNA abundance (Figure 7), we observed modestly higher goblet cell hyperplasia in mice with excess adiponectin (Figure 6).

Adiponectin overexpression caused a reduction in the number of cells emigrating into the airspaces after acute

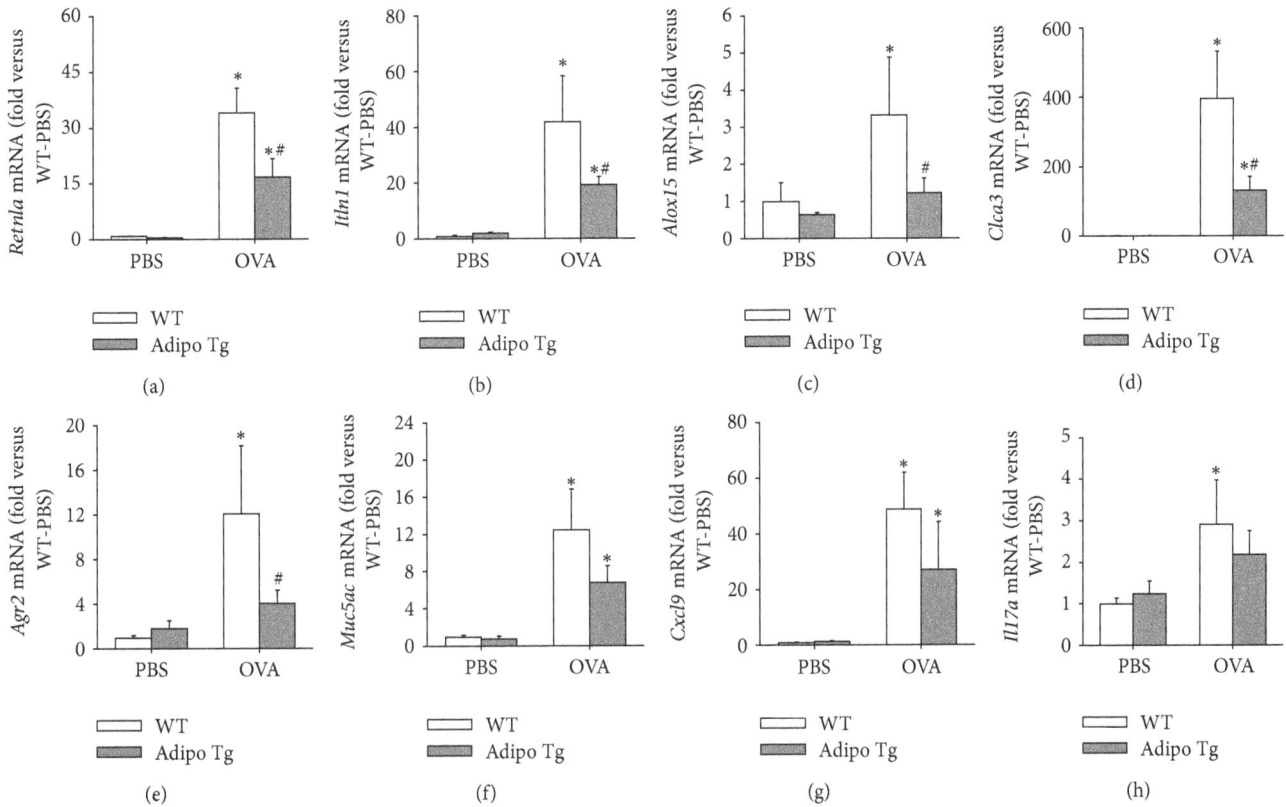

FIGURE 3: Pulmonary mRNA expression of *Retnla* (a), *Itln1* (b), *Alox15* (c), Clca3 (d), Agr2 (e), *Muc5ac* (f), *Cxcl9* (g), and *Il17a* (h) in wildtype (WT) and adiponectin transgenic (Adipo Tg) mice sensitized with ovalbumin (OVA) and exposed to aerosols of OVA or PBS every day for 3 days. Data shown are the means ± SEM of 5-6 mice/group. Data are normalized relative to 18S expression. *$P < 0.05$ versus PBS challenged mice of the same genotype; #$P < 0.05$ versus WT mice with the same challenge.

OVA challenge, consistent with previous observations using exogenous adiponectin administration and a similar allergen challenge model [13]. We also observed significant changes in BAL eotaxin in WT but not Adipo Tg mice after acute OVA challenge. Eotaxin has been shown to contribute to eosinophil recruitment following allergen challenge in mice [45]. OVA specific IgE was also increased by OVA exposure in WT but not Adipo Tg mice (Figure 2(e)). These data confirm results of previous studies that examined the impact of exogenous adiponectin administration [13, 14], albeit in a different strain of mice (C57BL/6 versus Balb/c). Thus, our findings provided proof of concept that the transgenic mice would be a useful model to use for a chronic allergen challenge protocol in which elevated serum adiponectin needed to be sustained for an extended period (see below).

Data from the acute challenge protocol extend results of previous studies by providing effects on expression of inflammatory genes relevant to allergic airways disease. For example, we observed a significant reduction in OVA-induced expression of *Retnla*, *Itln1*, *Clca3*, *Agr2,* and *Alox15* mRNA in Adipo Tg versus WT mice (Figure 3). Intelectin [37] and *Alox15* [42, 46] have each been shown to contribute to allergic airways inflammation in mice. Thus, our data suggest that adiponectin-dependent reductions in BAL cells

may have been secondary to changes in the expression of these genes. In contrast to the effects of adiponectin overexpression on *Retnla*, *Itln1*, *Alox15*, *Clca3*, and *Agr2* mRNA (Figures 3(a)–3(e)), we did not observe any effects of adiponectin on induction of either *Cxcl9* or *Il17a* following acute OVA challenge (Figures 3(g) and 3(h)). Induction of *Retnla*, *Itln1*, *Alox15*, *Clca3*, and *Agr2* by acute OVA challenge is dependent upon IL-13, whereas induction of *Cxcl9* and *Il17a* is not [38, 42, 44, 46, 47]. Nevertheless, we did not observe any significant change in BAL IL-13 in Adipo Tg versus WT mice nor was there any difference in lung IL-13 mRNA abundance (data not shown). Taken together, the data suggest that adiponectin may mediate its effects on expression of *Retnla*, *Itln1*, *Alox15*, *Clca3*, and *Agr2* downstream of IL-13 rather than directly impacting IL-13 expression.

We also examined the effects of adiponectin overexpression using a chronic OVA challenge protocol using weekly intranasal administration of OVA. We chose to examine this protocol because both inflammation and goblet cell hyperplasia require mast cells with this protocol [31], increasing the relevance to human asthma. In contrast, with the acute OVA challenge protocol, these outcomes are dependent upon T cells, but not mast cells [32]. Our data indicated that BAL inflammatory cells, IL-13, and eotaxin are reduced

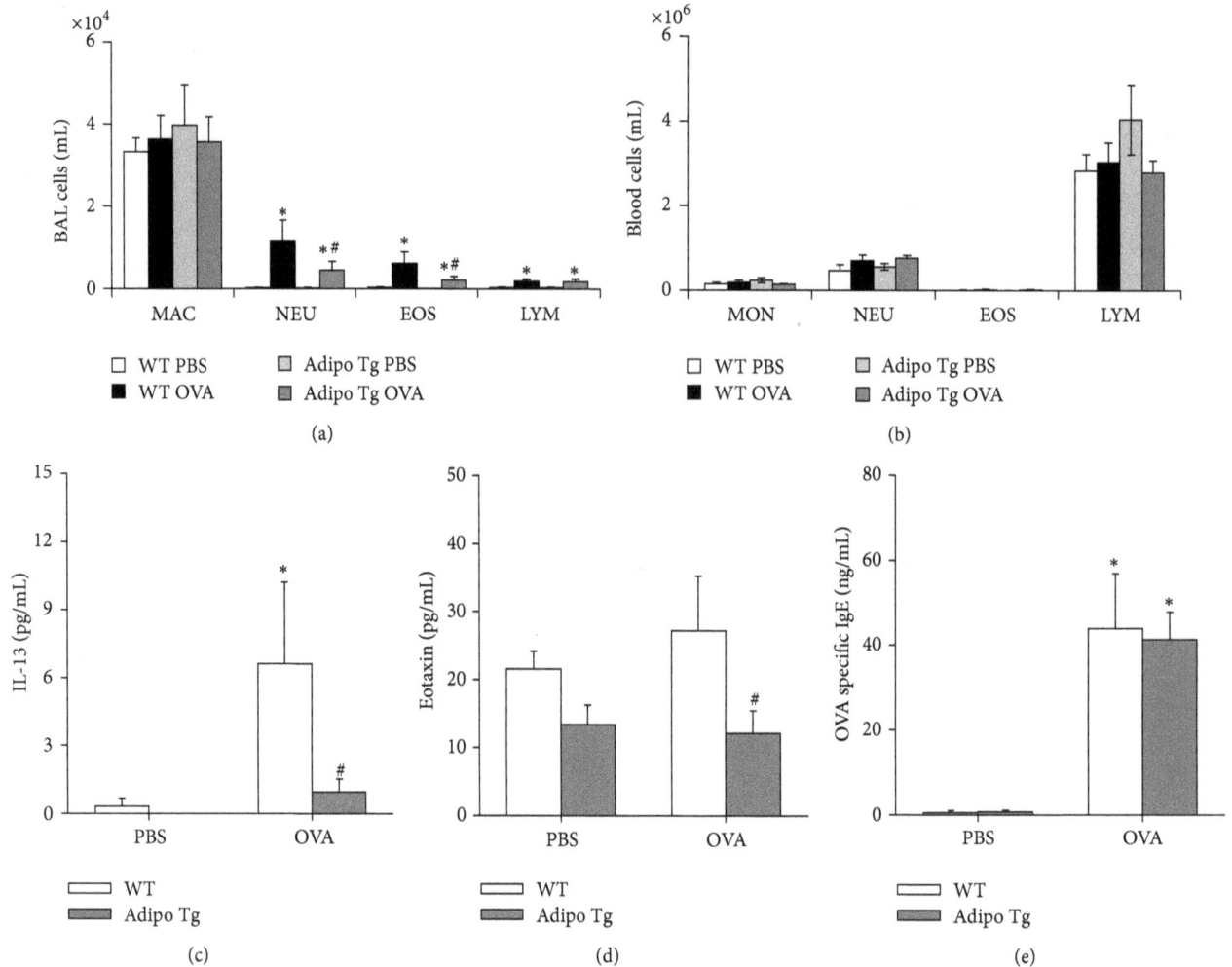

FIGURE 4: Leukocytes in BAL fluid (a) and blood (b), and BAL IL-13 (c), BAL eotaxin (d), and serum OVA-specific IgE (e) in wildtype (WT) and adiponectin transgenic (Adipo Tg) mice sensitized with ovalbumin (OVA) and challenged i.n. with OVA or PBS every week for 4 weeks. Data shown are mean $\pm$ SEM of 5–10 mice per group. $^*P < 0.05$ versus PBS challenged mice of the same genotype; $^\#P < 0.05$ versus WT mice with the same challenge. MAC: macrophages; NEU: neutrophils; EOS: eosinophils; LYM: lymphocytes; MON: mononuclear cells.

in Adipo Tg versus WT mice (Figure 4). These data are consistent with other reports showing that adiponectin deficiency increases allergic airways inflammation with this same challenge protocol [12]. Though our findings with respect to inflammation in chronic OVA-exposed mice (Figure 4) are similar to those from the acute OVA exposure mice (Figure 2), there were some differences. Whereas adiponectin overexpression reduced both inflammatory cell number and IL-13 in BAL in chronic OVA-exposed animals (Figure 4), we observed no difference in lung inflammatory gene expression (Figures 7 and 8). This contrasts with the marked reduction in gene expression induced by adiponectin overexpression with the acute OVA protocol (Figure 3). Consistent with the lack of effect on pulmonary gene expression in the chronic protocol, adiponectin overexpression had no effect on inflammation within the lung tissue: semi-quantitative analysis of airway inflammation from histological sections indicated no genotype-related effect (Figure 6). Taken together, the results

suggest that in the chronic OVA model, adiponectin may act to prevent inflammatory/immune cell transit across the airway epithelium.

We sought to determine whether transgenic expression of adiponectin might be effective in reducing the goblet cell metaplasia associated with allergic airways disease. Goblet cell metaplasia was induced in this chronic OVA challenge model (Figures 5 and 6), and there was also significant induction of genes involved in mucous cell metaplasia (*Muc5ac, Agr2, and Clca3*) (Figure 7). Nevertheless, we observed a modest but significant *increase* in goblet cells in Adipo Tg mice versus WT mice (Figures 5 and 6). To our knowledge, this is the first study examining effects of adiponectin on goblet cell metaplasia in the lungs, although others have reported significant reductions in other aspects of the remodeling process (pulmonary vascular and airway smooth muscle cell proliferation) in mice with elevated adiponectin [14, 48].

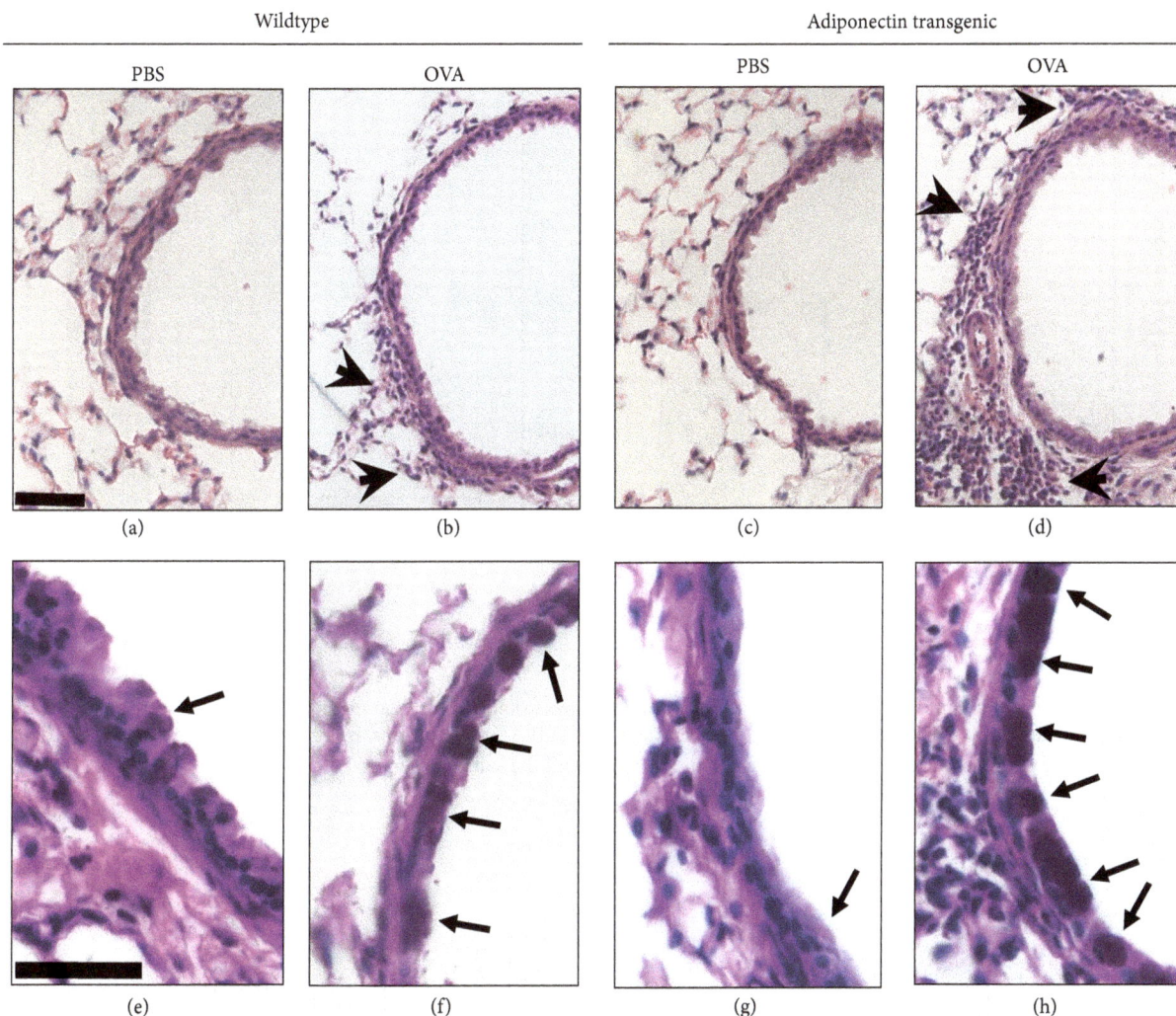

FIGURE 5: Histological sections of airways of wildtype (WT) and adiponectin transgenic (Adipo Tg) mice sensitized with ovalbumin (OVA) without alum and challenged intranasally with OVA or PBS every week for 4 weeks (chronic). Light micrographs showing H&E (panels (a)–(d)) or PAS (panels (e)–(h)) staining. Arrowheads in (a)–(d) indicate regions of inflammatory cell accumulation. Arrows in (e)–(h) indicate regions of "purple" staining that were recognized by Image Pro software (Olympus) during quantification of goblet cell abundance (see text). The bars in panels (a) and (e) = 10 μm and correspond to all images in the upper and lower row, respectively. PAS staining for mucous-containing goblet cells ((e)–(h)) is from medium sized peripheral airways.

We were somewhat surprised to find that adiponectin overexpression augmented goblet cell hyperplasia, especially since IL-13, which is widely considered to drive this phenotype, was reduced in the Adipo Tg mice (Figure 4(c)). It is conceivable that the apparent increase in goblet cells in Adipo Tg mice was the result of less release of mucus into the airways and consequent increased retention of mucus within the cells themselves. However, the observation that expression of *Agr2* and *Clca3* also tended to increase in Adipo Tg versus WT mice (Figure 7) suggests otherwise. Of note, *Agr2* is an endoplasmic reticulum protein required for production of mucous glycoproteins like Muc5ac [49], while *Clca3* (gob-5) is required for OVA-induced goblet cell metaplasia and airspace inflammation in mice [50]. The increased goblet cell numbers and the trend towards increased Agr2 and Clca3 mRNA abundance in the Adipo Tg versus WT mice

is consistent with the results of other investigators who have examined the impact of adiponectin on goblet cell hyperplasia in other organs [51, 52]. For example, Saxena et al. reported that adiponectin increases the differentiation of intestinal epithelial cells towards goblet cells [52]. Similarly, Li et al. reported that exogenous administration of adiponectin in the form of eye drops increased conjunctival goblet cell density in a mouse model of experimental dry eye [51].

In the Adipo Tg mice, adiponectin concentrations were extremely high both in the BAL fluid and the serum. It is possible that proinflammatory effects of adiponectin [18–20] impacted goblet cell numbers due to these sustained high concentrations. Contrary to this contention, we did observe reductions in both *Agr2* and *Clca3* mRNA in Adipo Tg versus WT mice upon acute OVA challenge. Others have used the chicken beta-actin promoter, cytomegalovirus enhancer that

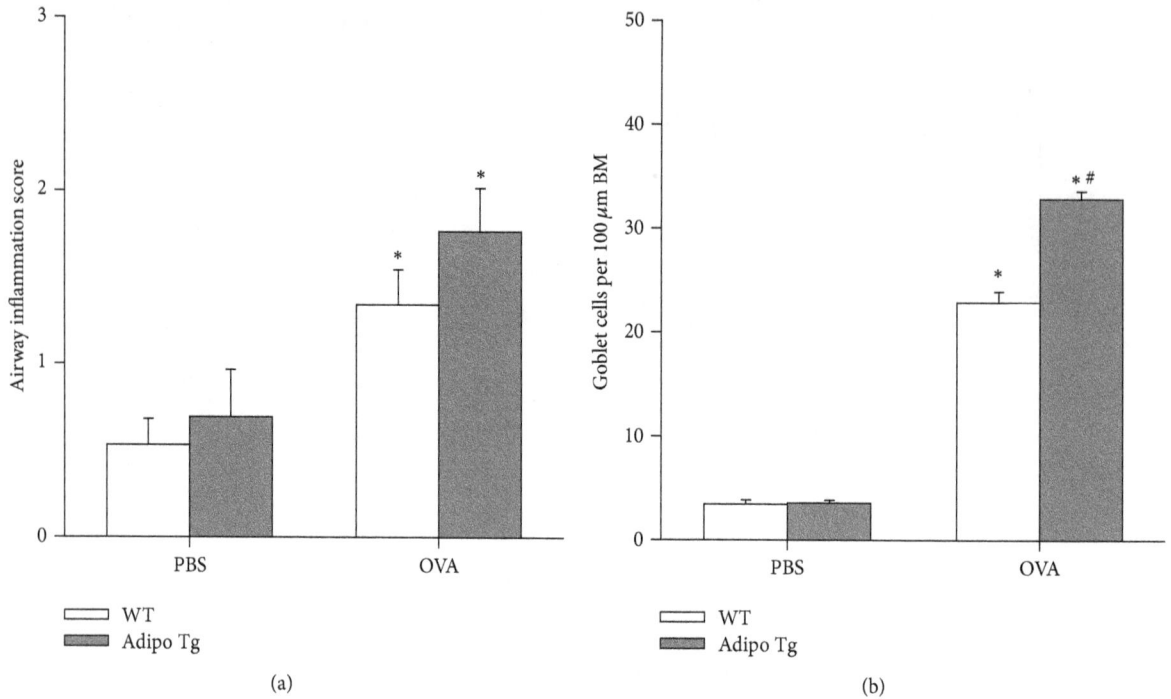

(a)

(b)

FIGURE 6: Quantitation of inflammatory cell accumulation around airways (a) and goblet cell metaplasia (b). Data shown are the means ± SEM of 4-5 mice/group in the PBS treated groups and 7 mice/group in the OVA treated groups. BM: basement membrane. $^*P < 0.05$ versus PBS challenged mice of the same genotype; $^\#P < 0.05$ versus WT mice with the same challenge.

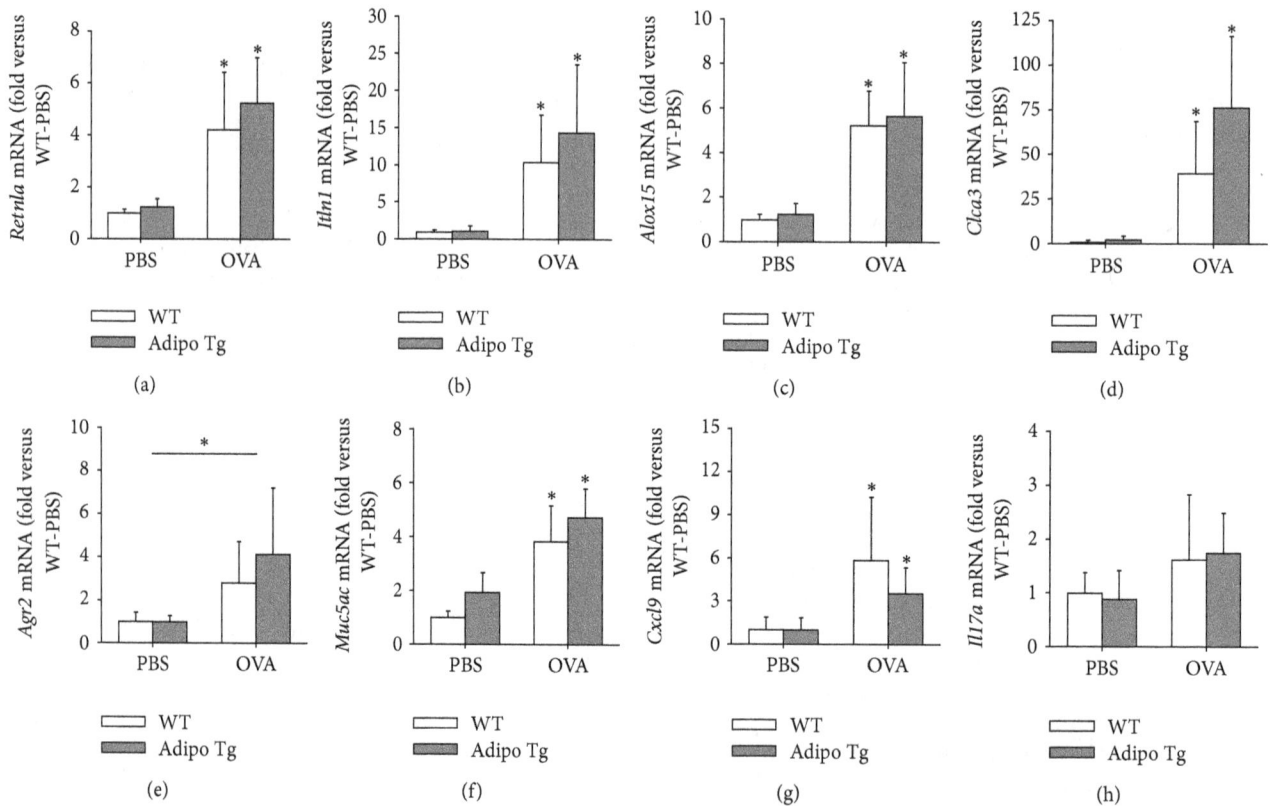

(a)

(b)

(c)

(d)

(e)

(f)

(g)

(h)

FIGURE 7: Pulmonary mRNA expression of *Retnla* (a), *Itln1* (b), Alox15 (c), Clca3 (d), Agr2 (e), *Muc5ac* (f), *Cxcl9* (g), and *Il17a* (h) in wildtype (WT) and adiponectin transgenic (Adipo Tg) mice sensitized with ovalbumin (OVA) and challenged i.n. with OVA or PBS once a week for 4 weeks. Data shown are the means ± SEM of 6–11 mice/group. Data are normalized relative to 18S expression. $^*P < 0.05$ versus PBS challenged mice of the same genotype.

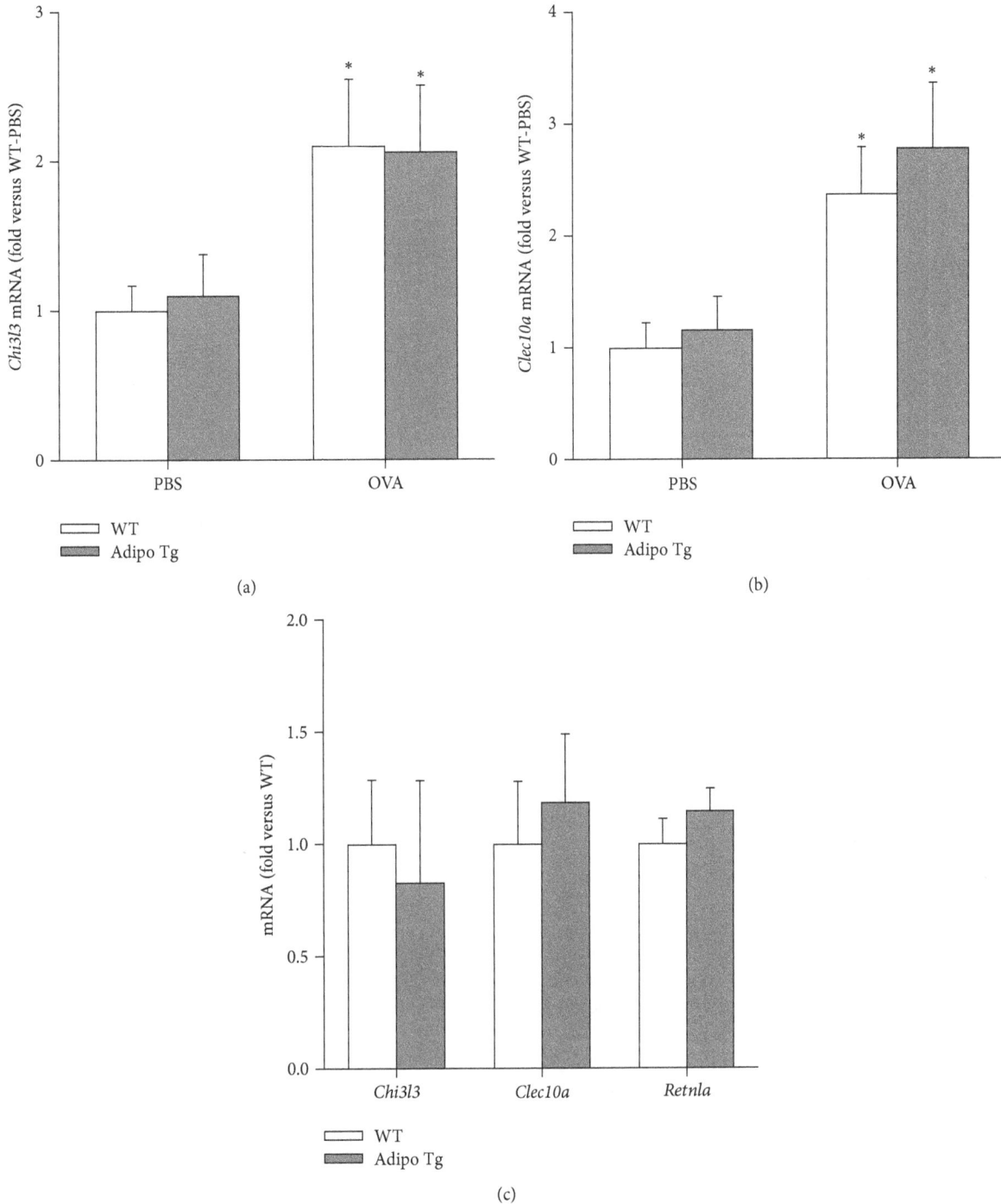

FIGURE 8: Pulmonary mRNA expression of *Chi3l3* (a) and *Clec10a* (b) in wildtype (WT) and adiponectin transgenic (Adipo Tg) mice sensitized with ovalbumin (OVA) and challenged i.n. with OVA or PBS. Data shown are the means ± SEM of 6–11 mice/group. $^{*}P < 0.05$ versus PBS challenged mice of the same genotype. (c) Expression of *Chi3l3*, *Clec10a*, and *Retnla* mRNA in alveolar macrophages harvested from naïve wildtype and Adipo Tg mice. Results are mean ± SEM of data from 5–8 mice in each group. Data were normalized relative to 18S expression.

drove adiponectin expression in these mice to drive EGFP [53]. In the lungs of the resulting "green" mice, EGFP is mostly observed in the airway epithelium. Hence, it is conceivable that the enhanced goblet cell numbers are a consequence of coexpression of a transgene within these cells, although mRNA expression of epithelial genes (i.e., *Itln1*, *Retnla*, *Agr2*, *Clca3*, and *Muc5ac*) was not affected (Figure 7). Further investigation will be required to identify the cellular and molecular mechanisms at play. Nonetheless, our observations suggest that the molecular mechanisms controlling goblet cell hyperplasia in response to sustained chronic allergen challenge may be regulated by mechanisms that are different from those that regulate immune cell accumulation within the airways.

Expression of *Retnla, Itln1, Alox15, Agr2, and Clca3* was not reduced in Adipo Tg versus WT mice after chronic OVA challenge (Figure 7), whereas adiponectin overexpression caused a marked reduction in these same genes following acute OVA challenge (Figure 3). The differences in these observations may relate to differences in the mast cell/T cell dependence of the two models, as discussed above. For example, the cell targeted by adiponectin in acute protocol may be T cells themselves. It is also important to note that the magnitude of the inflammation induced by chronic OVA challenge was substantially less than that induced by acute challenge (BAL eosinophilia in Figures 2 and 4, and gene expression in Figures 3 and 7). It is conceivable that with the more subdued inflammation in the chronic protocol, endogenous levels of adiponectin are sufficient to provide maximal inhibition of gene expression, and increasing adiponectin further has no effect. It is also possible that differences in the magnitude of inflammation induced in the two models contribute directly to differences in gene expression, since RNA was evaluated in whole lung: differences in lung gene expression may reflect the different cell populations in the lungs under the different conditions and the different gene expression profiles of these cells.

Our data do not support a role for adiponectin in alternative activation of *lung* macrophages. Firstly, we observed no difference in the expression of genes classically associated with M2 status in alveolar macrophages harvested from naïve Adipo Tg versus WT mice (Figure 8(c)), despite evidence that these macrophages normally exist in a microenvironment replete with excess adiponectin (Figure 1(b)). Secondly, adiponectin overexpression either had no effect on (Figures 7 and 8) or significantly reduced (Figure 3) OVA-induced increases in the expression of *Retnla, Chi3l3, and Clec10a.* In contrast, in macrophages from other sources, including peritoneal macrophages, adipose tissue macrophages, Kupffer cells, bone marrow or monocyte-derived macrophages, and macrophage cell lines, adiponectin augments the induction of these M2 genes either on its own or in conjunction with Th2 cytokines [27–29]. Effects of adiponectin on expression of M2 genes in lung macrophages has not previously been examined, although there is evidence that adiponectin deficiency increases M1 type activation of lung macrophages, as indicated by increased MHC class 2 expression and augmented TNFα production [26, 27]. However, adiponectin can also have proinflammatory effects on lung macrophages, since macrophages from adiponectin deficient mice produce less TNFα in response to cigarette smoke extract than wildtype mice [54].

5. Conclusions

In conclusion, transgenic overexpression of adiponectin in mice protected against the development of allergic airways inflammation and expression of IL-13 dependent genes after acute OVA challenge. Airspace inflammation was also reduced by adiponectin overexpression after chronic OVA. In contrast, inflammatory gene expression was not impacted by

adiponectin overexpression, and goblet cell hyperplasia was increased. The data indicate that the ability of adiponectin supplementation to ameliorate allergic airways disease is dependent on the nature of the model employed. From a clinical perspective, our data suggest that increasing circulating adiponectin in obese individuals or agonists that target adiponectin receptors would be expected to decrease allergic airway inflammation but would not be beneficial in reducing the mucous metaplasia characteristic of allergic asthma.

Acknowledgments

This study was supported by National Institutes of Health Grant HL-084044, HL-077499, and ES000002. Andrew J. Halayko is supported through the Canada Research Chairs Program.

References

[1] E. S. Ford, "The epidemiology of obesity and asthma," *Journal of Allergy and Clinical Immunology*, vol. 115, no. 5, pp. 897–910, 2005.

[2] B. Taylor, D. Mannino, C. Brown, D. Crocker, N. Twum-Baah, and F. Holguin, "Body mass index and asthma severity in the National Asthma Survey," *Thorax*, vol. 63, no. 1, pp. 14–20, 2008.

[3] K. L. Lavoie, S. L. Bacon, M. Labrecque, A. Cartier, and B. Ditto, "Higher BMI is associated with worse asthma control and quality of life but not asthma severity," *Respiratory Medicine*, vol. 100, no. 4, pp. 648–657, 2006.

[4] P. Saint-Pierre, A. Bourdin, P. Chanez, J. P. Daures, and P. Godard, "Are overweight asthmatics more difficult to control?" *Allergy*, vol. 61, no. 1, pp. 79–84, 2006.

[5] T. Kadowaki, T. Yamauchi, and N. Kubota, "The physiological and pathophysiological role of adiponectin and adiponectin receptors in the peripheral tissues and CNS," *FEBS Letters*, vol. 582, no. 1, pp. 74–80, 2008.

[6] N. Kubota, Y. Terauchi, T. Yamauchi et al., "Disruption of adiponectin causes insulin resistance and neointimal formation," *Journal of Biological Chemistry*, vol. 277, no. 29, pp. 25863–25866, 2002.

[7] A. R. Nawrocki, M. W. Rajala, E. Tomas et al., "Mice lacking adiponectin show decreased hepatic insulin sensitivity and reduced responsiveness to peroxisome proliferator-activated receptor γ agonists," *Journal of Biological Chemistry*, vol. 281, no. 5, pp. 2654–2660, 2006.

[8] K. Hotta, T. Funahashi, Y. Arita et al., "Plasma concentrations of a novel, adipose-specific protein, adiponectin, in type 2 diabetic patients," *Arteriosclerosis, Thrombosis, and Vascular Biology*, vol. 20, no. 6, pp. 1595–1599, 2000.

[9] D. A. Patel, S. R. Srinivasan, J. H. Xu, W. Chen, and G. S. Berenson, "Adiponectin and its correlates of cardiovascular risk in young adults: the Bogalusa Heart Study," *Metabolism*, vol. 55, pp. 1551–1557, 2006.

[10] M. Shargorodsky, M. Boaz, Y. Goldberg et al., "Adiponectin and vascular properties in obese patients: is it a novel biomarker of early atherosclerosis," *International Journal of Obesity*, vol. 33, no. 5, pp. 553–558, 2009.

[11] A. Sood, X. Cui, C. Quails et al., "Association between asthma and serum adiponectin concentration in women," *Thorax*, vol. 63, no. 10, pp. 877–882, 2008.

[12] B. D. Medoff, Y. Okamoto, P. Leyton et al., "Adiponectin deficiency increases allergic airway inflammation and pulmonary vascular remodeling," *The American Journal of Respiratory Cell and Molecular Biology*, vol. 41, no. 4, pp. 397–406, 2009.

[13] S. A. Shore, R. D. Terry, L. Flynt, A. Xu, and C. Hug, "Adiponectin attenuates allergen-induced airway inflammation and hyperresponsiveness in mice," *Journal of Allergy and Clinical Immunology*, vol. 118, no. 2, pp. 389–395, 2006.

[14] L. I. Ionescu, R. S. Alphonse, N. Arizmendi et al., "Airway delivery of soluble factors from plastic-adherent bone marrow cells prevents murine asthma," *The American Journal of Respiratory Cell and Molecular Biology*, vol. 46, pp. 207–216, 2012.

[15] S. Siddiqui and J. G. Martin, "Structural aspects of airway remodeling in asthma," *Current Allergy and Asthma Reports*, vol. 8, no. 6, pp. 540–547, 2008.

[16] M. Miller, J. Y. Cho, A. Pham, J. Ramsdell, and D. H. Broide, "Adiponectin and functional adiponectin receptor 1 are expressed by airway epithelial cells in chronic obstructive pulmonary disease," *Journal of Immunology*, vol. 182, no. 1, pp. 684–691, 2009.

[17] A. S. Williams, D. I. Kasahara, N. G. Verbout et al., "Role of the adiponectin binding protein, T-cadherin (Cdh13), in allergic airways responses in mice," *PLoS One*, vol. 7, Article ID e41088, 2012.

[18] F. Haugen and C. A. Drevon, "Activation of nuclear factor-κB by high molecular weight and globular adiponectin," *Endocrinology*, vol. 148, no. 11, pp. 5478–5486, 2007.

[19] E. A. Mcdonald and M. W. Wolfe, "The pro-inflammatory role of adiponectin at the maternal-fetal interface," *The American Journal of Reproductive Immunology*, vol. 66, no. 2, pp. 128–136, 2011.

[20] K. Kitahara, N. Kusunoki, T. Kakiuchi, T. Suguro, and S. Kawai, "Adiponectin stimulates IL-8 production by rheumatoid synovial fibroblasts," *Biochemical and Biophysical Research Communications*, vol. 378, no. 2, pp. 218–223, 2009.

[21] K. Furukawa, M. Hori, N. Ouchi et al., "Adiponectin downregulates acyl-coenzyme A: cholesterol acyltransferase-1 in cultured human monocyte-derived macrophages," *Biochemical and Biophysical Research Communications*, vol. 317, no. 3, pp. 831–836, 2004.

[22] N. Ouchi, S. Kihara, Y. Arita et al., "Adipocyte-derived plasma protein, adiponectin, suppresses lipid accumulation and class A scavenger receptor expression in human monocyte-derived macrophages," *Circulation*, vol. 103, no. 8, pp. 1057–1063, 2001.

[23] T. Yokota, K. Oritani, I. Takahashi et al., "Adiponectin, a new member of the family of soluble defense collagens, negatively regulates the growth of myelomonocytic progenitors and the functions of macrophages," *Blood*, vol. 96, no. 5, pp. 1723–1732, 2000.

[24] T. Masaki, S. Chiba, H. Tatsukawa et al., "Adiponectin protects LPS-induced liver injury through modulation of TNF-α in KK-Ay obese mice," *Hepatology*, vol. 40, no. 1, pp. 177–184, 2004.

[25] L. Tian, N. Luo, R. L. Klein, B. H. Chung, W. T. Garvey, and Y. Fu, "Adiponectin reduces lipid accumulation in macrophage foam cells," *Atherosclerosis*, vol. 202, no. 1, pp. 152–161, 2009.

[26] R. Summer, F. F. Little, N. Ouchi et al., "Alveolar macrophage activation and an emphysema-like phenotype in adiponectin-deficient mice," *The American Journal of Physiology*, vol. 294, no. 6, pp. L1035–L1042, 2008.

[27] K. Ohashi, J. L. Parker, N. Ouchi et al., "Adiponectin promotes macrophage polarization toward an anti-inflammatory phenotype," *Journal of Biological Chemistry*, vol. 285, no. 9, pp. 6153–6160, 2010.

[28] P. Mandal, B. T. Pratt, M. Barnes, M. R. McMullen, and L. E. Nagy, "Molecular mechanism for adiponectin-dependent m2 macrophage polarization link between the metabolic and innate immune activity of full-length adiponectin," *Journal of Biological Chemistry*, vol. 286, no. 15, pp. 13460–13469, 2011.

[29] F. Lovren, Y. Pan, A. Quan et al., "Adiponectin primes human monocytes into alternative anti-inflammatory M2 macrophages," *The American Journal of Physiology*, vol. 299, no. 3, pp. H656–H663, 2010.

[30] M. Zhu, C. Hug, D. I. Kasahara et al., "Impact of adiponectin deficiency on pulmonary responses to acute ozone exposure in mice," *The American Journal of Respiratory Cell and Molecular Biology*, vol. 43, no. 4, pp. 487–497, 2010.

[31] M. Yu, M. Tsai, S. Y. Tam, C. Jones, J. Zehnder, and S. J. Galli, "Mast cells can promote the development of multiple features of chronic asthma in mice," *Journal of Clinical Investigation*, vol. 116, no. 6, pp. 1633–1641, 2006.

[32] K. Takeda, E. Hamelmann, A. Joetham et al., "Development of eosinophilic airway inflammation and airway hyperresponsiveness in mast cell-deficient mice," *Journal of Experimental Medicine*, vol. 186, no. 3, pp. 449–454, 1997.

[33] G. W. Wong, S. A. Krawczyk, C. Kitidis-Mitrokostas et al., "Identification and characterization of CTRP9, a novel secreted glycoprotein, from adipose tissue that reduces serum glucose in mice and forms heterotrimers with adiponectin," *FASEB Journal*, vol. 23, no. 1, pp. 241–258, 2009.

[34] R. A. Johnston, M. Zhu, Y. M. Rivera-Sanchez et al., "Allergic airway responses in obese mice," *The American Journal of Respiratory and Critical Care Medicine*, vol. 176, no. 7, pp. 650–658, 2007.

[35] M. Zhu, P. Y. Liu, D. I. Kasahara et al., "Role of Rho kinase isoforms in murine allergic airway responses," *European Respiratory Journal*, vol. 38, pp. 841–850, 2011.

[36] K. Hamada, Y. Suzaki, A. Goldman et al., "Allergen-independent maternal transmission of asthma susceptibility," *Journal of Immunology*, vol. 170, no. 4, pp. 1683–1689, 2003.

[37] N. Gu, G. Kang, C. Jin et al., "Intelectin is required for IL-13-induced monocyte chemotactic protein-1 and -3 expression in lung epithelial cells and promotes allergic airway inflammation," *The American Journal of Physiology*, vol. 298, no. 3, pp. L290–L296, 2010.

[38] D. A. Kuperman, C. C. Lewis, P. G. Woodruff et al., "Dissecting asthma using focused transgenic modeling and functional genomics," *Journal of Allergy and Clinical Immunology*, vol. 116, no. 2, pp. 305–311, 2005.

[39] S. Schnyder-Candrian, D. Togbe, I. Couillin et al., "Interleukin-17 is a negative regulator of established allergic asthma," *Journal of Experimental Medicine*, vol. 203, no. 12, pp. 2715–2725, 2006.

[40] L. Zhang, M. Wang, X. Kang et al., "Oxidative stress and asthma: proteome analysis of chitinase-like proteins and FIZZ1 in lung tissue and bronchoalveolar lavage fluid," *Journal of Proteome Research*, vol. 8, no. 4, pp. 1631–1638, 2009.

[41] M. Z. Alimam, F. M. Piazza, D. M. Selby, N. Letwin, L. Huang, and M. C. Rose, "Muc-5/5ac mucin messenger RNA and protein expression is a marker of goblet cell metaplasia in murine airways," *The American Journal of Respiratory Cell and Molecular Biology*, vol. 22, no. 3, pp. 253–260, 2000.

[42] C. K. Andersson, H. E. Claesson, K. Rydell-Törmänen, S. Swedmark, A. Hällgren, and J. S. Erjefält, "Mice lacking 12/15-lipoxygenase have attenuated airway allergic inflammation and remodeling," *The American Journal of Respiratory Cell and Molecular Biology*, vol. 39, no. 6, pp. 648–656, 2008.

[43] E. Di Valentin, C. Crahay, N. Garbacki et al., "New asthma biomarkers: lessons from murine models of acute and chronic asthma," *The American Journal of Physiology*, vol. 296, no. 2, pp. L185–L197, 2009.

[44] C. C. Lewis, B. Aronow, J. Hutton et al., "Unique and overlapping gene expression patterns driven by IL-4 and IL-13 in the mouse lung," *Journal of Allergy and Clinical Immunology*, vol. 123, no. 4, pp. 795–804, 2009.

[45] M. E. Rothenberg, J. A. MacLean, E. Pearlman, A. D. Luster, and P. Leder, "Targeted disruption of the chemokine eotaxin partially reduces antigen-induced tissue eosinophilia," *Journal of Experimental Medicine*, vol. 185, no. 4, pp. 785–790, 1997.

[46] A. R. Lindley, M. Crapster-Pregont, Y. Liu, and D. A. Kuperman, "12/15-lipoxygenase is an interleukin-13 and interferon-γ counterregulated-mediator of allergic airway inflammation," *Mediators of Inflammation*, vol. 2010, Article ID 727305, 10 pages, 2010.

[47] P. Thai, Y. Chen, G. Dolganov, and R. Wu, "Differential regulation of MUC5AC/Muc5ac and hCLCA-1/mGob 5 expression in airway epithelium," *The American Journal of Respiratory Cell and Molecular Biology*, vol. 33, no. 6, pp. 523–530, 2005.

[48] M. Weng, M. J. Raher, P. Leyton et al., "Adiponectin decreases pulmonary arterial remodeling in murine models of pulmonary hypertension," *The American Journal of Respiratory Cell and Molecular Biology*, vol. 45, pp. 340–347, 2011.

[49] B. W. Schroeder, C. Verhaeghe, S. W. Park et al., "AGR2 is induced in asthma and promotes allergen-induced mucin overproduction," *The American Journal of Respiratory Cell and Molecular Biology*, vol. 47, pp. 178–185, 2012.

[50] A. J. Long, J. P. Sypek, R. Askew et al., "Gob-5 contributes to goblet cell hyperplasia and modulates pulmonary tissue inflammation," *The American Journal of Respiratory Cell and Molecular Biology*, vol. 35, pp. 357–365, 2006.

[51] Z. Li, J. M. Woo, S. W. Chung et al., "Therapeutic effect of topical adiponectin in a mouse model of desiccating stress-induced dry eye," *Investigative Ophthalmology and Visual Science*, vol. 54, pp. 155–162, 2013.

[52] A. Saxena, M. S. Baliga, V. Ponemone et al., "Mucus and adiponectin deficiency: role in chronic inflammation-induced colon cancer," *International Journal of Colorectal Disease*. In press.

[53] D. F. Ma, H. Tezuka, T. Kondo et al., "Differential tissue expression of enhanced green fluorescent protein in 'green mice'," *Histology and histopathology*, vol. 25, no. 6, pp. 749–754, 2010.

[54] M. Miller, A. Pham, J. Y. Cho, P. Rosenthal, and D. H. Broide, "Adiponectin-deficient mice are protected against tobacco-induced inflammation and increased emphysema," *The American Journal of Physiology*, vol. 299, no. 6, pp. L834–L842, 2010.

15

Immunochemical Characterization of *Acacia* Pollen Allergens and Evaluation of Cross-Reactivity Pattern with the Common Allergenic Pollens

Mohammad-Hosein Shamsbiranvand,[1,2] **Ali Khodadadi,**[1,2]
Mohammad-Ali Assarehzadegan,[2] **Seyed Hamid Borsi,**[3] **and Akram Amini**[2]

[1] *Cancer Research Center of Ahvaz Jundishapur University of Medical Sciences, Ahvaz, Iran*
[2] *Department of Immunology, Faculty of Medicine, Ahvaz Jundishapur University of Medical Sciences, Ahvaz 6135715794, Iran*
[3] *Department of Internal Medicine, Faculty of Medicine, Ahvaz Jundishapur University of Medical Sciences, Ahvaz, Iran*

Correspondence should be addressed to Mohammad-Ali Assarehzadegan; assarehma@gmail.com

Academic Editor: William E. Berger

Pollen from the *Acacia* has been reported as an important source of pollinosis in tropical and subtropical regions of the world. The aim of this study was to characterize the IgE binding protein of *Acacia farnesiana* pollen extract and evaluate cross-reactivity with the most allergenic pollens. In this study, pollen extract was fractionated by SDS-PAGE and the allergenic profile was determined by IgE-immunoblotting and specific ELISA using forty-two *Acacia* allergic patients. Potential cross-reactivity among *Acacia* and selected allergenic plants was evaluated with ELISA and immunoblotting inhibition experiments. There were several resolved protein fractions on SDS-PAGE which ranged from 12 to 85 kDa. Several allergenic protein bands with molecular weights approximately between 12 and 85 kDa were recognized by IgE-specific antibodies from *Acacia* allergic patients in the immunoblot assay. The inhibition by the *Prosopis juliflora* pollen extract was more than those by other pollen extracts. Moreover, the wheal diameters generated by the *Acacia* pollen extract were highly correlated with those of *P. juliflora* pollen extracts. The findings suggest that several proteins such as 15, 23, 45, and 50 kDa proteins could be used as diagnostic and therapeutic reagents for patients allergic to *A. farnesiana* and *P. juliflora*.

1. Introduction

Acacia farnesiana (*Vachellia farnesiana*), a member of the Fabaceae family, is common throughout tropical and subtropical regions of Asia, Africa, Australia, and America with hot and humid climates, where it is planted as a shade and/or ornamental tree or for binding sand [1, 2]. Pollens from the Fabaceae family have been reported as an important source of pollinosis in the United States, European countries, and Asia [1–3]. Moreover, the inhalation of *A. farnesiana* pollen is one of the main causes of respiratory allergic diseases in semiarid countries such as Iran, Saudi Arabia, and the United Arab Emirates, where the frequency of sensitization ranges from 25% to 48% [2, 4–7].

Howlett et al. reported a high level of cross-reactivity between *Acacia* (wattle) and *Lolium perenne* (rye grass) pollen using the radioallergosorbent test (RAST) [8]. The results showed that IgE molecules which bound to *Acacia* pollen proteins also bound to *L. perenne* pollen extracts. In spite of a high rate of sensitization to *Acacia* pollen in Iran and neighboring countries, to our knowledge, there are few studies about the characterization of *A. farnesiana* pollen extract, and cross-reactivity of this plant with the five most allergenic pollens in arid and semiarid areas (*Prosopis juliflora*, *Salsola kali*, *Amaranthus retroflexus*, *Chenopodium album*, and *Kochia scoparia*) is not well documented [2, 5, 9, 10].

The recognition of allergenic components of pollens is essential for component-resolved diagnosis, the design of patient-specific immunotherapy, and the explanation of sensitization mechanisms to various allergens [11, 12]. In this study, we evaluate proteins of *Acacia* pollen extract which are specifically reactive to the immunoglobulin E (IgE) of pollen-allergic patients and the IgE cross-reactivity among *A. farnesiana* and the selected plants using *in vivo* and *in vitro* assessments.

2. Materials and Methods

2.1. Preparation of Extract. Polleniferous materials were collected from *A. farnesiana's* flowers during February–May throughout Ahvaz city, a tropical region in southwest Iran with a tropical climate and a population of more than 1.4 million [2].

Collection and processing of pollen materials was done carefully by trained pollen collectors. Pollen grains were separated by passing the dried materials through different sieves (100, 200, and 300 meshes) successively. The final fine powder was subjected to a purity check for pollen content using a microscope. Pollen materials with more than 95% pollen and less than 5% floral parts of the same plant were taken for antigen extraction.

Pollen materials were defatted using repeated changes of diethyl ether. Pollen was extracted as described previously [10]. In brief, two grams of pollen was mixed with 10 mL phosphate-buffered saline (PBS) 0.01 M (pH 7.4) by continuous stirring for 18 h at 4°C. The extract was centrifuged at 16,000 g, filtered through a 0.22 μm membrane under sterile conditions, and dialyzed against 10 mM phosphate buffer. The extract was then freeze-dried. The protein content of the extract was measured by Bradford's method [13].

2.2. Patients and Skin Prick Test. Forty-two respiratory allergic patients were enrolled in this study presented to the Immunology and Allergy Department of Ahvaz Jundishapur University of Medical Sciences. The patients were asked to complete a detailed questionnaire. They were considered as having a history of allergy if they reported at least one eye, nasal, or respiratory symptom to common allergens such as house dust, domestic animals, food, or pollen. The patients were also evaluated by a clinical examination and a skin prick test (SPT) with common aeroallergens. Ten healthy subjects who presented negative SPTs and no specific IgE to the *A. farnesiana* pollen extract were assigned as negative controls. The human ethics committee of the institute approved the study protocol with informed written consent from each patient.

Skin prick tests were performed by an experienced nurse under physician's supervision. In this test, *A. farnesiana* and the most allergenic pollen extracts (*Prosopis juliflora, Salsola kali, Amaranthus retroflexus, Chenopodium album,* and *Kochia scoparia*) were put on the patients' inner forearms and irritation of the epidermis was caused by prick method. The result was observed after 15 minutes. Next, the mean diameter of wheal reaction in every patient was measured and compared with negative (glycerol saline) and positive (histamine, 10 mg/mL) controls. Patients with a wheal diameter >3 mm were considered positive compared to negative and

positive controls and were asked to donate a serum sample. Serum samples of patients were stored at −20°C before use.

2.3. Enzyme-Linked Immunosorbent Assays (ELISAs). Total serum IgE levels were measured by means of a commercially available ELISA kit according to the manufacturer's instructions (Radim, Italy).

To measure the levels of specific IgE to *A. farnesiana* pollen in patients' sera, an indirect ELISA was developed as described earlier [14]. Briefly, 0.2 μg of *A. farnesiana* pollen extract in 100 μL carbonate buffer (15 mM Na_2CO_3 and 35 mM $NaHCO_3$, pH 9.6) was incubated at 4°C overnight per well of a 96-well microtiter plate (Nunc MaxiSorp, Denmark). Each well was then blocked for 1 h at 37°C with 150 μL of 2% BSA in PBS followed by incubation for 3 h with 100 μL of serum at room temperature with shaking. Each well was then incubated for 2 h at room temperature with 1 : 1000 dilution of biotinylated goat anti-human IgE antibody (Nordic Immunology Co., Netherlands) in 1% BSA. Each incubation step was followed by five washes with PBS-T (PBS containing 0.05% Tween 20). Wells were added by 100 μL of a 1 : 5000 dilution of horseradish peroxidase-conjugated streptavidin (Bio-Rad, USA). Following five washes, 100 μL of chromogenic substrate was added to each well and the plate was incubated for 15 min in the dark. The plate was read at 450 nm with an ELISA reader. Optical density (OD_{450}) greater than four times the median values of the negative controls was considered to be positive.

2.4. Total Extract Preparation. Pollens from *P. juliflora* (mesquite), *S. kali, A. retroflexus, C. album,* and *K. scoparia* were prepared from polleniferous materials and then their extracts were prepared as described above [10]. The protein content of each extract was then determined using Bradford's method [13].

2.5. SDS-PAGE and IgE-Immunoblotting. Sodium dodecyl sulfate polyacrylamide gel electrophoresis (SDS-PAGE) of *Acacia* pollen extract (60 μg) was performed according to Laemmli [15] using 12.5% or 15% acrylamide separation gels under reducing and nonreducing conditions. Reducing and nonreducing sample buffers were the same except that the final reducing sample buffer contained 5% (vol/vol) 2-mercaptoethanol (2-ME). Separated protein bands from the electrophoresis of *A. farnesiana* pollen extract were electrotransferred to polyvinylidene difluoride (PVDF) membranes (Immobilon P, Millipore Corp., Bedford, MA, US), as described earlier [10]. In brief, after washing and blocking, membranes were incubated with a 1/5 dilution of serum pool or individual sera from patients with *A. farnesiana* allergy or with control sera (1 : 5 dilutions). Biotinylated anti-human IgE (Nordic Immunology Co., Netherlands) (1 : 500 v/v in 1% BSA) was added to the blotted membrane strips and incubated for 2 h at room temperature. The unbound antibodies were removed from blots by washing with PBS and followed by incubation with 1 : 10000 v/v in BSA1% HRP-linked streptavidin (Sigma-Aldrich, USA) for 2 h at room temperature. The bound enzymatic activity of horseradish peroxidase was

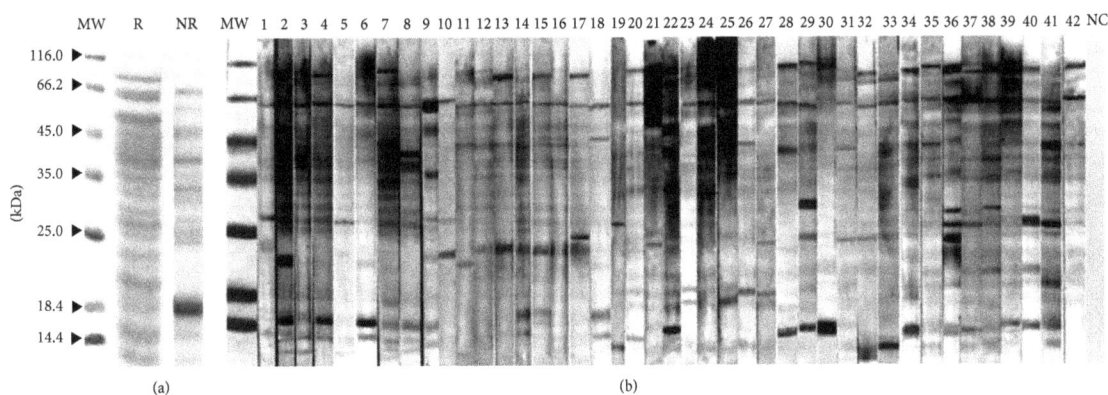

FIGURE 1: (a) Coomassie Brilliant Blue stained SDS-PAGE of the crude extract of *A. farnesiana* pollen in reducing and nonreducing conditions on 12.5% acrylamide gel. Lane MW, molecular weight marker (Fermentas, Lithuania); R, reducing condition; NR, nonreducing condition. (b) Immunoblotting of *Acacia* pollen extract (with reducing SDS-PAGE). Each strip was first blotted with *Acacia* pollen extract. All strips were then incubated with allergic patients' sera and detected for IgE reactive protein bands. Lane MW, low molecular weight. NC, negative control.

detected by high-sensitivity liquid diaminobenzidine (Liquid DAB$^+$) chromogen (DAKO, Denmark).

2.6. ELISA Inhibition.
ELISA inhibition assays were performed as described above, except that a pooled serum (1 : 2 v/v) from *A. farnesiana* allergic patients (numbers 2, 7, 21, 24, and 36) was preincubated for one hour at room temperature with either 1000, 100, 10, 1, 0.1, or 0.01 μg of the selected pollen extract (including *P. juliflora*, *S. kali*, *A. retroflexus*, *C. album*, and *K. scoparia*) as inhibitors or with BSA as a negative control. Percentage of inhibition was calculated using the following formula: (OD of sample without inhibitor − OD of sample with inhibitor/OD of sample without inhibitor) × 100.

2.7. IgE-Immunoblotting Inhibition.
To study the cross-reactivity between *A. farnesiana* pollen and selected allergenic plants, the IgE-immunoblot inhibition experiment was performed. Reducing SDS-PAGE resolved *A. farnesiana* pollen proteins were transferred to PVDF membrane. After blocking, membrane strips were kept for 3 h at room temperature with a mix of 100 μL of pooled sera (1 : 5 v/v) (from patients 2, 7, 21, 24, and 36) which were preincubated with pollen extracts from *P. juliflora*, *S. kali*, *A. retroflexus*, *C. album*, and *K. scoparia*, as well as BSA (as negative control).

3. Results

3.1. Patients.
Forty-two patients, 20 males and 22 females (mean age, 33.60 ± 14.47 years; age range 10–70 years) were included in the study (Table 1). All patients suffered from respiratory allergies and seasonal rhinitis without asthma. The patients were all positive by skin prick test with *A. farnesiana*, *P. juliflora*, *S. kali*, *A. retroflexus*, *C. album*, and *K. scoparia* extracts (Table 1). A serum pool of 5 nonallergic subjects was used as a negative control.

3.2. Skin Prick Test.
Mean diameters of positive wheal sizes were *A. farnesiana*: 6.69±1.17 mm, *P. juliflora*: 7.57±1.50 mm, *S. kali*: 9.95 ± 2.81 mm, *A. retroflexus*: 9.74 ± 4.79 mm,

C. album: 10.19 ± 3.79 mm, and *K. scoparia*: 8.9 ± 3.70 mm. Positive correlation coefficients were attained between the *A. farnesiana* and *P. juliflora* (r = 0.64, P < 0.01), *A. farnesiana* and *S. kali* (r = 0.07, P = 0.6), *A. farnesiana* and *A. retroflexus* (r = 0.1, P = 0.4), *A. farnesiana* and *C. album* (r = 0.06, P = 0.6), and *A. farnesiana* and *K. scoparia* (r = 0.007, P = 0.9) pollen extracts for wheal diameter on the SPT (ANOVA procedure).

3.3. Protein and Allergenic Profile.
The protein composition of *A. farnesiana* extract was analyzed by Coomassie Brilliant Blue staining (Figure 1(a)). The reducing SDS-PAGE separation of the pollen extract showed several resolved protein bands in the *A. farnesiana* extract with molecular weights in the range of approximately 12 to 85 kDa. The most prominent bands had MWs of approximately 50, 66, and 85 kDa. Other predominant bands were identified at 12, 15, 20, 23, 28, 37, and 45 kDa. Nonreducing SDS-PAGE of *Acacia* pollen extract showed eight prominent protein bands with estimated molecular weights between 15 and 66 kDa (Figure 1(a)).

IgE reactivity of the separated protein bands from the electrophoresis of *Acacia* pollen extract was determined via immunoblotting assays. Specific IgE binding fractions probed with sera from all forty-two allergic patients are shown in Figure 1(b). The results showed several IgE reactive bands ranging from about 12 to 85 kDa. Figure 1(b) shows the apparent MW of each protein fraction and the prevalence of each one among all forty-two allergic patients. The most frequent IgE reactive bands among the patients' sera were approximately 66 and 85 kDa. However, there were other IgE reactive protein bands among patients' sera with molecular weights 15, 20, 23, 28, 39, 45, and 50 kDa (Figure 1(b)). No band was detected when a negative control serum pool was assayed.

3.4. Specific IgE Levels and Inhibition ELISA.
The sera of forty-two allergic patients were evaluated for specific IgE binding to total *Acacia* pollen extract. All allergic patients had detectable specific IgE levels to the total extract of *Acacia* pollen (Table 1). These results are consistent with those

TABLE 1: Clinical characteristics, total and specific IgE values, and skin reactivity of allergic patients.

Sample number	Age (years)/sex[1]	Symptoms[2]	Acacia specific IgE[3] (OD)	Total IgE (IU/mL)	Diameters (mm) of the papules obtained by prick test[4]					
					A. farnesiana	P. juliflora	S. kali	A. retroflexus	C. album	K. scoparia
Patients										
1	34/M	L, N, E	0.9	181	7	5	8	9	10	9
2	41/M	N, E	2.33	453	8	9	10	30	11	11
3	39/F	L, N	2.71	156	5	7	16	11	10	9
4	14/F	L, N, E	1.11	165	7	9	7	5	14	11
5	12/M	L, N, E	1.10	123	5	6	4	3	2	0
6	10/M	L, N, E	1.19	313	6	5	10	10	9	8
7	29/F	L, N, E	1.89	345	7	8	8	7	11	5
8	43/F	N, E	1.98	234	6	7	10	12	11	12
9	21/M	N, E	2.07	381	7	9	10	10	12	11
10	26/F	N, E	0.89	225	5	7	10	9	10	11
11	26/F	L, N, E	1.02	468	5	5	10	7	12	8
12	23/F	L, N, E	0.85	265	6	8	13	9	10	10
13	30/M	N, E	1.63	167	7	7	10	7	8	9
14	21/F	L, N, E	1.50	275	7	9	10	10	11	12
15	70/M	L, N, E	1.97	187	6	6	12	11	15	10
16	43/F	N, E	1.85	212	8	7	12	8	11	10
17	32/F	L, N, E	1.94	250	6	8	10	11	13	15
18	46/F	L, N, E	1.52	261	5	7	10	7	9	10
19	34/F	N, E	1.42	301	5	6	5	5	4	0
20	13/M	N, E	2.01	463	8	9	12	5	8	6
21	22/M	N	2.21	280	9	8	8	8	6	7
22	17/F	L, N, E	2.02	302	8	10	8	7	5	5
23	61/M	N	1.04	186	5	6	9	10	9	10
24	66/M	L, N, E	2.10	293	10	12	9	8	6	7
25	10/M	L, N	1.83	220	8	7	4	4	5	0
26	33/M	L, N	1.55	214	7	7	10	10	9	9
27	40/F	L, N	1.65	122	5	5	10	9	11	9
28	53/F	N	1.87	200	7	9	8	8	9	10
29	46/M	N, E	1.91	192	7	6	10	9	10	10
30	43/M	L, N, E	2.15	284	7	7	8	7	9	5
31	19/F	L, N, E	1.92	187	8	7	9	8	9	6
32	36/F	L, N, E	1.89	156	7	8	15	23	25	15
33	19/F	L, N, E	1.29	360	7	10	10	9	10	10
34	37/F	N, E	1.93	267	7	8	12	12	11	11
35	32/M	N, E	1.87	228	7	9	8	9	10	10
36	51/M	N, E	2.11	358	7	8	14	13	11	12
37	28/F	L, N, E	1.60	294	6	8	12	11	11	10
38	29/M	L, N, E	1.96	304	6	7	18	16	18	14
39	44/M	N, E	2.02	418	6	8	10	8	9	9
40	40/M	N, E	2.12	315	8	9	13	18	16	17
41	38/F	N	2.09	480	7	8	8	9	9	6
42	40/F	N, E	1.72	257	6	7	8	7	9	5
Controls										
44	28/F	—	0.09	32	0	0	0	0	0	0
45	45/F	—	0.05	12	0	0	0	0	0	0
46	32/M	—	0.06	88	0	0	0	0	0	0
47	38/M	—	0.10	65	0	0	0	0	0	0
48	22/M	—	0.05	22	0	0	0	0	0	0

[1] M: male; F: female.
[2] L: lungs symptoms (breathlessness, tight chest, cough, wheeze); N: nose symptoms (sneezing, runny, blocked); E: eyes symptoms (itching, dry).
[3] Levels of specific IgE to *A. retroflexus* pollen extract by ELISA (optical density at 450 nm).
[4] The mean wheal diameters are displayed in mm. Histamine diphosphate (10 mg/mL) positive control; glycerin-negative control.

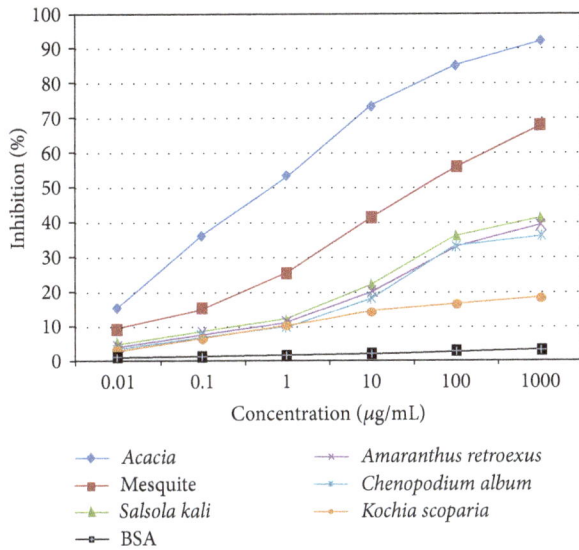

FIGURE 2: Inhibition of IgE binding to *Acacia* pollen extract by ELISA using pollen extract from the most allergenic plants, mesquite, *S. kali, A. retroflexus, C. album,* and *K. scoparia.* Control experiments were performed with BSA.

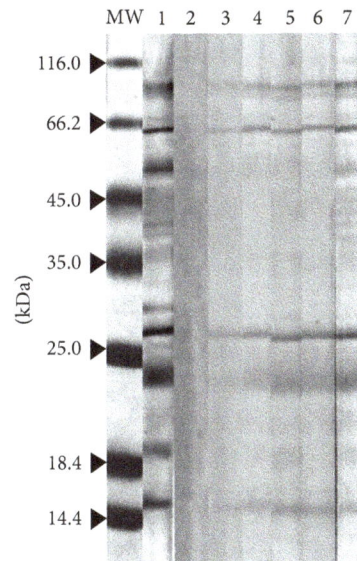

FIGURE 3: Immunoblotting inhibition assays. Lane MW, molecular weight marker (Fermentas, Lithuania). Lane 1, *Acacia* protein strip incubated with pooled serum without inhibitor (negative control). Lane 2, *Acacia* protein strip incubated with pooled serum containing 70 μg of *Acacia* pollen extract as inhibitor (positive control). Lane 3, *Acacia* protein strip incubated with pooled serum containing 70 μg *P. juliflora* as inhibitor. Lane 4, *Acacia* protein strip incubated with pooled serum containing 70 μg *S. kali* as inhibitor. Lane 5, *Acacia* protein strip incubated with pooled serum containing 70 μg *A. retroflexus* as inhibitor. Lane 6, *Acacia* protein strip incubated with pooled serum containing 70 μg *C. album* as inhibitor. Lane 7, *Acacia* protein strip incubated with pooled serum containing 70 μg *K. scoparia* as inhibitor.

obtained in the IgE-immunoblotting assays using the pollen extract of *Acacia* (Figure 1(b)). To investigate cross-reactivity and allergenic potency among *Acacia* and *P. juliflora, S. kali, A. retroflexus, C. album,* and *K. scoparia,* ELISA inhibition with their extracts was done (Figure 2). Almost complete inhibition was attained with 100 μg/mL of *Acacia* pollen extract as positive control. Preincubation of pooled serum with high concentration (1000 μg/mL) of *P. juliflora* revealed significant inhibition of IgE binding to allergenic proteins of *A. farnesiana* pollen extract (68%) (Figure 2).

3.5. Immunoblot Inhibition Assays.

In order to evaluate the IgE cross-reactivity between *Acacia* and five other allergenic pollen extracts, an immunoblot inhibition was carried out with the *Acacia* pollen extract as the solid phase. As shown in Figure 3, IgE reactivity to most of the allergenic proteins of *Acacia* pollen was inhibited when the *Acacia* pollen extract was used as an inhibitor (positive control Lane 2). Complete inhibition of IgE binding to 15, 23, 45, and 50 kDa components of *Acacia* extract occurred when the sera were preincubated with *P. juliflora* extract at 70 μg/mL. Meanwhile, the three bands at about 28, 66, and 85 kDa were partially inhibited. However, when *S. kali, A. retroflexus, C. album,* and *K. scoparia* pollen extracts were used as inhibitors, the 20, 39, 45, and 50 kDa bands were completely inhibited, whereas the 15, 23, 28, 66, and 85 kDa were not inhibited (Figure 3).

4. Discussion

Acacia is one of the major trees throughout arid and semiarid areas of Iran and neighboring countries along the Persian Gulf and the Sea of Oman [2, 16]. SDS-PAGE revealed several bands from the *Acacia* pollen extract with estimated MWs from 12 kDa to 85 kDa (Figure 1(a)). Among those bands, six IgE binding protein fractions with apparent MWs

of 85, 66, 39, 45, 28, 23, and 15 kDa were detected from the blot (Figure 1(b)). Moreover, the results of SDS-PAGE showed relative similarity patterns of migration by protein components of the five selected pollens, mainly those of 15–85 kDa (data not shown). In previous studies the proteins with apparent MWs 39, 45, 66, and 85 kDa have been the most allergenic proteins in the selected allergenic weeds in this study [10, 17–19].

In the current study, the immunoblot analysis with individual patient's serum demonstrated diverse IgE reactivity with seven proteins of 15, 23, 28, 39, 45, 66, and 85 kDa as major IgE binding components. However, immunoblots showed that in the allergenic profile of *Acacia* pollen extract the proteins with apparent MWs of 66 and 85 kDa are the major reactive proteins.

The results of SDS-PAGE revealed that the overall pattern of migration of *Acacia* pollen proteins changed under both reducing conditions. It was thus suggested that probable cysteine residues of the pollen proteins may be associated with interchain disulfide bonds. In previous studies, it was demonstrated that some proteins in pollen extract such as methionine synthase of *S. kali* or *A. retroflexus* were partially degraded into two fragments with approximate MWs of 45 and 39 kDa [19, 20]. Taken together, these observations suggested that some proteins in *Acacia* pollen extract are susceptible to degradation as a result of proteolysis or exposure to a reducing condition. Moreover, it is possible that the number or size of the products of these proteins' degradation depends on the conditions of pollen extract preparation and storage. Nevertheless, additional studies are required to elucidate the patterns of degradation and the number and the size of cleavage products.

Cross-reactivity among *Acacia* pollen components with *Lolium perenne* pollen allergens has been described [8].

Several studies reported that proteins with apparent MWs of 45 and 66 kDa are allergenic in the pollen extracts of mesquite [18] and the selected member of the Chenopodiaceae family [10, 19]. The results of immunoblotting inhibition revealed that the IgE binding reactivity of the allergenic proteins with 12, 20, 39, and 45 from the *A. farnesiana* pollen extract was partially inhibited by all four pollen extracts and also partially with *K. scoparia* pollen extract. As shown in Figure 3, IgE reactivity to most of the allergenic proteins of *A. farnesiana* pollen was inhibited when the *P. juliflora* pollen extract was used as an inhibitor. This indicates a significant IgE cross-reactivity between the two pollens and is also in line with the results of the SPTs (see below).

The results of SPTs indicated highly significant correlations between the wheal diameters from the *A. farnesiana* pollen extract and those from *P. juliflora* pollen extracts ($r = 0.64$, $P < 0.01$). These results suggest an extensive IgE cross-reactivity among these pollens and are concurrent with the results of immunoblotting and inhibition experiments. These results collectively suggest that in these pollen extracts, protein components with MWs range 45 to 66 kDa may play a greater role in cross-reactivity compared to others. Earlier studies had also indicated one of the most allergenic proteins of *S. kali* pollen, named Sal k 1, with a MW of 40–43 kDa [21, 22]. Sal k 1 displayed pectin methylesterase (PME) properties and is considered a major allergen of *S. kali* pollen [14, 21, 22].

In general, the knowledge of pollen cross-reactivity is crucial for diagnostics as well as formulation of immunotherapy vaccines. Cross-reactivity among pollens belonging to the same genus and/or different genera has been demonstrated earlier [23]. Some cross-reactive proteins have been genetically engineered and are found to have potential for use in immunotherapy [24].

Another dominant IgE binding protein band with an estimated MW of 15 kDa was also detected by immunoblotting of *Acacia* pollen extract (Figure 1(b)). Earlier, the allergens belonging to the profilin family with apparent MWs of 14 to 15 kDa were found from *S. kali* (Sal k 4), *A. retroflexus* (Ama r 2), and *C. album* (Che a 2) pollens [25–27]. It may be that the 15 kDa- protein of *Acacia* pollen is homologous with the 15-kDa IgE reactive band in these plants. However, further studies are required to prove the nature of this allergenic protein of *Acacia* pollen.

5. Conclusion

In conclusion, *A. farnesiana* pollen is a potent allergen source with several IgE binding components. The observations altogether suggest a close allergenic relationship between *Acacia* and mesquite. Regarding the extensive cross-reactivity between these two trees and the abundance of them in tropical and subtropical regions, identification and production of the recombinant forms of common allergens of these pollens may lead to the exploration of new guidelines for diagnostic, therapeutic, and preventive purposes. Efforts are now underway to clone cDNAs encoding allergenic cross-reactive proteins from *Acacia* pollen.

Disclosure

This paper is issued from thesis of Mr. Shams.

Conflict of Interests

The authors declare that there is no conflict of interests regarding the publication of this paper.

Acknowledgments

Financial support was provided by Ahvaz Jundishapur University of Medical Sciences (Grant no. CRC-9108). The authors would like to thank Dr. Afshin Arti, University of Toronto, for his critical reading of the paper.

References

[1] M. Caccavari and E. Dome, "An account of morphological and structural characterization of American Mimosoideae pollen. Part I: tribe Acacieae," *Palynology*, vol. 24, no. 1, pp. 231–248, 2000.

[2] M. A. Assarehzadegan, A. Shakurnia, and A. Amini, "The most common aeroallergens in a tropical region in Southwestern Iran," *World Allergy Organization Journal*, vol. 6, article 7, 2013.

[3] R. Ariano, R. C. Panzani, and J. Amedeo, "Pollen allergy to mimosa (*Acacia floribunda*) in a Mediterranean area: an occupational disease," *Annals of Allergy*, vol. 66, no. 3, pp. 253–256, 1991.

[4] A. Bener, W. Safa, S. Abdulhalik, and G. G. Lestringant, "An analysis of skin prick test reactions in asthmatics in a hot climate and desert environment," *Allergie et Immunologie*, vol. 34, no. 8, pp. 281–286, 2002.

[5] M. Fereidouni, R. Farid Hossini, F. Jabbari Azad, M. A. Assarehzadegan, and A. Varasteh, "Skin prick test reactivity to common aeroallergens among allergic rhinitis patients in Iran," *Allergologia et Immunopathologia*, vol. 37, no. 2, pp. 73–93, 2009.

[6] F. A. Suliaman, W. F. Holmes, S. Kwick, F. Khouri, and R. Ratard, "Pattern of immediate type hypersensitivity reactions in the Eastern Province, Saudi Arabia," *Annals of Allergy, Asthma & Immunology*, vol. 78, no. 4, pp. 415–418, 1997.

[7] M. A. Assarehzadegan, A. H. Shakurnia, and A. Amini, "Sensitization to common aeroallergens among asthmatic patients in a tropical region affected by dust storm," *Journal of Medical Sciences*, vol. 13, no. 7, pp. 592–597, 2013.

[8] B. J. Howlett, D. J. Hill, and R. B. Knox, "Cross-reactivity between Acacia (wattle) and rye grass pollen allergens. Detection of allergens in Acacia (wattle) pollen," *Clinical Allergy*, vol. 12, no. 3, pp. 259–268, 1982.

[9] A. Al-Dowaisan, N. Fakim, M. R. Khan et al., "Salsola pollen as a predominant cause of respiratory allergies in Kuwait," *Annals*

of Allergy, Asthma and Immunology, vol. 92, no. 2, pp. 262–267, 2004.

[10] M. A. Assarehzadegan, M. Sankin, F. Jabbari, R. Noorbakhsh, and A. Varasteh, "Allergy to *Salsola kali* in a Salsola incanescens-rich area: role of extensive cross allergenicity," *Allergology International*, vol. 58, no. 2, pp. 261–266, 2009.

[11] J. Mandal, I. Roy, S. Chatterjee, and S. Gupta-Bhattacharya, "Aerobiological investigation and in vitro studies of pollen grains from 2 dominant avenue trees in Kolkata, India," *Journal of Investigational Allergology and Clinical Immunology*, vol. 18, no. 1, pp. 22–30, 2008.

[12] R. Valenta and D. Kraft, "From allergen structure to new forms of allergen-specific immunotherapy," *Current Opinion in Immunology*, vol. 14, no. 6, pp. 718–727, 2002.

[13] M. M. Bradford, "A rapid and sensitive method for the quantitation of microgram quantities of protein utilizing the principle of protein dye binding," *Analytical Biochemistry*, vol. 72, no. 1-2, pp. 248–254, 1976.

[14] M. A. Assarehzadegan, M. Sankian, F. Jabbari, M. Tehrani, and A. Varasteh, "Expression of the recombinant major allergen of *Salsola kali* pollen (Sal k 1) and comparison with its low-immunoglobulin E-binding mutant," *Allergology International*, vol. 59, no. 2, pp. 213–222, 2010.

[15] U. K. Laemmli, "Cleavage of structural proteins during the assembly of the head of bacteriophage T4," *Nature*, vol. 227, no. 5259, pp. 680–685, 1970.

[16] S. Irian, A. Majd, A. Hoseinizadeh, and P. Jounobi, "A study on the allergenicity and ontogeny of *Acacia farnesiana* pollen grains in guinea pigs," *Aerobiologia*, vol. 29, no. 1, pp. 21–29, 2013.

[17] A. Dhyani, N. Arora, S. N. Gaur, V. K. Jain, S. Sridhara, and B. P. Singh, "Analysis of IgE binding proteins of mesquite (*Prosopis juliflora*) pollen and cross-reactivity with predominant tree pollens," *Immunobiology*, vol. 211, no. 9, pp. 733–740, 2006.

[18] A. Dhyani, B. P. Singh, N. Arora, V. K. Jain, and S. Sridhara, "A clinically relevant major cross-reactive allergen from mesquite tree pollen," *The European Journal of Clinical Investigation*, vol. 38, no. 10, pp. 774–781, 2008.

[19] M. Tehrani, M. Sankian, M. A. Assarehzadegan, R. Falak, F. Jabbari, and A. Varasteh, "Immunochemical characterization of *Amaranthus retroflexus* pollen extract: extensive cross-reactive allergenic components among the four species of Amaranthaceae/Chenopodiaceae," *Iranian Journal of Allergy, Asthma and Immunology*, vol. 9, no. 2, pp. 87–95, 2010.

[20] M. A. Assarehzadegan, M. Sankian, F. Jabbari, M. Tehrani, R. Falak, and A. Varasteh, "Identification of methionine synthase (Sal k 3), as a novel allergen of *Salsola kali* pollen," *Molecular Biology Reports*, vol. 38, no. 1, pp. 65–73, 2011.

[21] R. Barderas, J. García-Sellés, G. Salamanca et al., "A pectin methylesterase as an allergenic marker for the sensitization to Russian thistle (*Salsola kali*) pollen," *Clinical and Experimental Allergy*, vol. 37, no. 7, pp. 1111–1119, 2007.

[22] J. Carnés, E. Fernández-Caldas, A. Marina et al., "Immunochemical characterization of Russian thistle (*Salsola kali*) pollen extracts. Purification of the allergen Sal k 1," *Allergy*, vol. 58, no. 11, pp. 1152–1156, 2003.

[23] R. W. Weber, "Cross-reactivity of pollen allergens," *Current Allergy and Asthma Reports*, vol. 4, no. 5, pp. 401–408, 2004.

[24] V. Niederberger, F. Horak, S. Vrtala et al., "Vaccination with genetically engineered allergens prevents progression of allergic disease," *Proceedings of the National Academy of Sciences of the United States of America*, vol. 101, no. 2, pp. 14677–14682, 2004.

[25] A. Amini, M. Sankian, M. A. Assarehzadegan, F. Vahedi, and A. Varasteh, "Chenopodium album pollen profilin (Che a 2): homology modeling and evaluation of cross-reactivity with allergenic profilins based on predicted potential IgE epitopes and IgE reactivity analysis," *Molecular Biology Reports*, vol. 38, no. 4, pp. 2579–2587, 2011.

[26] M. A. Assarehzadegan, A. Amini, M. Sankian, M. Tehrani, F. Jabbari, and A. Varasteh, "Sal k 4, a new allergen of *Salsola kali*, is profilin: a predictive value of conserved conformational regions in cross-reactivity with other plant-derived profilins," *Bioscience, Biotechnology and Biochemistry*, vol. 74, no. 7, pp. 1441–1446, 2010.

[27] M. Tehrani, M. Sankian, M. A. Assarehzadegan et al., "Identification of a new allergen from amaranthus retroflexus pollen, ama r 2," *Allergology International*, vol. 60, no. 3, pp. 309–316, 2011.

16

Liposomal Nasal Spray versus Guideline-Recommended Steroid Nasal Spray in Patients with Chronic Rhinosinusitis: A Comparison of Tolerability and Quality of Life

Anna Eitenmüller,[1] Lisa Piano,[1] Myriam Böhm,[1] Kija Shah-Hosseini,[1] Andreas Glowania,[2] Oliver Pfaar,[3] Ralph Mösges,[1] and Ludger Klimek[3]

[1] Institute of Medical Statistics, Informatics and Epidemiology, University of Cologne, 50924 Cologne, Germany
[2] Ear, Nose and Throat Department, General Hospital Hietzing, 1130 Vienna, Austria
[3] Center for Rhinology and Allergology, 65183 Wiesbaden, Germany

Correspondence should be addressed to Anna Eitenmüller; anna.eitenmueller@web.de

Academic Editor: Desiderio Passali

Objective. To investigate the tolerability and impact on quality of life of liposomal nasal spray compared to guideline-recommended steroid-based therapy in patients with chronic rhinosinusitis. Symptom reduction and use of antisymptomatic medication were also examined. *Methods.* In this monocenter, prospective, controlled, open, and noninterventional study, 60 patients with chronic rhinosinusitis were treated with liposomal nasal spray and 30 patients received steroid-based therapy. The study comprised five visits occurring at intervals of two to four weeks. Efficacy was determined according to the sinusitis symptom score documented daily. The polyp score was recorded at the initial and final visits. Tolerability was determined through the Nasal Spray Evaluation Questionnaire, and quality of life was ascertained with the SNOT-20 Score. *Results.* Both treatments achieved a significant reduction of sinusitis symptoms ($P < 0.05$) and also rhinoscopic improvement ($P < 0.05$). The majority of patients assessed the treatments as "good" or "very good," and the quality of life improved significantly ($P < 0.05$). There was no significant difference in symptom reduction, QoL, and endoscopic exams between both treatments. *Conclusion.* The treatment of chronic rhinosinusitis with liposomal nasal spray results in a similar, significant reduction of symptoms and significant improvement in quality of life as guideline-recommended treatment and is therefore a comparable alternative.

1. Introduction

With a lifetime prevalence of about 5%, chronic rhinosinusitis (CRS) is one of the most frequently occurring chronic disorders worldwide [1, 2]. The German, European, and US-AWMF guidelines recommend as treatment the topical application of glucocorticoids since they represent an important treatment principle in addition to antibiotic treatment in conservative therapy [2, 3]. Nasal irrigation or sprays with hypertonic buffered solutions can also provide symptom relief in CRS disorders and are therefore recommended by guidelines. These sprays improve mucociliary clearance by liquefying nasal secretion and have been observed to have vasoconstrictive and decongestant effects [4].

Treatment alternatives should be pointed out to patients who have a critical view of guideline-recommended steroid-based therapy. One such alternative therapy concept is the nasal application of (phospholipid) liposomes. Several studies have already demonstrated the efficacy of this nonpharmacological mechanism of action in allergic rhinitis [5, 6]. Three precursor studies which investigated the application of a liposomal nasal spray in patients with seasonal allergic rhinitis showed significant symptom improvement and good tolerability of the liposomal nasal spray, also in comparison to guideline combination therapy with glucocorticoids and antihistamines [7–9].

Because the incidence of allergic rhinitis (AR) in adults with CRS is 40%–80%, liposome therapy therefore represents an interesting, steroid-free treatment alternative [10]. Since two-thirds of patients with AR alone have steroid phobia, the probability is high that the fear of medication containing cortisone also exists among patients with CRS [11]. The liposomes, produced from phosphatidylcholine, stabilize the surfactant film and prevent the moisture film lining the airways from tearing. A liposomal nasal spray (LN) therefore represents an entirely drug-free treatment concept [12]. The present study investigates symptom reduction after the application of a LN in patients with CRS. Tolerability and the impact on quality of life were also determined.

The study was carried out in compliance with the requirements for noninterventional studies [13]. Since both products can be purchased without a prescription, it was not necessary to seek approval from an ethics committee. Nevertheless, a consultation with the competent ethics committee with respect to professional regulations took place before the study commenced.

2. Methods

2.1. Study Design. This investigation was a monocenter, prospective, controlled, open, noninterventional study (NIS). Sixty patients with CRS symptoms were treated with LN, and 30 patients received guideline-recommended therapy with a steroid nasal spray. Patients were first offered the guideline-recommended therapy. Those patients having reservations towards pharmacological therapy were alternatively offered treatment with a liposomal nasal spray. No prior wash-out period was required. Patients 18 years or older were included who due to their disorder had already been undergoing treatment at the study center.

The NIS took place from 15 March 2011 to 31 January 2013 and consisted of five visits at intervals of two to four weeks within a total treatment period of three months. Efficacy was determined on the basis of the sinusitis symptom score (SSS), which was documented daily by the patients themselves in a patient diary; furthermore, the investigator recorded the SSS at every visit. For monitoring purposes, the investigator also determined the polyp score (PS) based on the size of polyps at the first and last visits [14]. The nasal spray sensory scale was used at the first and last visits to assess tolerability [15]. Quality of life (QoL) was determined at every visit by means of the SNOT-20 score [16].

2.2. Medication. The liposomal nasal spray *LipoNasal Pflege* (LN), manufactured by Optima Pharmazeutische GmbH, Moosburg/Wang, Germany, was applied in this study. The liposomes contained in this product consist of highly purified soy lecithin, which is composed of 94% phosphatidylcholine and a small proportion of other phospholipids. Other components of the nasal spray are sodium chloride, ethanol, dexpanthenol, vitamin A palmitate, tocopherol, and water for injection. Treatment was carried out according to leaflet instructions, with the spray being applied an average of 2-3 sprays per nostril daily.

The comparative treatment used in this study was *Livocab direkt mit Beclometason 0.05%* (LB), a corticoid having an anti-inflammatory effect for nasal application, manufactured by Orion Corporation Orion Pharma, Finland. This preparation is primarily applied short-term for seasonal allergic rhinitis. Its active ingredient is beclomethasone, which in this product is available as beclomethasone dipropionate. Beclomethasone is a synthetic glucocorticoid with vasoconstrictive, immunosuppressive, antiallergic, and anti-inflammatory properties that is used to treat asthma, allergic rhinitis, and sinusitis. Beclomethasone dipropionate is used as a prodrug and is subject to a first-pass effect in the liver, thereby limiting toxicity and systemic bioavailability.

Other components of the product are benzalkonium chloride, polysorbate 80, D-glucose, microcrystalline cellulose, carmellose sodium, purified water, sodium hydroxide, and hydrochloric acid for pH regulation.

One milliliter of nasal spray contains 0.555 mg (approx. 0.05%) beclomethasone dipropionate as the active ingredient.

One spray application (approx. 0.09 mL) contains 0.05 mg beclomethasone dipropionate.

The recommended dose for patients aged 12 years or older is 2 sprays per nostril and application. The maximum daily dosage is 4 sprays per nostril.

2.3. Study Protocol. On Day 1 of treatment (Visit 1), the investigator documented the detailed medical history and the SSS as well as the PS and conducted a regular rhinoscopy. Videoendoscopy and/or a smell test were optional.

Patients documented the number of sprays applied per nostril daily. They also specified when an onset of action occurred after the first-time application of the nasal spray (<5 min, 5–10 min, 10–30 min, 30–60 min, 1-2 h, 2–4 h, 4–8 h, >8 h, no onset of action).

Efficacy was recorded by means of the SSS, which was chosen based on the EPOS Paper [17]. The present study, however, implemented a slightly adapted version of the score to enable a direct comparison with another study that investigated steroid treatment of CRS [18]. The score was recorded at every visit by the physician as well as daily by the patient in a patient diary. The five main symptoms of rhinosinusitis (rhinorrhea, nasal obstruction, headache, facial pain, and postnasal drip) were evaluated on the basis of an ordinal scale from 0 to 3 (0 = no, 1 = mild, 2 = moderate, and 3 = severe), and the individual values were added together to obtain a sum score. Furthermore, a rhinoscopic examination was conducted at every visit to ensure an additional objective assessment of efficacy. In the process, the symptoms "edema," "secretion," and "redness" were evaluated on a 3-point scale (0 = no, 1 = mild, and 2 = severe), and the rhinoscopy score (RS) was calculated thereafter from the data obtained.

In addition, polyps were measured via endoscopy at the first and last visits to monitor polyp size. The PS was calculated from these data based on a 4-point scale (0 = no polyps, 1 = small polyps, 2 = medium-sized polyps, and 3 = large polyps) [14].

The tolerability of the nasal spray was determined by means of the Nasal Spray Sensory Scale [15]. Patients answered 14 questions pertaining to sensory parameters on a visual analog scale (0 = poor evaluation and 100 = good

TABLE 1: Demographic data.

	Female		Male		Valid		Missing	Total
	n	%	n	%	n	%	n	n
Liposomal nasal spray	35	58.3	25	41.7	60	100	0	60
Beclomethasone	16	53.3	14	46.7	30	100	0	30

TABLE 2: Distribution of allergies.

	Trees		Weeds		Grasses		Mites		Mold	
	n	%	n	%	n	%	n	%	n	%
Liposomal nasal spray										
Patients with allergy	14	24.1	2	3.4	16	27.6	8	13.8	3	5.2
Patients without allergy	44	75.9	56	96.6	42	72.4	50	86.2	55	94.8
Valid	58	100	58	100	58	100	58	100	58	100
Beclomethasone										
Patients with allergy	8	26.7	1	3.3	6	20	8	26.7	3	10
Patients without allergy	22	73.3	29	96.7	24	80	22	73.3	27	90
Valid	30	100	30	100	30	100	30	100	30	100

evaluation) immediately after applying the nasal spray as well as two minutes thereafter.

Quality of life was recorded using a validated questionnaire, the "Sino-Nasal Outcome Test German Adapted Version" (SNOT-20 GAV), which patients completed at every visit [19, 20]. This form consists of 20 individual questions relating to symptoms as well as social and emotional consequences, which the patient was able to assess on a 6-point scale (0 = no problem, 1 = very minor problem, 2 = small problem, 3 = moderate problem, 4 = severe problem, and 5 = it cannot get any worse). From these 20 individual questions, the patients were also able to choose the five items most important to them. In addition, the patients assessed their subjective condition daily on a visual analog scale (0 = very poor and 100 = very good).

At Visit 5, a final evaluation was made during which the investigator assessed the medication applied in terms of effect and tolerability. Patients were also able to evaluate tolerability and efficacy of the nasal spray at the end of the treatment period with a final diary entry.

2.4. Statistics. The program SPSS 21 for Windows was used to conduct the statistical analysis. To reduce any input errors, double data entry was carried out. Unreported values were treated as "missing values."

First, all data were analyzed descriptively and tested for normal distribution using the Kolmogorov-Smirnov test. In addition, the mean values of the variables from Visits 1 and 5 were compared with the aid of the t-test for paired samples. The level of significance was set at $\alpha = 0.05$.

3. Results

3.1. Homogeneity of Treatment Groups. Overall, 35 women and 25 men aged 18 to 77 years (mean age = 42 years) were included in the LN group, and 16 women and 14 men aged 22 to 74 years (mean age = 46 years) were in the comparison group. The statistical analysis and the comparison of the demographic data showed no relevant differences between the groups at the beginning of treatment (Table 1). The analysis of the symptom scores for the previous year revealed that most patients suffered from rhinoconjunctivitis complaints (LN = 55.2% and comparison group = 51.7%) and also from asthma, rhinoconjunctivitis, and conjunctivitis. Allergies were also frequent (LN = 54.2% and comparison group = 51.7%) (Table 2). Overall, 22% in the LN group and 30% in the comparison group suffered from polyps.

3.2. Onset of Action. In the LN group, the onset of action on Day 1 occurred within 30 minutes in 47.8% of the patients, with 39.1% not noticing any onset of action at all.

The onset of action on Day 1 in the beclomethasone group took place within 30 minutes in 20% of the patients, with 48% noticing no onset of action whatsoever.

3.3. Efficacy. The liposomal nasal spray and the steroid alternative were both able to improve sinusitis symptoms significantly, with rhinoscopy findings also demonstrating distinct improvement. The sinusitis symptom score in the LN group, for instance, declined from a baseline score from 6.61 (±2.668) to 3.88 (±3.674) and in the comparison group from 6.57 (±3.012) to 4.83 (±3.601) (see Table 3 and Figure 1). The sum score of the rhinoscopic evaluation also decreased in the LN group from 3.78 (±1.368) to 1.85 (±1.477) and in the steroid group from 4.26 (±1.096) to 2.30 (±1.222) (see Table 3). The analysis of the polyp scores showed no relevant change with respect to polyp size.

No relevant differences with regard to symptom reduction could be determined in the statistical analysis of the patient diaries.

Overall, the morning SSS, which consisted of the diary items "runny nose," "itching," "sneezing," "postnasal drip," "facial pain," "headache," and "nasal obstruction," was 4.06 in the LN group and 4.01 in the steroid group out of 15

TABLE 3: Sinusitis sum score (SSS), rhinoscopy sum score (RS), and SNOT-20 total score.

	V1	V2	V3	V4	V5	Improvement V1–V5
Liposomal nasal spray						
SSS						
MV	6.61	5.00	4.63	4.45	3.88	2.73
SD	*2,668*	*2.327*	*2.797*	*2.615*	*2.674*	*2.849*
RS						
MV	3.78	2.50	2.28	1.60	1.85	1.93
SD	*1.368*	*1.177*	*1.724*	*1.676*	*1.477*	*1.639*
SNOT						
MV	32.57	23.64	21.51	19.57	18.43	14,14
SD	*10.786*	*12.694*	*13.204*	*13.590*	*13.372*	*12,731*
Beclomethasone						
SSS						
MV	6.57	5.26	4.91	4.91	4.83	1.74
SD	*3.012*	*3.441*	*4.231*	*4.100*	*3.601*	*3.151*
RS						
MV	4.26	3.04	2.65	2.87	2.30	1.96
SD	*1.096*	*1.261*	*1.112*	*1.604*	*1.222*	*1.147*
SNOT						
MV	39.91	30.04	28.04	25.83	26.00	13.91
SD	*19.776*	*18.165*	*19.427*	*21.777*	*22.076*	*19.246*

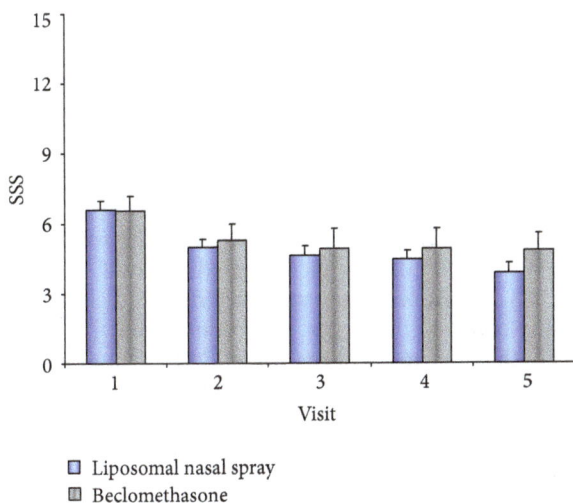

FIGURE 1: Sinusitis symptom score over the course of five visits in both groups.

possible points. Over the three-month observation period, the patients' daily documented sinusitis sum scores in both groups decreased from approximately 4 at baseline to 2.16 on Day 86. The difference between both groups was not significant.

At the final evaluation, the majority of the patients in both groups rated efficacy "good" or even "very good" (Table 7).

3.4. Tolerability and Safety. In the immediate evaluation of the Nasal Spray Sensory Scale, the steroid nasal spray group achieved somewhat better results than the LN group ($P = 0.178$), but ultimately there was no significant difference between both groups at V5 ($P = 0.564$) (Table 4).

In the evaluation after two minutes, both groups showed higher values, which means that the application was perceived as more pleasant. The value for the LN group was 80.4 at Visit 1 and 78.8 at Visit 5. In the group receiving beclomethasone, the value was 85.1 at Visit 1 and 78.3 at Visit 5. No significant difference existed between both nasal sprays comparing its tolerability immediately ($P = 0.594$) or after 2 minutes ($P = 0.815$), neither at V1 nor at V5 (Table 4).

In the final assessment of tolerability, the majority of evaluable patients in both groups rated both treatments "good" or even "very good" (Table 7).

Overall, both treatment modalities were tolerated well; no significant difference between both groups was observed ($P = 0.306$).

3.5. Dropouts and Adverse Events. Altogether, 20 patients from the LN group and seven patients from the cortisone group dropped out of the study. In most cases, the reasons for discontinuation remained unknown; only one patient from the LN group and two patients from the cortisone group dropped out of the study because of an adverse event (AE). AEs occurred in a total of 23 patients, 10 events of which were reported in the LN group and 13 in the group receiving the steroid nasal spray.

TABLE 4: Sensory evaluation immediately and two minutes after application.

	Immediately after application		Two minutes after application	
	V1	V5	V1	V5
Liposomal nasal spray				
MV	**75.25**	**72.42**	**80.39**	**78.81**
SD	*13.933*	*14.826*	*16.146*	*15.686*
Beclomethasone				
MV	**80.34**	**73.82**	**85.13**	**78.35**
SD	*13.549*	*16.714*	*11.2686*	*17.975*

One patient from the LN group and five patients from the beclomethasone group also experienced a second AE (Table 5).

None of these incidents were documented by the study investigators as serious adverse events in the serious adverse event (SAE) form. An association with the study drug could not be ruled out for five AEs in the beclomethasone and eight AEs in the LN group.

3.6. Quality of Life. The application of both preparations resulted in a significant improvement in quality of life as early as V2 ($P \leq 0.05$). The treatments themselves did not differ from each other significantly ($P \geq 0.05$).

In the LN group, therapy caused a drop in the total sum score of the SNOT-20 Quality of Life Scale from 32.57 ± 10.786 to 18.43 ± 13.372; the score decreased in the comparison group from 39.91 ± 19.776 to 26 ± 22.076 (see Table 3 and Figure 2). When dividing the SNOT-20 Quality of Life Scale into "primary nasal symptoms," "secondary rhinogenic symptoms," and "general quality of life," significant improvements could also be observed within these subareas ($P \leq 0.05$) (Table 6). No significant difference existed between the groups.

Besides the evaluation of the SNOT-20, patients recorded their subjectively perceived condition daily in a diary as a further parameter for determining quality of life.

Figure 3 shows the three-month course of the patients' mean subjective condition over the treatment period.

4. Discussion

Besides antibiotics, topical treatment with corticosteroids is the guideline-recommended treatment of choice for symptomatic CRS [2], although so-called "cortisone phobia" represents an increasing problem. This circumstance often results in lacking patient compliance and the change to an alternative steroid-free medication [21]. As demonstrated in previous studies on allergic rhinitis and rhinoconjunctivitis, therapy with a liposomal nasal spray is an equally effective and tolerable treatment alternative [7–9]. In terms of efficacy, it is assumed that the phospholipids supplemented via nasal spray stabilize or restore the impaired "nasal surfactant," thereby maintaining the natural moisture film protecting and moisturizing the nasal mucosa and as a basis of mucociliary

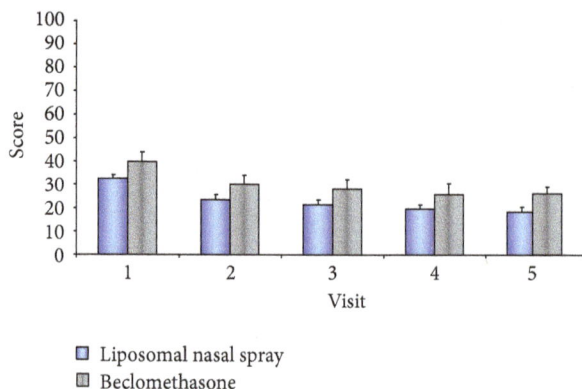

FIGURE 2: Course of the SNOT total score V1 to V5.

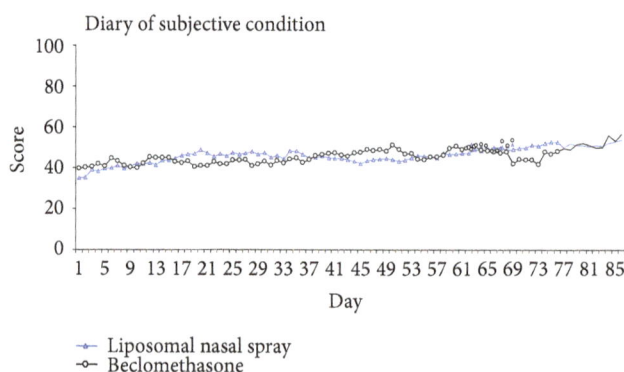

FIGURE 3: Diary assessment of the subjective condition of patients.

clearance [12]. The present study was able to illustrate that the application of liposomes also represents a promising treatment option for CRS. Since CRS is often accompanied by allergic rhinitis, a possible explanatory approach may also lie in the wound-healing and anti-inflammatory properties of liposomes [22]. The barrier function of the nasal mucus layer is impaired due to the inflamed mucosa. Liposomes primarily consist of phosphatidylcholine, which in terms of quantity make up the largest proportion of nasal surfactant and are thus able to stabilize the liquid film that moisturizes and protects the mucus membrane [12].

Since symptom scores can always be subjectively influenced [23] and to obtain the most objective evaluation of efficacy as possible, we chose a combination of investigator evaluation and patient evaluation. The symptoms for the SSS, which patients entered in their diaries and the physician filled out at the visits, were selected based on the EPOS Paper 2007 [17]; for better comparability with a steroid, however, the study implemented a slightly adapted score [18]. Ultimately, the items "nasal secretion," "postnasal drip," "facial pain," "headache," and "nasal obstruction" were used. Application of the liposomal nasal spray led to a significant improvement in the SSS of 2.7 from V1 to V5, corresponding to improvement by 41.4%; improvement in the comparison group was 26.5%. The sum score of the rhinoscopic evaluation also decreased significantly in the LN group from 3.78 to 1.85 (51% improvement) and in the steroid group from 4.26

TABLE 5: Adverse events.

	(1) Adverse event	(2) Adverse event
Beclomethasone	Acute sinusitis	Acute rhinitis
	Minor hemorrhoid bleeding	Acute viral rhinopharyngitis
	Cephalgia	Acute sinobronchitis
	Acute bacterial sinusitis	Acute bacterial sinusitis
	Rhinitis, cough	
	Acute viral rhinopharyngitis	
	Viral upper respiratory tract infection	
	Acute viral infection	
	Acute exacerbation of CRS	
	Gastroenteritis	Tonsillitis
	Acute viral rhinopharyngitis with rhinosinusitis	
	Bronchitis	
	Dysesthesia of nasal mucosa and facial pain	
Liposomal nasal spray	Recurrence of chronic lymphatic leukemia	
	Acute exacerbation of chronic rhinosinusitis	
	Acute bronchitis	
	Cephalgia	Fatigue
	Rhinitis	
	Infection of paranasal sinuses	
	Capsulitis DII right hand	
	Arthrosis of both hip joints	
	Acute exacerbation of chronic pansinusitis	
	Acute sinusitis	

TABLE 6: SNOT-20 subscales:primary nasal symptoms, secondary rhinogenic symptoms, and general quality of life.

	V1	V2	V3	V4	V5	Improvement V1–V5
Liposomal nasal spray						
Primary nasal symptoms						
MV	**40.24**	**31.02**	**28.57**	**26.20**	**24.90**	**15.34**
SD	14.976	13.204	17.531	18.295	18.042	−3.066
Secondary rhinogenic symptoms						
MV	**32.52**	**20.68**	**21.97**	**19.52**	**18.44**	**14.08**
SD	17.220	15.811	14.528	14.337	14.563	2.657
General quality of life						
MV	**29.22**	**21.42**	**18.39**	**16.78**	**15.70**	**13.52**
SD	16.726	17.451	16.341	16.217	15.634	1.092
Beclomethasone						
Primary nasal symptoms						
MV	**45.00**	**33.33**	**31.33**	**28.33**	**28.50**	**16.5**
SD	3.012	3.441	4.231	4.100	3.601	−0.589
Secondary rhinogenic symptoms						
MV	**35.00**	**28.89**	**27.64**	**25.14**	**24.86**	**10.14**
SD	19.009	17.629	20.489	20.990	21.714	−2.731
General quality of life						
MV	**40.10**	**29.18**	**26.57**	**25.51**	**25.99**	**14.11**
SD	24.255	21.496	22.267	25.662	25.806	−1.551

TABLE 7: Patients' final evaluation of efficacy and tolerability.

	Efficacy	Tolerability
Liposomal nasal spray		
Very good	17.8%	39.4%
Good	53.8%	50%
Satisfactory	17.9%	7.9%
Poor	10.3%	2.6%
Beclomethasone		
Very good	17.4%	26.1%
Good	47.8%	60.9%
Satisfactory	13%	4.3%
Poor	21.7%	8.7%

to 2.3 (46% improvement). In a precursor study on allergic rhinoconjunctivitis, the application of the liposomal nasal spray resulted in nasal symptom relief of 33.2% and global improvement of 41.4%, which support the results of the present study [9].

Overall, tolerability of the liposomal nasal spray was assessed positively; 50% of the valid percentages rated tolerability "good," 39.4% "very good," 7.9% "satisfactory," and only 2.6% evaluated tolerability "poor." Some patients commented on the smell of the liposomal spray. Since it was decided to deliberately forgo the addition of artificial aromas in the product to avoid possible allergic reactions or intolerances, the natural scent of lecithin (phospholipids) is perceptible.

4.1. Quality of Life. A study by Rudmik and Smith showed that CRS leads to a significant loss of quality of life, among other things due to symptoms such as sleeplessness, headache, and facial pain, and also emotional consequences such as sadness and a sense of shame [24]. In this study, a significant decrease resulted in the total sum score of the SNOT-20 Quality of Life Scale and in the subareas "primary nasal symptoms" and "secondary rhinogenic symptoms" as well as in the area "general quality of life." Thus, significant improvement in quality of life could be verified through the use of a nonpharmacological product in CRS. Both preparations, however, do not differ significantly.

5. Conclusion

All in all, both of the applied treatments led to significant improvement in the patients' condition, with no significant differences resulting between both study medications for the most part.

The values calculated in this study show that liposomal nasal spray is an effective treatment alternative for patients with CRS. Its application resulted in significant symptom reduction and improved quality of life. Furthermore, the majority of patients assessed its tolerability very positively. Liposomal nasal spray is therefore a suitable steroid-free method for treating CRS, particularly for patients who take a somewhat critical view of guideline-recommended therapy with cortisone.

Abbreviations

AE: Adverse event
AR: Allergic rhinitis
CRS: Chronic rhinosinusitis
LN: Liposomal nasal spray
LB: Livocab beclomethasone
NIS: Non-interventional study
PS: Polyp score
QoL: Quality of life
RS: Rhinoscopy score
SAE: Serious adverse event
SSS: Sinusitis symptom score.

Conflict of Interests

The authors declare that there is no conflict of interests regarding the publication of this paper.

Acknowledgments

The authors would like to thank Gena Kittel and Marie-Josefine Joisten for their editorial assistance. The study was funded and the medication was provided by Optima Pharmazeutische GmbH, Moosburg/Wang, Germany.

References

[1] M. S. Benninger, B. J. Ferguson, J. A. Hadley et al., "Adult chronic rhinosinusitis: definitions, diagnosis, epidemiology, and pathophysiology," *Otolaryngology: Head and Neck Surgery*, vol. 129, no. 3, pp. S1–S32, 2003.

[2] B. A. Stuck, C. Bachert, P. Federspil et al., "AWMF-Leitlinien-Register 017-049: Rhinosinusitis," 2011.

[3] R. Dahmen and R. Mösges, "Krankheitsbild und therapiekonzepte: sinusitis," *Symposium Medical*, pp. 4–7, 2002.

[4] L. Klimek, B. A. Stuck, O. Pfaar, and K. Hörmann, "Entzündliche erkrankungen der nase und der nasennebenhöhlen," *Atemwegs- und Lungenkrankheiten*, vol. 35, pp. 187–207, 2009.

[5] M. Andersson, L. Greiff, and P. Wollmer, "Nasal treatment with a microemulsion reduces allergen challenge-induced symptoms and signs of allergic rhinitis," *Acta Oto-Laryngologica*, vol. 128, no. 6, pp. 666–669, 2008.

[6] S. Schwetz, H. Olze, S. Melchisedech, A. Grigorov, and R. Latza, "Efficacy of pollen blocker cream in the treatment of allergic rhinitis," *Archives of Otolaryngology: Head and Neck Surgery*, vol. 130, no. 8, pp. 979–984, 2004.

[7] M. Böhm, G. Avgitidou, E. El Hassan, and R. Mösges, "Liposomes: a new non-pharmacological therapy concept for seasonal-allergic-rhinoconjunctivitis," *European Archives of Oto-Rhino-Laryngology*, vol. 269, no. 2, pp. 495–502, 2012.

[8] H. Meyer-Gutknecht and R. Mösges, "Wirkung eines neuartigen liposomalen nasensprays auf die symptome der saisonalen allergischen rhinitis," *HNO Kompakt Supplement*, vol. 1, pp. 1–5, 2008.

[9] L. Weston and R. Mösges, "Behandlung der saisonalen allergischen rhinokonjunktivitis mit einem liposomalen nasenspray," *Allergologie*, vol. 33, pp. 196–204, 2010.

[10] W. J. Fokkens, V. Lund, J. Mullol et al., "European position paper on rhinosinusitis and nasal polyps 2007," *Rhinology*, vol. 45, no. 20, pp. 1–136, 2007.

[11] "Verbreitung, Ursachen und Auswirkungen der Steroidphobie," 2008, http://www.bfarm.de/DE/Arzneimittel/zul/klinPr/nichtInterventPruef/_node.html.

[12] A. Glowania, R. Mösges, M. Böhm, A. Knopf, and L. Klimek, "Das surfactant-system—ein neuer Therapieansatz für die Schleimhaut der oberen Atemwege," *Atemwegs- und Lungenkrankheiten*, vol. 37, pp. 1–5, 2011.

[13] "Empfehlungen des Bundesinstituts für Arzneimittel und Medizinprodukte und des Paul-Ehrlich-Instituts zur Planung, Durchführung und Auswertung von Anwendungsbeobachtungen," 2010, http://www.bfarm.de/SharedDocs/Bekanntmachungen/DE/Arzneimittel/klinPr/bm-KlinPr-20100707-NichtinterventePr-pdf.pdf?__blob= publicationFile&v=4.

[14] M. Nonaka, A. Sakanushi, K. Kusama, N. Ogihara, and T. Yagi, "One-year evaluation of combined treatment with an intranasal corticosteroid and montelukast for chronic rhinosinusitis associated with asthma," *Journal of Nippon Medical School*, vol. 77, no. 1, pp. 21–28, 2010.

[15] R. Mösges, N. Pasch, A. Sayar, P. Schmalz, and J. Vent, "Survey of sensory perception and patients' subjective assessment of the application of nasal sprays—the nasal-spray-sensoric-scale," *Laryngo-Rhino-Otologie*, vol. 88, no. 9, pp. 587–591, 2009.

[16] I. Baumann, G. Blumenstock, H. DeMaddalena, J. F. Piccirillo, and P. K. Plinkert, "Quality of life in patients with chronic rhinosinusitis. Validation of the Sino-Nasal Outcome Test-20 German Adapted Version," *HNO*, vol. 55, no. 1, pp. 42–47, 2007.

[17] W. J. Fokkens, V. J. Lund, J. Mullol et al., "European position paper on nasal polyps 2007," *Rhinology*, vol. 45, pp. 1–139, 2007.

[18] E. O. Meltzer, C. Bachert, and H. Staudinger, "Treating acute rhinosinusitis: comparing efficacy and safety of mometasone furoate nasal spray, amoxicillin, and placebo," *Journal of Allergy and Clinical Immunology*, vol. 116, no. 6, pp. 1289–1295, 2005.

[19] I. Baumann, P. K. Plinkert, and H. de Maddalena, "Development of a grading scale for the Sino-Nasal Outcome Test-20 German Adapted Version (SNOT-20 GAV)," *HNO*, vol. 56, no. 8, pp. 784–788, 2008.

[20] J. F. Piccirillo, M. G. Merritt Jr., and M. L. Richards, "Psychometric and clinimetric validity of the 20-Item Sino-Nasal Outcome Test (SNOT-20)," *Otolaryngology: Head and Neck Surgery*, vol. 126, no. 1, pp. 41–47, 2002.

[21] O. Kaschke, "Allergische rhinitis: auswirkungen einer steroidphobie in Deutschland auf die therapie mit topischen glukokortikoiden," *MedReport*, vol. 17, article 10, 2008.

[22] H.-H. Homann, O. Rosbach, W. Moll et al., "A liposome hydrogel with polyvinyl-pyrrolidone iodine in the local treatment of partial-thickness burn wounds," *Annals of Plastic Surgery*, vol. 59, no. 4, pp. 423–427, 2007.

[23] A. Akerlund, M. Andersson, J. Leflein, T. Lildholdt, and N. Mygind, "Clinical trial design, nasal allergen challenge models, and considerations of relevance to pediatrics, nasal polyposis, and different classes of medication," *Journal of Allergy and Clinical Immunology*, vol. 115, no. 3, pp. S460–S482, 2005.

[24] L. Rudmik and T. L. Smith, "Quality of life in patients with chronic rhinosinusitis," *Current Allergy and Asthma Reports*, vol. 11, no. 3, pp. 247–252, 2011.

17

Serum Leptin and Adiponectin Levels in Obese and Nonobese Asthmatic School Children in relation to Asthma Control

Atqah Abdul Wahab,[1,2] **Muna M. Maarafiya,**[1] **Ashraf Soliman,**[1]
Noura B. M. Younes,[3] **and Prem Chandra**[4]

[1] *Department of Pediatrics, Hamad Medical Corporation, P.O. Box 3050, Doha, Qatar*
[2] *Weill Cornell Medical College, Doha, Qatar*
[3] *Laboratory Medicine and Pathology, Hamad Medical Corporation, P.O. Box 3050, Doha, Qatar*
[4] *Medical Research Center, Hamad Medical Corporation, P.O. Box 3050, Doha, Qatar*

Correspondence should be addressed to Atqah Abdul Wahab; atiqaaw@yahoo.com

Academic Editor: Harald Renz

There is growing evidence of a positive correlation between asthma and obesity in children and adults. Leptin and adiponectin regulate several metabolic and inflammatory functions. This study aims to evaluate serum leptin and adiponectin concentrations in asthmatic school children to investigate their association with obesity and the degree of asthma control. Obese asthmatic (OA) and nonobese asthmatic (NOA) children, aged 7 to 14, were randomly enrolled in this prospective study. Data on demographic, anthropometric, serum lipids, and spirometric measures and allergy status were collected and analyzed. Serum leptin was significantly higher (25.8 ± 11.1 versus 8.7 ± 11.1; $P < 0.0001$) and adiponectin levels were lower (2.5 ± 1.2 versus 5.4 ± 2.9; $P < 0.0001$) in OA compared to NOA children. The uncontrolled group had higher leptin and lower adiponectin levels compared to well and partially controlled asthma. BMI was positively correlated with leptin ($r = 0.79$; $P < 0.001$) and negatively with adiponectin ($r = -0.73$; $P < 0.001$). Mean BMI and leptin levels were observed to be higher in girls compared to boys. Stepwise multiple linear regression analysis showed that higher BMI and female gender had significant effect on serum leptin levels. Among asthmatic children higher serum leptin and lower adiponectin levels were significantly associated with obesity and showed no significant association with degree of asthma controls.

1. Introduction

Several epidemiological studies have shown that the prevalence of bronchial asthma and obesity is increasing concomitantly worldwide among children and young adults [1]. The mechanisms of these pathologies remain unclear despite a number of publications on the relationship between the two diseases [2, 3]. Multiple hypotheses have been proposed. Obesity may be associated with respiratory symptoms via cardio-respiratory deconditioning, physiological restriction of the chest wall by excess adipose tissue, or comorbidities, including gastroesophageal reflux and sleep-disordered breathing [4]. The disruption of immune tolerance mechanisms by obesity-associated adipokines and cytokines has been demonstrated to be involved in the association of obesity with asthma and autoimmune diseases [5].

Obesity is characterized by chronic low-grade systemic inflammation. Obese adipose tissue is infiltrated by macrophages that are a source of inflammatory cytokines [6]. More than 50 different adipokines are secreted by adipocytes. Adipokines are proteins that help regulate various body functions [7]. Leptin and adiponectin are two adipokines that are being studied to determine their association with asthma [8]. Serum leptin is proinflammatory that affects both innate and adaptive immune responses, and serum levels are markedly increased in obesity [7, 9]. Serum adiponectin has important anti-inflammatory effects in obesity that inhibits proinflammatory cytokines (TNF-a, IL-6, and nuclear factor-kB) and induces anti-inflammatory cytokines (IL-10 and IL-1 receptor antagonist) [7, 10]. Thus, leptin and adiponectin could have a role in the pathogenesis of asthma as supported by animal studies [11, 12], and only few studies have been done in humans to convincingly establish a link between adipokines and asthma [13–15].

The aim of the present study was to evaluate serum leptin and adiponectin concentrations in asthmatic school children and to investigate their association with obesity and degree of asthma control.

2. Methods

2.1. Study Population. This prospective cohort study was conducted at the Pediatric Pulmonary Clinic of the Department of Pediatrics, Hamad Medical Corporation (HMC). From April 2012 to November 2012, 60 children (31 nonobese asthmatics and 29 obese asthmatics) met inclusion criteria. The following inclusion criteria were used: (i) age between 7 to 14 years; (ii) the diagnosis of asthma was based on physician's diagnosis and according to American Thoracic Society (ATS) guidelines [16]. In addition in accordance with guidelines of the Global Initiative with the asthmatic patients that had history of recurrent chest symptoms such as coughing, dyspnea, and wheezing, which were relieved by bronchodilator treatment, they also demonstrated reversible airflow limitation. The International Study of Asthma and Allergy in Childhood (ISAAC) questionnaire was used to assess asthma-related symptoms [17]; (iii) patients visited as followup in the pediatric pulmonary clinics at HMC. Exclusion criteria were all of the children had been free of respiratory tract infections for more than 4 weeks prior to enrollment, healthy obese and nonobese subjects with any history of chronic lung disease such as cystic fibrosis (CF), non-CF bronchiectasis, chronic lung of prematurity (BPD), interstitial lung diseases, asthma exacerbation requiring systemic steroids within 4 weeks, secondary obesity with or without association with chromosomal or genetic anomalies. This study was reviewed and approved by the local ethics committee at Hamad Medical Corporation (number 12006/12).

During their initial visits, all asthmatic patients underwent skin prick tests and serum IgE. Allergic rhinitis (AR) was assessed based on the medical history including symptoms and a physical examination, in addition to skin prick tests and Serum IgE. Patients spirometric tests were performed in the respiratory laboratory unit in accordance with standards of the American Thoracic Society [16]. The highest of three technically appropriate measurements was recorded. Forced vital capacity (FVC; in liters), forced expiratory volume in 1 second (FEV1; in liters), and FEV1/FVC were measured using a flow-sensing spirometer (Sensor Medicus Model V6200, Germany). All-age predicted values for spirometry were used and Z-score was calculated [18].

Anthropometric measurements were performed using digital electronic platform scale and standing height measurement without shoes using a stadiometer. Body mass index (BMI) was calculated by dividing weight in kg by height squared in meters {weight (Kg)/(height (m))^2} and adjusted for age and gender. The standard deviation [Z] score for BMI was calculated. Normal weight was defined as BMI Z-score between −1.96 and +1.96 and obesity was defined as BMI Z-score >1.96. Data on demographic, anthropometric, serum lipids, spirometric measures, and allergy status were recorded and analyzed.

2.2. Biochemical and Hormonal Analysis. Blood samples were collected by a skilled and qualified technician at the outpatient clinic around 8 a.m. in the morning following an overnight fast. After collection, the blood samples were centrifuged for 10 minutes and stored at −70 C. The materials used for collection were disposable, adequately labeled, and of recognized quality. Leptin and adiponectin levels were measured using a commercially available enzyme-linked immunosorbent assay (ELISA) kit according to the manufacturer's instructions and standard guidelines.

2.3. Sample Size. The adequate sample was determined based on the primary outcome variables serum leptin and adiponectin levels between obese and nonobese asthmatic groups. As per literature review, the mean serum leptin levels in obese and nonobese asthmatic groups were found to be (16 ± 7.5 ng/mL and 8.5 ± 7.0 ng/mL) and adiponectin levels were observed to be (5.2 ± 2.5 ng/mL and 3.0 ± 2.0 ng/mL). With 90% power and at two sided 0.05 level of significance, the required sample size was 25 patients in each group. To account for the proportion of dropouts and nonparticipation it was planned to enroll 60 patients altogether.

2.4. Statistical Analysis. Categorical data was expressed as a frequency along with percentage and continuous data values presented in mean ± SD. Descriptive statistics were used to summarize all demographic anthropometric, serum lipids, and spirometric measures and other characteristics of the participants. Unpaired t-test was applied to compare mean of quantitative variables between the two independent groups (OA and NOA). Quantitative variables means between more than two independent groups (well controlled, partially controlled, and uncontrolled asthma) were analyzed using one way analysis of variance (ANOVA). The overall group was found to be significant, and Bonferroni multiple comparison test was performed for pair-wise comparison. For nonnormal or skewed data the corresponding nonparametric tests Mann-Whitney U and Kruskal-Wallis tests were performed. Associations between two or more qualitative variables were assessed using chi-square test. For small cell frequencies, chi-square test with continuity correction factor or Fisher's exact test was applied.

Pearson's correlation coefficient was used to assess the strength of linear relationship between two or more quantitative variables. Multiple liner regression was applied to examine and assess the effect of demographic, anthropometric, and spirometric measures and allergy status on serum leptin levels. Scatter plot was constructed and used to demonstrate the graphical presentation of the linear relationship between the two quantitative variables. A two-sided P value <0.05 was considered to be statistically significant. All statistical analyses were done using the statistical package SPSS 19.0 (SPSS Inc., Chicago, IL).

TABLE 1: Patients' demographic anthropometric, serum lipids, and spirometric measures between obese and nonobese asthmatics school children.

Variables	Obese asthmatic N = 29 (48.3%)	Nonobese asthmatic N = 31 (51.7%)	P value
Age (years)	10.9 ± 1.9 (10.7; 7.5–14.0)	11.3 ± 2.2 (11.2; 7–14)	0.432
Gender			
Male	22 (75.9%)	24 (77.4%)	0.887
Female	7 (24.1%)	7 (22.6%)	
BMI Z-score	3.9 ± 1.4 (3.6; 2.2–8.9)	0.38 ± 1.04 (−0.15; −0.95–1.96)	<0.0001
Regular daily inhaled corticosteroid (yes)	22 (75.9%)	23 (74.2%)	0.881
Steroid dose (μg/day)	301.1 ± 152.8 (250; 100–640)	299.7 ± 180.1 (250; 100–640)	0.975
Asthma control			
Well controlled	15 (48.4%)	17 (58.6%)	
Partially controlled	14 (45.2%)	10 (34.5%)	0.696
Uncontrolled	2 (6.5%)	2 (6.9%)	
Allergic rhinitis (yes)	18 (62.1%)	15 (48.4%)	0.287
Serum IgE	537.4 ± 545.4 (381; 15–2264)	445.6 ± 490.3 (208; 6–1663)	0.495
FEV1 Z-score	−0.77 ± 0.88 (−0.70; −2.3–1.1)	0.99 ± 1.0 (−0.89; −3.7–1.1)	0.399
FVC Z-score	−0.29 ± 0.77 (−0.09; −1.7–1.8)	−0.37 ± 1.13 (−0.45; −2.9–2.3)	0.775
FEV1/FVC Z-score	−0.87 ± 0.75 (−1.0; −2.5–0.67)	−0.88 ± 0.95 (−0.95; −2.5–0.69)	0.929
Serum leptin (ng/mL)	25.8 ± 11.1 (27.1; 4.6–46.8)	8.8 ± 11.1 (3.6; 0.32–48.9)	<0.0001
Serum adiponectin (ng/mL)	2.5 ± 1.2 (2.3; 0.75–4.9)	5.4 ± 2.9 (4.3; 1.9–12.0)	<0.0001

Values in parenthesis denote median and range.

3. Results

Between the periods from April 2012 to November 2012, a total of 60 asthmatic children, 29 with obesity and 31 without obesity, were enrolled in the study at the Pediatric Pulmonary Clinic, HMC. There were 14 (23.3%) girls and 46 (76.7%) boys and mean age in obese asthmatic children was 10.9 ± 1.9 years compared to nonobese asthmatic children 11.3 ± 2.2 years (P = 0.432). The percentage of patients with allergic rhinitis was higher in obese asthmatic children compared to nonobese asthmatic children (62.1% versus 48.4%; P = 0.287). The demographic, anthropometric, serum lipids, and spirometric measures, allergy status, and other characteristics of the study population are shown in Table 1. There were no significant differences between OA and NOA regarding age, sex, atopy serum total IgE, FEV1 Z-score, and FVC Z-score (P > 0.05).

As expected, serum leptin levels were significantly higher among OA children compared to NOA children (25.8 ± 11.1 ng/mL versus 8.7 ± 11.1 ng/mL; P < 0.0001) while serum adiponectin levels were significantly lower among OA children compared to NOA children (2.5 ± 1.2 ng/mL versus 5.4 ± 2.9 ng/mL; P < 0.0001). Mean steroid dose does not differ significantly between obese and nonobese asthmatic children (301.1 ± 152.8 versus 299.7 ± 180.1; P = 0.975) as presented in Table 1. Most of the patients were considered to have adequate asthma controls (53.3% well controlled and 40% partially controlled) and 6.7% uncontrolled asthma with their respective medications. Serum leptin levels in well controlled, partially controlled, and uncontrolled asthma groups

were found to be 17.01 ± 14 ng/mL, 16.04 ± 14.52 ng/mL, and 22.25 ± 12.37 ng/mL, respectively. The serum leptin concentration in the uncontrolled group was higher than that in the well and partly controlled, but the difference was not statistically significant (P = 0.719). The serum adiponectin concentration in the uncontrolled group was observed to be lower 2.3 ± 1.2 ng/mL compared to well controlled 3.8 ± 2.5 and partially controlled 4.6 ± 2.9 groups; however it did not differ significantly (P = 0.236). It is worth noting that the obesity was found to be similar across the asthma control groups. Lung function tests including FEV1 Z-score and FEV1/FVC Z-score ratio were strongly associated with degree of asthma controls. Mean FEV1/FVC Z-score was observationally higher among well controlled asthma −0.64 ± 0.81 compared to partially controlled −1.13 ± 0.84 and uncontrolled asthma −1.21 ± 0.83 (P = 0.099). No significant association was observed between age, gender, BMI Z-score, rhinitis, serum total IgE, and asthma controlled groups. The comparison in the serum leptin, adiponectin concentrations, and other parameters in the three groups of asthma control is shown in Table 2.

For the whole group of patients, BMI Z-score was positively correlated with serum leptin levels (r = 0.74; P < 0.001) and negatively correlated with adiponectin levels (r = −0.70, P < 0.001) as demonstrated in Figures 1 and 2. The leptin level showed a significant negative correlation with the adiponectin levels (r = −0.61; P < 0.001). No significant correlation was observed between leptin levels, IgE, and spirometric parameters (data not shown here). Mean BMI and leptin were found to be higher in girls (24.6 ± 5.9 ng/mL

TABLE 2: Association of demographic anthropometric, serum lipids, and spirometric measures with degree of asthma controls.

Variables	Asthma control			P value
	Well controlled $N = 32$ (53.3%)	Partially controlled $N = 24$ (40%)	Uncontrolled $N = 4$ (6.7%)	
Age (years)	10.75 ± 1.9	11.3 ± 2.3	12.5 ± 1.4	0.218
Gender				
Male	22 (68.7%)	22 (91.7%)	2 (50%)	0.181
Female	10 (31.3%)	2 (8.3%)	2 (50%)	
BMI Z-score ≤ 1.96	15 (46.9%)	14 (58.3%)	2 (50%)	0.769
BMI Z-score > 1.96	17 (53.1%)	10 (41.7%)	2 (50%)	
Regular daily inhaled corticosteroid (yes)	31 (96.9%)	12 (50%)	2 (50%)	<0.001
Allergic rhinitis (yes)	13 (40.6%)	17 (70.8%)	3 (75%)	0.132
Serum IgE	393.8 ± 529.8	618 ± 504.9	489.3 ± 369.9	0.208
FEV1 Z-score	-0.58 ± 0.89	-1.28 ± 1.03	-0.86 ± 0.86	0.052
FVC Z-score	-0.24 ± 0.86	-0.51 ± 1.04	0.08 ± 1.21	0.684
FEV1/FVC Z-score	-0.64 ± 0.81	-1.13 ± 0.84	-1.21 ± 0.83	0.099
Serum leptin (ng/mL)	17.01 ± 14.0	16.04 ± 14.5	22.25 ± 12.4	0.719
Serum adiponectin (ng/mL)	3.78 ± 2.5	4.60 ± 2.9	2.31 ± 1.2	0.236

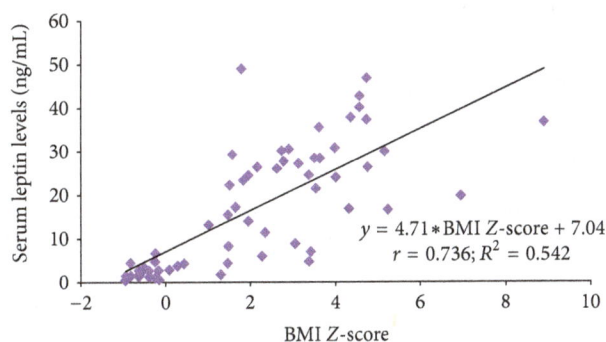

FIGURE 1: Relationship between serum leptin levels and BMI Z-score.

$y = 4.71 * \text{BMI } Z\text{-score} + 7.04$
$r = 0.736; R^2 = 0.542$

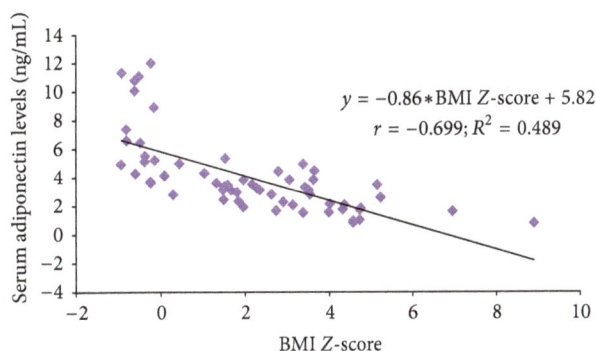

FIGURE 2: Relationship between serum adiponectin levels and BMI Z-Score.

$y = -0.86 * \text{BMI } Z\text{-score} + 5.82$
$r = -0.699; R^2 = 0.489$

versus 23.7 ± 7.2 ng/mL; $P = 0.687$) and (22.7 ± 14.2 ng/mL versus 15.2 ± 13.4 ng/mL; $P = 0.081$) compared to boys whereas mean adiponectin levels were significantly lower among girls compared to boys (2.6 ± 1.1 ng/mL versus 4.4 ± 2.8 ng/mL; $P = 0.028$). Stepwise multiple linear regression analysis showed that higher BMI (regression coefficient $\beta = 1.59$; $t = 10.3$; $P < 0.001$) and female gender (regression coefficient $\beta = 6.02$; $t = 2.41$; $P = 0.019$) have had significant effect on serum leptin levels accounting effect of other covariates such as age, rhinitis, IgE, FEV1 Z-score, and FVC Z-score.

4. Discussion

There has been intense interest in the potential role of adipose tissue in the development of asthma in obesity and in the pathogenesis of asthma. Whether activity restriction causes obesity or obesity by itself causes the development of asthma has been questioned. The possibility that asthma may lead to obesity is less controversial, because of fear of exercise or inability to exercise regularly. The adipose tissue in obese subjects leads to a systemic inflammatory state which produces a rise in the serum concentrations of several proinflammatory cytokines, chemokines, and adipokines, such as leptin as proinflammatory and adiponectin as anti-inflammatory. As body weight increases, more leptin is produced as expected in our study population, where serum leptin levels show positive correlation with BMI Z-Score with higher levels in OA children in our study population. This is in agreement with the previous studies [19, 20]. Adiponectin demonstrated a strong negative correlation with BMI Z-Score with lower levels in OA children, in contrast to a recent study where serum leptin levels were not elevated in obese asthmatics compared to nonobese asthmatics or controls but were only significantly raised in obese children without asthma [21]. Although the relationship among obesity, asthma, and leptin cannot be adequately addressed in this study, we found that BMI is determining factor for leptin; however it did not have a significant association with asthma controls.

The role of adipokines quite likely varies between different asthma inflammatory processes and reported data are inconclusive regarding the independent association between serum leptin or adiponectin and the risk of asthma. Adipocytes in the white adipose tissue are the main source of leptin, but adipocytes also secrete cytokines like TNF-α, IL-6, and IL-10. TNF-α stimulates the production of Th2 type cytokines. In summary, a common inflammatory pathway in both, obesity and asthma, is orchestrated by TNF. Similar to leptin human data on the independent association between serum adiponectin concentration and asthma are currently inconclusive [22]. In a recent study there were no significant differences between cell counts in induced sputum (eosinophils, macrophages, lymphocytes, and neutrophils) between obese and nonobese asthmatic patients [23]. Asthma is often considered as a single disease entity, but it is actually a syndrome with many different pathological pathways ultimately leading to quite similar clinical presentation: variable airway obstruction with chest tightness, wheezing, and cough [24]. Previously, conflicting results on the levels of adipokines in patients with asthma have been published including childhood asthma. Leptin has been reported to be increased [14, 25] or normal [26, 27] and adiponectin either decreased [28, 29] or normal [26, 27]. The conflicting results are likely explained by differences in patient selection. In addition, there are patient-related contributing factors like age, sex, and fat distribution. In this study, we did not find any correlation between leptin levels and IgE or spirometric parameters although FEV1 is considered a measure of asthma severity; it is not consistently related to inflammation or symptoms and is affected by multiple factors.

This study examined the association of serum leptin and adiponectin in OA and NOA children in relation with asthma control and we found that serum leptin and adiponectin concentrations did not differ among well controlled, partial controlled, and uncontrolled asthma groups suggesting that serum leptin levels may not have a major role among asthma control groups with obesity. In a recent study, where serum leptin levels were compared in intermittent, mild persistent, and moderate persistent asthma groups and found an increase in leptin levels correlated with the increase in the clinic severity of asthma, suggesting that serum leptin levels may reflect clinic severity of asthma, BMI Z-score also did not differ significantly among the asthma control groups. These findings were supported by Stanford et al. that enrolled 2238 outpatient adults and 2429 children across the United States and found that high BMI was not a predictor of controlled asthma in children (OR 1.54) [30].

We found that in obese and nonobese female asthmatic children, the levels of leptin were higher and adiponectin levels were lower than boys. The influence of leptin on increasing asthma risks varied by gender has been reported [31]. Among asthmatic children, higher serum leptin levels were shown to have stronger associations with female gender [32]. On the other hand, in a case control study conducted in 102 prepubertal asthmatic children, significant difference was observed in serum leptin levels between asthmatic and healthy children. However, this difference was confined entirely to boys [25]. Our study obviously has some

limitations. First, small percentages of the subjects enrolled were girls. To our knowledge this is the first study of this kind to report leptin and adiponectin levels in OA and NOA children in relation to the degree of asthma control. Though, we have small percentage of patients in the uncontrolled asthma group and our data did not demonstrate a significant association between obesity and the degree of asthma control. This can be explored and validated in another larger study.

5. Conclusion

In conclusion, our study findings indicate that among asthmatic school children higher serum leptin and lower adiponectin levels were significantly associated with obesity. Serum leptin and adiponectin levels did not show significant effect on the degree of asthma controls. Other factors should be sought for a better understanding of the connection between serum leptin and adiponectin levels with obesity and asthma controls. Further, larger prospective study with adequate statistical power needs to be conducted for generalization of the above findings.

Conflict of Interests

The authors declare that there is no conflict of interests regarding the publication of this paper.

References

[1] E. S. Ford, "The epidemiology of obesity and asthma," *Journal of Allergy and Clinical Immunology*, vol. 115, no. 5, pp. 897–910, 2005.

[2] D. A. Beuther, S. T. Weiss, and E. R. Sutherland, "Obesity and asthma," *American Journal of Respiratory and Critical Care Medicine*, vol. 174, no. 2, pp. 112–119, 2006.

[3] S. A. Shore, "Obesity and asthma: implications for treatment," *Current Opinion in Pulmonary Medicine*, vol. 13, no. 1, pp. 56–62, 2007.

[4] C. S. Farah and C. M. Salome, "Asthma and obesity: a known association but unknown mechanism," *Respirology*, vol. 17, no. 3, pp. 412–421, 2012.

[5] L.-G. Hersoug and A. Linneberg, "The link between the epidemics of obesity and allergic diseases: does obesity induce decreased immune tolerance?" *Allergy*, vol. 62, no. 10, pp. 1205–1213, 2007.

[6] K. E. Wellen and G. S. Hotamisligil, "Obesity-induced inflammatory changes in adipose tissue," *Journal of Clinical Investigation*, vol. 112, no. 12, pp. 1785–1788, 2003.

[7] N. A. Assad and A. Sood, "Leptin, adiponectin and pulmonary diseases," *Biochimie*, vol. 94, no. 10, pp. 2180–2189, 2012.

[8] K. W. Kim, Y. H. Shin, K. E. Lee, E. S. Kim, M. H. Sohn, and K.-E. Kim, "Relationship between adipokines and manifestations of childhood asthma," *Pediatric Allergy and Immunology*, vol. 19, no. 6, pp. 535–540, 2008.

[9] D. A. De Luis, J. L. Perez Castrillón, and A. Dueñas, "Leptin and obesity," *Minerva Medica*, vol. 100, no. 3, pp. 229–236, 2009.

[10] A. M. Wolf, D. Wolf, H. Rumpold, B. Enrich, and H. Tilg, "Adiponectin induces the anti-inflammatory cytokines IL-10 and IL-1RA in human leukocytes," *Biochemical and Biophysical Research Communications*, vol. 323, no. 2, pp. 630–635, 2004.

[11] S. A. Shore, R. D. Terry, L. Flynt, A. Xu, and C. Hug, "Adiponectin attenuates allergen-induced airway inflammation and hyperresponsiveness in mice," *Journal of Allergy and Clinical Immunology*, vol. 118, no. 2, pp. 389–395, 2006.

[12] S. A. Shore, I. N. Schwartzman, M. S. Mellema, L. Flynt, A. Imrich, and R. A. Johnston, "Effect of leptin on allergic airway responses in mice," *Journal of Allergy and Clinical Immunology*, vol. 115, no. 1, pp. 103–109, 2005.

[13] X.-M. Mai, M. F. Böttcher, and I. Leijon, "Leptin and asthma in overweight children at 12 years of age," *Pediatric Allergy and Immunology*, vol. 15, no. 6, pp. 523–530, 2004.

[14] A. Sood, E. S. Ford, and C. A. Camargo Jr., "Association between leptin and asthma in adults," *Thorax*, vol. 61, no. 4, pp. 300–305, 2006.

[15] S. A. Shore and J. J. Fredberg, "Obesity, smooth muscle, and airway hyperresponsiveness," *Journal of Allergy and Clinical Immunology*, vol. 115, no. 5, pp. 925–927, 2005.

[16] American Thoracic Society, "Guidelines for assessing and managing asthma risk at work, school, and recreation," *American Journal of Respiratory and Critical Care Medicine*, vol. 169, no. 7, pp. 837–881, 2004.

[17] S. K. Weiland, B. Björkstén, B. Brunekreef, W. O. Cookson, E. von Mutius, and D. P. Strachan, "International study protocol: international study of asthma and allergies in childhood (ISAAC): rationale and methods," *European Respiratory Journal*, vol. 24, no. 3, pp. 406–412, 2004.

[18] P. H. Quanjer, S. Stanojevic, T. J. Cole et al., "Multi-ethnic reference values for spirometry for the 3–95-yr age range: the global lung function 2012 equations," *European Respiratory Journal*, vol. 40, no. 6, pp. 1324–1343, 2012.

[19] H. Shimizu, Y. Shimomura, R. Hayashi et al., "Serum leptin concentration is associated with total body fat mass, but not abdominal fat distribution," *International Journal of Obesity*, vol. 21, no. 7, pp. 536–541, 1997.

[20] R. V. Considine, M. K. Sinha, M. L. Heiman et al., "Serum immunoreactive-leptin concentrations in normal-weight and obese humans," *The New England Journal of Medicine*, vol. 334, no. 5, pp. 292–295, 1996.

[21] M. E. Jensen, P. G. Gibson, C. E. Collins, and L. G. Wood, "Airway and systemic inflammation in obese children with asthma," *European Respiratory Journal*, vol. 24, no. 4, pp. 1012–1019, 2013.

[22] M.G. Niedoszytko, S. Małgorzewicz, M. Niedoszytko, M. Gnacińska, and E. Jassem, "The influence of obesity on inflammation and clinical symptoms in asthma," *Advances in Medical Sciences*, vol. 58, no. 1, pp. 15–21, 2013.

[23] A. Lessard, H. Turcotte, Y. Cormier, and L.-P. Boulet, "Obesity and asthma: a specific phenotype?" *Chest*, vol. 134, no. 2, pp. 317–323, 2008.

[24] G. P. Anderson, "Endotyping asthma: new insights into key pathogenic mechanisms in a complex, heterogeneous disease," *The Lancet*, vol. 372, no. 9643, pp. 1107–1119, 2008.

[25] N. Guler, E. Kirerleri, U. Ones, Z. Tamay, N. Salmayenli, and F. Darendeliler, "Leptin: does it have any role in childhood asthma?" *Journal of Allergy and Clinical Immunology*, vol. 114, no. 2, pp. 254–259, 2004.

[26] T. Jartti, L. Saarikoski, L. Jartti et al., "Obesity, adipokines and asthma," *European Journal of Allergy and Clinical Immunology*, vol. 64, no. 5, pp. 770–777, 2009.

[27] K. W. Kim, Y. H. Shin, K. E. Lee, E. S. Kim, M. H. Sohn, and K.-E. Kim, "Relationship between adipokines and manifestations of childhood asthma," *Pediatric Allergy and Immunology*, vol. 19, no. 6, pp. 535–540, 2008.

[28] A. Sood, X. Cui, C. Quails et al., "Association between asthma and serum adiponectin concentration in women," *Thorax*, vol. 63, no. 10, pp. 877–882, 2008.

[29] A. Sood, C. Quails, J. Seagrave et al., "Effect of specific allergen inhalation on serum adiponectin in human asthma," *Chest*, vol. 135, no. 2, pp. 287–294, 2009.

[30] R. H. Stanford, A. W. Gilsenan, R. Ziemiecki, X. Zhou, W. R. Lincourt, and H. Ortega, "Predictors of uncontrolled asthma in adult and pediatric patients: analysis of the asthma control characteristics and prevalence survey studies (ACCESS)," *Journal of Asthma*, vol. 47, no. 3, pp. 257–262, 2010.

[31] Y. C. Chen, G. H. Dong, K. C. Lin, and Y. L. Lee, "Gender difference of childhood overweight and obesity in predicting the risk of incident asthma: a systematic review and meta-analysis," *Obesity Reviews*, vol. 14, no. 3, pp. 222–231, 2013.

[32] Y.-W. Quek, H.-L. Sun, Y.-Y. Ng et al., "Associations of serum leptin with atopic asthma and allergic rhinitis in children," *American Journal of Rhinology and Allergy*, vol. 24, no. 5, pp. 354–358, 2010.

Proteolytic Activity Present in House-Dust-Mite Extracts Degrades ENA-78/CXCL5 and Reduces Neutrophil Migration

Laura Keglowich,[1] **Michael Tamm,**[2] **Jun Zhong,**[1] **Nicola Miglino,**[1] **and Pieter Borger**[1]

[1] *Department of Biomedicine, University Hospital Basel, Hebelstrasse 20, 4031 Basel, Switzerland*
[2] *Department of Pulmonology, University Hospital Basel, Petersgraben 2, 4031 Basel, Switzerland*

Correspondence should be addressed to Pieter Borger; pieter.borger@unibas.ch

Academic Editor: Kurt Blaser

Background. Bronchial smooth muscle cells (BSMC) are a major source of proinflammatory and proangiogenic cytokines and chemokines, including VEGF and CXC-chemokines. CXC-chemokines act primarily on neutrophils, mediating their recruitment to and activation at the site of inflammation. In humans, house-dust mite (HDM) allergens can cause asthmatic exacerbations and trigger an inflammatory response through protease-dependent mechanisms. *Objective.* We investigated the effect HDM extract on the release of pro-angiogenic and proinflammatory cytokines from BSMC. *Methods.* Human primary BSMC were stimulated with HDM extract in the absence or presence of fetal calf serum (FCS). Twenty angiogenic cytokines were detected by a specific antibody array and modified protein levels were confirmed by ELISA. Neutrophil migration was measured using a 96-well Boyden chamber. *Results.* ENA-78/CXCL5 protein levels in conditioned medium of BSMC stimulated with HDM extract were significantly reduced ($n = 10$, $P < 0.05$) but restored in the presence of 5% FCS. HDM extracts did not affect ENA-78/CXCL5 mRNA levels. Recombinant ENA-78/CXCL5 was degraded after incubation with HDM extracts ($n = 7$, $P < 0.05$) but restored after the addition of the serine protease AEBSF. Neutrophil migration towards recombinant ENA-78/CXCL5 was also reduced in the presence of HDM extract. *Conclusion.* HDM proteases degrade ENA-78/CXCL5. Thus exposure to HDM allergens may alter ENA-78/CXCL5 levels in the lungs and may affect angiogenesis and the inflammatory response in the airways of asthma patients.

1. Introduction

House-dust mites (HDM) (*Dermatophagoides pteronissinus*) allergens are among the most potent stimuli of asthma attacks [1, 2]. HDM excretions contain a plethora of biologically active compounds, which have allergenic potential that prompts IgE response in sensitized subjects. The same HDM compounds also have proinflammatory properties, which are independent of the IgE response. In asthma, neoangiogenesis of the airway wall is a recently recognized pathology, which contributes to airway wall thickness [3–5]. There is also evidence from animal models that HDM and other allergens can induce neovascularization of the inflamed airway [6, 7]. However, the effects of HDM allergens on asthma related angiogenesis remain incompletely understood.

HDM extracts have been shown to disrupt the tight junctions between epithelial cells and lead to the complete desquamation of the epithelial cell layer, hence facilitating the passage of allergens across the epithelial air-tissue border [8–10]. The major HDM allergen, Der *p1*, is a cysteine protease [11–13] and may be responsible for the observed epithelial cell desquamation, for the release of cytokines, and facilitates the transport of allergens across cultured epithelial cell layers [9–11, 14–16]. In consequence, the desquamation of the protective epithelium may allow allergenic compounds to penetrate deeper into the airway wall, thereby facilitating airway hyper-sensitization.

Proteases present in HDM excrements also exerted a direct modulatory effect on regulatory proteins in cultured human bronchial smooth muscle cells (BSMC) that affect the cell's ability to proliferate and to secrete cytokines [17]. In particular, BSMC exposed to HDM extract increased interleukin (IL)-6 production and cell proliferation through the protease-activated receptor 2 [17]. Hence, HDM exposure contributes to inflammation and airway wall remodeling in a mechanism independent of the immune system by direct interaction with BSMC. Furthermore, proteolytic activities present in fungal and bacterial extracts have been shown to specifically and dose-dependently degrade human interleukin (IL)-6 and IL-8/CXCL8 [18], as well as RANTES, monocyte chemotactic protein (MCP)-1, and epithelial-derived neutrophil attractant (ENA)-78/CXCL5 [19], hence reducing the bioavailability of these cytokines. Together, these data imply that the exposure of the airways to external factors with intrinsic proteolytic activity affects the relative level of immuno-modulatory cytokines, which may affect inflammation and microvessel formation and airway remodeling. In the present study, we analyzed the effect of HDM extract on the release and degradation of a panel of cytokines that have proinflammatory and angiogenic activity and are implicated in airway wall remodeling. Our data show that the proteolytic activity present in HDM extract degraded ENA-78/CXCL5 and reduced the migration of neutrophils. These findings imply that HDM allergens may have the capacity to modify the development of an eosinophil dominated inflammatory response in the lung.

2. Methods

2.1. Isolation of Primary Bronchial Smooth Muscle Cells.
BSMC were obtained from endobronchial biopsies obtained by flexible bronchoscopy or from therapeutically resected bronchial tissue obtained from the Department of Internal Medicine and Pneumology (University Hospital Basel, Basel, Switzerland) with the approval of the local ethical committee (EK: 05/06) and written informed consent of all patients. Patients with mild to moderate asthma had reversible airway obstruction documented in the past, with a median FEV1 of 70.5% of the predicted value (ranging from 45.3% to 84.6%). The samples used as nonasthmatic controls participating in this study were either from healthy organ donors whose lungs were deemed unfit for use in a transplant procedure or from the healthy part of lung resection material obtained after lung surgery.

Isolation of BSMC was performed as described earlier [20, 21]. BSMC bundles were dissected from the surrounding tissue by microscopy and pure muscle bundles were plated in a 25 cm^2-flask prewetted with 1 mL of Dulbecco's modified Eagle's medium (DMEM) containing GlutaMax 4.5 g/L glucose (Gibco, Bioconcept, Allschwil, Switzerland), 5% FCS, 1x antibiotics-antimycotics, and 1x modified Eagle's medium vitamin mix (Invitrogen, Lubio, Luzern, Switzerland). BSMC were characterized by immunostaining as described earlier [22].

2.2. Generation of Conditioned Medium (CM).
BSMC were grown in BSMC-growth medium (GM): RPMI 1640 supplemented with 5% fetal calf serum (FCS), 8 mM L-glutamine, 20 mM hydroxyethyl piperazine ethane sulfonic acid, 1x antibiotics-antimycotics, and 1x modified Eagle's medium vitamin mix (Invitrogen, Lubio, Luzern, Switzerland) under normoxic conditions (21% O_2, 5% CO_2, and 37°C). BSMC were seeded and kept in BSMC-GM for 24 h before they were serum deprived for 24 h prior to stimulation. A stock solution (1 mg/mL) of HDM extract (gift from: Peter Adler Wurtzen, Alk Abello's Research Department, Hørsholm, Denmark) was prepared in RPMI 1640 medium and diluted in RPMI 1640 to the final concentration (20, 10, and 2 μg/mL), which was then sterilized by filtration (0.22 mm) (MN Sterilizer PES; Macherey-Nagel AG, Oensingen, Switzerland). 10 ng/mL of colistin (Roth, Arlesheim, Switzerland) was to avoid effects of lipopolysacchrids (LPS) in HDM extract. To obtain HDM-CM, BSMC were incubated for 72 h (37°C) with HDM extract (2 and 10 μg/mL) or without HDM extract in the presence or absence of 5% FCS.

2.3. Angiogenesis Antibody Array.
The human angiogenesis antibody array G 1000 (Raybiotech, Lucerna-Chem, Luzern, Switzerland) was used to detect the release of 20 angiogenesis-related cytokines and growth factors in CM obtained from BSMC stimulated with HDM extract or unstimulated BSMC. 100 μL of undiluted CM collected after 72 h was applied to each array and the angiogenesis related factors were evaluated according to the manufacturer instructions. Cy3 fluorescence was measured by a NimbleGen MS 200 microarray scanner (Roche, Basel, Switzerland) and signal intensity was analyzed by AIDA software (Raytest, Straubenhardt, Germany).

2.4. Cytokine-ELISA.
Enzyme linked immunosorbent assay (ELISA) kits for IL-8/CXCL8 (sensitivity: 7.5 pg/mL), ENA-78/CXCL5 (sensitivity: 15 pg/mL), and VEGF (sensitivity: 9 pg/mL) were purchased from R & D (Abingdon, UK) and ELISA was performed according to the manufacturer's instructions. 100 μL of CM obtained from BSMC was measured undiluted (VEGF), 1 : 5 diluted (ENA-78/CXCL5), or 1 : 50 diluted (IL-8/CXCL8).

2.5. ENA-78/CXCL5 mRNA Expression by RT-PCR.
To induce mRNA, BSMC were grown in absence and presence of HDM extract (20 μg/mL) for 6 h. Total RNA was extracted from 10^6 cells ($t = 0$ h, and $t = 6$ h) by Trizol method (Gibco, Bioconcept, Allschwil, Switzerland). Then, 5 μg of total RNA was converted into cDNA. Semiquantitative PCR (94°C, 65°C, and 72°C) was performed for 28 cycles using a Thermo Hybaid PCR Express (Catalys, Wallisellen, Switzerland) as described elsewhere [23]. The primers for ENA-78/CXCL5 were forward: 5′-ATC TCC GCT CCT CCA CCC AGT-3′ and reverse: 5′-TTC TTG TCT TCC CTG GGT-3′ generating a PCR fragment of 493 bp. The primers GAPDH were forward: 5′-CCA AAG GGT CAT CAT CTC TGC-3′ and GAPDH reverse: 5′-ATT TGG CAG GTT TTT CTA-3′ generating a PCR fragment of 417 bp.

2.6. Neutrophil Migration Assay.
Polymorphonuclear cells (PMNC) isolation and neutrophil chemotaxis anticoagulated blood was obtained from the local blood bank (Blutspendezentrum, Basel, Switzerland) after written informed consent of all donors. PMNC were isolated using PolymorphprepTM separation medium as recommended by the manufacturer (Axis-Shield, Axonlab, Baden, Switzerland). Chemotaxis was assessed using 96-well Boyden chamber

(Neuroprobe, Gaithersburg, USA) as previously described [24]. The lower compartments of the 96-well chamber were filled with either 100 ng/mL recombinant ENA-78/CXCL5, or 10 ng/mL recombinant ENA-78/CXCL5 (stimulated for 24 h with or without 10 μg/mL HDM extract), or 10 μg/mL HDM extract in RPMI 1640, or RPMI 1640 alone, and then covered with a 5 μm pore-sized polycarbonate filter (Neuroprobe, Gaithersburg, USA). Next, 200 μL of neutrophil suspension (2×10^6 cells/mL) was added to the upper compartments. After 2 h of incubation (37°C, 5% CO_2) the upper compartment was removed and the filter was fixed and stained with Differential Quik Staining Kit (Polyscience, Brunschwig, Basel, Switzerland). The membrane was scanned with a desktop scanner, and the intensity of spots was analyzed using Image J software.

2.7. Statistics. Cytokine data are presented as mean ± S.E.M. Migration analysis is shown as mean ± S.E.M. after densitometric image analysis (Image J software, National Institute of Mental Health, Bethesda, Maryland, USA). Unpaired Student's t test was performed and P values < 0.05 were considered significant.

3. Results

3.1. HDM Extract Downregulated ENA-78/CXCL5 Protein Levels. To identify proteins that are affected by the addition of HDM extract to BSMC, CM of stimulated and unstimulated BSMC was applied to an antibody array. Comparing the protein expression patterns of 2 independent angiogenesis arrays, the expression of ENA-78/CXCL5 was consistently reduced in CM collected from BSMC that had been stimulated with HDM extract (Figures 1(a) and 1(b)). The panel of proangiogenic proteins of the array is shown in Figure 1(c). We then confirmed this finding with an ENA-78/CXCL5 ELISA in CM collected from BSMC stimulated with HDM extract for 24 and 72 h. As shown in Figure 1(d), HDM extract (10 μg/mL) significantly decreased the concentration of ENA-78/CXCL5 in CM of stimulated BSMC (P < 0.05; n = 10). In contrast, using ELISA, we observed that HDM extract (10 μg/mL) did not significantly alter the levels of IL-8/CXCL8 or VEGF protein (Figures 1(e) and 1(f)).

3.2. HDM Extract Did Not Affect ENA-78/CXCL5 mRNA Levels. To determine whether the HDM-dependent reduction of ENA-78/CXCL5 protein levels were associated with reduced gene transcription RT-PCR was performed using total RNA extracted after 0 and 6 h from BSMC grown in the absence and presence of HDM extract (20 μg/mL). As shown in Figure 2, exposure to HDM extract did not significantly affect RNA levels of ENA-78/CXCL5.

3.3. HDM Extract Specifically Degraded ENA-78/CXCL5 Protein. The observation that HDM extract stimulation decreased ENA-78/CXCL5 protein levels while ENA-78/CXCL5 mRNA levels were unchanged indicated that the ENA-78/CXCL5 protein may be degraded by proteolytic activities of the HDM extract. Therefore, we incubated

BSMC with 5% FCS which has strong antiproteolytic activity in the presence of HDM extract (2 and 10 μg/mL). As shown in Figure 1(d), HDM extract reduced the ENA-78/CXCL5 protein level in CM collected from BSMC. In the presence of 5% FCS, this effect was completely abrogated (Figure 3(a)), suggesting a protease-dependent mechanism of ENA-78/CXCL5 degradation. Next, we tested the effect of HDM extract on the basal concentration of ENA-78/CXCL5 in CM from BSMC (n = 7) grown in the absence of FCS for 24 and 72 h. After collection of the CM, we incubated with either HDM extract alone or a combination of HDM extract + 5% FSC. In the absence of FCS, the addition of HDM extract significantly reduced the basal concentration of ENA-78/CXCL5 in CM. FCS abrogated this effect (Figure 3(b)). We confirmed the proteolytic activity of HDM extract and the antiproteolytic effect of FCS on ENA-78/CXCL5 degradation with recombinant ENA-78/CXCL5. Furthermore, we assessed the effect of the serine protease inhibitor AEBSF and the cysteine protease inhibitor E64 on the degradation of recombinant ENA-78/CXCL5 by HDM extract. Incubation with E64 (0.5 μM, 5 μM, and 10 μM) did not prevent ENA-78/CXCL5 degradation by HDM extract in any of the used concentrations (data not shown). In contrast, the addition of AEBSF led to a significant increase in ENA-78/CXCL5 concentration compared to control condition (without AEBSF) (Figure 3(c)).

3.4. HDM-CM Reduced Chemotaxis of Neutrophils. Finally, we tested the effect of HDM extract-dependent ENA-78/CXCL5 degradation in regard to the chemotactic capacity of ENA-78/CXCL5. As shown in Figure 4, ENA-78/CXCL5 alone dose-dependently induced neutrophil migration compared to medium only, while HDM extract alone had no significant effect on the induction of migration when combined HDM extract reduced the neutrophil migratory effect of ENA-78/CXCL5.

4. Discussion

In our study, we demonstrated for the first time that the CXCR2 ligand ENA-78/CXCL5 was degraded upon exposure to HDM extract, whereas a second CXCR2 ligand IL-8/CXCL8 was not affected. CXCR2 ligands have been suggested to play a crucial role in inflammation and angiogenesis, in particular in directing neovascularization in tumors [25]. We recently showed that angiogenic CXCR2 ligands are produced by human BSMC directing sprout outgrowth from endothelial cell spheroids [unpublished data, manuscript submitted]. In addition to its angiogenic characteristics, ENA-78/CXCL5 exerts strong chemotactic properties for neutrophils [26]. Several neutrophil attracting chemokines are present in the lung, including IL-8/CXCL8, growth related proteins (GRO/CXCL1-α, β, γ), and ENA-78/CXCL5 [27, 28]. Although ENA-78/CXCL5 and IL-8/CXCL8 share some properties, each cytokine has its own specific effects [29–33]. Comparing these studies, ENA-78/CXCL5 seems to be more important in chronic than in acute immunological responses.

The observation that FCS completely blocked the degradation of ENA-78/CXCL5 protein demonstrated that

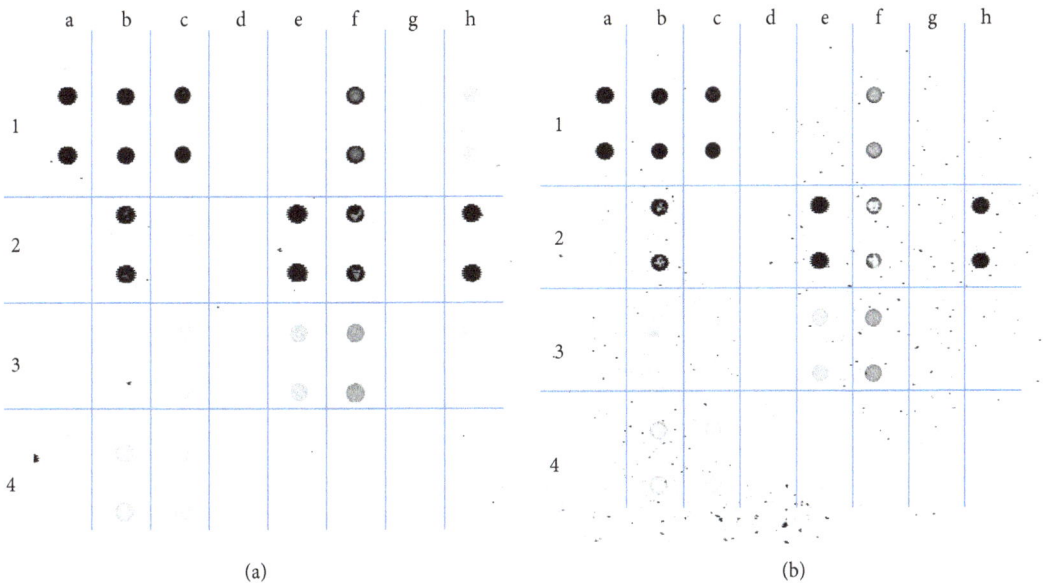

(a)   (b)

	a	b	c	d	e	f	g	h
1	Pos	Pos	Pos	Neg	Neg	Angio-genin	EGF	ENA-78
2	bFGF	GRO	IFN-g	IGF-1	IL-6	IL-8	Leptin	MCP-1
3	PFGF-BB	PIGF	RANTES	TGF-beta	TIMP-1	TIMP-2	Thrombo-poeitin	VEGF
4	VEGF-D	IC1	IC2	IC3	Neg	Neg	Neg	Neg

(c)

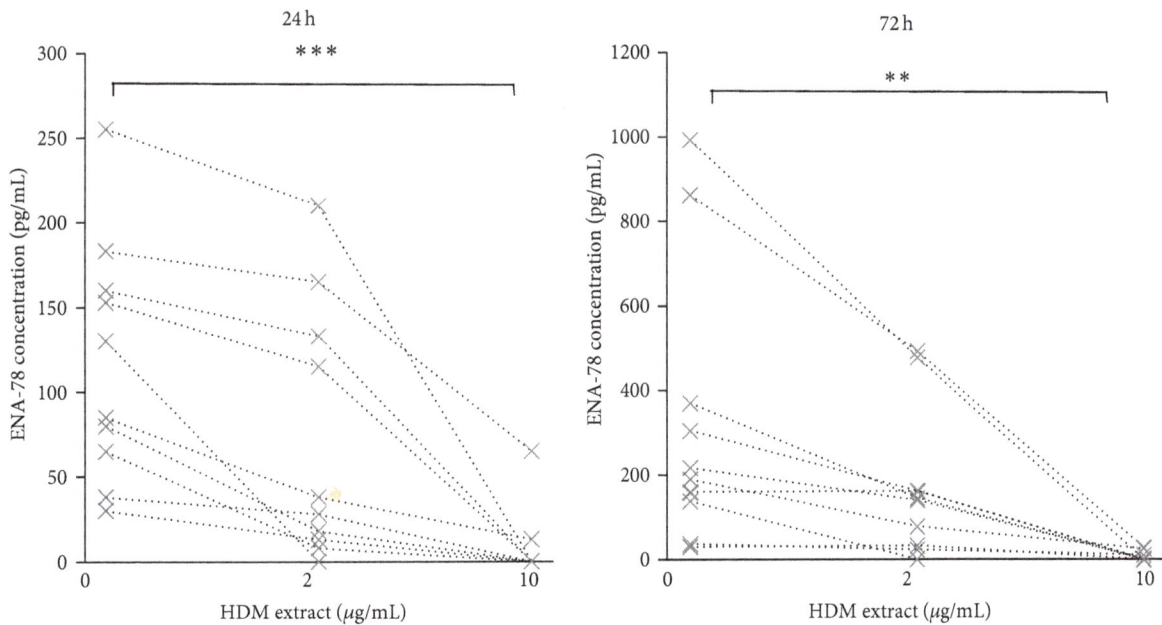

(d)

FIGURE 1: Continued.

(e)

(f)

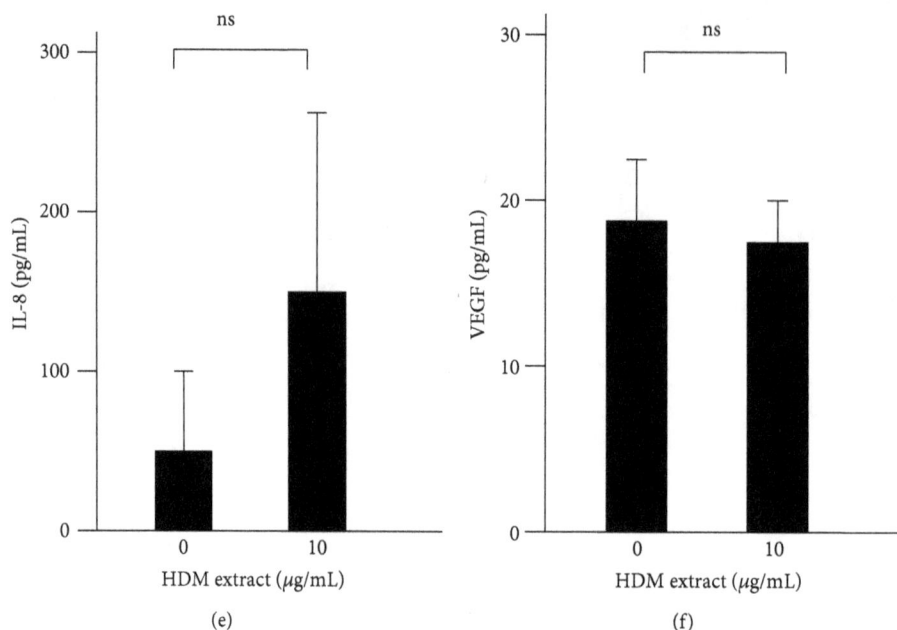

FIGURE 1: *Effect of HDM extract (HDME) on the release of angiogenic factors.* Typical examples of angiogenesis antibody arrays incubated with conditioned medium (CM) of unstimulated BSMC (a) and with CM of BSMC that were stimulated with 10 μg/mL HDME (b). For identification purposes, the corresponding antibody array map is presented in (c). Angiogenic factors are identified by a letter-number code (e.g., IL-8/CXCL8 = f2, ENA78/CXCL5 = h1, VEGF = h3, etc.). Pos = positive control; Neg = negative control; IC1-IC3 = internal controls 1–3, and standard abbreviations are used for the detected angiogenic factors. (d) Time- and dose-dependent reduction of ENA-78/CXCL5 in the presence of CM of BSMC that were stimulated with 2 concentrations of HDM extract (n = 10) for either 24 or 72 hours. The same CM did not significantly affect IL-8/CXCL8 (e) and VEGF (f) levels. $^{**}P < 0.005$; $^{***}P < 0.001$; ns = not significant.

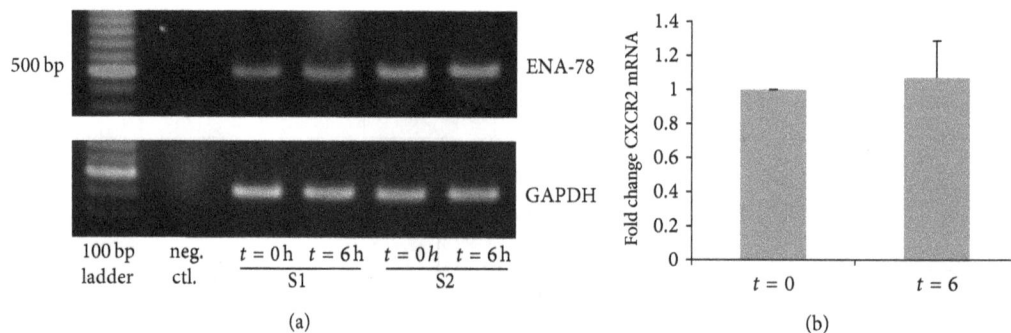

(a)

(b)

FIGURE 2: *Detection of ENA-78/CXCL5 mRNA by RT-PCR.* (a) Typical experiment showing ENA-78/CXCL5 (fragment size: 493 bp) and GAPDH (fragment size: 417 bp) RT-PCR products in BSM cells of 2 subjects (S1 = subject 1; S2 = subjects 2). (b) Densitometric analysis of RT-PCR as mean ± SEM. For details, see text.

the degradation was due to the proteolytic activity present in the HDM extract and this was confirmed by the protective effect of the serine protease inhibitor AEBSF. In contrast, the cysteine protease inhibitor E64 did not prevent HDM extract-dependent ENA-78/CXCL5 degradation; therefore, we conclude that one mechanism of ENA-78/CXCL5 degradation is dependent on serine proteases present in HDM extract. Proteolytic activities present in HDM extracts have been extensively studied and several HDM allergens have been identified as proteases [34]. A major effect of these proteases is the selective reduction of the bioavailability of cytokines, since not all cytokines are equally prone to

proteolytic degradation [19]. Diminished bioavailability of cytokines due to proteolytic degradation has been associated with opportunistic fungi, in particular *Aspergillus fumigatus* [18], as well as with pathogenic bacteria, such as *Pseudomonas aeruginosa* [19]. Characteristic for both organisms is the secretion of a wide range of proteolytic enzymes intended for growth and existence. Present in the lung, these enzymes may help the microorganisms to penetrate into deeper areas of the airway wall. In addition, their protease-activity may change the relative quantities of cytokines of the airways and skew the immune system. Proteolytic modifications of ENA-78/CXCL5 protein have been shown to reduce and to

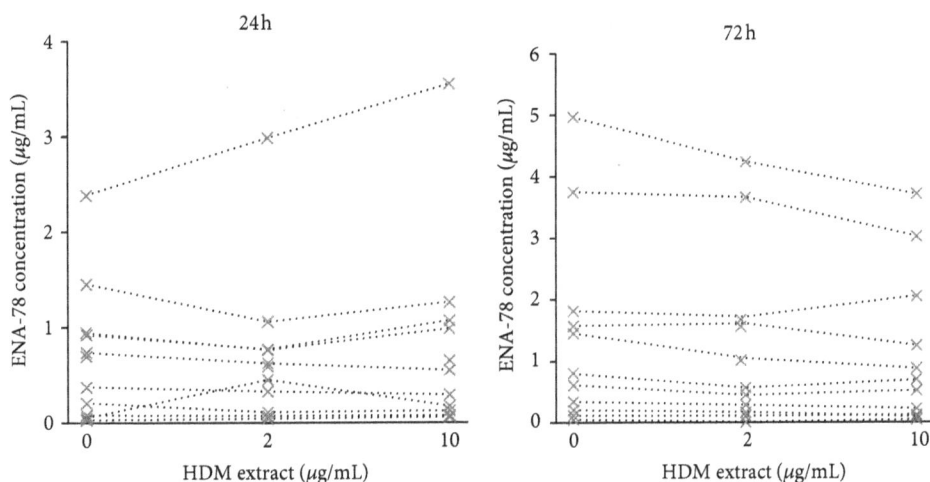

(a)

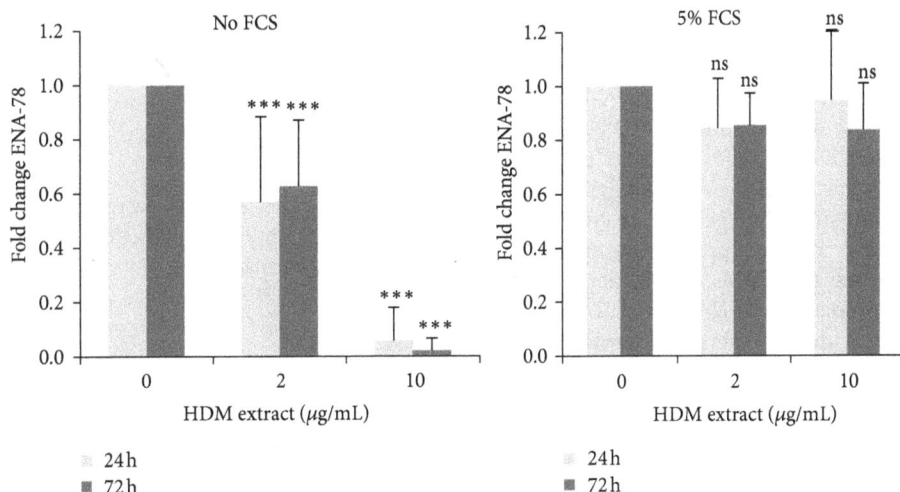

(b)

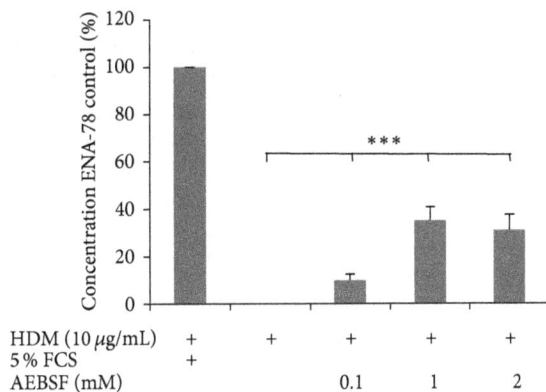

(c)

FIGURE 3: *FCS and AEBSF block the effect of HDM extract.* (a) Effect of HDM extract (2 and 10 μg/mL) on ENA-78 levels in the presence of 5% FCS. ENA78/CXCL5 levels were measured in different HDM containing CM preparations after 24 h (left panel) and 72 h (right panel). (b) Effect of FCS (5%) on HDM extract-induced reduction of ENA-78/CXCL5 levels ($n = 5$; $^{***}P < 0.001$ comparing HDM extract stimulated CM to unstimulated CM). (c) Degradation of recombinant ENA-78/CXCL5 by HDM extract is inhibited by the addition of the serine proteases inhibitor AEBSF or FCS ($n = 3$, measured as duplicates; bars represent the mean $\pm$ SEM, $^{***}P < 0.001$ relative to the rescue effect of AEBSF on HDM extract-induced ENA-78/CXCL5 degradation).

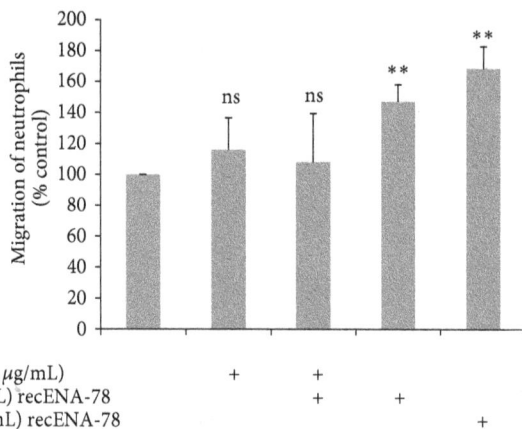

HDM (10 µg/mL)		+	+	
10 (ng/mL) recENA-78			+	+
100 (ng/mL) recENA-78				+

FIGURE 4: *HDM extract reduces recombinant ENA-78/CXCL5-induced neutrophil migration.* Migrated cells were stained with Diff Quick staining kit, scanned with a desktop scanner and densitometric analysis was performed with Image J. Values are expressed as mean ± SEM. $^{**}P < 0.005$; $n = 3$ (neutrophils from 1 healthy subject in triplicate).

enhance its biological activity. Cleavage of ENA-78/CXCL5 by MMP, MMP2, or the aminopeptidase CD13 has been shown to enhance its activity [35, 36], whereas proteolytic modifications caused by metalloproteases from *Pseudomonas aeruginosa* were accompanied by the loss of chemotactic activity [19]. We were able to provide evidence that proteolytic modifications by HDM extract abrogate the neutrophil-attracting properties of ENA-78/CXCL5.

Our data provide evidence that HDM proteases may directly affect the proinflammatory and proangiogenic cytokine response through proteolytic degradation of ENA-78/CXCL5 protein. Produced by epithelial cells, ENA-78/CXCL5 was first described as a chemoattractant for neutrophils [31]. We have recently reported that not only epithelial cells but also BSMC release high levels of ENA-78/CXCL8 [37]. Continuous exposure to HDM allergens may reduce the bioavailability of ENA-78/CXCL5 due to proteolytic degradation and lower the number of neutrophils that infiltrate the asthmatic airway. This may alter the immune response in favor of eosinophilic inflammation, as it is often observed in the lungs of asthmatic patients and thought of as the main histopathology of the asthmatic lung [38–40]. It should be noted, however, that asthma sometimes is associated with neutrophilia. In a sheep model of asthma, HDM extracts induced neutrophil infiltration at 6 h, followed by eosinophils and activated lymphocytes into the lung tissue and BAL, similar to the late-phase allergic response seen in human asthma [41]. It is currently unknown whether or not an association exists between exposure to HDM allergens and eosinophilia. However, selective degradation of ENA-78/CXCL5 by proteases present in HDM extract might provide a partial explanation.

Our experiments with the Boyden chamber showed that chemotactic migration of neutrophils towards ENA-78/CXCL5 is reduced in the presence of HDM extract. The microenvironment–such as the presence of serum (e.g., due

to increased vascular leakage), as well as the relative presence of cytokines and chemotactic factors–will ultimately determine the immunological response. A common pathological feature of inflammatory airway diseases is an imbalance of proteases and antiproteases present in the lining fluid of the lungs. The presence of serum-derived antiproteases may further delineate a balanced equilibrium between proteases and antiproteases, as bystander effects neutralize the protease-activity of inhaled compounds. An external addition of foreign proteases, which may be derived from fungi, bacteria, or HDM, may distort this intricate balance and lead to irreversible impairment of airway function and disease.

Taken together, our data demonstrate that the ENA-78/CXCL5 protein is susceptible to degradation by proteases present in HDM extract. Although reduced bioavailability of ENA-78/CXCL5 could potentially cause atypical immunological characteristics *in vivo*, the biological relevance of this observation remains to be established.

Conflict of Interests

The authors declare that there is no conflict of interests regarding the publication of this paper.

Acknowledgment

House-dust-mite extracts were kindly provided by Peter Adler Wurtzen, Alk Abello's Research Department, Hørsholm, Denmark.

References

[1] R. P. Nelson Jr., R. DiNicolo, E. Fernández-Caldas, M. J. Seleznick, R. F. Lockey, and R. A. Good, "Allergen-specific IgE levels and mite allergen exposure in children with acute asthma first seen in an emergency department and in nonasthmatic control subjects," *The Journal of Allergy and Clinical Immunology*, vol. 98, no. 2, pp. 258–263, 1996.

[2] W. R. Thomas, B. J. Hales, and W.-A. Smith, "House dust mite allergens in asthma and allergy," *Trends in Molecular Medicine*, vol. 16, no. 7, pp. 321–328, 2010.

[3] S. Al-Muhsen, J. R. Johnson, and Q. Hamid, "Remodeling in asthma," *The Journal of Allergy and Clinical Immunology*, vol. 128, no. 3, pp. 451–462, 2011.

[4] A. Detoraki, F. Granata, S. Staibano, F. W. Rossi, G. Marone, and A. Genovese, "Angiogenesis and lymphangiogenesis in bronchial asthma," *Allergy*, vol. 65, no. 8, pp. 946–958, 2010.

[5] J. W. Wilson and T. Kotsimbos, "Airway vascular remodeling in asthma," *Current Allergy and Asthma Reports*, vol. 3, no. 2, pp. 153–158, 2003.

[6] J. van der Velden, D. Barker, G. Barcham, E. Koumoundouros, and K. Snibson, "Increased vascular density is a persistent feature of airway remodeling in a sheep model of chronic asthma," *Experimental Lung Research*, vol. 38, no. 6, pp. 307–315, 2012.

[7] M. V. Avdalovic, L. F. Putney, E. S. Schelegle et al., "Vascular remodeling is airway generation-specific in a primate model of chronic asthma," *The American Journal of Respiratory and Critical Care Medicine*, vol. 174, no. 10, pp. 1069–1076, 2006.

[8] H. Wan, H. L. Winton, C. Soeller et al., "Quantitative structural and biochemical analyses of tight junction dynamics following exposure of epithelial cells to house dust mite allergen Der p 1," *Clinical and Experimental Allergy*, vol. 30, no. 5, pp. 685–698, 2000.

[9] H. Wan, H. L. Winton, C. Soeller et al., "Der p 1 facilitates transepithelial allergen delivery by disruption of tight junctions," *The Journal of Clinical Investigation*, vol. 104, no. 1, pp. 123–133, 1999.

[10] H. L. Winton, H. Wan, M. B. Cannell et al., "Cell lines of pulmonary and non-pulmonary origin as tools to study the effects of house dust mite proteinases on the regulation of epithelial permeability," *Clinical and Experimental Allergy*, vol. 28, no. 10, pp. 1273–1285, 1998.

[11] R. J. Simpson, E. C. Nice, R. L. Moritz, and G. A. Stewart, "Structural studies on the allergen Der p1 from the house dust mite *Dermatophagoides pteronyssinus*: similarity with cysteine proteinases," *Protein Sequences & Data Analysis*, vol. 2, no. 1, pp. 17–21, 1989.

[12] K. Y. Chua, G. A. Stewart, W. R. Thomas et al., "Sequence analysis of cDNA coding for a major house dust mite allergen, Der p 1: homology with cysteine proteases," *The Journal of Experimental Medicine*, vol. 167, no. 1, pp. 175–182, 1988.

[13] C. R. A. Hewitt, H. Horton, R. M. Jones, and D. I. Pritchard, "Heterogeneous proteolytic specificity and activity of the house dust mite proteinase allergen Der p I," *Clinical and Experimental Allergy*, vol. 27, no. 2, pp. 201–207, 1997.

[14] C. King, S. Brennan, P. J. Thompson, and G. A. Stewart, "Dust mite proteolytic allergens induce cytokine release from cultured airway epithelium," *Journal of Immunology*, vol. 161, no. 7, pp. 3645–3651, 1998.

[15] C. Robinson, N. A. Kalsheker, N. Srinivasan et al., "On the potential significance of the enzymatic activity of mite allergens to immunogenicity. Clues to structure and function revealed by molecular characterization," *Clinical and Experimental Allergy*, vol. 27, no. 1, pp. 10–21, 1997.

[16] H. F. Kauffman, M. Tamm, J. A. B. Timmerman, and P. Borger, "House dust mite major allergens Der p 1 and Der p 5 activate human airway-derived epithelial cells by protease-dependent and protease-independent mechanisms," *Clinical and Molecular Allergy*, vol. 4, article 5, 2006.

[17] N. Miglino, M. Roth, M. Tamm, and P. Borger, "House dust mite extract downregulates C/EBPα in asthmatic bronchial smooth muscle cells," *The European Respiratory Journal*, vol. 38, no. 1, pp. 50–58, 2011.

[18] H. F. Kauffman, J. F. Christomee, M. A. van de Riet, A. J. B. Timmerman, and P. Borger, "Protease-dependent activation of epithelial cells by fungal allergens leads to morphologic changes and cytokine production," *The Journal of Allergy and Clinical Immunology*, vol. 105, no. 6, part 1, pp. 1185–1193, 2000.

[19] K. G. Leidal, K. L. Munson, M. C. Johnson, and G. M. Denning, "Metalloproteases from *Pseudomonas aeruginosa* degrade human RANTES, MCP-1, and ENA-78," *Journal of Interferon & Cytokine Research*, vol. 23, no. 6, pp. 307–318, 2003.

[20] P. R. A. Johnson, C. L. Armour, D. Carey, and J. L. Black, "Heparin and PGE2 inhibit DNA synthesis in human airway smooth muscle cells in culture," *The American Journal of Physiology—Lung Cellular and Molecular Physiology*, vol. 269, no. 4, part 1, pp. L514–L519, 1995.

[21] P. R. A. Johnson, M. Roth, M. Tamm et al., "Airway smooth muscle cell proliferation is increased in asthma," *The American*

[22] P. Seidel, M. Roth, Q. Ge, I. Merfort, C. T. S'ng, and A. J. Ammit, "IκBα glutathionylation and reduced histone H3 phosphorylation inhibit eotaxin and RANTES," *The European Respiratory Journal*, vol. 38, no. 6, pp. 1444–1452, 2011.

[23] R. A. Fillmore, S. E. Nelson, R. N. Lausch, and J. E. Oakes, "Differential regulation of ENA-78 and GCP-2 gene expression in human corneal keratocytes and epithelial cells," *Investigative Ophthalmology and Visual Science*, vol. 44, no. 8, pp. 3432–3437, 2003.

[24] S. Henness, E. Van Thoor, Q. Ge, C. L. Armour, J. M. Hughes, and A. J. Ammit, "IL-17A acts via p38 MAPK to increase stability of TNF-α-induced IL-8 mRNA in human ASM," *The American Journal of Physiology—Lung Cellular and Molecular Physiology*, vol. 290, no. 6, pp. L1283–L1290, 2006.

[25] R. M. Strieter, M. D. Burdick, J. Mestas, B. Gomperts, M. P. Keane, and J. A. Belperio, "Cancer CXC chemokine networks and tumour angiogenesis," *European Journal of Cancer*, vol. 42, no. 6, pp. 768–778, 2006.

[26] M. Baggiolini, B. Dewald, and B. Moser, "Interleukin-8 and related chemotactic cytokines—CXC and CC chemokines," *Advances in Immunology*, vol. 55, pp. 97–179, 1994.

[27] S. Kikuchi, I. Kikuchi, Y. Takaku et al., "Neutrophilic inflammation and CXC chemokines in patients with refractory asthma," *International Archives of Allergy and Immunology*, vol. 149, supplement 1, pp. 87–93, 2009.

[28] K. Nakagome, S. Matsushita, and M. Nagata, "Neutrophilic inflammation in severe asthma," *International Archives of Allergy and Immunology*, vol. 158, supplement 1, pp. 96–102, 2012.

[29] R. M. Strieter, S. W. Chensue, M. A. Basha et al., "Human alveolar macrophage gene expression of interleukin-8 by tumor necrosis factor-alpha, lipopolysaccharide, and interleukin-1 beta," *The American Journal of Respiratory Cell and Molecular Biology*, vol. 2, no. 4, pp. 321–326, 1990.

[30] A. Walz, P. Schmutz, C. Mueller, and S. Schnyder-Candrian, "Regulation and function of the CXC chemokine ENA-78 in monocytes and its role in disease," *Journal of Leukocyte Biology*, vol. 62, no. 5, pp. 604–611, 1997.

[31] A. Walz, R. Burgener, B. Car, M. Baggiolini, S. L. Kunkel, and R. M. Strieter, "Structure and neutrophil-activating properties of a novel inflammatory peptide (ENA-78) with homology to interleukin 8," *The Journal of Experimental Medicine*, vol. 174, no. 6, pp. 1355–1362, 1991.

[32] T.-A. Imaizumi, K. H. Albertine, D. L. Jicha, T. M. McIntyre, S. M. Prescott, and G. A. Zimmerman, "Human Endothelial Cells Synthesize ENA-78: relationship to IL-8 and to Signaling of PMN Adhesion," *The American Journal of Respiratory Cell and Molecular Biology*, vol. 17, no. 2, pp. 181–192, 1997.

[33] S. Schnyder-Candrian and A. Walz, "Neutrophil-activating protein ENA-78 and IL-8 exhibit different patterns of expression in lipopolysaccharide- and cytokine-stimulated human monocytes," *The Journal of Immunology*, vol. 158, no. 8, pp. 3888–3894, 1997.

[34] W. R. Thomas, W.-A. Smith, B. J. Hales, K. L. Mills, and R. M. O'Brien, "Characterization and immunobiology of house dust mite allergens," *International Archives of Allergy and Immunology*, vol. 129, no. 1, pp. 1–18, 2002.

[35] J. Song, C. Wu, X. Zhang, and L. M. Sorokin, "In vivo processing of CXCL5 (LIX) by matrix metalloproteinase (MMP)-2 and

MMP-9 promotes early neutrophil recruitment in IL-1beta-induced peritonitis," *The Journal of Immunology*, vol. 190, no. 1, pp. 401–410, 2013.

[36] A. Mortier, T. Loos, M. Gouwy, I. Ronsse, J. van Damme, and P. Proost, "Posttranslational modification of the NH2-terminal region of CXCL5 by proteases or peptidylarginine deiminases (PAD) differently affects its biological activity," *The Journal of Biological Chemistry*, vol. 285, no. 39, pp. 29750–29759, 2010.

[37] L. Keglowich, M. Roth, M. Philippova et al., "Bronchial Smooth Muscle Cells of Asthmatics Promote Angiogenesis through Elevated Secretion of CXC-Chemokines (ENA-78, GRO-α, and IL-8)," *PLoS ONE*, vol. 8, no. 12, Article ID e81494, 2013.

[38] A. B. Kay, "The role of eosinophils in the pathogenesis of asthma," *Trends in Molecular Medicine*, vol. 11, no. 4, pp. 148–152, 2005.

[39] C. Lemière, P. Ernst, R. Olivenstein et al., "Airway inflammation assessed by invasive and noninvasive means in severe asthma: eosinophilic and noneosinophilic phenotypes," *The Journal of Allergy and Clinical Immunology*, vol. 118, no. 5, pp. 1033–1039, 2006.

[40] S. E. Wenzel, "Eosinophils in Asthma—closing the loop or opening the door?" *The New England Journal of Medicine*, vol. 360, no. 10, pp. 1026–1028, 2009.

[41] R. J. Bischof, K. Snibson, R. Shaw, and E. N. T. Meeusen, "Induction of allergic inflammation in the lungs of sensitized sheep after local challenge with house dust mite," *Clinical and Experimental Allergy*, vol. 33, no. 3, pp. 367–375, 2003.

19

The Compatible Solute Ectoine Reduces the Exacerbating Effect of Environmental Model Particles on the Immune Response of the Airways

Klaus Unfried,[1] Matthias Kroker,[1] Andrea Autengruber,[1] Marijan Gotić,[2] and Ulrich Sydlik[1]

[1] *IUF Leibniz Research Institute for Environmental Medicine, Auf'm Hennekamp 50, 40225 Düsseldorf, Germany*
[2] *Department of Material Chemistry, Ruđer Bosković Institute, Bijenička cesta 54, 10000 Zagreb, Croatia*

Correspondence should be addressed to Klaus Unfried; klaus.unfried@uni-duesseldorf.de

Academic Editor: Ralph Mösges

Exposure of humans to particulate air pollution has been correlated with the incidence and aggravation of allergic airway diseases. In predisposed individuals, inhalation of environmental particles can lead to an exacerbation of immune responses. Previous studies demonstrated a beneficial effect of the compatible solute ectoine on lung inflammation in rats exposed to carbon nanoparticles (CNP) as a model of environmental particle exposure. In the current study we investigated the effect of such a treatment on airway inflammation in a mouse allergy model. Ectoine in nonsensitized animals significantly reduced the neutrophilic lung inflammation after CNP exposure. This effect was accompanied by a reduction of inflammatory factors in the bronchoalveolar lavage. Reduced IL-6 levels in the serum also indicate the effects of ectoine on systemic inflammation. In sensitized animals, an aggravation of the immune response was observed when animals were exposed to CNP prior to antigen provocation. The coadministration of ectoine together with the particles significantly reduced this exacerbation. The data indicate the role of neutrophilic lung inflammation in the exacerbation of allergic airway responses. Moreover, the data suggest to use ectoine as a preventive treatment to avoid the exacerbation of allergic airway responses induced by environmental air pollution.

1. Introduction

The exposure of humans to particulate air pollution has been correlated with the incidence of atopic allergies [1]. In particular, traffic-related air pollution is strongly linked to allergic diseases including asthmatic bronchitis [2]. It is hypothesized that an adjuvant effect of inhaled particles may influence either the process of sensitization or the immune response, at the level of the disease outcome [3]. In asthma patients, such adverse effects of particulate air pollution can be observed as an acute exacerbation of allergic lung inflammation [4–6].

Current research is focusing on the molecular mechanisms by which such a toxic potential of environmental particles is mediated. As one common denominator of particle-induced adverse health effects, oxidative stress in the airways has been identified [7]. Reactive oxygen species may

be triggered by the intrinsic oxidative potential of inhaled particulate matter which depends on chemical properties like elemental composition and surface charges. But also via indirect cell mediated pathways oxidative stress is generated in the airways. Upon cell contact, in particular ultrafine or nano-sized particles may interact with cellular components and organelles which can contribute to the production of reactive oxygen species [8]. Additionally, the induction of an inflammatory response, which is a typical reaction to the inhalation of poorly soluble material, can lead to an oxidative burst from inflammatory cells like macrophages and neutrophilic granulocytes [9].

So far, it is not clear whether all these potential mechanisms contribute to the exacerbation of immune reactions of the airways or whether one of these pathways dominates the adverse effects and might therefore be a useful target for preventive and therapeutic approaches. In the system of ovalbumin (OVA)-sensitized mice this problem was addressed by inhalation studies with pure carbon nanoparticles (CNP). Such particles are considered model particles for combustion-derived recent particulate air pollution. Inhalation of these particles prior to OVA challenge led to an aggravation of the allergic airway responses including infiltration of inflammatory cells and excretion of cytokines [10]. An intervention study employing antioxidants in this scenario demonstrated that a reduction of the oxidative stress prevents the exacerbation of the airway response [11]. Using this experimental system, it should be possible to test the preventive value of compounds for individuals who suffer from atopic asthma, which might be exacerbated after inhalation of particulate matter.

In our earlier studies, we were able to demonstrate that the compatible solute ectoine is able to reduce the neutrophilic inflammatory response of the airways after exposure to pure (CNP). In the system of particle-exposed rats, the neutrophilic lung inflammation was significantly reduced when ectoine was present during exposure [12]. At a mechanistic level, we were able to demonstrate that ectoine prevents the activation of proinflammatory reactions in lung epithelial cells by stabilizing membrane signalling platforms which are addressed by oxidative cell stress coming by the particles [13]. In this context, it has been shown that ectoine does not interact with the particles themselves. The stabilizing mechanism of ectoine was investigated by a number of "proof of principle" experiments, which demonstrated that the mechanism is not based on antioxidant properties of the substance. Additionally, investigating the effect of ectoine during an ongoing neutrophilic inflammation, we observed the prevention of antiapoptotic and therefore proinflammatory reactions of neutrophils in the inflammatory environment by ectoine [14]. This effect was observed not only in the animal system, where it led to an accelerated resolution of the inflammation, but also in the human system employing peripheral neutrophils from patients suffering from chronic obstructive pulmonary disease (COPD).

The possibility to reduce neutrophilic lung inflammation without directly interfering with the oxidative potential of the nanoparticles offers the possibility to investigate the relevance of the neutrophilic inflammation for the exacerbation of allergic lung inflammation. Ectoine is a highly compatible substance which is tolerated by higher organisms without any known side effects. Therefore, the system might give indications for possible therapeutic value for asthma patients. For that purpose, the experimental system of CNP-induced neutrophilic lung inflammation was adopted to C57/Bl6 mice and the effect of ectoine application was evaluated in these organisms. The influence of ectoine of local and systemic cytokines with immune relevance was tested. In a second step, the system was applied to OVA-sensitized mice which were challenged in the presence of CNP and ectoine.

2. Materials and Methods

2.1. Particle Suspensions. Carbon nanoparticles (CNP, Printex 90) were obtained from Degussa (Essen, Germany). Stock suspensions (1 mg/mL) of particles were prepared in phosphate buffered saline (PBS) by sonication for 60 min. Particles and particle suspensions were characterized by (i) scanning electron microscopy (JSM 7000F, JEOL Ltd., Japan), (ii) BET using FlowSorb II 2300 analyzer (Micromeritics, Norcross, USA), and (iii) light scattering using ZetratracTM NPA152 (Microtrac, Montgomeryville, PA, USA). Particle suspension characteristics were as described previously [13].

2.2. Animal Experiments. Female C57BL/6JRj mice (8 weeks old, Janvier, France) were treated with particle suspensions or control solutions via pharyngeal aspiration with a volume of 50 μL, under inhalation anaesthesia (isoflurane, 5% in synthetic air, 1-2 min). Animals were sensitized by repetitive intraperitoneal injection of 1 μg OVA/alum. At the indicated time point, mice were challenged by aerosol inhalation (1% OVA in PBS) for 30 min using a Pari-Boy Nebuliser (Pari, Starnberg, Germany). Animals were sacrificed by exsanguination under anaesthesia after the indicated exposure times. Serum was prepared from blood samples taken prior to exsanguination. Bronchoalveolar lavage was taken using 4 × 1 mL PBS. All animal experiments were performed after relevant permission according to German animal protection laws.

2.3. Lavage Parameters. Differential cell counts were performed from Giemsa/May-Grünwald stainings of lavage cells. Cell free lavage fluids were subjected either to solid-phase ELISA in order to determine KC and IL-6 (R&D systems, Minneapolis, MN) or to Mouse Cytokine Antibody Arrays (RayBiotech, Inc., Norcross, CA) according to the respective manufacturer's instructions. Signal strengths of the arrays were determined densitometrically from autoradiographs using Quantity One software (version 4.1, Biorad, Hercules, CA, USA). IL-6 serum content was determined using the above-mentioned ELISA system.

2.4. Statistical Analyses. Statistical calculations were performed using IBM SPSS statistics 22. Significant values were calculated either by ANOVA analyses with Tukey's HSD post hoc testing or by comparison of individual groups by Mann-Whitney U-test. Dose response relationships were analysed by Pearson correlations. Except for the boxplot in Figure 1, mean values with standard errors are given. Power calculations for the design of animal experiments were performed using G*Power version 3.1.5 (University of Kiel, Germany).

3. Results and Discussion

With the current studies we aimed at investigating the effect of ectoine in an in vivo experimental system suitable as a model for allergic airway diseases. In a first approach, lung inflammation in C57/Bl6 mice was investigated with respect to dose response after 24 h (Figure 1). Analyses of bronchoalveolar lavage (BAL) demonstrate a dose dependent increase of inflammatory cells. The neutrophil influx is reflected by the increase of the neutrophil recruiting cytokine KC. The effect of ectoine was then tested in a time course experiment in which animals were exposed for 12 h, 24 h,

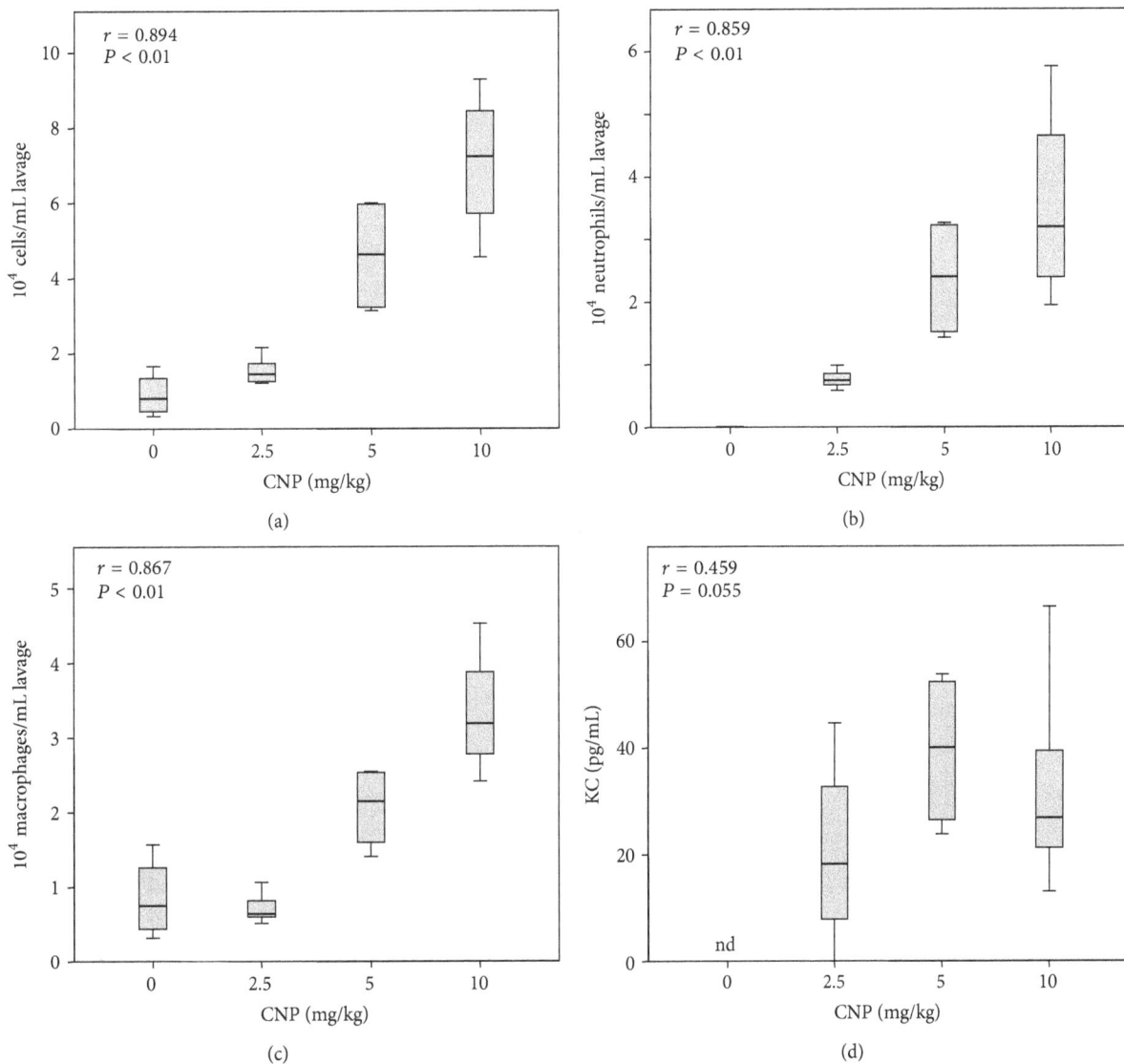

FIGURE 1: Lung inflammation induced by increasing doses of CNP. Female C57/Bl6 mice (8 weeks old) were exposed once to the indicated dose of CNP suspended in PBS. Animal numbers were 0 mg/kg $n = 4$, 2.5 mg/kg $n = 5$, 5 mg/kg $n = 4$, and 10 mg/kg $n = 5$. Inflammation parameters were determined 24 h after exposure. (a) Total number of cells per mL BAL; (b) total number of neutrophilic granulocytes per mL BAL; (c) total number of macrophages and monocytes per mL BAL; (d) pg/mL of KC in BAL. r, correlation coefficient of Pearson correlation; P, two sided significance; nd, not detectable.

and 48 h with 5 mg/kg CNP in the presence or absence of ectoine (Figure 2). Control animals were exposed with saline (PBS) or ectoine solution for 24 h. After a maximum of total cell counts as well as neutrophil numbers in BAL after 12 h, the inflammatory parameters attenuated during the observation period. The reduction of neutrophils was counteracted by the increase of macrophages, which help to clear the lung from apoptotic neutrophils. In the presence of 1 mM ectoine, the kinetics of the neutrophilic inflammation were mirrored at a lower level, indicating the preventive potential of the substance in the mouse system with the most striking statistical significance after 12 h.

The consequences of this reaction were furthermore tested at the level of cytokines and chemokines using membrane arrays for two BAL samples from each 12 h exposure group (Figure 3(a)). Although the differences in cytokine patterns are based on a low number of individuals, the general reduction of the selected inflammatory markers by the ectoine is obvious. In addition to these analyses, the potential of ectoine to reduce systemic inflammation was investigated by measuring IL-6 in BAL and in serum of exposed animals (Figures 3(b) and 3(c)). IL-6 levels in control animals were not detectable. The application of ectoine together with CNP led to a significant reduction of cytokine levels both in BAL and in serum of the animals. In particular, the reduction of IL-6 in the serum of the animals treated with ectoine in addition to CNP highlights the potential of this kind of treatment to reduce systemic effects of the lung inflammation. IL-6 has been discussed as a serum marker for asthma which also might be involved in the pathogenesis of asthma [15]. This

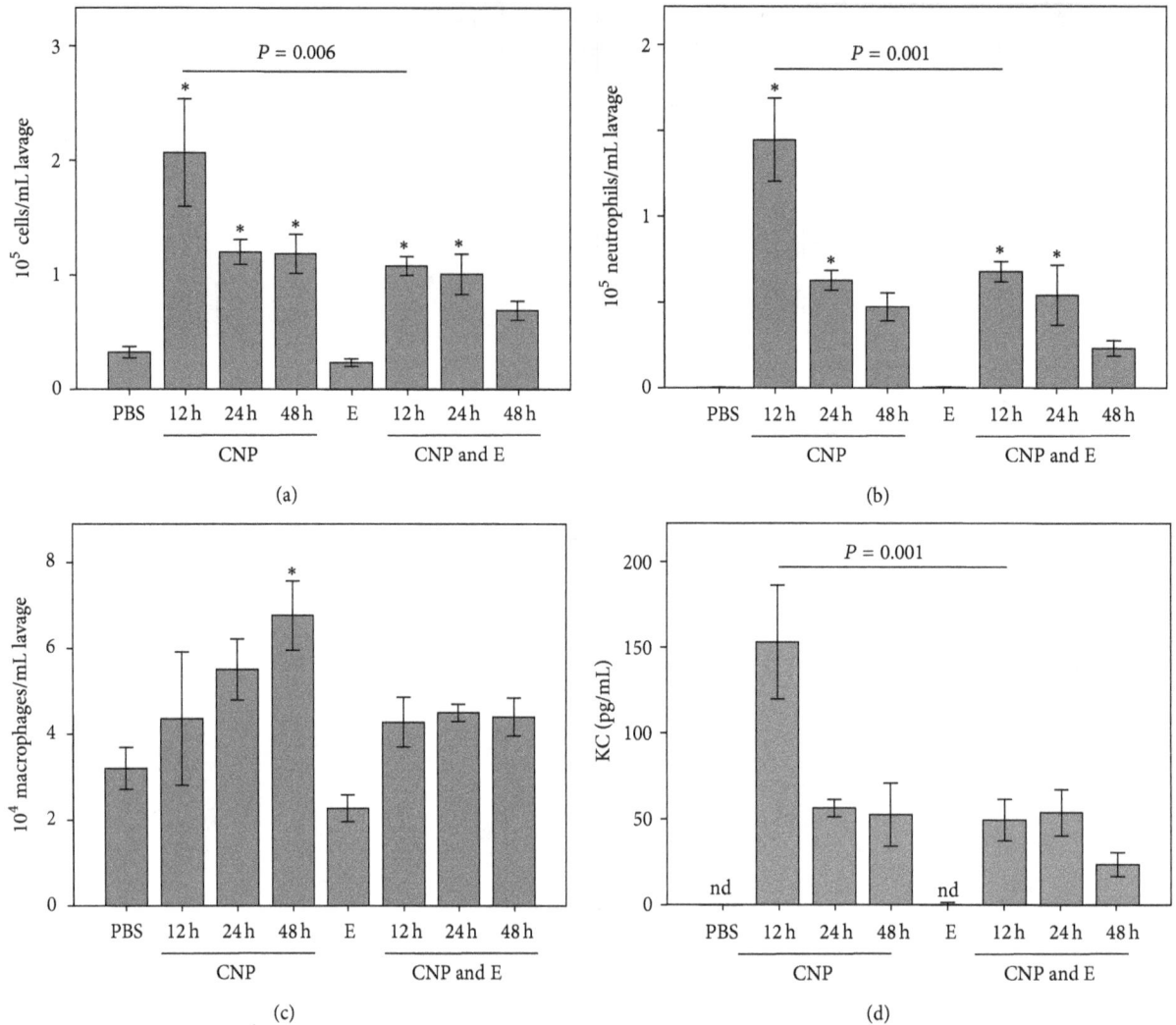

FIGURE 2: Time course of lung inflammation after single application of 5 mg/kg CNP in the presence or absence of ectoine (1 mM). Animals ($n = 5$) were analysed after the indicated time points. (a) Total number of cells per mL BAL; (b) total number of neutrophilic granulocytes per mL BAL; (c) total number of macrophages and monocytes per mL BAL; (d) pg/mL of KC in BAL. *, significantly different to the respective control (PBS or ectoine) after Tukey's HSD post hoc testing considering multiple testing; E, ectoine; nd, not detectable.

result may be an indication that ectoine has also beneficial effects with respect to the allergic sensitization which might be boosted by environmental pollution.

The potential of ectoine to reduce the exacerbation of the immune reaction by the neutrophilic lung inflammation was then tested in animals which were sensitized for 12 weeks by repetitive injection of the model allergen ovalbumin (OVA). Animals were challenged 12 h after the application of particles in the presence or absence of ectoine (Figure 4(a)). Inflammatory parameters in the lung of the animals were investigated 24 h after the provocation. At this time point, all sensitized animals exhibited elevated cell numbers in BAL which were highest in CNP-exposed animals (Figure 4(b)). This reaction proved to be significantly reduced when ectoine was applied together with the particles. The differential analysis of the cells revealed that the exacerbating effect of the particles as well as the preventive effect is mostly due to the changes in neutrophilic granulocytes. Remarkably, the

same effects are observed at the level of lymphocytes and eosinophils which are considered relevant for the allergic response (Figure 4(e)). Due to the very low number of these cells and the overwhelming number of neutrophils, these cell types were analysed together (other cells). Although exhibiting high heterogeneity, macrophage numbers were elevated in all challenged animals irrespective of an existing inflammation during the provocation. As observed in earlier experiments, this effect was not influenced by the ectoine treatment (Figure 4(d)).

Considering that ectoine itself has no antioxidant capacity the current data may give an indication for the mechanisms by which environmental particles contribute to asthma exacerbation. In this scenario, ectoine significantly reduces the neutrophilic inflammation induced by the particles at the time point of the onset of the antigen provocation. Ectoine is known not to interact with the particles and it does not scavenge reactive oxygen species. It is therefore plausible that

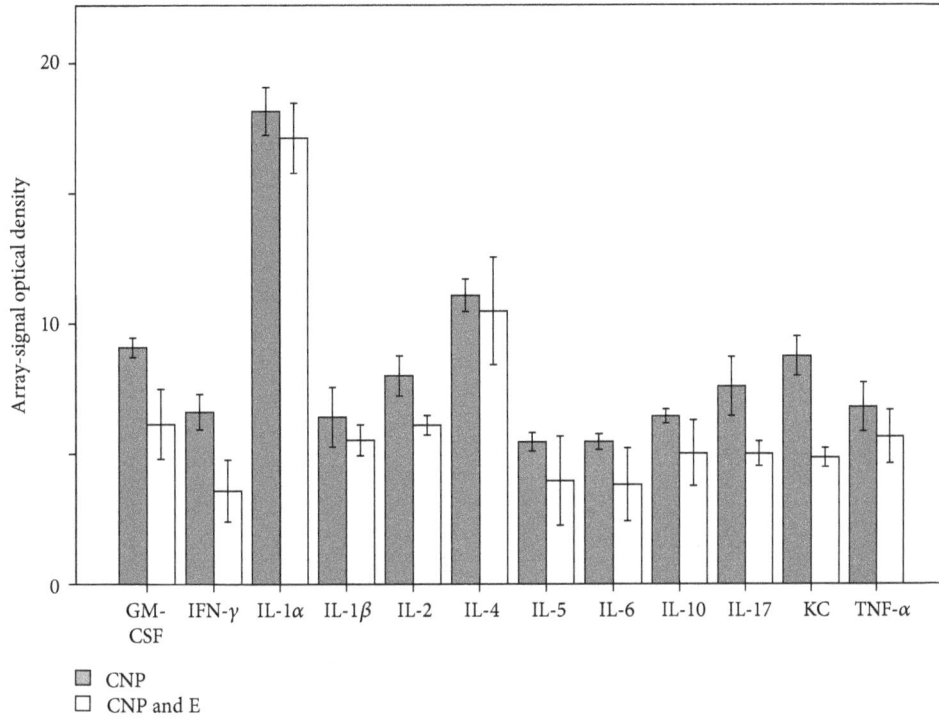

(a)

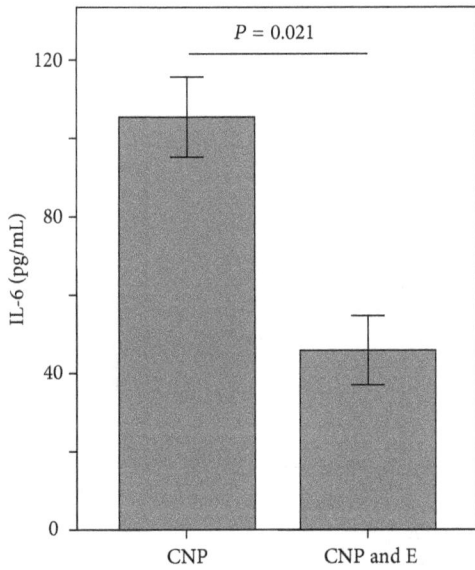

(b)

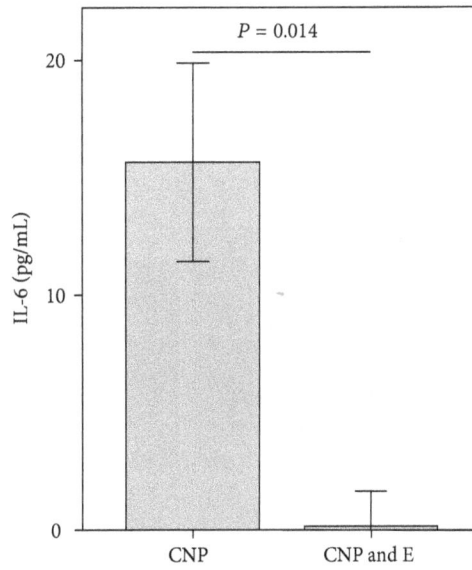

(c)

Figure 3: Effect of ectoine treatment on inflammatory mediators 12 h after exposure. (a) BAL analyses of two animals from each group. Given error bars are based on duplicates from both measurements. Significant values cannot be calculated. (b) IL-6 in BAL of 5 animals; (c) IL-6 in serum of 5 animals. CNP, 5 mg/kg carbon nanoparticles; E, 1 mM ectoine. Significant values (two sided) in (b) and (c) were calculated by Mann-Whitney U-test.

the exacerbating effect of combustion-derived nanoparticles is mediated by the proinflammatory trigger which can be observed at the level of neutrophil influx and the respective proinflammatory mediators.

Due to the molecular mechanisms by which ectoine acts, the substance in a first line was suggested to be used as a preventive agent against environmental particulate air

pollution. Ectoine in epithelial cells has been shown to prevent typical effects of cell stress triggered by combustion-derived nanoparticles [16]. This strategy however was not designed to replace attempts to improve ambient air quality but was rather considered for predisposed persons who may suffer from chronic lung inflammation or from allergic diseases of the airways. It was therefore important to test

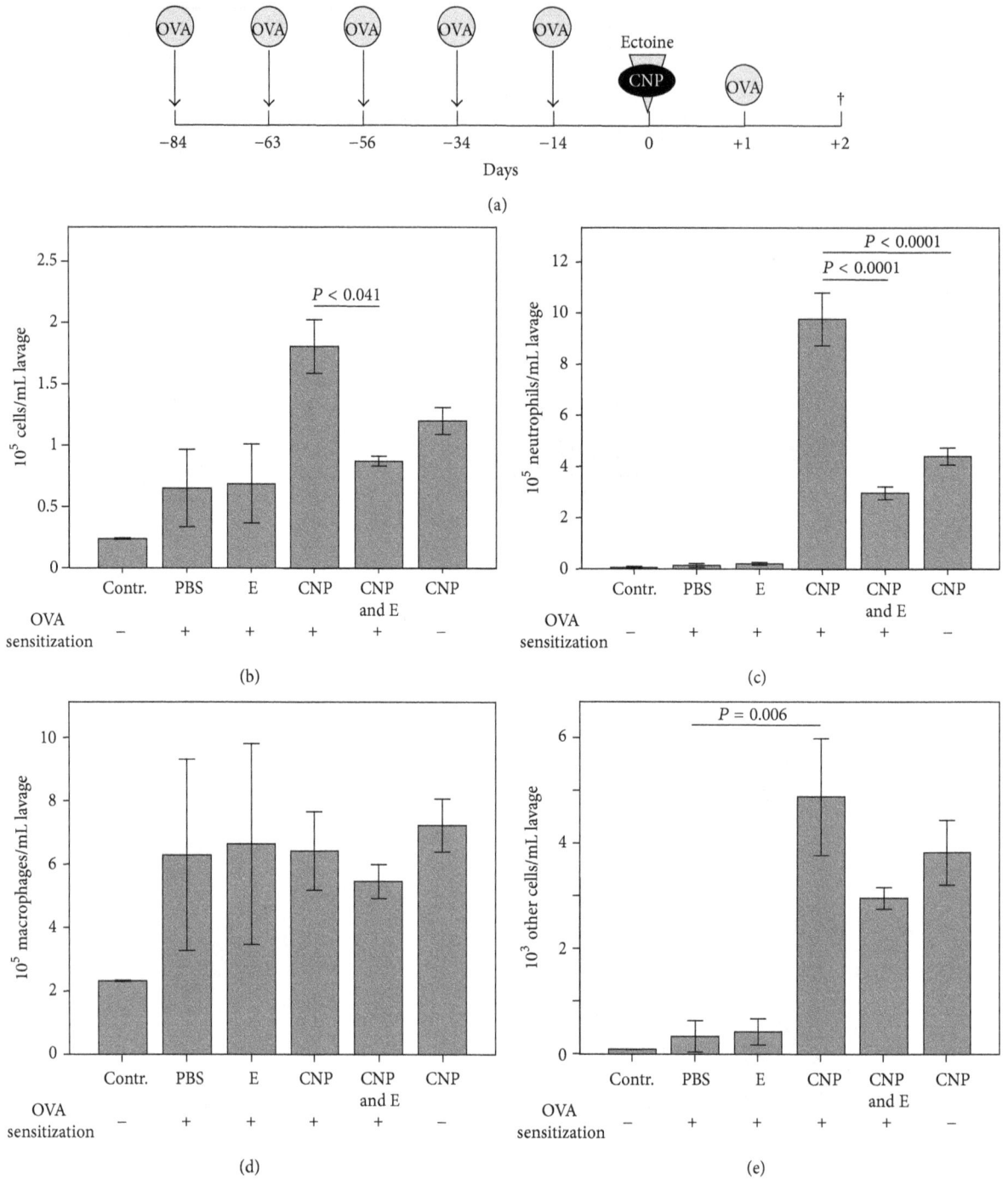

FIGURE 4: Effect of CNP and ectoine on OVA provocation-induced lung inflammation in sensitized animals (control groups $n = 3$ and exposure groups $n = 5$). (a) Experimental design. Animals were sensitized by repetitive intraperitoneal OVA application. At day 0, 5 mg/kg CNP in the presence or absence of 1 mM ectoine was applied to the animals. OVA provocation by inhalation (1%, 30 min) was performed 12 h after treatment. Measurements were made 24 h after challenge. (b) Total number of cells per mL BAL; (c) total number of neutrophilic granulocytes per mL BAL; (d) total number of macrophages and monocytes per mL BAL; (e) total number of other cells including lymphocytes and eosinophilic granulocytes.

whether in the situation of an immune response which is exacerbated by the presence of environmental model particles the inflammatory outcome can be reduced by ectoine. The data show significant differences in neutrophil numbers 36 h after the challenge, indicating that the number of neutrophils

recruited by the immune response on OVA provocation can be reduced. At this time point eosinophilic infiltration has just started. Other studies observe elevated levels of these cell types later after the challenge [17]. Therefore the analysis of other cell types in our system has to deal with very low absolute numbers. Although statistically not significant, a trend in the reduction of these cell types by ectoine can also be observed. In order to investigate the effect of ectoine on this particular immune reaction, long-term experiments have to performed. It has to be tested whether one single ectoine application is sufficient to reduce the accumulation of eosinophils in the lung or whether repetitive treatments are necessary.

In humans different immunological phenotypes of asthma are described. Besides asthma which is characterised by eosinophilic granulocytes, neutrophilic asthma as probably environmentally induced disease is observed [18]. Like COPD, this disease is dominated by a stable chronic neutrophilic lung inflammation which often is not sensitive to the treatment with glucocorticoids [19]. Together with our earlier studies, which demonstrate an effect of ectoine on neutrophils in vivo and ex vivo [14], the current data suggest that ectoine might also be efficient in the treatment of neutrophilic asthma and should be tested in this context.

4. Conclusions

From the data presented here, we conclude that ectoine has beneficial effects on the exacerbation of airway immune responses by environmental particulate air pollution. After having revealed deeper insight into the value and mechanisms of ectoine in chronic neutrophilic lung inflammation, the recent data can be considered the first approach to apply this preventive strategy to predisposed persons like asthmatics. Furthermore, the study indicates the mechanistic importance of neutrophilic lung inflammation in the exacerbation of allergic airway diseases.

Conflict of Interests

The authors declare that there is no conflict of interests regarding the publication of this paper.

References

[1] H. S. Koren, "Environmental risk factors in atopic asthma," *International Archives of Allergy and Immunology*, vol. 113, no. 1–3, pp. 65–68, 1997.

[2] V. Morgenstern, A. Zutavern, J. Cyrys et al., "Atopic diseases, allergic sensitization, and exposure to traffic-related air pollution in children," *The American Journal of Respiratory and Critical Care Medicine*, vol. 177, no. 12, pp. 1331–1337, 2008.

[3] S. H. Gavett and H. S. Koren, "The role of particulate matter in exacerbation of atopic asthma," *International Archives of Allergy and Immunology*, vol. 124, no. 1–3, pp. 109–112, 2001.

[4] E. Samoli, P. T. Nastos, A. G. Paliatsos, K. Katsouyanni, and K. N. Priftis, "Acute effects of air pollution on pediatric asthma exacerbation: evidence of association and effect modification," *Environmental Research*, vol. 111, no. 3, pp. 418–424, 2011.

[5] K. Evans, J. S. Halterman, P. K. Hopke, M. Fagnano, and D. Q. Rich, "Increased utrafine particles and carbon monoxide concentrations are associated with asthma exacerbation among urban children," *Environmental Research*, vol. 129, pp. 11–19, 2014.

[6] W. Lin, W. Huang, T. Zhu et al., "Acute respiratory inflammation in children and black carbon in ambient air before and during the 2008 Beijing Olympics," *Environmental Health Perspectives*, vol. 119, no. 10, pp. 1507–1512, 2011.

[7] M. A. Riedl and A. E. Nel, "Importance of oxidative stress in the pathogenesis and treatment of asthma," *Current Opinion in Allergy and Clinical Immunology*, vol. 8, no. 1, pp. 49–56, 2008.

[8] K. Unfried, C. Albrecht, L. Klotz, A. von Mikecz, S. Grether-Beck, and R. P. F. Schins, "Cellular responses to nanoparticles: target structures and mechanisms," *Nanotoxicology*, vol. 1, no. 1, pp. 52–71, 2007.

[9] P. J. Barnes, "Reactive oxygen species and airway inflammation," *Free Radical Biology and Medicine*, vol. 9, no. 3, pp. 235–243, 1990.

[10] F. Alessandrini, H. Schulz, S. Takenaka et al., "Effects of ultrafine carbon particle inhalation on allergic inflammation of the lung," *Journal of Allergy and Clinical Immunology*, vol. 117, no. 4, pp. 824–830, 2006.

[11] F. Alessandrini, I. Beck-Speier, D. Krappmann et al., "Role of oxidative stress in ultrafine particle-induced exacerbation of allergic lung inflammation," *The American Journal of Respiratory and Critical Care Medicine*, vol. 179, no. 11, pp. 984–991, 2009.

[12] U. Sydlik, I. Gallitz, C. Albrecht, J. Abel, J. Krutmann, and K. Unfried, "The compatible solute ectoine protects against nanoparticle-induced neutrophilic lung inflammation," *The American Journal of Respiratory and Critical Care Medicine*, vol. 180, no. 1, pp. 29–35, 2009.

[13] H. Peuschel, U. Sydlik, S. Grether-Beck et al., "Carbon nanoparticles induce ceramide- and lipid raft-dependent signalling in lung epithelial cells: a target for a preventive strategy against environmentally-induced lung inflammation," *Particle and Fibre Toxicology*, vol. 9, article 48, 2012.

[14] U. Sydlik, H. Peuschel, A. Paunel-Görgülü et al., "Recovery of neutrophil apoptosis by ectoine: a new strategy against lung inflammation," *European Respiratory Journal*, vol. 41, no. 2, pp. 433–442, 2013.

[15] M. Rincon and C. G. Irvin, "Role of IL-6 in asthma and other inflammatory pulmonary diseases," *International Journal of Biological Sciences*, vol. 8, no. 9, pp. 1281–1290, 2012.

[16] H. Peuschel, U. Sydlik, J. Haendeler et al., "C-Src-mediated activation of Erk1/2 is a reaction of epithelial cells to carbon nanoparticle treatment and may be a target for a molecular preventive strategy," *Biological Chemistry*, vol. 391, no. 11, pp. 1327–1332, 2010.

[17] I. Beck-Speier, E. Karg, H. Behrendt, T. Stoeger, and F. Alessandrini, "Ultrafine particles affect the balance of endogenous pro- and anti-inflammatory lipid mediators in the lung: in-vitro and in-vivo studies," *Particle and Fibre Toxicology*, vol. 9, article 27, 2012.

[18] C. L. Ordoñez, T. E. Shaughnessy, M. A. Matthay, and J. V. Fahy, "Increased neutrophil numbers and IL-8 levels in airway secretions in acute severe asthma: clinical and biologic significance," *The American Journal of Respiratory and Critical Care Medicine*, vol. 161, no. 4, pp. 1185–1190, 2000.

[19] S. E. Wenzel, "Asthma: defining of the persistent adult phenotypes," *The Lancet*, vol. 368, no. 9537, pp. 804–813, 2006.

20

The Effectiveness of Acupuncture Compared to Loratadine in Patients Allergic to House Dust Mites

Bettina Hauswald,[1] **Christina Dill,**[1] **Jürgen Boxberger,**[1] **Eberhard Kuhlisch,**[2] **Thomas Zahnert,**[1] **and Yury M. Yarin**[1]

[1] *Clinic of Otorhinolaryngology, Department of Medicine, University Hospital Dresden, Fetscherstraße 74, 01307 Dresden, Germany*
[2] *Institute for Medical Informatics and Biometry, Department of Medicine, University Hospital Dresden, Fetscherstraße 74, 01307 Dresden, Germany*

Correspondence should be addressed to Yury M. Yarin; yury.yarin@uniklinikum-dresden.de

Academic Editor: Ralph Mösges

Background. The aim of this work was to evaluate the clinical effectiveness of acupuncture and its impact on the immune system in comparison to loratadine in the treatment of persistent allergic rhinitis caused by house dust mites. *Methods*. In this study, 24 patients suffering from persistent allergic rhinitis induced by house dust mites were treated either with acupuncture ($n = 15$) or with loratadine ($n = 9$). The evaluation of the data was based on the subjective and the objective rhinoconjunctivitis symptom scores, specific and total IgE, and interleukins (IL-4, IL-10, and IFN-γ) as markers for the activity of Th1 or Th2 cells. *Results*. The treatments with acupuncture as well as with loratadine were considered effective in the patients' subjective assessment, whereby the effect of the acupuncture tended to be assessed as more persistent after the end of treatment. A change in the specific or the total IgE was not detectable in either group. The interleukin profile showed the tendency of an increasing IL-10 value in the acupuncture group. The results of the study show that the effectiveness of acupuncture is comparable to that of loratadine. *Conclusion*. Acupuncture is a clinically effective form of therapy in the treatment of patients suffering from persistent allergic rhinitis. The results indicate the probability of an immunomodulatory effect.

1. Introduction

With a prevalence of 20 to 30%, allergic rhinitis is one of the most frequent atopic diseases in Western Europe [1–3]. It leads to a decrease of the patients' quality of life [4] and causes great cost for medication and social benefits [5].

House dust mites, namely, *Dermatophagoides pteronyssinus* and *D. farinae*, are two of the most common persistent allergens. In 30% of all house dust mite allergies, a development of allergic bronchial asthma with coexisting nasal symptoms is expected. Especially in patients suffering from untreated allergic rhinitis, an exacerbation usually follows 5–15 years after the first occurrence of nasal symptoms [6].

Traditional Chinese medicine (TCM), of which acupuncture is a part, gains in importance as an addition to conventional therapies. According to a report of the World Health Organization of 2002 [7] and to clinical studies [8], acupuncture is ranked among the sufficient methods for the treatment of allergic rhinitis and further allergic diseases such as bronchial asthma [9, 10]. Despite the conventional forms of therapy, 64% of patients suffering from persistent allergic rhinitis (PER) desire acupuncture as an alternative form of therapy [11]. Two of the latest multicentre and randomised trials found evidence for a significant improvement of symptoms and the quality of life through acupuncture in patients with allergic rhinitis [1, 12].

Acupuncture, which is described as immunomodulatory therapy [13, 14], has already been examined for its effect and tested for cellular [15] and humoral [10] components of the immune system. In the last decade, numerous findings concerning the key role of CD4+ cells were made. Depending on the subtype, very different cytokines are produced. These can be regarded as prospective markers for the effectiveness of the therapy. Th1 cells mainly express the cytokine interleukin-2

(IL-2) and interferon- (IFN-)γ, which cause a cellular immune response, while Th2 cells release interleukins (IL) 4, 5, 10, and 13, which control the maturation of B lymphocytes to cells producing antibodies and their total IgE [16–19].

Examinations show that IL-10 can be considered as markers in the course of the therapy [20]. In several studies on bronchial asthma [10, 21, 22] and allergic rhinitis [23–25], it was possible to show in animal testing as well as in patients that the cytokine profile of IL-10 can be modulated through acupuncture. At the same time, an improvement of the symptoms could be observed. Only fragmentary data are available on the effect of acupuncture on interleukins 4 (IL-4) and 5 (IL-5) and INF-γ which are involved in the Th1/Th2 equilibrium [10, 24].

It was the objective of this investigation to prove the effectiveness of acupuncture in the treatment of PER by comparing it with the effectiveness of antihistaminic loratadine as well as to gain a better understanding of the mechanisms of action of acupuncture through the examination of the interleukin profile.

2. Material and Methods

Patients in the outpatient department for allergy of the ENT clinic in Dresden suffering from PER were included in this study if a house dust mite allergy was ascertained by means of specific symptoms, skin prick test, and the assessment of the allergen specific IgE. With regard to the skin prick test (Allergopharma Joachim Ganzer KG, Reinbek), a sensitisation to *Dermatophagoides pteronyssinus* or *D. farinae* was then given if the diameter of the wheal measured $\geq$3 mm after 20 minutes [4]. The CAP-FEIA system of Pharmacia & Upjohn Diagnostics AB, Uppsala, Sweden, was used for the allergological in vitro diagnostics for the determination of the total and the specific IgE. A total IgE of more than 100 kU/L as well as a specific IgE of more than 0.70 kU/L (CAP class 2) [5, 26, 27] was used to verify a sensitisation.

The cytokine profile was examined through the interleukins 4 (IL-4) and 10 (IL-10) and IFN-γ using the ELISA technique by Quantikine Immunoassay, Firma R&D Systems, Wiesbaden-Nordenstadt, Germany.

Exclusion criteria were pregnancy, continuous immunotherapy, other therapies influencing the immune system like glucocorticoids or chemotherapeutics, or the use of additional antiallergic medication.

2.1. Study Design. This study included 30 patients. The data of 24 patients could be collected fully until the end of the study and were evaluated accordingly (acupuncture group: $n = 15$ and loratadine group: $n = 9$). The average age of the patients was 16.5 ± 9.8 years. The mean duration of the disease was 7.8 ± 6.1 years. Table 1 shows the mean age of both treatment groups.

2.2. Therapy Groups. The patients were randomly assigned to the different treatment groups. Patients being treated with acupuncture received twelve acupuncture sessions in total, two sessions a week, using the same acupuncture points for every patient. Sterile, disposable needles made of stainless

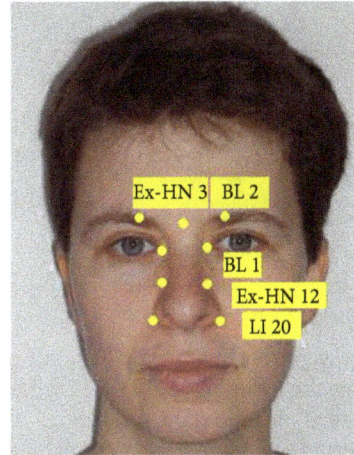

FIGURE 1: Standardised point chart for facial acupuncture.

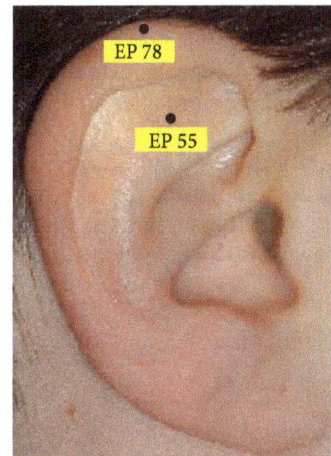

FIGURE 2: Standardised point chart for ear acupuncture.

TABLE 1: Demographic structure.

	Acupuncture $n = 15$	Loratadine $n = 9$
Male/female	9/6	3/6
Age (years)	28.1 (±9.9)	24.9 (±9.6)
Duration of disease (years)	7.3 (±6.7)	8.6 (±5.1)

Demographic data: illustration of gender, age, and duration of disease (mean values ± standard deviations) within the groups; n: number of patients.

steel (Seirin, Dreieich/Germany) were used for body (0.3 × 0.3 mm in strength) and for face and ear acupuncture (0.2 × 0.15 mm in strength).

To allow for standardisation and comparability, all patients were acupunctured at the same points which were chosen in accordance with the rules of TCM. Needles were inserted unilaterally or bilaterally at the following points: LI 20, Ex-HN 12, Ex-HN 3, BL 1, BL 2, LI 4, LI 11, ear pont 78, and ear point 55 (Figures 1, 2, and 3). In addition, all patients werde acupuntured at LU 20, GB 20, SI 3, and ST 36 (not shown).

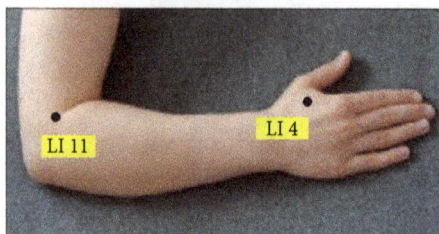

FIGURE 3: Standardised point chart for "extraordinary" points on the forearm.

The needles were kept in place for 20 minutes. All patients were treated by the same physician throughout the whole study in order to allow for a standardisation.

Patients treated with loratadine took 10 mg of loratadine (Lisino, Essex Pharma GmbH) in the morning of each day over the treatment period of 21 days.

2.3. Course of the Study. The patients were examined three times during this study. The first examination took place before the treatment (t_1), the second at the day after the end of treatment (t_2), and the third after an interval of 10 weeks without therapy (t_3).

At all three points, the clinical examination included anterior rhinoscopy, an estimation of the current nasal symptoms by use of the symptom score, and a blood sample (one tube for heparinised whole blood and one for serum each time).

2.4. Symptom Scores. All symptom scores were recorded on a 5-point scale (FPS).

2.4.1. Objective Symptom Scores. For the anterior rhinoscopy, the condition of the mucosa and the size of the nasal concha were recorded by the physician. Mucosal reddening and swelling of the inferior nasal concha were rated in the following score: 0 = normal, 1 = slightly changed, 2 = moderately changed, 3 = severely changed, and 4 = most severely changed.

2.4.2. Subjective Symptom Scores. While the objective nasal symptoms and findings were recorded three times in the course of the study, subjective symptoms (complaints) were determined retrospectively in the form of patient interviews. Nasal obstruction and secretion were evaluated using the following scale: 0 = free of symptoms, 1 = slight but noticeable symptoms, not interfering with daily activities, 2 = moderate symptoms, hardly interfering with daily activities and sleep, 3 = severe symptoms, clearly interfering with daily activities and sleep, and 4 = most severe symptoms, substantially interfering with daily activities and sleep.

The assessment of sneezing attacks was classified into 3 categories: 0 = no sneezing attacks, 1 = rare sneezing attacks, 1-2 sneezing attacks per day, and 2 = frequent sneezing attacks with more than 3 attacks per day.

2.4.3. Total Symptom Score. All symptom scores were summed up to a total symptom score in order to elucidate the therapeutic effect.

2.5. Subjective Estimation of the Therapeutic Effect. At examinations t_2 and t_3, the subjective state of health was evaluated by comparing the afflictions prior to the therapy with the current ones (1 = improved and 2 = unchanged or worsened).

2.6. Statistics. The data collected were evaluated using the statistical software SPSS Version 21 for Microsoft Windows. The results were given in form of mean ± standard deviation or standard error of the mean. The study was planned as repeated measures design and consequently evaluated by means of an analysis of variance. A significance level of $P < 0.005$ was considered statistically significant.

3. Results

In the acupuncture group, 87% of the patients reported an improvement of their afflictions at the end of therapy (t_1). 13% did not notice a change at all at t_2 and still not at t_3, 10 weeks after the end of therapy. At t_3, 20% did not notice a change in comparison to the beginning of therapy (t_1) anymore. In the loratadine group, 67% of the patients stated an improvement at t_2, while 33% did not detect an improvement. At t_3 none of the patients treated with loratadine noticed an improvement in comparison to t_1 (see Figure 4).

3.1. Total Sum Score. Looking at the subjective and objective symptoms separately, there is no significant difference noticeable, neither in the course of the therapy nor between the groups. The total sum score, however, showed significant changes in the time course of the therapy. Both in the acupuncture and the loratadine group, a significant improvement was gained under therapy. In the ten-week period following the therapy, a significant deterioration which led to the recurrence of the allergic symptoms was shown in the loratadine group, while the significant improvement of the symptoms persisted in the acupuncture group (multivariate tests $P < 0.005$). Comparing both groups, no significance was ascertainable (see Figure 5).

3.2. Allergic Parameter (Total IgE; Specific IgE Dermatophagoides pteronyssinus/D. farinae). Neither the acupuncture nor the loratadine group showed a significant difference in the specific IgE or the total IgE.

3.3. Interleukin Profile (IL-4 and IFN-γ). The intermediate IL-4 level in the acupuncture group slightly increased during therapy, between t_1 and t_2, from 0.182 pg/mL to 0.185 pg/mL. It then decreased to 0.177 pg/mL during the period without treatment, between t_2 and t_3. Contrarily, in the loratadine group, the IL-4 level already decreased during therapy from 0.13 pg/mL (t_1) to 0.112 (t_2) and increased then to 0.126 pg/mL s (t_3).

In the acupuncture group, the serum level of IFN-γ increased between t_1 and t_2 from 4.799 pg/mL to 5.844 pg/mL and decreased between t_2 and t_3 to 4.399 pg/mL. The intermediate IFN-γ level of the loratadine group showed a similar course. After the increase from 5.186 pg/mL to 5.664 pg/mL at the beginning of therapy, the IFN-γ serum level decreased to 5.504 pg/mL (t_3).

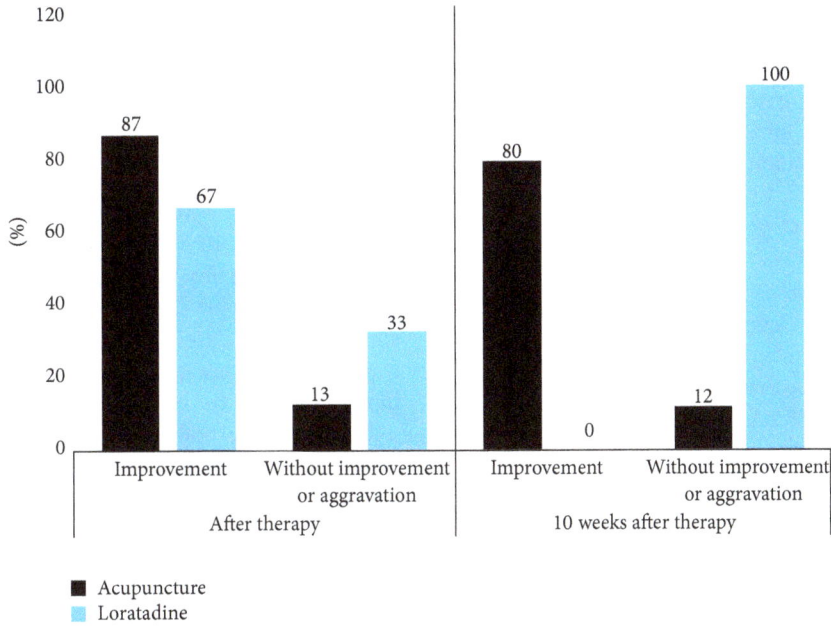

FIGURE 4: Subjective evaluation of rhinitis symptoms on the day after the end of therapy and after the 10-week therapy-free interval in comparison to the state of health immediately before the beginning of therapy (percentage frequencies in relation to the total patient numbers within the treatment groups).

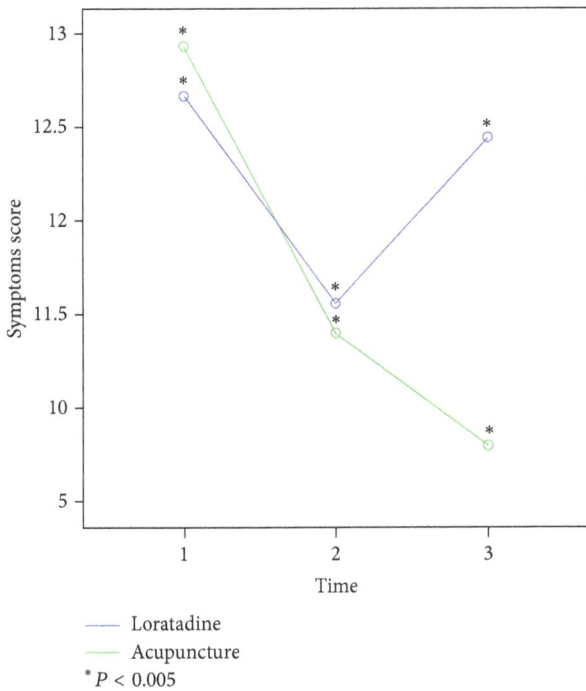

FIGURE 5: Change in the total symptom scores in both groups during the study period.

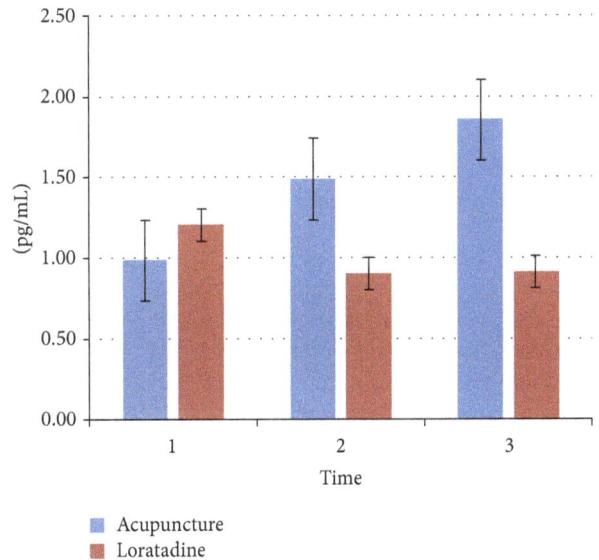

FIGURE 6: Change in interleukin-10 level in serum; mean values ± standard mean of error at the three examination times.

None of the observed differences of the IL-4 and IFN-γ were significant.

3.4. Interleukin Profile IL-10. For the IL-10 serum level, an increase from 1.001 pg/mL (t_1) to 1.49 pg/mL (t_2) was observed in the acupuncture group. Also, after the end of therapy, an increase to 1.857 pg/mL (t_3) was shown. In the loratadine group, the IL-10 also increased from 1.84 pg/mL (t_1) to 2.013 pg/mL (t_2) but decreased after the end of treatment to 1.909 pg/mL (t_1).

Even though the increase of the IL-10 serum level was not significant, it showed a distinct tendency to increase in the partial eta squared values (Figure 6).

4. Discussion

In order to prove that acupuncture can serve as complementary form of therapy in the treatment of PER, its effectiveness was compared to that of loratadine. It was also examined whether acupuncture has a long-term effect beyond the end of the treatment period. Furthermore, the theory according to which the therapy effect of acupuncture is based on an immunomodulatory effect was checked.

The role of IL-10 in the pathogenesis of allergic diseases during treatment and its level changes in the serum are currently the subject of controversial discussion [20]. It was shown that the IL-10 is able to obstruct the histamine release of activated mast cells [28]. In addition, an increased IL-10 level in the nasal mucosa led to a definite reduction of nasal allergy symptoms of patients with dust mite allergy after nasal provocation [29]. Thus, the IL-10 level could function as a marker for the effectiveness of antiallergic therapy. Some reasearchers suggest that the interleukin levels, especially that of IL-10, change under acupuncture [10, 21, 24].

In our study, we were likewise able to observe that the IL-10 level tends to increase in the acupuncture group. This observation could be an indication for the immunomodulatory effect of acupuncture. Due to the small number of patients, however, it was not possible to show a significance.

Even though there is information that the level of the other cytokines investigated here, namely, IL-4 and IFN-γ, can change during acupuncture [10, 21, 24], this was not observed in our study, which might be due to the small sample size.

In a number of studies, the effectiveness of acupuncture in regard to quality of life and the reduction of medication as well as significant improvements of the clinical symptoms has already been shown [1, 8, 12, 30, 31]. Even though our results did not show any significant differences of the single symptoms, a significant improvement of the symptoms was observed in the total sum scores in both the acupuncture and loratadine groups during the course of the treatment. This outcome correlates with the patients' subjective assessment of their state of health recorded immediately at the end of treatment. The difference between both groups develops within the 10-week period without treatment, between t_2 and t_3. While the patients in the acupuncture group still experienced improvement in symptoms (a significant improvement in comparison to the beginning of therapy), the symptoms of the loratadine group started to increase again after the end of treatment. Nevertheless, this difference between both groups was not significant.

Modern medicine requires an evidence-based, double-blind, and placebo-controlled study design in order to prove effectiveness. This is, however, hardly applicable for acupuncture studies. Especially blinding and placebo control present an unsolved problem. Theoretically, a blinding would be possible for laser acupuncture but a comparability of the effectiveness of needle acupuncture with laser acupuncture has not yet been proven. A placebo treatment with acupuncture needles founders on the circumstance that the so-called sham acupuncture, where acupuncture needles are inserted in the acupuncture points, can still have a physiological impact or an effect on the immune system. As the skin is related to internal organs and body systems by the principle of segmental innervations [32], it is not possible to exclude an impact of the skin irritation on the examined effect.

In our study, we tried to prove the effectiveness of acupuncture in PER through changes in the interleukin level in the serum. However, parameters depending on interleukin can be strongly influenced by factors such as autoimmune diseases, inflammations, or even the weather. It might be for this reason that no significant changes in the interleukin level in the serum could be found. Furthermore, a larger number of participants are necessary to prove significance of the treatment effects. The small number of patients allows in many cases only a statistical tendency to increase.

Despite these limitations, the results at hand make it possible to conclude that acupuncture itself and the acupuncture points used are effective in the treatment of PER. Acupuncture, therefore, presents a suitable alternative for patients with drug intolerance or pregnancy. Further studies with a larger patient collective are necessary to confirm these positive results of the mode of action of acupuncture and to examine the effectiveness of further TCM acupoints.

5. Conclusion

Acupuncture is an effective, well-tolerated form of therapy in the treatment of patients suffering from dust mite allergy with its effect being comparable to loratadine.

Although the theory that the mechanism of action of acupuncture is based on immunomodulation could not be proven significantly, it was possible to show a tendential increase of the IL-10 level in the serum under acupuncture. For a definite assessment of this issue, further studies with larger numbers of patients are necessary.

Acupuncture can function as an effective therapeutic alternative for patients having a contraindication to specific immunotherapy or to a medicinal symptomatic therapy.

Abbreviations

EP: Ear point
PER: Persistent allergic rhinitis
TCM: Traditional Chinese medicine
FPS: Five-point scale.

Consent

The tested subjects were first informed about the studies and their written consents were obtained. The Institutional Review Board considered investigations as safe and in agreement with the principles of the Declaration of Helsinki.

Conflict of Interests

The authors declare that there is no conflict of interests regarding the publication of this paper.

Authors' Contribution

Bettina Hauswald was the principal investigator of the study and contributed to the protocol design together with Christina Dill, Thomas Zahnert, and Yury M. Yarin. Bettina Hauswald and Christina Dill carried out the acupuncture treatment. Yury M. Yarin and Jürgen Boxberger critically revised the paper. Eberhard Kuhlisch performed the statistical analysis under the guidance of Yury M. Yarin. All authors read and approved the final paper.

References

[1] S. M. Choi, J.-E. Park, S.-S. Li et al., "A multicenter, randomized, controlled trial testing the effects of acupuncture on allergic rhinitis," *Allergy: European Journal of Allergy and Clinical Immunology*, vol. 68, no. 3, pp. 365–374, 2013.

[2] R. Mösges and L. Klimek, "Today's allergic rhinitis patients are different: new factors that may play a role," *Allergy: European Journal of Allergy and Clinical Immunology*, vol. 62, no. 9, pp. 969–975, 2007.

[3] V. Bauchau and S. R. Durham, "Prevalence and rate of diagnosis of allergic rhinitis in Europe," *European Respiratory Journal*, vol. 24, no. 5, pp. 758–764, 2004.

[4] J. Bousquet, P. Van Cauwenberge, and N. Khaltaev, "Allergic rhinitis and its impact on asthma," *Journal of Allergy and Clinical Immunology*, vol. 108, no. 5, pp. S147–S334, 2001.

[5] P. Van Cauwenberge, C. Bachert, G. Passalacqua et al., "Consensus statement on the treatment of allergic rhinitis," *Allergy: European Journal of Allergy and Clinical Immunology*, vol. 55, no. 2, pp. 116–134, 2000.

[6] H. P. Zenner, *Allergologie in Der Hals-Nasen-Ohren-Heilkunde*, Springer, Berlin, Germany, 1993.

[7] WHO, *Acupuncture—Review and Analysis of Reports on Controlled Clinical Trials*, WHO, Geneva, Switzerland, 2002.

[8] C. C. Xue, R. English, J. J. Zhang, C. Da Costa, and C. G. Li, "Effect of acupuncture in the treatment of seasonal allergic rhinitis: a randomized controlled clinical trial," *American Journal of Chinese Medicine*, vol. 30, no. 1, pp. 1–11, 2002.

[9] P. A. Christensen, L. C. Laursen, E. Taudorf, S. C. Sørensen, and B. Weeke, "Acupuncture and bronchial asthma," *Allergy: European Journal of Allergy and Clinical Immunology*, vol. 39, no. 5, pp. 379–385, 1984.

[10] S. Joos, C. Schott, H. Zou, V. Daniel, and E. Martin, "Immunomodulatory effects of acupuncture in the treatment of allergic asthma: a randomized controlled study," *Journal of Alternative and Complementary Medicine*, vol. 6, no. 6, pp. 519–525, 2000.

[11] T. Schäfer, A. Riehle, H.-E. Wichmann, and J. Ring, "Alternative medicine in allergies—prevalence, patterns of use, and costs," *Allergy: European Journal of Allergy and Clinical Immunology*, vol. 57, no. 8, pp. 694–700, 2002.

[12] B. Brinkhaus, M. Ortiz, C. M. Witt et al., "Acupuncture in patients with seasonal allergic rhinitis a randomized trial," *Annals of Internal Medicine*, vol. 158, no. 4, pp. 225–234, 2013.

[13] O. Mastalier, "Möglichkeiten der Akupunktur zur Stimulation des Immunsystems," *Aga Khan University*, vol. 21, pp. 19–28, 1993.

[14] W. Stör, "Immunmodulierende wirkung der akupunktur," *Aga Khan University*, vol. 22, no. 3, pp. 188–193, 1994.

[15] T. Lundeberg, S. V. Eriksson, and E. Theodorsson, "Neuroimmunomodulatory effects of acupuncture in mice," *Neuroscience Letters*, vol. 128, no. 2, pp. 161–164, 1991.

[16] F. Annunziato and S. Romagnani, "Heterogeneity of human effector CD4$^+$ T cells," *Arthritis Research and Therapy*, vol. 11, no. 6, article 257, 2009.

[17] J. A. Woodfolk, "Cytokines as a therapeutic target for allergic diseases: a complex picture," *Current Pharmaceutical Design*, vol. 12, no. 19, pp. 2349–2363, 2006.

[18] J. A. Woodfolk, "T-cell responses to allergens," *Journal of Allergy and Clinical Immunology*, vol. 119, no. 2, pp. 280–294, 2007.

[19] A. Cutler and F. Brombacher, "Cytokine therapy," *Annals of the New York Academy of Sciences*, vol. 1056, pp. 16–29, 2005.

[20] J. A. Woodfolk, "Selective roles and dysregulation of interleukin-10 in allergic disease," *Current Allergy and Asthma Reports*, vol. 6, no. 1, pp. 40–46, 2006.

[21] E. R. Carneiro, R. A. N. Xavier, M. A. P. D. Castro, C. M. O. D. Nascimento, and V. L. F. Silveira, "Electroacupuncture promotes a decrease in inflammatory response associated with Th1/Th2 cytokines, nitric oxide and leukotriene B4 modulation in experimental asthma," *Cytokine*, vol. 50, no. 3, pp. 335–340, 2010.

[22] H.-J. Jeong, B.-S. Kim, J. G. Oh, K.-S. Kim, and H.-M. Kim, "Regulatory effect of cytokine production in asthma patients by SOOJI CHIM," *Immunopharmacology and Immunotoxicology*, vol. 24, no. 2, pp. 265–274, 2002.

[23] B. Hauswald, C. H. Schmidt, J. Knothe, K. B. Hüttenbrink, and T. H. Zahnert, "Effects of acupuncture in treatment of perennial allergic rhinitis in comparison to antihistaminic medication," *Deutsche Zeitschrift für Akupunktur*, vol. 52, no. 3, p. 31, 2009.

[24] F. B. Petti, A. Liguori, and F. Ippoliti, "Study on cytokines IL-2, IL-6, IL-10 in patients of chronic allergic rhinitis treated with acupuncture," *Journal of Traditional Chinese Medicine*, vol. 22, no. 2, pp. 104–111, 2002.

[25] Y. Q. Rao and N. Y. Han, "Therapeutic effect of acupuncture on allergic rhinitis and its effects on immunologic function," *Chinese Acupuncture & Moxibustion*, vol. 26, no. 8, pp. 557–560, 2006.

[26] L. Klimek, J. Saloga, W. Mann, and J. Knop, *Allergische Rhinitis—Einführung in Diagnostik Und Therapie*, Schattauer, Stuttgart, Germany, 1998.

[27] V. L. Lund, D. Aaronson, J. Bousquet et al., "International consensus report on the diagnosis and management of rhinitis," *Allergy: European Journal of Allergy and Clinical Immunology, Supplement*, vol. 49, no. 19, pp. 1–34, 1994.

[28] B. Royer, S. Varadaradjalou, P. Saas, J. J. Guillosson, J. P. Kantelip, and M. Arock, "Inhibition of IgE-induced activation of human mast cells by IL-10," *Clinical and Experimental Allergy*, vol. 31, no. 5, pp. 694–704, 2001.

[29] B. Muller, E. J. J. De Groot, I. J. M. Kortekaas, W. J. Fokkens, and C. M. Van Drunen, "Nasal endothelial interleukin-10 expression is negatively correlated with nasal symptoms after allergen provocation," *Allergy: European Journal of Allergy and Clinical Immunology*, vol. 64, no. 5, pp. 738–745, 2009.

[30] B. Hauswald and H. Langer, "Akupunktur und Laserpunktur bei Rhinopathia pollinosa—ergebnisse einer klinisch kontrollierten Studie," *Akupunktur-Theorie Und Praxis*, vol. 17, pp. 14–21, 1989.

[31] H. Langer and B. Hauswald, "Langzeitstudie über die Therapie der Rhinitis pollinosa mittels Akupunktur beziehungsweise Laserakupunktur," *Erfahrungsheilkunde*, vol. 4, pp. 262–267, 1992.

[32] H. Head, *Die Sensibilitätsstörungen Der Haut Bei Viszeralerkrankungen*, Verlag Hirschwald, Berlin, Germany, 1898.

21

Growth Parameters Impairment in Patients with Food Allergies

Larissa Carvalho Costa, Erica Rodrigues Rezende, and Gesmar Rodrigues Silva Segundo

Pediatrics Department, Federal University of Uberlândia, Campus Umuarama, Avenida Para 1720, 38400-920 Uberlândia, MG, Brazil

Correspondence should be addressed to Gesmar Rodrigues Silva Segundo; gesmar@bol.com.br

Academic Editor: Ting Fan Leung

Background and Aims. Food allergy (FA) is a common disease that is rapidly increasing in prevalence for reasons that remain unknown. *Objective.* The aim of this study was to analyze the clinical characteristics and anthropometric data of patients with food allergies followed in a tertiary centre of allergy and immunology. *Methods.* A retrospective study was performed that assessed the data records of patients with food allergy diagnosis, covering a period from February 2009 to February 2012. *Results.* 354 patients were evaluated in the period; 228 (69.1%) patients had a confirmed FA diagnosis. The z-scores for weight-for-age, height-for-age, and body mass indices-for-age showed lower significant values in the FA group compared with the non-FA group by Mann-Whitney test, with significance values of $P = 0.0005$, $P = 0.0030$, and $P = 0.0066$, respectively. There were no statistical differences in sex, gestational age, birth type, breastfeeding period, and age of introduction of complementary formulas based on cow milk protein between groups. *Conclusion.* FA patients had a lower growth rate in comparison with patients without FA. The early recognition of food allergies with the establishment of protein-implicated diet exclusion, in association with an adequate nutrient replenishment, is important to reduce the nutritional impact of food allergies.

1. Introduction

Food allergy (FA) is a common disease that is rapidly increasing in prevalence for reasons that remain unknown. Recent estimates suggest that around 17 million people in Europe suffer from allergies triggered by foods such as milk, eggs, peanuts, tree nuts, or seafood, and an increasing number are seeking treatment through primary care and hospital emergency departments [1]. A recent national survey of allergies in the United States showed an increase in the prevalence of food allergies from 3.4% in 1997–1999 to 5.1% in 2009–2011 [2].

FA can have a significant effect on an individual's quality of life and physical functioning and can also be costly in terms of medical visits and treatments [1]. Food allergies manifest various symptoms in the skin, gastrointestinal tract, and airways as a result of adverse responses to a food protein via IgE-mediated or non-IgE-mediated immune mechanisms.

Allergic responses to food present as inflammation due to cellular responses activated against the food allergen [3].

There is a lack of information on the role of nutrition versus only food avoidance in the management and natural history of food allergy. Little information is also known about the effect of a nutrition consultation in this process. Furthermore, the role of the dietician and the diagnostic and therapeutic value of the elimination diet has not been established and extensively investigated [4].

The aim of the present study is analyze the clinical characteristics and nutritional status of patients with food allergies followed in a tertiary centre of allergy and immunology.

2. Methods

This was a retrospective study that assessed the data records of patients who were evaluated in the food allergy out-patient clinic of the Clinical Hospital of Federal University of Uberlandia, between February 2009 and February 2012.

Data from age, sex, gestational age, delivery birth type, breastfeeding period, age of introduction of complementary formulas based on cow milk protein, anthropometric parameters, and foods implicated in allergies were obtained from the patient records.

The diagnosis routine of food allergy was performed based on the history and laboratory tests (specific IgE, skin prick test). Since there are no effective laboratory methods for the diagnosis of non-IgE-mediated FA, suspected in patients with symptoms suggestive of proctocolitis and enterocolitis, or in patients with diagnosis of eosinophilic esophagitis and atopic dermatitis moderate to severe, an elimination diet without a suspected allergenic protein and subsequent oral food challenge, which was open for children younger than 3 years and double-blind for children above 3 years, was used for diagnosis [5, 6].

The anthropometric data of patients seen for the first time was evaluated according to z-scores for weight-for-age, height-for-age, and body mass index (BMI). WHO-Antro software version 3.2.2, January 2011, available from (http://www.who.int/childgrowth/software/en/) was used to calculate z-scores and the World Health Organization growth charts were used as reference values [7].

The Kolmogorov-Smirnov test was used to determine whether variables were normally distributed. For continuous variables, groups were compared using the Mann-Whitney test. The Fisher exact test and Chi-square for trend were used for categorical variables. The level of significance for all statistical tests was 2-sided, $P < 0.05$. All analyses were conducted using Graph Pad Prism 5.0 (La Jolla, California, USA). The study was approved by the Human Research Ethics Committee of Federal University of Uberlandia.

3. Results

In the period studied, the medical files showed that 389 different patients were evaluated in the out-patient clinic of food allergy. Of these, 35 patients did not undergo any consultation or medical records did not present data regarding the query. Among the 354 patients that were evaluated by physicians in our unit, 228 (69.1%) had a confirmed diagnosis of food allergy, while the diagnosis of food allergy was excluded in the remaining 126 (30.9%).

The median age of patients with an FA diagnosis was 10 months (1–193 months) while the group without FA was 36.5 months (1–216 months). There was a significant difference between the ages of the groups ($P < 0.0001$ by Mann-Whitney test). There were no statistical differences in sex, gestational age, birth type, breastfeeding period, and age of introduction of complementary formulas based on cow milk protein, as shown in Table 1.

The most frequent symptoms in patients with food allergy were nausea and vomiting in 118 (51.7%), abdominal pain in 104 (45.6%), diarrhea in 73 (32.0%), fresh rectal bleeding in 71 (31.1%), failure to thrive in 55 (24.1%), urticaria in 50 (21.9%), constipation in 19 (8.3%), dysphagia in 8 (3.5%), and

food aversion in 8 (3.5%). The diagnosis of non-IgE-mediated allergy was performed in 168 (73.68%), while the diagnosis of IgE-mediated food allergy was performed in 75 (32.89%). The diagnosis of mixed IgE and non-IgE-mediated food allergy was done in 15 (6.57%). The foods implicated in food allergies are presented in Table 2.

The z-scores for weight-for-age, height-for-age, and body mass indices- (BMI-) for-age showed less significant values in the FA group compared with the non-FA group by Mann-Whitney test, with values of $P = 0.0005$, $P = 0.0030$, and $P = 0.0066$, respectively (Table 1).

Indeed, 18.4% presented with a low weight-for-age z-score (<-2.0 standard deviation (SD)), 15.9% with a low height-for-age z-score (<-2.0 SD), and 15.4% with a low BMI-for-age z-score (<-2.0 SD). A significant difference in low levels (<-2.0 SD) by Fisher exact test was found between the FA and non-FA groups only in height-for-age z-score ($P = 0.0189$), although the weight-for-age z-score analysis showed a P value that was close to significance ($P = 0.0549$). When we separated the groups with z-score less than -2 and up, there is no difference relative to the numbers of implicated food allergens. In BMI-for-age z-score less than -2, 16 (51.61%) of patients had one food allergy, 9 (29.03%) had two foods involved, and 6 (19.36%) had three or more foods, while in group with z-scores up -2, 117 (59.40%) had one food implicated, 36 (18.28%) had two foods, and 44 (22.32%) had three or more foods.

Figure 1 represents the comparison between z-scores of food allergy patients and a reference curve of growth in childhood. Food allergy patient curve is lower and presents a left variation in evaluation with reference to the three parameters (weight-for-age, height-for-age, and BMI-for-age) demonstrating the impairment in growth parameters.

4. Discussion

The incidence and prevalence of food allergies are believed to be increasing in several countries. Dietary antigens induce a local hypersensitivity reaction impairing the intestine's barrier function, leading to the continuation of inflammation. The consequences of inflammatory responses may be severe and manifest as impaired growth, increased symptoms, and poor quality of life [4].

We did not find an association between sex, gestational age, delivery birth type, breastfeeding period, and age of introduction of complementary formulas based on cow milk protein with the development of FA. However, the number of medical records without any analyzed data was a limiting factor in data analysis. Approximately one-third of the patients did not have the studied data clearly outlined in their medical report, indicating that it is important to improve the completion of data in documents.

In the present study, cow's milk protein was responsible for FA in more than 90% of patients with non-IgE-mediated disease and more than 78% in patients with an IgE-mediated mechanism. Similarly to other studies, besides cow's milk, the foods most commonly implicated with allergy in infants were hen's eggs, soy, and wheat. In contrast to that found in

TABLE 1: Data from patients evaluated in food allergy out-patient clinic from Clinical Hospital of Federal University of Uberlandia, Brazil.

Data	Groups		P value
	Food allergy (*n*: 228)	Nonfood allergy (*n*: 126)	
Age (median in months)	10	36.5	<0.0001*
Sex—male (%)	120 (52.63)	75 (59.53)	0.5067**
Birth delivery—*n* (%)			
Vaginal	24 (10.53)	13 (10.32)	
Cesarean	128 (56.14)	59 (46.82)	0.1882***
ND	76 (33.33)	54 (42.86)	
Gestational age—*n* (%)			
Preterm	36 (15.79)	13 (10.32)	
Term	87 (38.16)	50 (39.68)	0.2235***
Postterm	1 (0.44)	0 (0.00)	
ND	104 (45.61)	63 (50.00)	
Breastfeeding—*n* (%)			
No breastfeed	37 (16.23)	9 (7.14)	
<1 month	54 (23.68)	25 (19.84)	
1–6 months	92 (40.35)	34 (26.98)	0.5363***
>6 months	3 (1.32)	2 (1.59)	
Only breastfeed	1 (0.44)	1 (0.80)	
ND	41 (17.98)	55 (43.65)	
Onset use of complementary formulas—*n* (%)			
<1 month	81 (35.53)	24 (19.04)	
1–6 months	73 (32.02)	23 (18.25)	
6–12 months	20 (8.77)	7 (5.56)	0.1154***
>12 months	2 (0.88)	0 (0.00)	
No use	8 (3.51)	7 (5.56)	
ND	44 (19.29)	65 (51.59)	
z-score weight × age			
Median (interval)	−0.95 (−5.30–2.25)	−0.30 (−4.77–4.80)	0.0005*
z-score height × age			
Median (interval)	−0.41 (−5.04–2.81)	−0.01 (−4.78–2.55)	0.0030*
z-score BMI × age			
Median (interval)	−0.85 (−6.20–3.59)	−0.33 (−3.06–6.55)	0.0053*

*Mann-Whitney test.
**Fisher's exact test.
***Chi-square test for trend.
BMI: body mass indices.

TABLE 2: Food implicate with Non-IgE- and IgE-mediated food allergens in patients evaluated in food allergy out-patient clinic from Clinical Hospital of Federal University of Uberlandia, Brazil.

Food implicate	Allergy type		Total (*n*: 228)
	Non-IgE-mediated (*n*: 168)	IgE-mediated (*n*: 75)	
Cow's milk	152 (90.48%)	59 (78.67%)	211 (92.54%)
Hen's egg	23 (13.69%)	38 (50.67%)	61 (26.75%)
Soy	29 (17.26%)	13 (17.33%)	42 (18.42%)
Wheat	19 (11.31%)	10 (13.33%)	29 (12.72%)
Corn	23 (13.69)	8 (10.67%)	31 (13.59%)
Chicken	4 (2.38%)	2 (2.67%)	6 (2.63%)
Beef	3 (1.78%)	2 (2.67%)	5 (2.19%)
Pork	2 (1.19%)	2 (2.67%)	4 (1.75%)
Fish	2 (1.19%)	—	2 (0.88%)
Other foods	11 (6.55%)	6 (8.00%)	17 (7.46%)

(a) Weight-for-age

(b) Length/height-for-age

(c) BMI-for-age

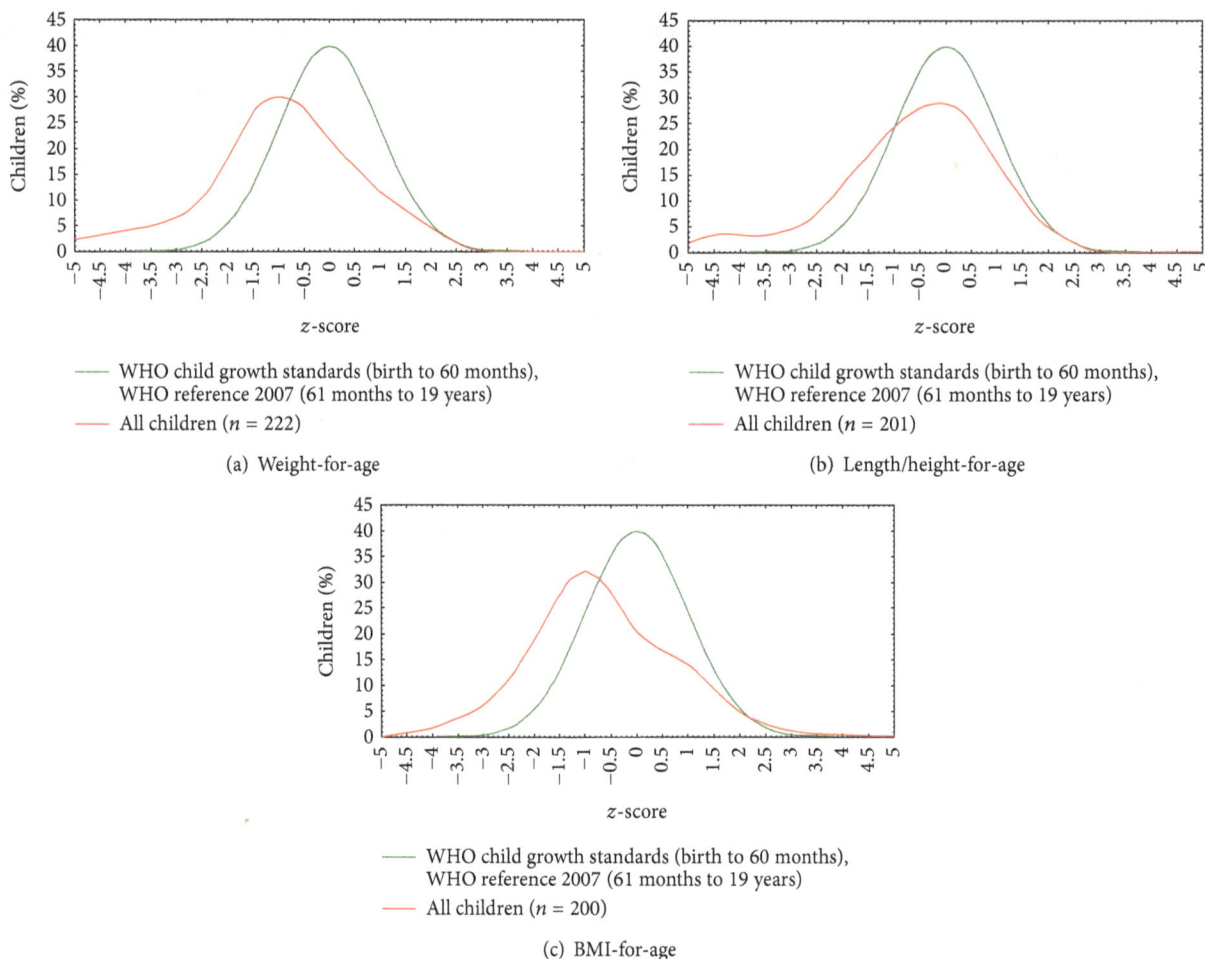

FIGURE 1: Comparison between z-scores reference curve from World Health Organization and patients with food allergy evaluated in the food allergy out-patient clinic from Clinical Hospital of Federal University of Uberlandia, Brazil. (a) Weight-for-age, (b) length/height-for-age, and (c) BMI- (body mass index-) for-age.

other studies, allergy to corn protein was found in 13.59% of patients, demonstrating a peculiarity of this region where there is intense corn consumption due to cultural factors. Several patients had more than one food sensitization.

One study performed in Brazil and focused on infants with cow milk allergies showed that, among the 159 patients seen at first evaluation, 15.1% presented with a low weight-for-age z-score (<-2.0 SD), 8.7% with a low weight-for-height z-score (<-2.0 SD), and 23.9% with a low height-for-age z-score (<-2.0 SD) [8]. We also found similar data in the present study, as shown in the Results section. Another study conducted on 99 patients with food allergies showed that patients with a milk allergy or multiple food allergies are at greater risk of developing growth problems or inadequate nutrient intake.

In the present study, the control group was filled by patients that looked for the out-patient clinic with FA suspicion; then it is possible that patients could have another clinical disorder that affected their growth data and express less significant differences between FA and control group. Because of that, the comparative evaluation with WHO growth reference curves is important. The curves showed

a clear impact in growth data found in FA group in all scores in comparison with reference values.

More than 25% of children in both groups consumed less than 67% of the dietary reference intakes for calcium, vitamin D, and vitamin E [9]. According to previous data, the present study showed lower z-scores in FA patients related to non-FA patients, suggesting difficulties in receiving adequate nutrient intake when a necessity to avoid specific proteins exists. This difficulty in establishing a diet and the presence of levels of z-score less than -2 apparently were related with absence of medical and nutritional information, once there are no significant correlation with number of the implicated foods in allergy.

We also believe that the presence of non-IgE-mediated FA promotes intestinal inflammation that can lead to difficulties in the absorption of other nutrients, which justifies the meeting of nutritional changes or even the admission of patients to hospital. These difficulties in a phase of life where there is a large increase in height and weight probably contributed to the difference in z-scores observed in patients with food allergies [10].

One limitation of this study in respect to nutritional status is the use only of height, weight, and BMI, but these are only data possible in medical charts. Another limitation of this study is the retrospective format. The cohort studies will effectively show more accurate data, but that does not cut the value of the present study.

In conclusion, FA patients had a lower growth rate in comparison with patients without FA. The early recognition of food allergies with the establishment of a diet excluding the implicated protein, in association with an adequate nutrient replenishment, is important to reduce the nutritional impact of food allergies.

Ethical Approval

The study was approved by the Human Research Ethics Committee of Federal University of Uberlandia (Institutional Review Board).

Conflict of Interests

The authors declare that there is no conflict of interests regarding the publication of this paper.

Acknowledgments

Thanks are due to all physicians, nutritionists, and patients of food allergy out-patient clinic, who made it possible to perform this study.

References

[1] European Academy of Allergy and Clinical Immunology, *17 Million Europeans Allergic to Food; Allergies in Children Doubled in the Last 10 Years*, EAACI, Zurich, Switzerland, 2011.

[2] K. D. Jackson, L. D. Howie, and L. J. Akinbami, "Trends in allergic conditions among children: United States, 1997–2011," *NCHS Data Brief*, no. 121, pp. 1–8, 2013.

[3] H.-N. Cho, S. Hong, S.-H. Lee, and H.-Y. Yum, "Nutritional status according to sensitized food allergens in children with atopic dermatitis," *Allergy, Asthma and Immunology Research*, vol. 3, no. 1, pp. 53–57, 2011.

[4] C. Venter, K. Laitinen, and B. Vlieg-Boerstra, "Nutritional aspects in diagnosis and management of food hypersensitivity-the dietitians role," *Journal of Allergy*, vol. 2012, Article ID 269376, 11 pages, 2012.

[5] H. A. Sampson, R. Gerth van Wijk, C. Bindslev-Jensen et al., "Standardizing double-blind, placebo-controlled oral food challenges: American Academy of Allergy, Asthma & Immunology-European Academy of Allergy and Clinical Immunology PRACTALL consensus report," *The Journal of Allergy and Clinical Immunology*, vol. 130, no. 6, pp. 1260–1274, 2012.

[6] E. R. Rezende, C. P. Barros, L. H. Ynoue, A. T. Santos, R. M. Pinto, and G. R. Segundo, "Clinical characteristics and sensitivity to food and inhalants among children with eosinophilic esophagitis," *BMC Research Notes*, vol. 7, article 47, 2014.

[7] World Health Organization, *Physical Status: The Use and Interpretation of Anthropometry*, Technical Report Series no. 854, WHO, Geneve, Switzerland, 1995.

[8] M. C. Vieira, M. B. Morais, J. V. N. Spolidoro et al., "A survey on clinical presentation and nutritional status of infants with suspected cow's milk allergy," *BMC Pediatrics*, vol. 10, article 25, 2010.

[9] L. Christie, R. J. Hine, J. G. Parker, and W. Burks, "Food allergies in children affect nutrient intake and growth," *Journal of the American Dietetic Association*, vol. 102, no. 11, pp. 1648–1651, 2002.

[10] J. M. Tiainen, O. M. Nuutinen, and M. P. Kalavainen, "Diet and nutritional status in children with cow's milk allergy," *European Journal of Clinical Nutrition*, vol. 49, no. 8, pp. 605–612, 1995.

22

Diagnosis of Asthma in Primary Health Care: A Pilot Study

Karin C. Ringsberg,[1,2] **Paula Bjärneman,**[2] **Ronny Larsson,**[3]
Elisabeth Wallström,[3] **and Olle Löwhagen**[2]

[1] *Nordic School of Public Health, 402 42 Gothenburg, Sweden*
[2] *Sahlgrenska Academy, University of Gothenburg, 413 90 Gothenburg, Sweden*
[3] *Kungsten Health Care Centre, 414 74 Gothenburg, Sweden*

Correspondence should be addressed to Karin C. Ringsberg; karin.ringsberg@gu.se

Academic Editor: Steven Nordin

Some patients with an asthma diagnosis have a poor controlled asthma. One explanation may be an incorrect diagnosis. *Aim.* The aim of the study was to diagnose and classify patients with non-infectious lower respiratory tract problems in primary health care using internationally applied diagnostic criteria and diagnostic tests. *Patients and Methods.* New adult patients visiting a primary health care centre due to lower airway problems were included. The diagnostic tests included FEV_1, FVC, PEF, two questionnaires, methacholine test, and skin prick test. *Results.* The patients ($n = 43$) could be divided into four groups: asthma (28%), asthma-like disorder (44%), idiopathic cough (12%), and a nonreversible bronchial obstructive group (16%). The asthma and asthma-like groups showed similar patterns of airway symptoms and trigger factors, not significantly separated by a special questionnaire. Phlegm, heavy breathing, chest pressure/pain, cough, and wheezing were the most common symptoms. Physical exercise and scents were the dominating trigger factors. *Conclusions.* Nonobstructive asthma-like symptoms seem to be as common as bronchial asthma in primary health care. Due to the similarities in symptoms and trigger factors the study supports the hypothesis that asthma and nonobstructive asthma-like disorders are integrated in the same "asthma syndrome," including different mechanisms, not only bronchial obstruction.

1. Introduction

Bronchial asthma is a common disease worldwide and good treatment could often be offered [1]. Its prevalence in the adult population in Sweden is up to 10% [2], being the highest in the north part and in younger people. The diagnosis is based on the presence of episodic breathing troubles and variable and reversible airway obstruction [1, 3]. Most cases are not difficult to diagnose and treat; however, some patients respond poorly to asthma treatment despite ongoing asthma-like symptoms. In those cases, other diagnoses must be considered [4–15]. Disorders with asthma-like symptoms mentioned in the literature are dysfunctional breathing [11, 16–18], vocal cord dysfunction [19], pseudoasthma [20], cough variant asthma [8], multiple chemical sensitivity [21], and airway sensory hyperreactivity (SHR) [22]. In GINA, the international guidelines for asthma diagnostics and treatment [1], two disorders with asthma-like symptoms are

mentioned, vocal cord dysfunction (VC) [19] and hyperventilation syndrome (HVS) [7]. As the above conditions are presented under different names, it is not possible to know the prevalence. However, Marklund et al. found that every third asthmatic had been given a wrong diagnosis [14]. They also found that the older the patients, the greater the risk of an incorrect diagnosis [14]. Johansson et al. [23] estimated the prevalence of airway sensory hyperreactivity to be about 6% in the adult population. These patients often seek primary care because of asthma-like symptoms and poor quality of life [5]. Using factor analysis in a general population sample Bonde et al. [18] identified five groups of breathing-related disorders, dysfunctional breathing, odour intolerance, asthma, bronchitis, and a group with mixed symptoms. These groups should therefore be considered when investigating patients in the primary care.

In this study, an operational definition of asthma-like disorder is used, meaning symptoms that most physicians associate with asthma but where abnormal lung function cannot be demonstrated [10]. The term asthma-like disorder is henceforth used.

Aim. The aim of this pilot study, preceding a larger study, was to diagnose and classify adult patients with noninfectious lower respiratory tract problems in primary health care by using international applied diagnostic criteria.

2. Patients and Methods

The study was performed at a primary health care centre in Sweden in a city with about half a million inhabitants. The health care centre served about 12,000 inhabitants with intermediate to high incomes. Four GPs and five nurses worked at the centre. One of the nurses and one of the physicians were specially trained in asthma and respiratory diseases.

2.1. Patients. Consecutive patients who visited the health care centre for the first time over a period of one year were included.

2.1.1. Inclusion Criteria. Inclusion criteria included the following:

(1) male or female, age ≥17,

(2) respiratory symptoms from lower airways persisting for more than one month in order to exclude patients with short term symptoms,

(3) not earlier diagnosed for these symptoms.

2.1.2. Exclusion Criteria. Exclusion criteria included the following:

(1) previously diagnosed airway disease (asthma, COPD, alveolitis, bronchiectasis, sarcoidosis, etc.),

(2) ongoing airway infection,

(3) other diseases that could influence the lower airways and chest mobility (heart disease, systemic immunological disease, osteoporosis, pulmonary emboli, etc.).

2.2. Methods

2.2.1. Lung Function Test. Lung function test included the following:

(1) FEV_1 before and after inhalation of salbutamol 0.8 mg (reversibility) [1],

(2) PEF morning and evening, before and after inhaled salbutamol 0.4 mg over a period of two weeks (variability) [1],

(3) FVC and VC (obstruction) [1].

FEV% was calculated as FEV1/FVC or FEV1/VC (if VC was higher than FVC) after bronchodilation [24].

Lung function was measured by volume-dependent spirometry (Vitalograph) with normal reference values from Standardization of Lung Function Tests (Bull Europ. Physiopath. Resp.1983:19 suppl). PEF was measured by a Mini wright peak flow meter. All tests were performed in the same way in each patient.

As the patients included in the study were new patient they had no treatment, neither before nor during the investigation. They were prescribed therapy after completed investigation.

2.2.2. Skin Prick Test. The skin prick test was performed on patients who reported a suspected allergy history. A standard panel of 10 allergen extracts (Soluprick SQ ALK Copenhagen) was used (two mites, two moulds, birch, mugwort, timothy, cat, dog, horse).

2.2.3. Methacholine Test. Patients with unclear lung function data or values close to pathological limit were referred to an asthma-allergy clinic for a methacholine inhalation test. A positive test was defined as PC_{20} (provocation concentration at 20% fall in $FEV_1 \leq 4$ mg/mL) [25].

2.2.4. Questionnaire. Two questionnaires were used. One general questionnaire, number 1 (see Tables 2 and 5), used for several years in the clinic included common symptoms (cough, wheezing, heavy breathing, phlegm, and chest pressure/pain) and common trigger factors (cold air, physical exercise, smoke, strong scents, emotional stress, and allergens). The patients were asked to answer yes or no. The second questionnaire, number 2, included 21 symptoms and 7 trigger factors (see Tables 3 and 6) and had earlier been designed to separate asthma from asthma-like disorders in patients referred to a special clinic for asthma and allergy [26]. The patient was asked to rate the frequency of symptoms on a five-point Likert scale: 1 = never, 2 = occasionally, 3 = once a month, 4 = once a week, and 5 = daily and the severity of the trigger factors on a five-point Likert scale: 1 = not at all, 2 = some, 3 = rather a lot, 4 = much, and 5 = very much. One question in the original version of questionnaire number 2 (strong scents) was excluded as it was also included as a trigger factor. Symptoms presented in questionnaire number 2 (Table 3) were grouped into five subsets of symptoms [26]: "upper airways nose throat", "lower airways-chest", "general symptoms", "stomach", and "sleep".

2.2.5. Diagnostic Criteria. For bronchial asthma, COPD, and chronic cough, international approved criteria were used [1, 24, 25]. For asthma-like disorders, criteria were set up on the basis of earlier studies [4, 9–11, 14, 15].

Bronchial Asthma [1]. Bronchial asthma included the following:

(1) episodic lower airway symptoms (breathing complaints, wheezing, coughing, phlegm, chest tightness, or chest pain/pressure) [1],

TABLE 1: Age, sex, lung function, and classification of patients.

Group	Age median (range)	Sex male/female	FEV$_1$ % predicted mean (range)	FEV$_1$ reversibility mean % (range)	PEF variability mean % (range)
(I) Asthma $N = 12$	44 (36–83)	0/12	99 (76–123)	6 (0–13)	24 (8–52)
(II) Asthma-like $N = 19$	47 (19–76)	3/16	103 (91–122)	2 (0–8)	10 (7–19)
(III) Idiopathic cough $N = 5$	50 (39–57)	0/5	103 (95–107)	3 (0–7)	11 (2–15)
(IV) Nonreversible bronchial obstructive $N = 7$	59 (17–66)	2/5	79 (73–86)	4 (0–11)	11 (5–16)

(2)

(a) reversibility of FEV$_1$ ≥ 12% [1],

(b) variability in PEF ≥ 20% [1].

Asthma-Like Disorders [4, 9–11, 14, 15, 26]. Asthma-like disorders include the following:

(1) episodic lower airway symptoms (breathing complaints, wheezing, coughing, phlegm, chest tightness, or chest pain/pressure),

(2) reversibility in FEV$_1$ < 12%,

(3) FEV$_1$ ≥ 90% of normal predicted value,

(4) variability in PEF < 20% [4, 9].

COPD [24]. COPD included the following:

(1) lower airway symptoms (breathing complaints, wheezing, coughing, phlegm, chest tightness, and chest pain/pressure),

(2) reversibility in FEV$_1$ < 12%,

(3) variability in PEF < 20%,

(4) FEV% < 70% (FEV$_1$/FVC or FEV$_1$/VC if VC was higher than FVC) after bronchodilation.

Chronic Idiopathic Cough [27]. Chronic idiopathic cough included the following:

(1) dominant cough lasting ≥ 8 weeks,

(2) FEV$_1$ ≥ 90% of predicted normal value,

(3) reversibility in FEV$_1$ < 12%,

(4) variability in PEF < 20%.

2.3. Statistics. Within-group comparisons in questionnaire number 1 (yes/no answers) were analysed using the chi-square test. The statistical analysis focused on the difference between asthma and asthma-like disorders. For differences between groups, nonparametric methods were used; for

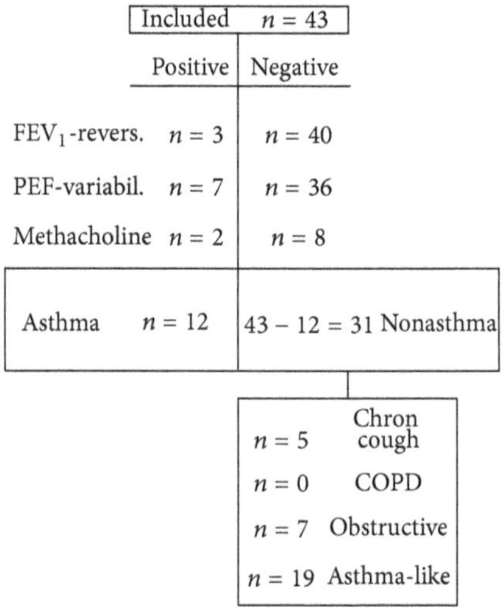

FIGURE 1: Flow chart. Classification to different groups (see Section 3) depending on FEV$_1$-reversibility, PEF-variability, and methacholine test.

questionnaire number 2, the Wilcoxon signed-ranks test was used and for comparisons between Group I and II, Mann Whitney's test was used. $P < 0.05$ was considered to be statistically significant.

3. Results

Of the 537 patients visiting the centre because of airway symptoms eight percent ($n = 43$) fulfilled the inclusion criteria for the study. Characteristics are shown in Table 1 and Figure 1 (flow chart).

3.1. Classification. Based on the diagnostic criteria above, the patients (38 women and 5 men, aged 17–83, median 54) were divided into four groups; (Group I) asthma (28%), (Group II) asthma-like (44%), (Group III) chronic idiopathic cough (12%), and (Group IV) nonreversible bronchial obstructive group (16%). No patient fulfilled the criteria for COPD. The median age was the highest in Group IV (59 years) and the lowest in Group I (44 years). The dominant

TABLE 2: The five most reported symptoms based on questionnaire no. 1. Group I–IV.

	Group I N = 12	Group II N = 19	Group III N = 5	Group IV N = 7
Phlegm	12 (100%)	18 (95%)	4 (80%)	7 (100%)
Heavy breathing	9 (75%)	16 (84%)	0 (0%)	4 (58%)
Chest pressure/pain	9 (75%)	9 (47%)	0 (0%)	2 (29%)
Cough	2 (16%)	12 (63%)	5 (100%)	3 (29%)
Wheezing	6 (50%)	7 (37%)	0 (0%)	3 (43%)

TABLE 3: Frequency of single symptoms scored on questionnaire no. 2.

Symptom	Group I N = 12 Median (range)	Group II N = 19 Median (range)	Group III N = 5 Median (range)	Group IV N = 7 Median (range)
(1) Dry eyes	1.0 (1–4)	1.0 (1–4)	1.0 (1-1)	1.0 (1-1)
(2) Dry mucus in nose	2.0 (1–5)	2.0 (1–5)	1.0 (1–4)	2.0 (1–5)
(3) Dry mucus in throat	2.0 (1–5)	2.0 (1–5)	1.0 (1–5)	3.0 (2–5)
(4) Taste of blood	1.0 (1-2)	1.0 (1–4)	1.0 (1-2)	1.0 (1-1)
(5) Difficulty in getting air	2.0 (1–5)	3.0 (1–5)	1.0 (1–4)	2.0 (1–3)
(6) Difficulty in taking deep breaths	2.0 (1–5)	2.0 (1–5)	2.0 (1–4)	2.0 (1–5)
(7) Wheezing	2.0 (1–5)	2.0(1–5)	1.0 (1-2)	1.0 (1–4)
(8) Hissing	2.0 (1–5)	2.0 (1–5)	1.0 (1-2)	1.0 (1–4)
(9) Feeling of sore airways	2.0 (1–5)	2.0 (1–5)	1.0 (1–4)	2.0 (1–5)
(10) Irritating cough	5.0 (1–5)	3.0 (2–5)	5.0 (1–5)	3.0 (2–5)
(11) Nausea	1.0 (1–3)	2.0 (1–5)	1.0 (1–4)	2.0 (1–4)
(12) Sensation of bloated abdomen	1.0 (1–4)	2.0 (1–4)	1.0 (1–5)	1.0 (1-2)
(13) Waking up due to nasal congestion	2.0 (1–5)	2.0 (1–5)	2.0 (1–5)	2.0 (1–5)
(14) Abnormal tiredness, weakness after psychological stress	2.0 (1–5)	2.0 (1–5)	1.0 (1–4)	2.0 (1–4)
(15) A sore throat	2.0 (1–5)	2.0 (1–5)	1.0 (1–4)	2.0 (1–5)
(16) Headaches	2.0 (1–4)	2.0 (1–5)	3.0 (2–4)	2.0 (1–3)
(17) Feeling of confusion	1.0 (1–4)	1.0 (1–4)	1.0 (1-1)	2.0 (1–3)
(18) Cold hands and feet	2.0 (1–5)	2.5 (1–5)	2.0 (1–5)	2.0 (1–4)
(19) Feeling of tenseness in the body	2.0 (1–5)	3.0 (1–5)	2.0 (1–3)	2.5 (1–3)
(20) Difficulty in concentrating	2.0 (1–4)	2.5 (1–5)	2.0 (1–4)	2.0 (1–5)

sex was female in all groups. Men were only represented in Groups II and IV (Table 1).

Group I. Twelve patients (28%) fulfilled the diagnostic criteria for bronchial asthma. Two patients (with borderline reversibility or variability) were classified as belonging to this group on the basis of a positive methacholine tests (threshold dose ≤ 4 mg/Ml). Four patients had a positive skin prick test.

Group II. Nineteen patients (44%) fulfilled the criteria for an asthma-like disorder. All patients had a FEV_1, reversibility, and PEF variability within normal range. A methacholine test was performed in six cases, and all tests were negative (threshold dose > 16 mg/mL).

Group III. Five patients (12%) fulfilled the criteria for a chronic idiopathic cough. The duration of the cough varied from four months to 10 years. In none of the patients were there clinical signs of a reflux, rhinitis, or sinusitis.

Group IV. Seven patients (16%) had a bronchial obstruction, varying in FEV_1 from 73% to 86% predicted; however, without reversibility or variability. None of them was a smoker, none had an allergy, and none fulfilled the criteria for COPD. One patient was classified as belonging to this group on the basis of a negative methacholine test. The investigation of these obstructive patients continued and ended with the following final diagnoses: two patients with infection-induced asthma, one with asthma and lung cancer, one with probable asthma and unclear resting dyspnea, one with bronchiectasis, one with asthma, diaphragmatic hernia, and reflux, and one patient with obstruction, chronic cough, and phlegm.

3.2. Skin Prick Test. Eleven patients reported a positive allergy history with airway complaints. Five of these patients had a negative skin prick test and were considered nonallergic. Of the six patients with a positive test, four were found

TABLE 4: Subsets of symptoms scored in questionnaire no. 2.

Subsets of symptoms (questions number)	Group I N = 12 Median (range)	Group II N = 19 Median (range)	Group III N = 5 Median (range)	Group IV N = 7 Median (range)
Upper airways, eyes, nose, throat (1, 2, 3, 4)	2.0 (1–5)	1.0 (1–5)	1.0 (1–5)	1.0 (1–5)
Lower airways (5, 6, 7, 8, 9, 10)	2.0 (1–5)	2.0 (1–5)	1.0 (1–5)	2.0 (1–5)
General symptoms (16, 17, 18, 19, 20)	2.0 (1–5)	2.0 (1–5)	2.0 (1–5)	2.0 (1–5)
Stomach (11, 12)	1.0 (1–4)	2.0 (1–5)	1.0 (1–5)	1.0 (1–4)
Sleep (13, 14)	2.0 (1–5)	2.0 (1–5)	2.0 (1–5)	2.0 (1–5)

in Group I (pollen, cat, dog, and mite) and two in Group II (pollen, cat, and dog). The results of the skin prick test did not change the classification of the patients.

3.3. Symptoms

Questionnaire Number 1. The most common symptom reported in all groups was phlegm (Table 2). Cough was, by definition, the most common symptom in Group III. The second most common symptom was chest pressure/pain (Group I) and heavy breathing (Groups II and IV). Wheezing, often considered to be a criterion for asthma, was reported by 50% of Group I and by 37% of Group II. There were no significant differences between Groups I and II for any of the five most common symptoms.

Questionnaire Number 2. There were no significant differences in symptoms of breathing troubles (wheezing, hissing, difficulty in getting air, and difficulty in taking deep breaths) between Groups I and II (Table 3).

When symptoms in questionnaire number 2 were grouped into five subsets of symptoms [26]: "upper airways" (eye, nose, throat), "lower airways", "general symptoms", "stomach", and "sleep", no significant differences between Groups I and II were found (Table 4).

3.4. Trigger Factors

Questionnaire Number 1. The most common trigger factor in all the groups was physical exercise (walking up hills/stairs) and cold air (Table 5). There were no statistically significant differences between Groups I and II for any of these seven factors.

Questionnaire Number 2. The total median score of trigger factors in questionnaire number 2 (Table 6) for Group I was 1.7, for Group II 1.6, for Group III 1.1, and for Group IV 2.5. Thus, there was no difference between Groups I and II. The highest median score was seen in Group IV, "some" to "rather a lot."

4. Discussion

Most patients with respiratory complaints in Sweden are first visiting the primary health care, which has good access to practical and reliable diagnostic methods. The number of new

patients in this one-year study was in line with a reported incidence of 2% of adult asthma [28] in this area. Accordingly, we believe that the results could be generalized to a larger population. Bronchial asthma and COPD are reported to be the most common chronic lower airway diseases [1, 3, 24]. In this clinical study in primary health care, the picture was different. A clear bronchial asthma was found in 28% while the majority had other respiratory complaints, asthma-like (44%), chronic idiopathic cough (12%), and nonreversible bronchial obstruction (16%). If five patients (possibly asthma) in the unclear obstructive group were added to the asthma group, the prevalence of asthma and asthma-like disorders was approximately the same. Similar findings are reported in another study in the primary care [14]. The results are also supported by a recent epidemiological study by Bonde et al. [18]. By use of factor analysis five groups of breathing related symptoms were identified, asthma, bronchitis, dysfunctional breathing, odour intolerance, and a mixed group. As the patients included in the study were new patients they had no treatment, neither before nor during the investigation. The patients were prescribed therapy after completing the investigation.

An asthma-like disorder may be an early stage of bronchial asthma or bronchial asthma in a temporary symptom-free stage with normal lung function. However, it has been shown that a disorder with asthma-like symptoms and normal lung function may persist for more than 5 years [29, 30]. New cases of COPD were not found during this study period which was somewhat unexpected. However, this may be explained by the low percentage of smokers in this area, 10%, compared to 18% in national epidemiological studies [18]. One or more patients in the obstructive group (group IV) may have incipient COPD but did not fulfil the diagnostic criteria. The non-COPD diagnosis was supported by the fact that none of the patients was a smoker. Another explanation could be obstruction due to remodelling. The extended investigation of the unclear group showed complicated and combined diseases were asthma could be suspected in 5 of the 7 cases.

In international guidelines [1, 3] two asthma-like disorders are mentioned as the most common differential diagnoses, vocal cord dysfunction [19], and hyperventilation syndrome [7, 31]. In this study there were no clear indications of these diseases. Based on the questionnaires and records, no patient reported inspiratory stridor or upper airway symptoms typical of VCD. Hyperventilation syndrome

TABLE 5: Most reported symptom-inducing trigger factors based on questionnaire no. 1.

Trigger factor	Group I N = 12 n (%)	Group II N = 19 n (%)	Group III N = 5 n (%)	Group IV N = 7 n (%)
Walking up hills/stairs	10 (83)	10 (53)	2 (40)	6 (86)
Cold air	7 (58)	8 (42)	3 (60)	4 (57)
Mental stress	3 (25)	4 (21)	1 (20)	4 (57)
Tobacco smoke	3 (25)	7 (37)	1 (20)	4 (57)
Flowers	3 (25)	4 (21)	0 (0)	5 (71)
Perfume	3 (25)	0 (0)	0 (0)	5 (71)
Exhaust gases	3 (25)	3 (16)	0 (0)	2 (29)

TABLE 6: Severity of symptom induced trigger factors based on questionnaire no. 2.

Trigger factor	Group I N = 12 Median (range)	Group II N = 19 Median (range)	Group III N = 5 Median (range)	Group IV N = 7 Median (range)
(1) Warm weather	1.0 (1–5)	1.0 (1–4)	1.0 (1–2)	1.5 (1–4)
(2) Conflicting situations	1.5 (1–4)	1.0 (1–4)	1.0 (1–3)	1.5 (1–4)
(3) Strong scents	2.5 (1–5)	2.0 (1–4)	1.0 (1–1)	3.0 (2–5)
(4) Exhaust gases	2.0 (1–5)	2.0 (1–4)	1.0 (1–3)	3.0 (2–5)
(5) Stuffy air	2.0 (1–4)	2.0 (1–3)	1.0 (1–1)	3.0 (1–5)
(6) Smell of tobacco	2.0 (1–5)	2.0 (1–5)	2.0 (1–4)	3.5 (2–5)
(7) Dust from detergent	1.0 (1–4)	1.0 (1–3)	1.0 (1–1)	2.0 (1–5)

$P = \leq 0.05$.

[7, 31] is a well-known asthma-like disorder since many years, but its existence in a chronic form has been contested [31, 32]. However, as it has been clearly demonstrated in acute studies hyperventilation it is still of interest [12, 13, 16, 17, 20, 31, 33–36]. By using the Nijmegen questionnaire, often used for identifying hyperventilation syndrome, Thomas et al. [16] recently found that every third woman with an asthma diagnosis had a positive score (≥ 23). The disorder that was identified in this way was not called hyperventilation but dysfunctional breathing. Dysfunctional breathing has also been described in other studies [7, 17, 36]. Some symptoms listed in the Nijmegen questionnaire are also included in questionnaire number 2 [26]: "difficulty in taking deep breaths," "sensation of bloated abdomen," "feeling of confusion," "cold hands and feet," and "feeling of tenseness in the body." Thus, it is likely that the asthma-like disorder found in our study overlaps with the above described dysfunctional breathing. In 1998 the asthma-like disorder airway sensory hyperreactivity (SHR) was described by use of the capsaicin inhalation test [22]. Its prevalence has been reported to be about 6% [23], which can be compared with the prevalence of asthma of 6–10% in the same area [2]. This disorder may well be found in Group II in our study, but capsaicin inhalation test is still not available in the primary care.

International guidelines of respiratory diseases focus on asthma and COPD [1, 3]. This study points to the importance of also seeing other nonvariable and nonobstructive asthma-like disorders. The symptoms and trigger factors are very similar to asthma, which makes the differential diagnosing difficult. Bronchial obstruction,

reversible and variable, is one mechanism but there might be more forming an "asthma syndrome". This hypothesis is supported by a recent study by Bonde et al. [18]. It is important not to ignore asthma-like disorders even if they do not fit into any diagnostic criterion. The patients are often complaining of poor quality of life and that their symptoms are seen "just as psychological problems". For the moment no medical treatment can be offered. However, alternative treatment inspired by cognitive behavioural therapy has been successful [37–39].

5. Conclusions

In conclusion, this study shows that asthma-like symptoms with or without reversible bronchial obstruction are equally common in patients seeking primary health care. The similarities in symptoms and trigger factors support the hypothesis that asthma and nonobstructive asthma-like disorders are integrated in the same "asthma syndrome", which might include different mechanisms, not only bronchial obstruction.

Ethical Approval

All diagnostic tests were included in the clinical routine at the centre. This pilot study is included in a larger planned study whose design was approved by the local ethical committee (reference no. 615-11). The rules of the Helsinki Declaration were followed. Both patients and doctors were carefully informed.

Conflict of Interests

The authors declare that there is no conflict of interests regarding the publication of this paper.

Acknowledgment

The authors would like to thank Inger Winberg at the Asthma and Allergy Centre, Sahlgrenska University Hospital, for performing the methacholine tests.

References

[1] Global Initiative for Asthma (GINA), National Institutes of Health. National Heart, Lung, and Blood Institute. Revised 2004, http://www.ginasthma.com.

[2] B. Lundbäck, "Epidemiology of rhinitis and asthma," *Clinical and Experimental Allergy*, vol. 28, no. 2, pp. 3–10, 1998.

[3] M. L. Levy, M. Fletcher, D. B. Price, T. Hausen, R. J. Halbert, and B. P. Yawn, "International Primary Care Respiratory Group (IPCRG) Guidelines: diagnosis of respiratory diseases in primary care," *Primary Care Respiratory Journal*, vol. 15, no. 1, pp. 20–34, 2006.

[4] O. Löwhagen, "Asthma and asthma-like disorders," *Respiratory Medicine*, vol. 93, pp. 851–855, 1999.

[5] K. C. Ringsberg, K. Segesten, and I. Åkerlind, "Walking around in circles—the life situation of patients with asthma-like symptoms but negative asthma tests," *Scandinavian Journal of Caring Sciences*, vol. 11, no. 2, pp. 103–112, 1997.

[6] P. J. Barnes and A. J. Woolcock, "Difficult asthma," *European Respiratory Journal*, vol. 12, no. 5, pp. 1209–1218, 1998.

[7] H. Folgering, "The pathophysiology of hyperventilation syndrome," *Monaldi Archives for Chest Disease*, vol. 54, no. 4, pp. 365–372, 1999.

[8] S. A. Antoniu, T. Mihaescu, and C. F. Donner, "Pharmacotherapy of cough-variant asthma," *Expert Opinion on Pharmacotherapy*, vol. 8, no. 17, pp. 3021–3028, 2007.

[9] O. Löwhagen, "Functional respiratory disorders as significant differential diagnosis in asthma," *Lakartidningen*, vol. 86, no. 1-2, pp. 57–59, 1989.

[10] K. C. Ringsberg, "Patients with asthma-like symptoms but negative asthma tests and patients with bronchial asthma. Physiological, psychological and social characteristics," Medical Dissertations 522, Linköping University, 1997.

[11] K. C. Ringsberg, O. Löwhagen, and T. Sivik, "Psychological differences between asthmatics and patients suffering from an asthma-like condition, functional breathing disorder: a comparison between the two groups concerning personality, psychosocial and somatic parameters," *Integrative Physiological and Behavioral Science*, vol. 28, no. 4, pp. 358–367, 1993.

[12] K. C. Ringsberg, H. Wetterqvist, O. Löwhagen, and T. Sivik, "Physical capacity and dyspnea in patients with asthma-like symptoms but negative asthma tests," *Allergy*, vol. 52, no. 5, pp. 532–540, 1997.

[13] K. C. Ringsberg and I. Åkerlind, "Presence of hyperventilation in patients with asthma-like symptoms but negative asthma test responses: provocation with voluntary hyperventilation and mental stress," *Journal of Allergy and Clinical Immunology*, vol. 103, no. 4, pp. 601–608, 1999.

[14] B. Marklund, A. Tunsäter, and C. Bengtsson, "How often is the diagnosis bronchial asthma correct?" *Family Practice*, vol. 16, no. 2, pp. 112–116, 1999.

[15] O. Lowhagen, "Asthma—a disease difficult to define," *Läkartidningen*, vol. 102, pp. 3875–3878, 2005.

[16] M. Thomas, R. K. McKinley, E. Freeman, and C. Foy, "Prevalence of dysfunctional breathing in patients treated for asthma in primary care: Cross sectional survey," *British Medical Journal*, vol. 322, no. 7294, pp. 1098–1100, 2001.

[17] M. Thomas, R. K. McKinley, E. Freeman, C. Foy, and D. Price, "The prevalence of dysfunctional breathing in adults in the community with and without asthma," *Primary Care Respiratory Journal*, vol. 14, no. 2, pp. 78–82, 2005.

[18] E. Bonde, E. Andersson, J. Brisman, M. Eklöf, K. C. Ringsberg, and K. Torén, "Dissociation of dysfunctional breathing and odour intolerance among adults in a general-population study," *The Clinical Respiratory Journal*, vol. 7, no. 2, pp. 176–182, 2013.

[19] A. H. Bahrainwala and M. R. Simon, "Wheezing and vocal cord dysfunction mimicking asthma," *Current Opinion in Pulmonary Medicine*, vol. 7, no. 1, pp. 8–13, 2001.

[20] A. H. Hammo and M. M. Weinberger, "Exercise-induced hyperventilation: a pseudoasthma syndrome," *Annals of Allergy, Asthma and Immunology*, vol. 82, no. 6, pp. 574–578, 1999.

[21] I. R. Bell, C. S. Miller, and G. E. Schwartz, "An olfactory-limbic model of multiple chemical sensitivity syndrome: possible relationships to kindling and affective spectrum disorders," *Biological Psychiatry*, vol. 32, no. 3, pp. 218–242, 1992.

[22] E. Millqvist, M. Bende, and O. Löwhagen, "Sensory hyperreactivity—a possible mechanism underlying cough and asthma-like symptoms," *Allergy*, vol. 53, no. 12, pp. 1208–1212, 1998.

[23] Å. Johansson, E. Millqvist, S. Nordin, and M. Bende, "Relationship between self-reported odor intolerance and sensitivity to inhaled capsaicin: proposed definition of airway sensory hyperreactivity and estimation of its prevalence," *Chest*, vol. 129, no. 6, pp. 1623–1628, 2006.

[24] "Global Initiative for Chronic Obstructive Lung Disease. Global Strategy for the Diagnosis, Management and Prevention of Chronic Obstructive Pulmonary Disease," NHLBI/WHO Workshop Report 2701: 1—100, Bethesda, National Heart, Lung and Blood Institute, 2001.

[25] L. Löwhagen, "Some procedures used to assess clinical airway hyperreactivity," *European Journal of Respiratory Diseases*, vol. 131, pp. 215–239, 1983.

[26] K. C. Ringsberg, P. Bjärneman, O. Löwhagen, A. Odén, and K. Torén, "Differences in trigger factors and symptoms between patients with asthma-like symptoms and patients with asthma: development of a basis for a questionnaire," *Respiratory Medicine*, vol. 96, no. 5, pp. 305–311, 2002.

[27] A. H. Morice, "Chronic cough," *Breathe*, vol. 3, pp. 165–174, 2006.

[28] K. Torén, T. Gislason, E. Omenaas et al., "A prospective study of asthma incidence and its predictors: the RHINE study," *European Respiratory Journal*, vol. 24, no. 6, pp. 942–946, 2004.

[29] O. Löwhagen, M. Arvidsson, and K. Pettersson, "Asthma and asthma-like disorder, a 5-year follow-up study," *Respiratory Medicine*, vol. 96, no. 12, pp. 1040–1044, 2002.

[30] E. Ternesten-Hasséus, O. Lowhagen, and E. Millqvist, "Quality of life and capsaicin sensitivity in patients with airway symptoms induced by chemicals and scents: a longitudinal study,"

Environmental Health Perspectives, vol. 115, no. 3, pp. 425–429, 2007.

[31] W. N. Gardner, "The pathophysiology of hyperventilation disorders," *Chest*, vol. 109, no. 2, pp. 516–534, 1996.

[32] H. Hornsveld and B. Garssen, "Hyperventilation syndrome: an elegant but scientifically untenable concept," *Netherlands Journal of Medicine*, vol. 50, no. 1, pp. 13–20, 1997.

[33] O. Löwhagen, M. Arvidsson, P. Bjärneman, and N. Jörgensen, "Exercised-induced respiratory symptoms are not always asthma.," *Respiratory Medicine*, vol. 93, no. 10, pp. 734–738, 1999.

[34] S. Jack, H. B. Rossiter, M. G. Pearson, S. A. Ward, C. J. Warburton, and B. J. Whipp, "Ventilatory responses to inhaled carbon dioxide, hypoxia, and in idiopathic hyperventilation," *The American Journal of Respiratory and Critical Care Medicine*, vol. 170, no. 2, pp. 118–125, 2004.

[35] E. Ternesten-Hasséus, E. L. Johansson, M. Bende, and E. Millqvist, "Dyspnea from exercise in cold air is not always asthma," *Journal of Asthma*, vol. 45, no. 8, pp. 705–709, 2008.

[36] J. van Dixhoorn and H. J. Duivenvoorden, "Efficacy of Nijmegen questionnaire in recognition of the hyperventilation syndrome," *Journal of Psychosomatic Research*, vol. 29, no. 2, pp. 199–206, 1985.

[37] "Socialstyrelsens riktlinjer för förebyggande, diagnostik, behandling och rehabilitering av astma och KOL," Artikelnummer 2203-102-4, 2003.

[38] K. C. Ringsberg, M. Lepp, and B. Finnström, "Experiences by patients with asthma-like symptoms of a problem-based learning health education programme," *Family Practice*, vol. 19, no. 3, pp. 290–293, 2002.

[39] K. C. Ringsberg and T. Timpka, "Clinical health education for patients with asthma-like symptoms but negative asthma tests," *Allergy*, vol. 56, no. 11, pp. 1049–1054, 2001.

23

Human Lung Mast Cell Products Regulate Airway Smooth Muscle CXCL10 Levels

H. Alkhouri,[1] V. Cha,[1] K. Tong,[1] L. M. Moir,[2] C. L. Armour,[2] and J. M. Hughes[1]

[1] Faculty of Pharmacy, The University of Sydney, Sydney, NSW 2006, Australia
[2] Discipline of Pharmacology and Woolcock Institute of Medical Research, The University of Sydney, Sydney, NSW 2006, Australia

Correspondence should be addressed to J. M. Hughes; margaret.hughes@sydney.edu.au

Academic Editor: William E. Berger

In asthma, the airway smooth muscle (ASM) produces CXCL10 which may attract CXCR3$^+$ mast/T cells to it. Our aim was to investigate the effects of mast cell products on ASM cell CXCL10 production. ASM cells from people with and without asthma were stimulated with IL-1β, TNF-α, and/or IFNγ and treated with histamine (1–100 μM) ± chlorpheniramine (H1R antagonist; 1 μM) or ranitidine (H2R antagonist; 50 μM) or tryptase (1 nM) ± leupeptin (serine protease inhibitor; 50 μM), heat-inactivated tryptase, or vehicle for 4 h or 24 h. Human lung mast cells (MC) were isolated and activated with IgE/anti-IgE and supernatants were collected after 2 h or 24 h. The supernatants were added to ASM cells for 48 h and ASM cell CXCL10 production detected using ELISA (protein) and real-time PCR (mRNA). Histamine reduced IL-1β/TNF-α-induced CXCL10 protein, but not mRNA, levels independent of H1 and H2 receptor activation, whereas tryptase and MC 2 h supernatants reduced all cytokine-induced CXCL10. Tryptase also reduced CXCL10 levels in a cell-free system. Leupeptin inhibited the effects of tryptase and MC 2 h supernatants. MC 24 h supernatants contained TNF-α and amplified IFNγ-induced ASM cell CXCL10 production. This is the first evidence that MC can regulate ASM cell CXCL10 production and its degradation. Thus MC may regulate airway myositis in asthma.

1. Introduction

In asthma, airway smooth muscle (ASM) cells may play a significant role in supporting inflammation locally. They produce a wide range of chemokines and growth factors *in vitro* in response to proinflammatory cytokines, which are elevated in asthma following release by activated inflammatory cells and other airway structural cells [1–3].

Degranulating mast cells (MC) are present in higher numbers in the ASM bundles of people with asthma than people without asthma [4–7]. MC numbers are further increased in allergic compared with nonallergic asthma [5] and thus may be a specific feature of eosinophilic asthma. There is conflicting evidence about the presence of MC in the ASM in severe asthma, which is often associated with neutrophilia and steroid resistance. Carroll et al. [4] found that degranulating MC numbers were highest in the ASM layer in fatal asthma, whereas Balzar et al. [8] found no evidence of them in the ASM in biopsies from a severe asthma cohort.

MC activation by allergen mediated cross-linking of IgE results in the release of a variety of preformed and newly synthesised mediators [9, 10]. These include the major granule-derived mediators histamine and tryptase and newly synthesised cysteinyl leukotrienes, whose effects on ASM contractility are well established. MC also produce other proteases, arachidonic acid metabolites, and a wide range of cytokines and growth factors [9, 10]. The relative balance of these mediators in the vicinity of the ASM cell will determine the overall effect MC have on ASM production of a certain chemokine. What role that chemokine plays in airway inflammation will depend on its quantity and activity locally.

To date, the effects of many MC products on ASM chemokine production are unknown. When studied individually, some MC mediators directly affect ASM chemokine production and thus may regulate inflammation locally. For example, interleukin (IL-)1β or tumour necrosis factor (TNF-)α alone [11] and IL-4 or IL-13 alone and in combination with IL-1β [12], induce ASM release of the potent eosinophil chemoattractant CCL11 (eotaxin), while we and others have shown that MC proteases cleave CCL11 [13, 14]. We have also shown that histamine enhances IL-1β-induced granulocyte-macrophage colony stimulating factor (GM-CSF) release but strongly inhibits CCL5 (RANTES) release by ASM cells from people with and without asthma [15]. Further studies are needed to investigate the pro- and anti-inflammatory effects of MC and whether or not they can regulate their own recruitment to the ASM and survival there.

Increased localization of MC to the ASM layer could be controlled by many ASM cell derived chemokines, as human lung MC (HLMC) express a range of chemokine receptors [16]. However MC in the ASM of people with asthma are CXCR3 positive, whereas less than half of the MC elsewhere in the airway submucosa express CXCR3. Further, ASM in biopsies from people with asthma are often (~50%) immunoreactive for the CXCR3 ligand CXCL10, whereas the ASM in biopsies from people without asthma are not [17]. *In vitro* we have established that asthmatic ASM cells produce CXCL10 more rapidly than nonasthmatic ASM cells under Th1 inflammatory conditions [18] and MC chemotaxis towards medium from the asthmatic ASM cells is driven by CXCL10 activating CXCR3 on the MC [17]. Whether or not MC can regulate ASM CXCL10 production and activity is not known.

Thus, the aims of this study were to investigate the effects of MC products on CXCL10 production by ASM cells from people with and without asthma. The effects of the granule-derived products histamine and tryptase, as well as the overall effects of human lung MC products released in the first 2 h or 2–24 h after activation, on ASM CXCL10 production were examined.

2. Methods

2.1. Agents. Recombinant Human IFNγ (BD Biosciences, Australia), IL-1β, and TNFα (R&D Systems, Minneapolis, MN) were reconstituted in sterile PBS containing 0.1% bovine serum albumin (BSA). Histamine, chlorpheniramine, and ranitidine (Sigma-Aldrich, Sydney, Australia) were reconstituted in water for irrigation (Baxter, Sydney, Australia). Human lung tryptase ($\geq$5,000 mU/mg/mL of vehicle consisting of 1 M NaCl, 50 mM sodium acetate, 0.01% sodium azide, and 50 μM heparin) was obtained from Calbiochem (La Jolla, CA, USA). BSA and leupeptin were purchased from Sigma-Aldrich. All agents were stored in aliquots at -20°C, except for IFNγ which was stored at -80°C.

2.2. Airway Smooth Muscle. ASM cell cultures were established from lung samples donated by 16 people with a doctor diagnosis of mild to moderate asthma (mean age 36 y and range 23–62 y) and 17 people without asthma (mean age 55 y and range 29–83 y). The lung samples were either bronchial biopsies or resected lung tissue obtained from people undergoing surgery for thoracic malignancies or lung transplantation. All samples were obtained with the donor's informed consent and approval from Sydney South West Area Health Service or Australian Red Cross. Approval for this

study was granted by The University of Sydney Human Ethics Committee.

2.3. Airway Smooth Muscle Cell Culture. ASM bundles were dissected out from macroscopically normal lung samples and grown as explants. The cells from people who had no doctor diagnosis of asthma are referred to as nonasthmatic. ASM cells were maintained in culture as previously described [19] in Dulbecco's Modified Eagle's Medium (DMEM) (Sigma-Aldrich) supplemented with 10% v/v heat-inactivated foetal bovine serum (FBS), 100 units/mL penicillin G, 100 μg/mL streptomycin sulphate, 25 μg/mL amphotericin B, 4 mM L-glutamine, and 20 mM HEPES, at pH 7.4 (growth medium) and grown at 37°C in a humidified 5% CO_2 in air atmosphere. The cells adopted a "hill and valley" growth pattern and were positive for α-smooth muscle actin and h-calponin using immunofluorescence [19, 20]. ASM cells harvested between passages 4 and 7 were used in experiments.

2.4. Histamine and Tryptase Effects on ASM Cell CXCL10 Production. To investigate the effects of histamine and tryptase on ASM cell CXCL10 production, ASM cells were seeded into the wells of 6- or 24-well plates at 1×10^4 cells/cm^2 in growth medium. After 7 days growth, the cells were serum-deprived for 48 h in FBS-free DMEM supplemented as described above and also with 0.1% v/v bovine serum albumin (BSA) (serum-free medium). The well cultures were left untreated or treated with histamine (1, 10, or 100 μM), tryptase (0.2, 1.0, or 5.0 nM), or the vehicle for tryptase and heparin (50 μM), as used previously [15]. Immediately afterwards the cytokines IL-1β, TNF-α, and IFNγ, alone and in combination (cytomix), were added to untreated and treated wells. The cytokines were each used at 10 ng/mL and all treatments were performed in duplicate.

To investigate which histamine receptor was involved in the effects of histamine on ASM cell CXCL10 release, the cells were treated in duplicate with either the H1 receptor antagonist chlorpheniramine at 1 μM [15, 21] or the H2 receptor antagonist ranitidine at 50 μM [15, 22], for 30 minutes prior to the addition of histamine followed by the cytokines.

To investigate whether the proteolytic activity of tryptase was involved in its effects on ASM cell CXCL10 release, an aliquot of the same tryptase batch was first heat-inactivated at 56°C for 30 minutes and then immediately added to the ASM cells, or the serine protease inhibitor leupeptin (50 μM) [15] was added to tryptase-treated ASM cells 3 h after the addition of the cytokines.

After 4 hours cytokine stimulation, the cells in the well cultures were washed and total RNA was extracted using the guanidine thiocyanate/phenol chloroform method [23]. The RNA was reverse transcribed using RevertAid First Strand cDNA Synthesis Kit (Fermentas Life Sciences, Hanover, MD, USA) and the cDNA amplified by PCR using FAM-labeled human CXCL10 and VIC labeled 18srRNA TaqMan probes on an ABI Prism 7500 (Applied Biosystems) as described previously [18].

Alternatively, the ASM well cultures were incubated with the cytokines for 24 hours and then the culture medium (CM) was collected and stored at −20°C for later analysis of CXCL10 levels using the CXCL10 Duo-set ELISA kit and protocol (R&D Systems, Minneapolis, MN, USA).

2.5. Tryptase Effects on Recombinant Human CXCL10.

To investigate whether tryptase can cleave CXCL10, recombinant human CXCL10 diluted in serum-free medium to 250, 500, and 1000 pg/mL, or the same volume of CM from cytokine-stimulated ASM cells, was added to a series of wells in microwell plates. Tryptase (1 nM), heat-inactivated tryptase, or tryptase followed by leupeptin (50 μM) 3 hours later, was added to duplicate wells containing CXCL10 or the ASM cell CM and the plates were incubated at 37°C for 24 hours and then CXCL10 was detected using ELISA.

2.6. Human Lung Mast Cell Isolation and Activation.

MC were isolated from macroscopically normal lung tissue dissected immediately by a pathologist from lung samples donated by 6 people undergoing surgery for thoracic malignancies. The MC were isolated within 24 hours of resection as previously described [14, 24]. Briefly, the lung parenchyma was chopped finely, washed, and digested with collagenase (7.5 mg/g tissue) and hyaluronidase (3.75 mg/g tissue) for 90 minutes at 37°C. MC in the cell suspension were positively selected using sheep anti-mouse IgG-coated magnetic beads (Dynal, Oslo, Norway), which were coated with a second anti-human CD117 (clone YB5B8; Bioscientific, Sydney, Australia) antibody (5 μg/mL) just before use and resuspended at 1 × 10^6 cells /mL in growth medium. The HLMC were activated with IgE (2.5 μg/mL) and goat anti-human IgE (1 μg/mL) (Calbiochem, CA, USA) immediately or left unstimulated. The HLMC culture supernatants (SN) were collected after 2 hours (MC 2 h SN) and fresh growth medium was added to the HLMC. This medium was collected 24 hours after the HLMC were first activated (MC 24 h SN). The MC 2 h and 24 h SN were stored at −20°C until immediately before use in the experiments described below.

2.7. ASM Cell Treatment with Human Lung Mast Cell Products.

To investigate the effects of HLMC products released at different times after activation on ASM cell CXCL10 production, harvested ASM cells were placed in the wells of 96-well plates at a density of 3200 cells/100 uL/well in growth medium and incubated as described above. After 24 hours the cells were serum-deprived in serum-free medium for 72 hours. Then the ASM cells were stimulated with growth medium ± IFNγ (10 ng/mL) and, after 30 minutes, treated in triplicate or quadruplicate with the MC 2 h or 24 h SN (prepared as described above) at 0, 20, or 40% v/v in growth medium in the presence of the same concentration of IFNγ, or left untreated. This order was used to ensure that the ASM cells were activated by IFNγ as it induces CXCL10 production and the effects of the MC SN directly on its activity were not known. After 48 hours of treatment, the medium was collected from each ASM culture and stored at −20°C for later measurement of CXCL10 levels using ELISA. ASM cell

CXCL10 release in response to growth medium ± IgE/anti IgE was also determined.

2.8. Protease Involvement in the Effects of HLMC Products Released by 2 h.

To establish whether or not MC proteases were involved in modulating ASM CXCL10 release, 2 h MC SN or the same SN already pretreated for 30 minutes with 50 μM leupeptin were added at 40% v/v in growth medium to the ASM cell well cultures. After 3 hours coincubation at 37°C, leupeptin was added to some of the wells containing untreated MC SN and the incubation was continued. All the culture medium was collected from each well after 48 hours and CXCL10 levels were quantified using ELISA.

To investigate if the effects of 24 h MC SN on cytokine-induced ASM CXCL10 could be due to TNF-α produced by MC, TNF-α levels were measured in the MC SN using ELISA. Then serum-deprived ASM cells were stimulated with IFN-γ (10 ng/mL), with and without a similar range of TNF-α concentrations to those detected in the MC SN, and made up in growth medium. After 24 h incubation at 37°C, the culture SN were collected and CXCL10 levels in them were quantified as above.

The effects of 2 h MC SN, β-tryptase, or leupeptin on the CXCL10 ELISA capture antibody were also investigated. Wells were coated with CXCL10 capture antibody and washed ready for use as usual; then either 40% v/v 2 h MC SN, 1 nM β-tryptase, 50 μM leupeptin, or vehicle, in growth medium or growth medium alone, was added to the wells already containing capture antibody. After incubation together for 1 hour at 37°C, the wells were washed and doubling dilutions of CXCL10 standards were added and the remainder of the ELISA protocol was completed without modification.

2.9. Data Analysis.

CXCL10 mRNA or protein levels from replicate treatments were averaged. The results for each experiment were expressed as a percentage of the cytokine control. The mean ± SEM was then calculated for the asthmatic and non-asthmatic cell lines and for each treatment. Statistical analyses were performed on all data using Statview (SAS Institute, Cary, North Carolina) or Prism 5.03 (Graph-Pad, La Jolla, CA) and significance ($P < 0.05$) was determined using 1-way or 2-way analysis of variance (ANOVA) with the Bonferroni correction for multiple comparisons or using the Student's t-test as appropriate.

3. Results

3.1. Histamine Effects on ASM Cell CXCL10 Production.

In preliminary experiments we established that histamine did not induce ASM cell CXCL10 release. The levels of CXCL10 released by untreated ASM cells from people with and without asthma were very low (Table 1). Histamine treatment at 1, 10, or 100 μM for 24 h did not alter CXCL10 release by the ASM cells (data not shown).

Similar to previous reports, cytokine stimulation increased ASM cell CXCL10 production. IL-1β, TNF-α and IFNγ, alone and in combination (cytomix), stimulated

TABLE 1: Cytokine-induced CXCL10 release by ASM cells.

Cytokine Treatment	CXCL10 Release (ng/mL, mean ± SEM)	
	Asthmatic $(n = 5)^1$	Non-asthmatic $(n = 5)$
Unstimulated	0.16 ± 0.04 $(n = 6)$	0.10 ± 0.03 $(n = 7)$
IL-1β	$1.34 \pm 0.27^*$	$7.35 \pm 3.53^*$
TNF-α	$6.45 \pm 1.56^*$	$20.71 \pm 9.44^*$
IFNγ	$17.06 \pm 11.57^*$ $(n = 6)$	$13.27 \pm 10.0^*$ $(n = 7)$
Cytomix	$49.57 \pm 16.21^{**}$	$66.56 \pm 14.44^{**}$

^{1}Except where indicated; $^*P \leq 0.01$ and $^{**}P < 0.001$ compared to unstimulated, paired t-test.

TABLE 2: The effects of tryptase on cytokine-induced CXCL10 release.

Cytokine Stimulus	CXCL10 Release (% cytokine control, mean ± SEM)	
	Asthmatic $(n = 4)$	Non-asthmatic $(n = 7\text{-}8)$
IL-1β	$22.8 \pm 14.5^*$	$9.0 \pm 3.6^*$
TNF-α	$36.3 \pm 14.4^*$	$25.2 \pm 5.1^*$
IFNγ	$11.1 \pm 4.3^*$	$13.6 \pm 3.5^*$
Cytomix	$65.8 \pm 15.8^*$	$42.8 \pm 9.4^*$

$^*P < 0.01$ compared to cytokine control, paired t-test.

significant CXCL10 release from the asthmatic and non-asthmatic ASM cells (Table 1).

Histamine had much greater inhibitory effects on IL-1β- and TNF-α-induced CXCL10 release than cytomix-induced release from both asthmatic and non-asthmatic ASM cells. The inhibitory effects of 1, 10, and 100 μM histamine on IL-1β-, and TNF-α-induced CXCL10 were all significant and concentration-related (Figures 1(a) and 1(b)). Histamine at the highest concentration (100 μM) reduced IL-1β-induced release from asthmatic ($n = 3$, $P < 0.0001$) and non-asthmatic ($n = 4$, $P < 0.0001$) ASM cells to a similar extent ($35.7 \pm 3.3\%$ and $37.5 \pm 6.5\%$ of the IL-1β control, resp.) (Figure 1(a)). Whereas it reduced TNF-α-induced release from asthmatic ($n = 3$, $P < 0.0001$) and non-asthmatic ($n = 4$, $P = 0.0013$) ASM cells down to $39.6 \pm 3.7\%$ and $61.0 \pm 7.9\%$ of the TNF-α control, respectively, (Figure 1(b)), but this difference in effects on asthmatic and non-asthmatic cells did not achieve statistical significance. In contrast, histamine had no effect on IFNγ-induced CXCL10 release from asthmatic and non-asthmatic ASM cells (Figure 1(c)) but at each concentration did reduce cytomix-induced release from non-asthmatic cells very slightly (Figure 1(d)).

Although IL-1β and TNF-α both induced significant increases in CXCL10 gene expression over 4 hours, histamine 10 μM did not affect CXCL10 mRNA levels induced by either cytokine (Figure 2(a)), even though it significantly reduced CXCL10 release. Further, the effects of 10 μM histamine on CXCL10 release were not reversed by pretreating the asthmatic and non-asthmatic ASM cells with the H1 and H2 receptor antagonists chlorpheniramine and ranitidine, respectively, or with the cell membrane permeable adenylate cyclase inhibitor SQ 22,536 (Figures 2(b) and 2(c)).

3.2. Tryptase Effects on ASM Cell CXCL10 Production. Neither tryptase (0.2, 1, or 5 nM) nor the vehicle (heparin 50 μM) induced CXCL10 release from ASM cells from people with and without asthma. The levels of CXCL10 were similar to those in the untreated controls (asthmatic: 0.15 ± 0.06 ng/mL, $n = 3$; non-asthmatic: 0.15 ± 0.07 ng/mL, $n = 4$).

Tryptase reduced the levels of CXCL10 detected in CM from asthmatic and non-asthmatic ASM cells. When tryptase (1 nM) was added to the ASM cells 30 minutes after the

cytokines IL-1β, TNF-α, IFNγ, or cytomix, the CXCL10 levels detected in non-asthmatic and asthmatic ASM cell CM were very much lower than the respective cytokine control (Table 2). The heparin vehicle for tryptase did not affect cytokine-induced CXCL10 levels (data not shown).

To investigate whether tryptase proteolytic activity was involved, the effects of tryptase and the same tryptase either heat-inactivated just before use or in the presence of the serine protease inhibitor leupeptin were compared. Untreated tryptase again markedly reduced nonasthmatic and asthmatic ASM cell cytokine-induced CXCL10 levels, whereas heat-inactivated tryptase did not affect them (Figures 3(a)–3(d)). Similarly, tryptase did not reduce CXCL10 levels when leupeptin (50 μM) was added 3 hours after the cytokine(s). However asthmatic ASM cell CXCL10 levels were more variable in the presence of leupeptin. CXCL10 levels in CM from asthmatic IL-1β-, TNF-α-, or IFNγ-stimulated cells treated with tryptase followed by leupeptin were higher than levels in the presence of the same tryptase which had been heat-inactivated, but the differences were not significant (Figures 3(a)–3(d)).

3.3. Tryptase Effects on Recombinant Human CXCL10. The proteolytic effects of tryptase on CXCL10 were investigated further in a cell-free system. Significantly less CXCL10 was detected in wells containing human recombinant CXCL10 (500–1000 pg/mL in serum-free medium) following treatment for 24 hours at 37°C with 1 nM tryptase than with its vehicle (Figure 4). CXCL10 levels were not reduced in wells treated with heat-inactivated tryptase and were even increased in those treated with tryptase followed by leupeptin (50 μM) 3 hours later. Similarly, tryptase treatment after-collection also markedly reduced detectable CXCL10 levels in culture medium collected from cytokine-stimulated ASM cells when compared to the vehicle-treated controls (data not shown). The capacity of the antibody from the Duo-set kit to capture CXCL10 standards was not affected by direct incubation with tryptase, its vehicle, or leupeptin at the concentrations used above (data not shown).

3.4. Effects of Human Lung Mast Cell Products on ASM Cell CXCL10. Asthmatic and non-asthmatic ASM cells responded in a similar way to the products released by human lung MC, but the effects of the 2 h and 24 h MC SN on ASM cell CXCL10 production differed. Although 10% FBS did not induce ASM cell CXCL10 release, IFNγ induced substantial

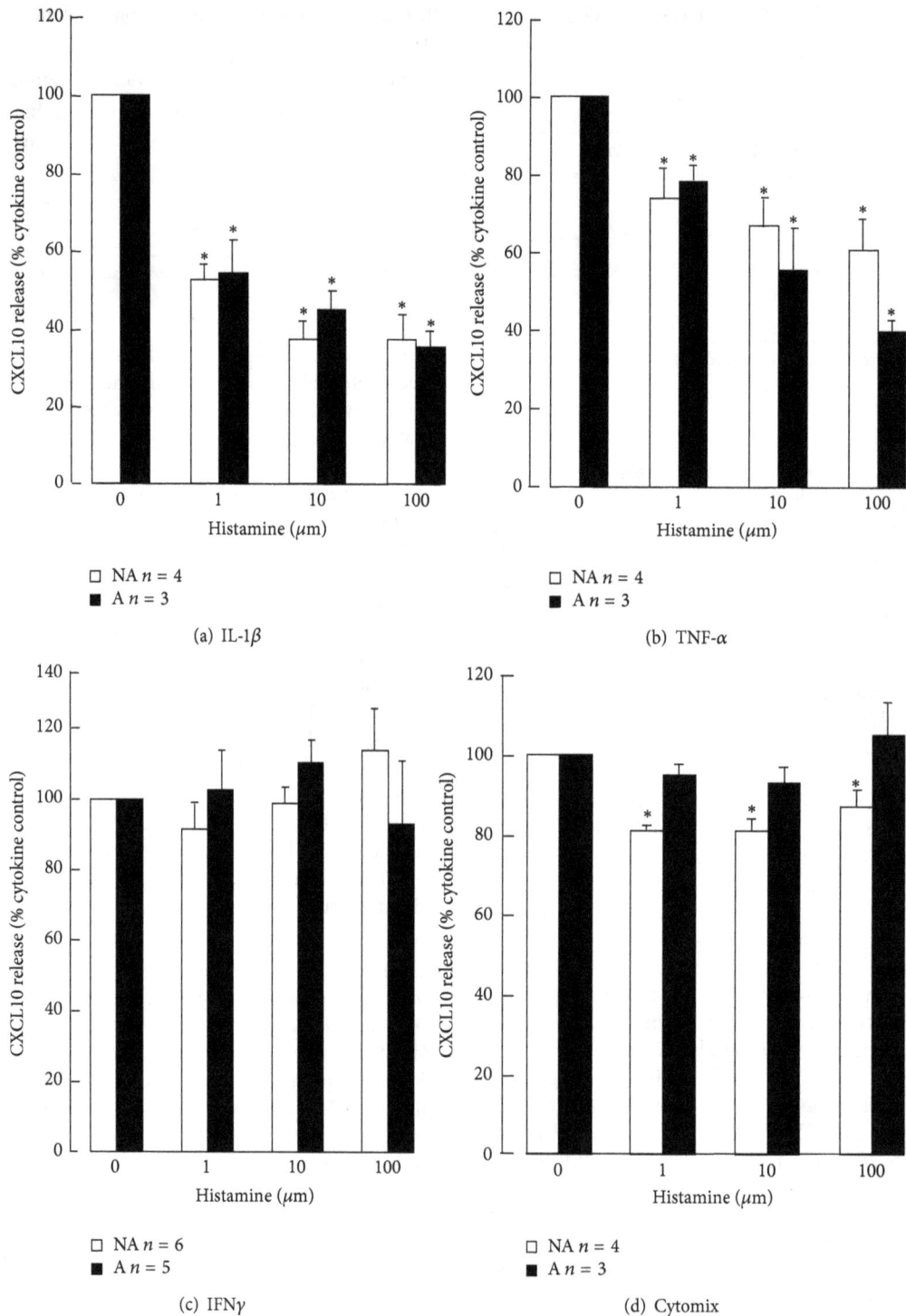

FIGURE 1: The effects of histamine on CXCL10 production by asthmatic (A) and nonasthmatic (NA) ASM cells. Confluent serum-deprived ASM cells were stimulated with the individual cytokines (a) IL-1β, (b) TNFα, (c) IFNγ, or (d) cytomix for 24 h and CXCL10 released into the culture medium quantified using ELISA. $^*P < 0.05$ compared with the cytokine control, ANOVA.

release in its presence over the 48 hour incubation. CXCL10 release was generally greater from asthmatic ASM cells (9.3 ± 2.4 ng/mL, $n = 6$) than non-asthmatic ASM cells (5.4 ± 2.0 ng/mL, $n = 6$), but the difference was not statistically significant. ASM cell CXCL10 release was not affected by the presence of IgE/anti-IgE (Figure 5(a)).

The MC 2 h SN markedly reduced asthmatic and non-asthmatic ASM cell CXCL10 levels following IFNγ stimulation. At 20% v/v, the MC 2 h SN significantly reduced non-asthmatic ASM cell CXCL10 levels down to 47 ± 12% of the FBS-IFNγ control and at 40% v/v significantly reduced asthmatic ASM cell CXCL10 levels to 46 ± 15% of control

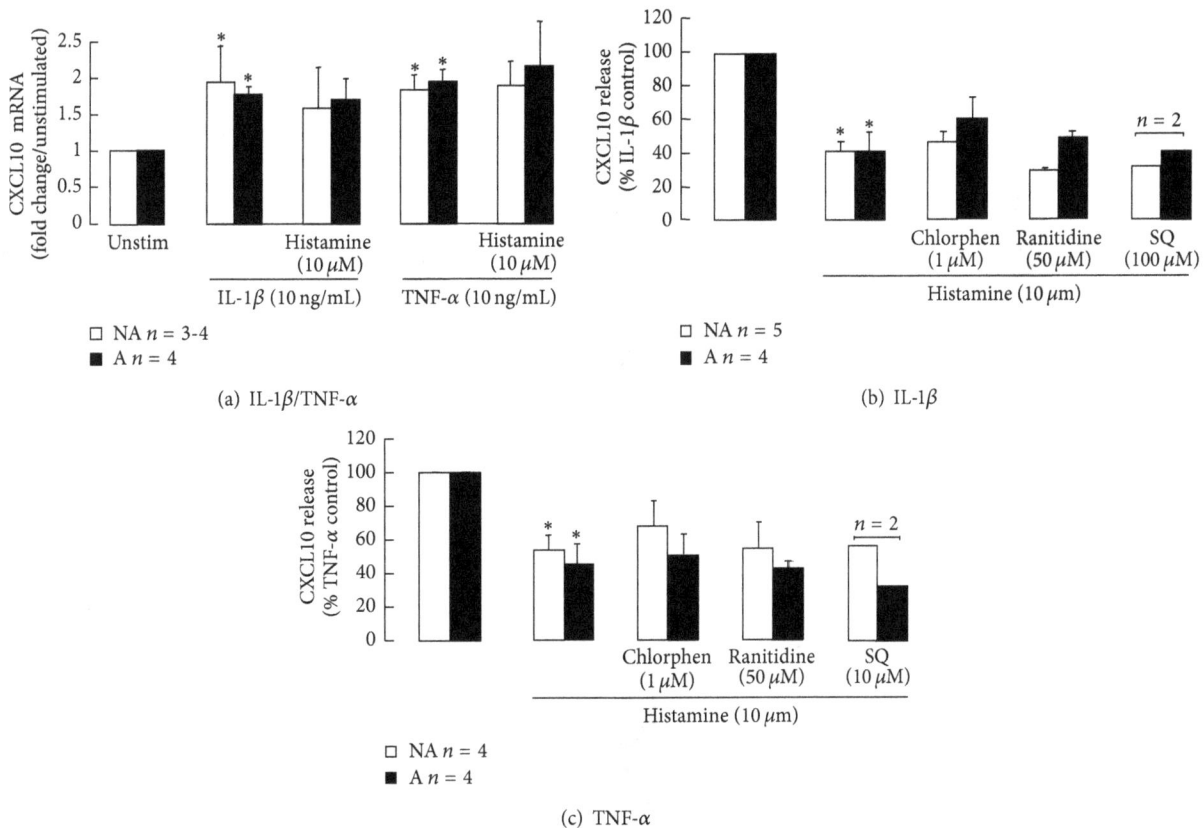

(a) IL-1β/TNF-α

(b) IL-1β

(c) TNF-α

FIGURE 2: The effects of histamine on cytokine-induced (a) CXCL10 gene expression and (b) H1/H2 receptor involvement. Asthmatic (A) and nonasthmatic (NA) confluent serum-deprived ASM cells were left untreated or treated with the H1 or H2 receptor antagonists chlorpheniramine and ranitidine, respectively, for 45 minutes prior to and during stimulation with IL-1β or TNF-α. After 4 or 24 h stimulation cells were lysed and CXCL10 mRNA levels were measured using real-time RT PCR or CXCL10 in the culture medium quantified using ELISA, respectively. $^{*}P < 0.05$ compared with (a) unstimulated cells (unstim) or (b) and (c) the cytokine control, ANOVA.

(Figure 5(b)). To investigate whether this effect was due to MC protease activity affecting early events leading to CXCL10 production or affecting CXCL10 after new gene transcription had commenced, leupeptin (50 μM) was added at two different steps. Leupeptin inhibited the effects of the MC 2 h SN irrespective of whether the SN were treated with it before they were added to the ASM cells (0 h), or it was added to the ASM cultures 3 hours after the SN (3 h) (Figure 5(c)). When the CXCL10 capture antibody was incubated with the MC 2 h SN there was no effect as detection of human recombinant CXCL10 in the ELISA remained the same as with the vehicle-treated and untreated capture antibody controls (data not shown).

In contrast, the MC 24 h SN increased asthmatic and non-asthmatic ASM cell IFNγ-induced CXCL10 release. The MC 24 h SN at 20% and 40% v/v significantly increased IFNγ-induced CXCL10 release from asthmatic cells up to 157 ± 28% and 137 ± 16% and from non-asthmatic cells up to 155 ± 22% and 170 ± 32% of the FBS-IFNγ control, respectively (Figure 6(a)). As TNF-α acts synergistically with IFNγ to increase CXCL10 production, the levels of TNF-α in MC SN were quantified. The MC 2 h and 24 h SN contained TNF-α at 227 ±

79 and 434 ± 87 pg/mL, respectively (Figure 6(b)). TNF-α over those concentrations increased ASM cell IFNγ-induced CXCL10 release by ≥5fold (Figure 6(c)).

4. Discussion

In asthma, the ASM produces the chemokine CXCL10 which we have previously shown induces MC chemotaxis through CXCR3 engagement [17]. CXCL10 may also mediate CXCR3^{+}T lymphocyte recruitment to the ASM in severe asthma and following allergen challenge [25]. Thus CXCL10 may be critical in asthma because it can induce airway myositis. This is the first study to examine the effects of MC products on CXCL10 production by ASM cells from people with and without asthma. The effects of individual granule-derived MC products and all the products released by human lung MC in the first 2 or 2–24 hours following IgE receptor activation were investigated. The key granule-derived product histamine reduced ASM cell CXCL10 release induced by the proinflammatory cytokines IL-1β and TNF-α. As well, the proteolytic activity of tryptase, or the leupeptin-sensitive serine proteases released by human lung MC within

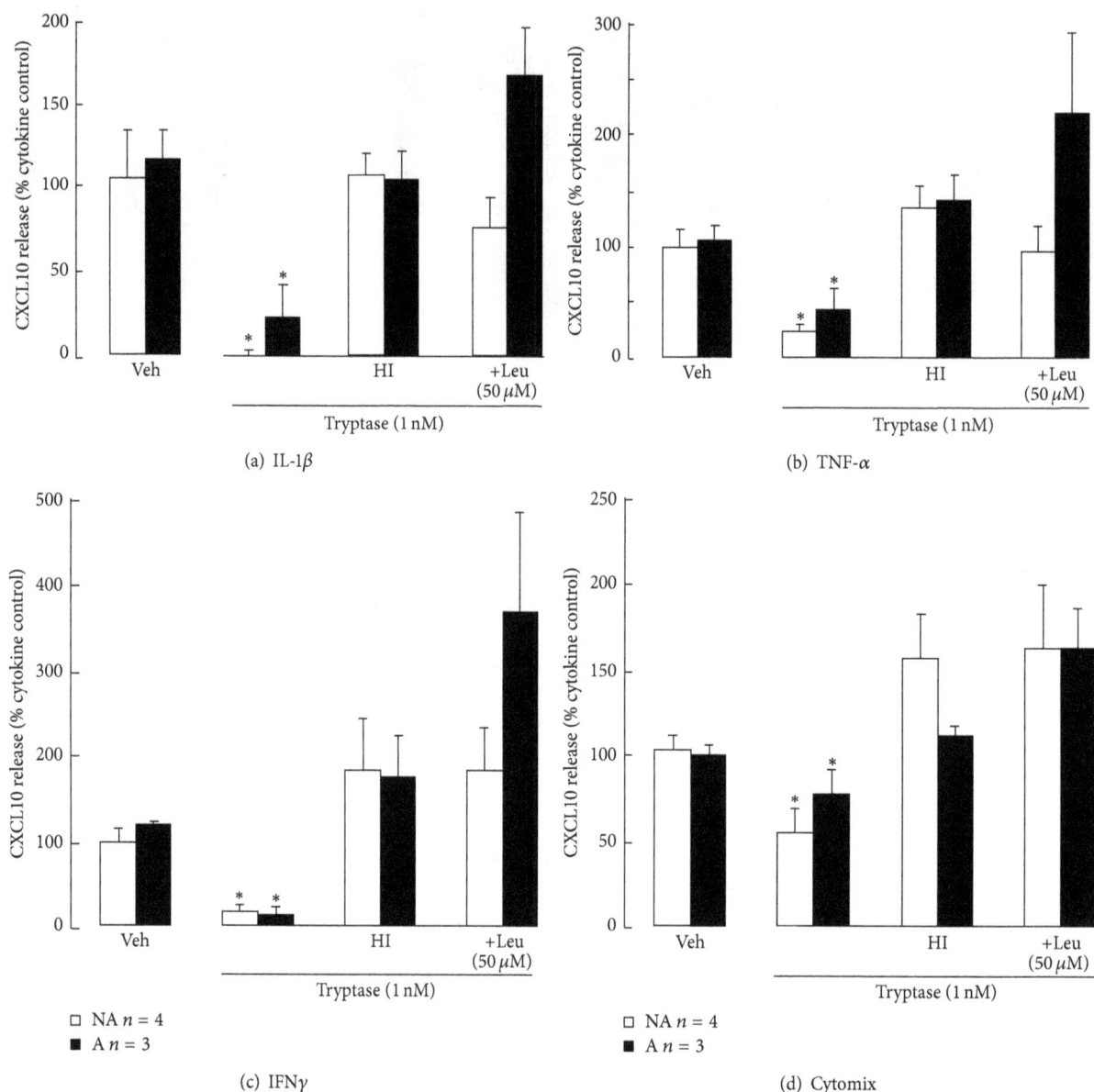

FIGURE 3: The proteolytic effects of tryptase on cytokine-induced CXCL10 production by asthmatic (A) and non-asthmatic (NA) ASM cells. Confluent serum-deprived ASM cells were stimulated with (a) IL-1β, (b) TNFα, (c) IFNγ, or (d) cytomixfor 30 minutes prior to and during treatment with tryptase, heat-inactivated tryptase (HI), or its vehicle (veh) for 24 h. Leupeptin (Leu) was added to some cell cultures 3 h after the cytokines. CXCL10 in the culture supernatants was detected using ELISA. $^*P < 0.05$ compared with the vehicle control, ANOVA.

two hours of activation, markedly reduced CXCL10 levels released following ASM cell cytokine stimulation. In contrast, human lung MC products synthesised and released later increased ASM CXCL10 release and levels of human lung MC-derived TNF-α were sufficient to amplify IFNγ-induced CXCL10 production. These findings are evidence that mast cells are able to regulate ASM cell CXCL10 production and degradation and thus may regulate their own and/or T cell recruitment to the ASM in asthma.

Following MC activation histamine, along with other products also stored in the granules, is released rapidly (reviewed in [10]). Histamine has a very broad spectrum of activities and histamine levels are high in the bronchoalveolar

lavage fluid of people with asthma and correlate with airway hyperresponsiveness [26]. The contractile effects of histamine on ASM are well characterised and mediated via its H1 and H2 receptors, which are highly expressed on ASM. Histamine binding to the H1 receptor primarily activates phospholipase C-inositol triphosphate-diacylglycerol signalling and leads to Ca^{2+} release from intracellular stores and protein kinase C activation, both of which can also upregulate cAMP [27]. Signalling via H2 receptors activates adenylate cyclase to directly generate cyclic adenosine monophosphate (cAMP), but H2 receptors are also coupled to the phosphoinositide system [27]. Through the H1 receptor, histamine can also activate NFκB [28, 29] and thus might be expected to

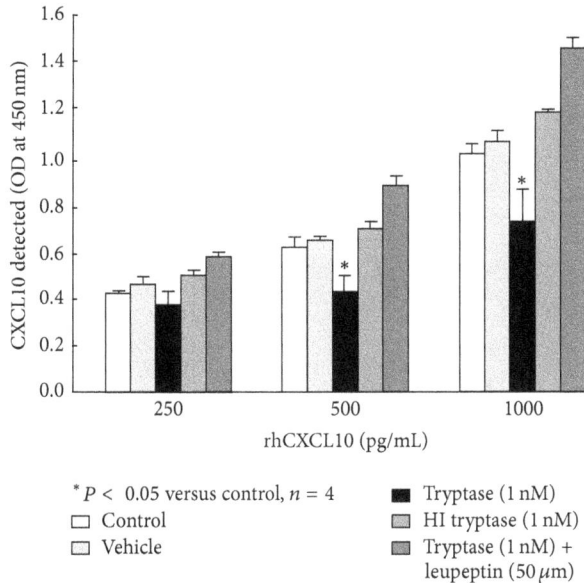

FIGURE 4: The proteolytic effects of tryptase on rhCXCL10 in a cell free system. The rhCXCL10 made up in serum-free DMEM supplemented with 0.1% BSA was placed in 96-well culture plates and incubated with tryptase ± leupeptin, heat-inactivated tryptase (HI), or its vehicle for 24 h under the same conditions as the ASM cells. CXCL10 was detected using ELISA. $^*P < 0.05$ compared with the vehicle control, ANOVA.

enhance proinflammatory gene transcription. Histamine also modulates the activity of the coactivator cAMP response element-binding protein (CREB/CBP) to mediate some of its effects on gene expression [30, 31]. However in this study histamine reduced IL-1β- and TNF-α-induced CXCL10 release, but not gene expression, which is mediated via the transcription factor NFκB [18, 32]. Neither the H1 nor the H2 receptor antagonists chlorpheniramine and ranitidine, respectively, prevented the inhibition of CXCL10 release.

Nevertheless, differences in transcriptional pathways following ASM cell stimulation with the individual cytokines and cytomix may contribute to the differential effects of histamine indirectly. In contrast to ASM CXCL10 production induced by IL-1β and TNF-α, IFNγ-induced production was not affected by histamine. Although Smith et al. [33] demonstrated that IFNγ, but not TNF-α, significantly increases histamine-induced inositol-phosphate signalling and H1R mRNA expression, those IFNγ effects do not match with the observations reported here. IFNγ activates the JAK$_2$-STAT-1 pathway predominantly and NFκB only weakly in non-asthmatic ASM cells to induce CXCL10 production [34]. As observed here and previously [18, 34], IFNγ synergistically increases CXCL10 production when used with IL-1β and/or TNF-α, but Clarke et al. [34] did not observe any effects on NFκB or STAT-1 activation and DNA binding. Rather they found that the combined cytokines synergistically increase the recruitment of CREB binding protein (CBP) and RNA polymerase II to the CXCL10 promoter. Such IFNγ-induced increases in CREB binding to the CXCL10 promoter may overwhelm any inhibitory effects of histamine. Further, we

have observed in asthmatic compared with non-asthmatic ASM cells that NFκB activation is stronger and STAT-1 activation is weaker in response to the three cytokines combined (cytomix) [35], which may underlie the small inhibitory effect of histamine in the non-asthmatic ASM cells. Interestingly CXCL10 production induced by IFNγ or cytomix is also not inhibited by current asthma therapies such as fluticasone and/or salmeterol, whereas IL-1β- and TNF-α-induced release is markedly reduced by these agents [34, 36].

Histamine and cytokines may have opposing effects on intracellular (Ca^{2+}) levels in human ASM cells. Mitochondria buffer cytosolic (Ca^{2+}) levels [37] and histamine causes a rapid increase in both cytosolic and mitochondrial (Ca^{2+}) levels. Whereas TNF-α decreases mitochondrial (Ca^{2+}) levels through the mitochondrial Na$^+$/Ca^{2+} exchanger, while increasing cytosolic (Ca^{2+}) levels [37]. As indicated above, TNF-α also induces NFκB mediated CXCL10 gene transcription [18, 32], whereas histamine does not. NFκB mediated gene transcription is inhibited by SERCA pump inhibition [38], including CXCL10 production, especially in asthmatic ASM cells [35]. If histamine modulated TNF-α-induced changes in mitochondrial and cytosolic (Ca^{2+}) levels to limit ASM cell CXCL10 production, reduced CXCL10 mRNA levels in histamine-treated cells would have been observed in this study but they were not.

The lack of effect of the H1 and H2 receptor antagonists was surprising in view of our previous findings. Firstly, chlorpheniramine prevented histamine-induced changes in ASM cell GM-CSF and RANTES release following stimulation by IL-1β or TNF-α [15]. Secondly, the long acting β_2-adrenoceptor agonist salmeterol which, like histamine, increases cAMP levels also inhibited ASM cell CXCL10 release induced by these cytokines [36]. Further, the effects of histamine appeared to be posttranscriptional, as cytokine-induced CXCL10 gene expression was not affected. Posttranscriptional effects of histamine on keratinocytes have been reported but were mediated via the H1 receptor [39]. To our knowledge, H3 receptors are expressed on cholinergic nerves, but not ASM in the airways [40]. Gantner and colleagues [41] used specific primers for receptors H1-4 and detected mRNA expression for H1, H2, and H4 receptors, but not for H3 receptors. Perhaps the indirect inhibitory effects of histamine observed in this study were mediated via the Gi/o coupled H4 receptors. H4 receptors play an important role in the regulation of immune responses, including chemokine production, in the skin [42] and so might also regulate ASM cell chemokine production. Further studies of cytokine-stimulated ASM cell CXL10 production in the presence of histamine are needed to determine the molecular mechanisms underlying its effects and histamine receptor involvement. Recently developed selective agonists (e.g., 4-methylhistamine) and antagonists (e.g., JNJ7777120) for H4 receptors would be useful to clarify its role [43].

ASM cells also express the organic cation transporter 3 (OCT3 or EMT) in addition to histamine receptors [44]. Histamine is a good substrate for OCT3 [45] and so it is possible that histamine entered the ASM cells stimulated with IL-1β and TNF-α via OCT 3 and affected posttranscriptional

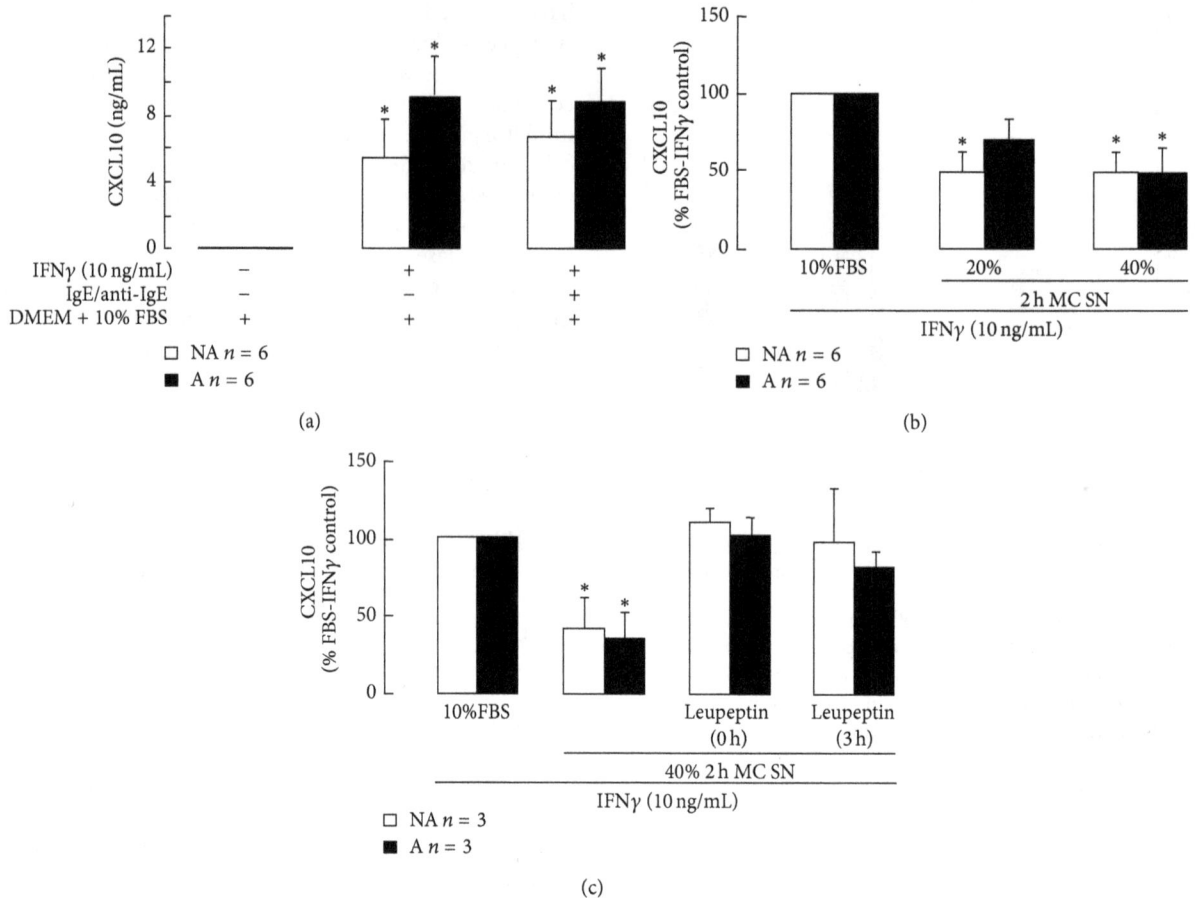

FIGURE 5: The effects of human lung mast cell products released early after activation on asthmatic (A) and non-asthmatic (NA) ASM cell CXCL10 production. Mast cells (MC) were isolated from human lung and immediately activated with IgE/anti-IgE in culture medium (DMEM + 10% FBS) and the culture supernatants collected after 2 hours (2 h MC SN). The MC SN were added at 20% and 40% v/v to ASM cells stimulated with IFNγ and CXCL10 levels were quantified after 48 hours stimulation using ELISA. $^*P < 0.05$ compared with the DMEM + 10% FBS control (a) or FBS-IFNγ control ((b) and (c)), ANOVA.

events involved in CXCL10 protein synthesis/release. Further studies are needed to investigate the above possibilities and the mechanisms involved in any effects of histamine.

Importantly, this study is the first demonstration that CXCL10 is susceptible to digestion by serine proteases such as tryptase. The levels of CXCL10 released following cytokine stimulation were reduced by tryptase, which is stored in the granules as a tetrameric complex with proteoglycans such as heparin and released at the same time as histamine. Unlike histamine, tryptase reduced detectable CXCL10 levels irrespective of the individual cytokine used to stimulate the ASM cells. This effect was due to tryptase protease activity as it was prevented by heat-inactivation and the serine protease inhibitor leupeptin. Further it was likely due, at least in part, to direct tryptase proteolysis of CXCL10, as tryptase reduced the levels of CXCL10 detected in a cell-free system. In addition, leupeptin added 3 h after any of the cytokines, when there is already a substantial increase in CXCL10 mRNA expression [18], completely prevented the reduction in cytokine-induced CXCL10 levels. These findings add CXCL10 to the chemokines CCL11 (eotaxin) and CCL5 (RANTES) that are also produced by ASM cells and cleaved

by tryptase *in vitro* [13] or by ASM cell cocullture with MC [46].

Although other studies have investigated the effect of MC products individually on ASM cell synthetic function as above, this is the first study to also examine the overall effects of MC products released at different times after MC activation on asthmatic and non-asthmatic ASM cell CXCL10 production. As ASM cells do not release CXCL10 constitutively, or in response to FBS, IFNγ was used to induce CXCL10 release so the effects of the MC products on it could be assessed. The effects of rapidly released human lung MC products (2 h SN) on ASM cell CXCL10 levels complement the effects obtained with tryptase. Early MC products reduced asthmatic and non-asthmatic ASM cell IFNγ-induced CXCL10 levels by a similar amount. These effects were also prevented by leupeptin added later, indicating that serine proteases were involved, but do not affect early CXCL10 gene transcription.

As well, a role for histamine cannot be completely dismissed. MC supernatants generated in the manner used here contain significant amounts of histamine [47], which would have been ineffective against the IFNγ-induced CXCL10 production used in this study. Early release of histamine

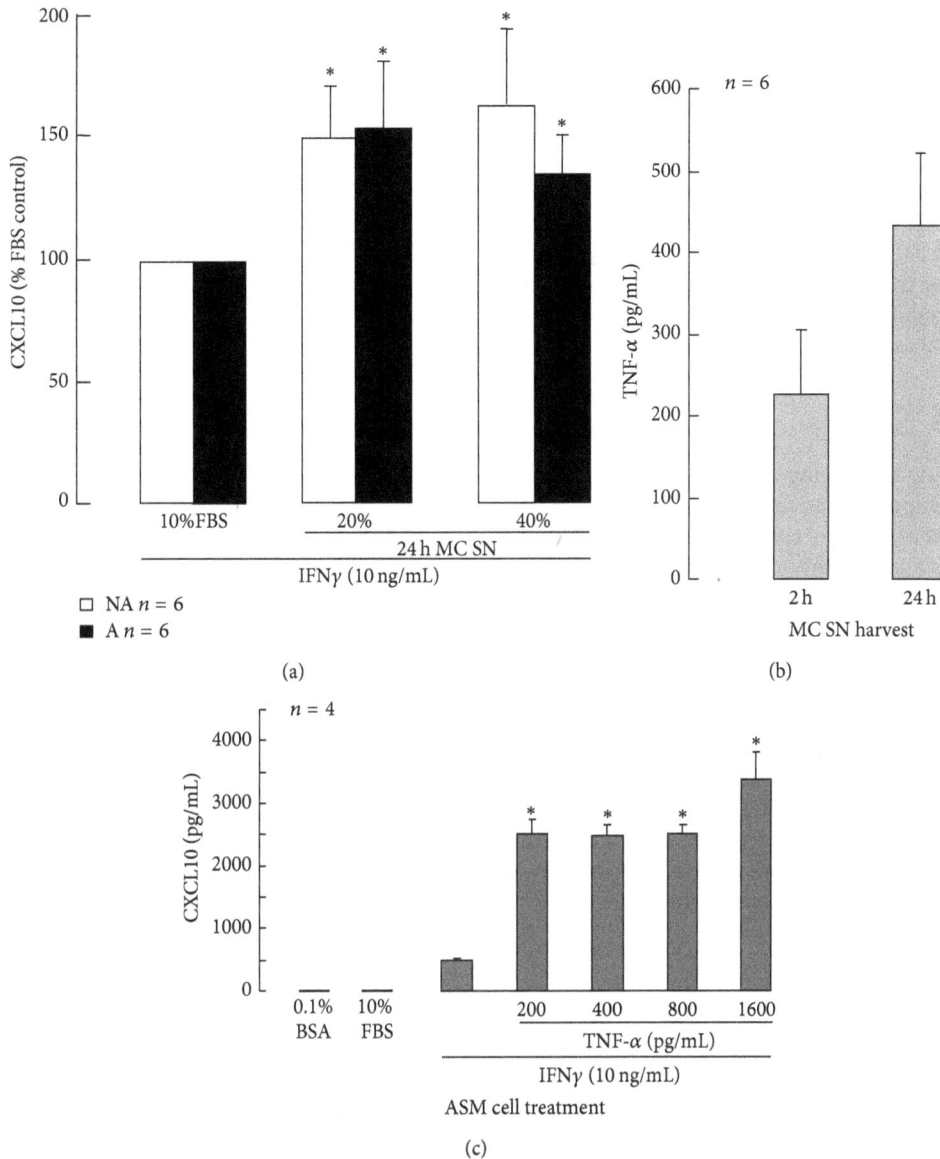

FIGURE 6: The effects of human lung mast cell products released later after activation (2–24 h) on asthmatic (A) and non-asthmatic (NA) ASM cell CXCL10 production. Mast cells (MC) were isolated from human lung and immediately activated with IgE/anti-IgE in culture medium (DMEM + 10% FBS). After 2 hours the culture supernatants were collected (2 h MC SN) and replaced by fresh medium. Further supernatants were collected at 24 hours (24 h MC SN). The 24 h MC SN were added at 20% and 40% v/v to IFNγ-stimulated ASM cells and after 48 hours CXCL10 levels were quantified using ELISA (a). TNF-α levels in the 2 h and 24 h MC SN were quantified using ELISA (b) and the effects of these low concentrations of TNF-α on IFNγ-induced CXCL10 production by ASM cells in DMEM + 10% FBS quantified (c). $^{*}P < 0.05$ compared with the DMEM + 10% FBS control ((a) and (c)), ANOVA.

may limit CXCL10 production generated under different inflammatory conditions when IFNγ is absent.

In contrast to the effects of the MC products released early, newly synthesised products released sometime later (24 h SN) increased IFNγ-induced CXCL10 levels. Again the proportional effects of the MC products on ASM cells from people with and without asthma were similar. MC produce TNF-α [48], which synergistically increases IFNγ-induced CXCL10 production by ASM cells *in vitro* [18, 32, 34]. This study has extended those findings by providing evidence that products released from human lung MC activated by IgE

also increase CXCL10 release and include sufficient TNF-α to cause such an increase. Although TNF-α levels in MC SN collected early were half those in the SN collected later, they were still sufficient to amplify IFNγ-induced CXCL10 release. However no increase was observed, probably because the granule-derived proteases present in the SN cleaved the CXCL10 after it was released and thus reduced the amount of protein detected.

In this study, the effects of MC products released together, either early or later, after IgE receptor activation were examined *in vitro* on ASM cells obtained from people with and without asthma. The MC could only be isolated from larger lung samples as they became available and were all from people without asthma. The effects of MC from people with asthma on asthmatic ASM cell CXCL10 production may be different. However different percentages of the MC SN were used to reflect what occurs *in vivo*, where activated MC are present in the ASM layer in different numbers in asthma [4, 5, 7]. Thus not all ASM cells are in direct contact with a MC, but they have been observed in close proximity to each other [6, 7]. Given this proximity, it is apparent from our study that MC products could still affect ASM chemokine production in the absence of cell-cell contact.

5. Conclusions

This is the first study to examine the effects of MC products on CXCL10 production by ASM cells. Activated MC numbers are increased in the ASM in eosinophilic asthma and T-lymphocytes are present in the ASM in severe asthma and following allergen challenge. ASM-derived CXCL10 production may play a role in the recruitment of these cells to the ASM as both cell types express the CXCL10 receptor receptor CXCR3. In this study we have demonstrated that MC products released from granules soon after cell activation, or newly synthesized and then released later, differentially modulated levels of CXCL10 released by ASM cells from donors with and without asthma. Thus mast cells in the ASM have the potential to up- and downregulate chemokine levels locally and thereby affect their own recruitment and that of other inflammatory cells to the ASM in asthma.

Conflict of Interests

The authors declare that there is no conflict of interests regarding the publication of this paper.

Acknowledgments

The authors acknowledge the collaborative effort of the SSWAHS Theatre and Pathology Staff, Dr. M. Baraket and Associate Professor G. King (Woolcock Institute of Medical Research, Sydney), Professor I. Young (Royal Prince Alfred Hospital, Sydney), the Cardiopulmonary Transplant Team at St. Vincent's Hospital, and their RRG colleagues who helped with lung sample/biopsy collection. This study was funded by project grants from the NHMRC of Australia.

References

[1] M. Saetta and G. Turato, "Airway pathology in asthma," *European Respiratory Journal*, vol. 18, no. 34, pp. 18s–23s, 2001.

[2] P. Bradding, A. F. Walls, and S. T. Holgate, "The role of the mast cell in the pathophysiology of asthma," *Journal of Allergy and Clinical Immunology*, vol. 117, no. 6, pp. 1277–1284, 2006.

[3] J. Bousquet, P. K. Jeffery, W. W. Busse, M. Johnson, and A. M. Vignola, "Asthma: from bronchoconstriction to airways inflammation and remodeling," *The American Journal of Respiratory and Critical Care Medicine*, vol. 161, no. 5, pp. 1720–1745, 2000.

[4] N. G. Carroll, S. Mutavdzic, and A. L. James, "Distribution and degranulation of airway mast cells in normal and asthmatic subjects," *European Respiratory Journal*, vol. 19, no. 5, pp. 879–885, 2002.

[5] K. Amin, C. Janson, G. Boman, and P. Venge, "The extracellular deposition of mast cell products is increased in hypertrophic airways smooth muscles in allergic asthma but not in nonallergic asthma," *Allergy*, vol. 60, no. 10, pp. 1241–1247, 2005.

[6] H. Begueret, P. Berger, J.-M. Vernejoux, L. Dubuisson, R. Marthan, and J. M. Tunon-De-Lara, "Inflammation of bronchial smooth muscle in allergic asthma," *Thorax*, vol. 62, no. 1, pp. 8–15, 2007.

[7] C. E. Brightling, P. Bradding, F. A. Symon, S. T. Holgate, A. J. Wardlaw, and I. D. Pavord, "Mast-cell infiltration of airway smooth muscle in asthma," *New England Journal of Medicine*, vol. 346, no. 22, pp. 1699–1705, 2002.

[8] S. Balzar, M. L. Fajt, S. A. A. Comhair et al., "Mast cell phenotype, location, and activation in severe asthma: data from the Severe Asthma Research Program," *The American Journal of Respiratory and Critical Care Medicine*, vol. 183, no. 3, pp. 299–309, 2011.

[9] I. G. Reischl, W. R. Coward, and M. K. Church, "Molecular consequences of human mast cell activation following immunoglobulin E-high-affinity immunoglobulin E receptor (IgE-FcεRI) interaction," *Biochemical Pharmacology*, vol. 58, no. 12, pp. 1841–1850, 1999.

[10] S. Page, A. J. Ammit, J. L. Black, and C. L. Armour, "Human mast cell and airway smooth muscle cell interactions: implications for asthma," *The American Journal of Physiology—Lung Cellular and Molecular Physiology*, vol. 281, no. 6, pp. L1313–L1323, 2001.

[11] O. Ghaffar, Q. Hamid, P. M. Renzi et al., "Constitutive and cytokine-stimulated expression of eotaxin by human airway smooth muscle cells," *The American Journal of Respiratory and Critical Care Medicine*, vol. 159, no. 6, pp. 1933–1942, 1999.

[12] S. J. Hirst, M. P. Hallsworth, Q. Peng, and T. H. Lee, "Selective induction of eotaxin release by interleukin-13 or interleukin-4 in human airway smooth muscle cells is synergistic with interleukin-1β and is mediated by the interleukin-4 receptor α-chain," *The American Journal of Respiratory and Critical Care Medicine*, vol. 165, no. 8, pp. 1161–1171, 2002.

[13] L. Pang, M. Nie, L. Corbett, A. Sutcliffe, and A. J. Knox, "Mast cell β-tryptase selectively cleaves eotaxin and RANTES and abrogates their eosinophil chemotactic activities," *Journal of Immunology*, vol. 176, no. 6, pp. 3788–3795, 2006.

[14] H. Alkhouri, F. Hollins, L. M. Moir, C. E. Brightling, C. L. Armour, and J. M. Hughes, "Human lung mast cells modulate the functions of airway smooth muscle cells in asthma," *Allergy*, vol. 66, no. 9, pp. 1231–1241, 2011.

[15] J. Chhabra, Y.-Z. Li, H. Alkhouri et al., "Histamine and tryptase modulate asthmatic airway smooth muscle GM-CSF and RANTES release," *European Respiratory Journal*, vol. 29, no. 5, pp. 861–870, 2007.

[16] C. E. Brightling, D. Kaur, P. Berger, A. J. Morgan, A. J. Wardlaw, and P. Bradding, "Differential expression of CCR3 and CXCR3 by human lung and bone marrow-derived mast cells: implications for tissue mast cell migration," *Journal of Leukocyte Biology*, vol. 77, no. 5, pp. 759–766, 2005.

[17] C. E. Brightling, A. J. Ammit, D. Kaur et al., "The CXCL10/CXCR3 axis mediates human lung mast cell migration to asthmatic airway smooth muscle," *The American Journal of Respiratory and Critical Care Medicine*, vol. 171, no. 10, pp. 1103–1108, 2005.

[18] Y. Alrashdan, H. Alkhouri, E. Chen et al., "Asthmatic airway smooth muscle CXCL10 production: mitogen-activated protein kinase JNK involvement," *The American Journal of Physiology—Lung Cellular and Molecular Physiology*, vol. 302, pp. L1118–L1127, 2012.

[19] M. B. Sukkar, A. J. Stanley, A. E. Blake et al., "'Proliferative' and "synthetic" airway smooth muscle cells are overlapping populations," *Immunology and Cell Biology*, vol. 82, no. 5, pp. 471–478, 2004.

[20] H. Marsumoto, L. M. Moir, B. G. G. Oliver et al., "Comparison of gel contraction mediated by airway smooth muscle cells from patients with and without asthma," *Thorax*, vol. 62, no. 10, pp. 848–854, 2007.

[21] L. M. Ruck, C. A. Rizzo, J. C. Anthes et al., "Synergistic antiallergic activity of combined histamine H_1- and cysteinyl leukotrienel-receptor blockade in human bronchus," *Life Sciences*, vol. 68, no. 25, pp. 2825–2834, 2001.

[22] D. A. Knight, G. A. Stewart, and P. J. Thompson, "Histamine tachyphylaxis in human airway smooth muscle: the role of H_2-receptors and the bronchial epithelium," *The American Review of Respiratory Disease*, vol. 146, no. 1, pp. 137–140, 1992.

[23] P. Chomczynski and N. Sacchi, "Single-step method of RNA isolation by acid guanidinium thiocyanate-phenol-chloroform extraction," *Analytical Biochemistry*, vol. 162, no. 1, pp. 156–159, 1987.

[24] A. Sutcliffe, D. Kaur, S. Page et al., "Mast cell migration to Th2 stimulated airway smooth muscle from asthmatics," *Thorax*, vol. 61, no. 8, pp. 657–662, 2006.

[25] D. Ramos-Barbón, R. Fraga-Iriso, N. S. Brienza et al., "T cells localize with proliferating smooth muscle α-actin+ cell compartments in asthma," *The American Journal of Respiratory and Critical Care Medicine*, vol. 182, no. 3, pp. 317–324, 2010.

[26] N. N. Jarjour, W. J. Calhoun, L. B. Schwartz, and W. W. Busse, "Elevated bronchoalveolar lavage fluid histamine levels in allergic asthmatics are associated with increased airway obstruction," *The American Review of Respiratory Disease*, vol. 144, no. 1, pp. 83–87, 1991.

[27] S. J. Hill, C. R. Ganellin, H. Timmerman et al., "International union of pharmacology. XIII. Classification of histamine receptors," *Pharmacological Reviews*, vol. 49, no. 3, pp. 253–278, 1997.

[28] M. Dy and E. Schneider, "Histamine-cytokine connection in immunity and hematopoiesis," *Cytokine and Growth Factor Reviews*, vol. 15, no. 5, pp. 393–410, 2004.

[29] R. A. Bakker, S. B. J. Schoonus, J. Smit, H. Timmerman, and R. Leurs, "Histamine H_1-receptor activation of nuclear factor-kappaB: roles for Gbeta gamma- and Galpha(/11)-subunits in constitutive and agonist-mediated signalling," *Molecular Pharmacology*, vol. 60, pp. 1133–1142, 2001.

[30] D. Zocco, J. P. McMorrow, and E. P. Murphy, "Histamine modulation of peripheral CRH receptor type 1α expression is dependent on Ca^{2+} signalling and NF-κB/p65 transcriptional activity," *Molecular Immunology*, vol. 47, no. 7-8, pp. 1426–1437, 2010.

[31] K. Hegyi, A. Falus, and S. Toth, "Elevated CREB activity in embryonic fibroblasts of gene-targeted histamine deficient mice," *Inflammation Research*, vol. 56, no. 8, pp. 339–344, 2007.

[32] E. L. Hardaker, A. M. Bacon, K. Carlson et al., "Regulation of TNF-alpha- and IFN-gamma-induced CXCL10 expression: participation of the airway smooth muscle in the pulmonary inflammatory response in chronic obstructive pulmonary disease," *The FASEB Journal*, vol. 18, no. 1, pp. 191–193, 2004.

[33] N. Smith, C. A. Browning, N. Duroudier et al., "Salmeterol and cytokines modulate inositol-phosphate signalling in Human airway smooth muscle cells via regulation at the receptor locus," *Respiratory Research*, vol. 8, article 68, 2007.

[34] D. L. Clarke, R. L. Clifford, S. Jindarat et al., "TNFα and IFNγ synergistically enhance transcriptional activation of CXCL10 in human airway smooth muscle cells via STAT-1, NF-κB, and the transcriptional coactivator CREB-binding protein," *Journal of Biological Chemistry*, vol. 285, no. 38, pp. 29101–29110, 2010.

[35] X. Tan, Y. A. Alrashdan, H. Alkhouri, B. G. G. Oliver, C. l. Armour, and J. M. Hughes, "Airway smooth muscle CXCR3 ligand production: regulation by JAK-STAT1 and intracellular calcium," *The American Journal of Physiology—Lung Cellular and Molecular Physiology*, vol. 304, pp. L790–L802, 2013.

[36] P. Seidel, H. Alkhouri, D. J. Lalor, J. K. Burgess, C. L. Armour, and J. M. Hughes, "Thiazolidinediones inhibit airway smooth muscle release of the chemokine CXCL10: in vitro comparison with current asthma therapies," *Respiratory Research*, vol. 13, article 90, 2012.

[37] P. F. Delmotte, B. Yang, M. A. Thompson, C. M. Pabelick, Y. S. Prakash, and G. C. Sieck, "Inflammation alters regional mitochondrial calcium in human airway smooth muscle cells," *The American Journal of Physiology—Cell Physiology*, vol. 303, pp. C244–C256, 2012.

[38] Y. Amrani, A. L. Lazaar, R. Hoffman, K. Amin, S. Ousmer, and R. A. Panettieri Jr., "Activation of p55 tumor necrosis factor-α receptor-1 coupled to tumor necrosis factor receptor-associated factor 2 stimulates intercellular adhesion molecule-1 expression by modulating a thapsigargin-sensitive pathway in human tracheal smooth muscle cells," *Molecular Pharmacology*, vol. 58, no. 1, pp. 237–245, 2000.

[39] N. Kanda and S. Watanabe, "Histamine enhances the production of granulocyte-macrophage colony-stimulating factor via protein kinase Cα and extracellular signal-regulated kinase in human keratinocytes," *Journal of Investigative Dermatology*, vol. 122, no. 4, pp. 863–872, 2004.

[40] M. Ichinose and P. J. Barnes, "Inhibitory histamine H_3-receptors on cholinergic nerves in human airways," *European Journal of Pharmacology*, vol. 163, no. 2-3, pp. 383–386, 1989.

[41] F. Gantner, K. Sakai, M. W. Tusche, W. W. Cruikshank, D. M. Center, and K. B. Bacon, "Histamine H_4 and H_2 receptors control histamine-induced interleukin-16 release from human CD8+ T cells," *Journal of Pharmacology and Experimental Therapeutics*, vol. 303, no. 1, pp. 300–307, 2002.

[42] C. A. Akdis, "Immune regulation by histamine H_4 receptors in skin," *Journal of Investigative Dermatology*, vol. 128, no. 7, pp. 1615–1616, 2008.

[43] H. D. Lim, R. M. Van Rijn, P. Ling, R. A. Bakker, R. L. Thurmond, and R. Leurs, "Evaluation of histamine H_1-, H_2-, and H_3-receptor ligands at the human histamine H_4 receptor: identification of 4-methylhistamine as the first potent and selective H 4 receptor agonist," *Journal of Pharmacology and Experimental Therapeutics*, vol. 314, no. 3, pp. 1310–1321, 2005.

[44] G. Horvath, E. S. Mendes, N. Schmid et al., "The effect of corticosteroids on the disposal of long-acting β2-agonists by airway smooth muscle cells," *Journal of Allergy and Clinical Immunology*, vol. 120, no. 5, pp. 1103–1109, 2007.

[45] D. Gründemann, G. Liebich, N. Kiefer, S. Köster, and E. Schömig, "Selective substrates for non-neuronal monoamine transporters," *Molecular Pharmacology*, vol. 56, no. 1, pp. 1–10, 1999.

[46] R. Saunders, A. Sutcliffe, L. Woodman et al., "The airway smooth muscle CCR3/CCL11 axis is inhibited by mast cells," *Allergy*, vol. 63, no. 9, pp. 1148–1155, 2008.

[47] F. Hollins, D. Kaur, W. Yang et al., "Human airway smooth muscle promotes human lung mast cell survival, proliferation, and constitutive activation: cooperative roles for CADM1, stem cell factor, and IL-6," *Journal of Immunology*, vol. 181, no. 4, pp. 2772–2780, 2008.

[48] Y. Ohkawara, K. Yamauchi, Y. Tanno et al., "Human lung mast cells and pulmonary macrophages produce tumor necrosis factor-alpha in sensitized lung tissue after IgE receptor triggering," *The American Journal of Respiratory Cell and Molecular Biology*, vol. 7, no. 4, pp. 385–392, 1992.

24

Apgar Score Is Related to Development of Atopic Dermatitis: Cotwin Control Study

Vibeke Naeser,[1] Niklas Kahr,[1] Lone Graff Stensballe,[2] Kirsten Ohm Kyvik,[3] Axel Skytthe,[4] Vibeke Backer,[1] Charlotte Giwercman Carson,[5] and Simon Francis Thomsen[6]

[1] *Department of Respiratory Medicine, Bispebjerg Hospital, 2400 Copenhagen, Denmark*
[2] *Danish Epidemiology Science Centre, Statens Serum Institut, 2300 Copenhagen, Denmark*
[3] *Institute of Regional Health Services Research & Odense Patient Data Explorative Network,*
  University of Southern Denmark, 5000 Odense, Denmark
[4] *The Danish Twin Registry, University of Southern Denmark, 5000 Odense, Denmark*
[5] *Danish Pediatric Asthma Center, Gentofte Hospital, 2900 Hellerup, Denmark*
[6] *Department of Dermato-Allergology, Gentofte Hospital, 2900 Hellerup, Denmark*

Correspondence should be addressed to Simon Francis Thomsen; sft@city.dk

Academic Editor: S. L. Johnston

Aim. To study the impact of birth characteristics on the risk of atopic dermatitis in a twin population. *Methods.* In a population-based questionnaire study of 10,809 twins, 3–9 years of age, from the Danish Twin Registry, we identified 907 twin pairs discordant for parent-reported atopic dermatitis. We cross-linked with data from the Danish National Birth Registry and performed cotwin control analysis in order to test the impact of birth characteristics on the risk of atopic dermatitis. *Results.* Apgar score, OR (per unit) = 1.23 (1.06–1.44), $P = 0.008$, and female sex, OR = 1.31 (1.06–1.61), $P = 0.012$, were risk factors for atopic dermatitis in cotwin control analysis, whereas birth anthropometric factors were not significantly related to disease development. Risk estimates in monozygotic and dizygotic twins were not significantly different for the identified risk factors. *Conclusions.* In this population-based cotwin control study, high Apgar score was a risk factor for atopic dermatitis. This novel finding must be confirmed in subsequent studies.

1. Introduction

Atopic dermatitis is a chronic relapsing skin disease with a lifetime prevalence of around 20%. The disease has an early onset with 60% being affected during the first year of life and 85% before the age of five [1]. Atopic dermatitis is characterized by recurrent episodes of itching and eczema occurring at typical sites such as the face and extensor aspects of the arms and legs in early childhood, flexures in later childhood, and head and neck as well as the hands in adulthood. Atopic dermatitis is highly heritable and individual susceptibility to the disease is attributable particularly to mutations in the filaggrin gene [2], although other genetic variants [3] as well as environmental factors have been implicated. Previous studies have shown that the prevalence

of atopic dermatitis has increased both in developed [4, 5] and developing countries [6] in recent years, but the causes for this increase are still poorly understood.

The onset of atopic dermatitis early in life implies that risk factors for the disease exert their effect already in utero or in very early childhood. However, previous studies of the association between perinatal factors and the risk of atopic dermatitis are conflicting. With regard to alcohol intake during pregnancy, results indicate an increased risk for atopic dermatitis in children of mothers who consume alcohol during pregnancy [7, 8]. Contrary to this, smoking during pregnancy has been inversely related to development of atopic dermatitis in the offspring [9, 10]. The association between exclusive breastfeeding/increased duration of breastfeeding and atopic dermatitis varies; while some studies show a positive association [11] others show a negative [12] or no [13] association. Some studies [9, 14] but not all [15] have found that high birth weight increases the risk of atopic dermatitis, whereas other studies have found that a higher gestational age increases the risk of atopic dermatitis [16]. Mallen et al. investigated the association between six birth-related exposures (birth weight, mode of delivery, artificial commencement of labor, prematurity, neonatal intensive care unit admission, and fetal distress) and asthma, allergic rhinitis, eczema, and hay fever in adulthood [17]. No statistically significant association was demonstrated between any of the birth-related exposures and the four allergic conditions studied, although some nonsignificant trends were noted for those born by Caesarean section and those exposed to fetal distress during labor.

The cotwin control study design is a matched case-control study that utilizes twin pairs discordant for an exposure or an outcome. Particularly, because twin pairs are inherently matched on several confounding factors relating to early life and upbringing, this type of study design is ideal to tease out causative relationships in complex diseases. In the present study we use the cotwin control design to identify birth-associated risk factors for atopic dermatitis in twin pairs discordant for the disease.

2. Methods

The study population comprised all live-born twins in Denmark between 1994 and 2000 included in the Danish Twin Registry. In 2003 when the twins were 3–9 years of age the twins' parents responded to a two-page questionnaire concerning atopic diseases, diabetes, febrile and epileptic seizures, and mental health attributes. Atopic dermatitis was diagnosed by the question "has your child ever had eczema in the folds of the elbows or knees?" Zygosity was determined by information regarding the twins' similarity to family, friends, teachers, and relations. This method determines zygosity correctly in more than 95% of the cases compared with genetic marker information [18]. We cross-linked the information from the questionnaire with data from the Danish National Birth Registry where data on birth weight, birth length, maternal smoking during pregnancy, gestational age, mode of delivery (Caesarean section versus vaginal delivery), and Apgar score were obtained.

A total of 10,809 twin subjects participated in the questionnaire study (participation rate 68%). Of these, complete information on atopic dermatitis was available for 5399 intact twin pairs: 850 monozygotic (MZ) twin pairs, 2,279 dizygotic (DZ) twin pairs of the same sex, 1,999 DZ twin pairs of opposite sex, and 271 twin pairs of unknown zygosity. There were 907 twin pairs discordant for atopic dermatitis, and of these 58 and 827 were monozygotic (MZ) and dizygotic (DZ) pairs, respectively.

2.1. Statistical Analysis. First, the relationship between birth-associated risk factors and atopic dermatitis was examined in the whole population using unpaired t-tests and chi-square tests, ignoring the familial relationship between the twins.

Next, the risk factors that were unshared between the twins within the pair were examined in a 1:1 matched conditional logistic regression analysis (cotwin control analysis) in order to determine the effect of these risk factors on atopic dermatitis. The factors entered into this analysis were birth weight, birth length, Apgar score, and sex. The matching was done with the affected (atopic dermatitis) twin in each pair being the case and the unaffected twin being the control. DZ same-sex and DZ opposite-sex twin pairs were considered together in the analysis. The matching of the twins in the cotwin control design allows an inherent adjustment for other factors that would otherwise confound the association between birth factors and atopic dermatitis such as genetic factors, atopic predisposition, maternal smoking during pregnancy, gestational age, mode of delivery, and current age, as well as effects of the rearing environment. Therefore the estimated risk of atopic dermatitis can be assumed to reflect more precisely the influence of birth factors, for example, Apgar score. The following predictions can be made for the cotwin control analysis (Figure 1): if the association between birth factors and atopic dermatitis is mediated via genetics, then we do not expect to find any significant risk of atopic dermatitis among discordant MZ twin pairs, because MZ twins are concordant for early rearing environmental and genetic factors. Alternatively, an increased risk of atopic dermatitis in discordant DZ twin pairs would suggest that genetic factors underlie the association, because DZ twins share the same rearing environment, but only half their genetic variants. Finally, a direct (causal) effect of birth factors, for example, Apgar score, on atopic dermatitis would be suggested by the finding that both discordant MZ and DZ twin pairs are also discordant on, for example, Apgar score, as the association can neither be reflected by environmental nor genetic factors [19]. Data were analyzed with the statistical package SPSS 18.0 (SPSS Inc., Chicago, IL).

3. Results

The proportions of girls and boys in the population were 48.9% and 51.1%, respectively. The mean age was 5.9 years with no difference between girls and boys. The overall prevalence of atopic dermatitis was 14.9%, 14.0% in boys and 16.0% in girls, $P = 0.003$. Increasing birth length ($P = 0.038$), nonsmoking of the mother during pregnancy ($P = 0.002$), and monozygosity (0.012) were also significant predictors for atopic dermatitis in the whole sample when ignoring the familial relationship between the twins (Table 1).

Within twin pairs discordant for atopic dermatitis, the affected twin had, on average, a higher Apgar score and was smaller at birth compared with the unaffected twin (Table 2). In multiple conditional logistic regression comparing the affected with the unaffected twin, Apgar score, OR (per unit) = 1.23 (1.06–1.44), $P = 0.008$, and female sex, OR = 1.31 (1.06–1.61), $P = 0.012$, were significantly predisposing factors for atopic dermatitis, whereas birth anthropometric factors were not significantly related to development of atopic dermatitis. Risk estimates in discordant MZ and DZ twins were not significantly different (Table 3).

TABLE 1: Characteristics of subjects with and without atopic dermatitis in a sample of Danish twin pairs, 3–9 years of age.

	Atopic dermatitis		OR (95% CI)	P value
	Yes N = 1614	No N = 9195		
Birth weight, g	2593	2571	22 (−9–52)	0.167
Birth length, cm	48.24	48.05	0.19 (0.01–0.38)	0.038
Apgar score	9.76	9.73	0.03 (−0.02–0.09)	0.172
Gestational age, days	254.9	254.6	0.32 (−0.61–1.26)	0.496
Caesarean section	14.4	15.3	0.93 (0.84–1.04)	0.220
Maternal smoking	12.9	15.5	0.80 (0.70–0.92)	0.002
Sex				
Boys	14.0	86.0	1.00	
Girls	16.0	84.0	1.17 (1.05–1.30)	0.003
Age, years	5.92	5.86	0.06 (−0.05–0.17)	0.257
Zygosity				
DZ	14.4	85.6	1.00	
MZ	16.8	83.2	1.20 (1.04–1.38)	0.012

Means and proportions are calculated from available data for the individual variables.
OR is mean difference for birth weight, birth length, Apgar score, gestational age, and age.

TABLE 2: Distribution of perinatal risk factors for atopic dermatitis in 907 twin pairs, 3–9 years of age, discordant for atopic dermatitis.

	All twin pairs (n = 907)		MZ twin pairs (n = 58)		DZ twin pairs (n = 827)	
	Affected twins	Unaffected twins	Affected twins	Unaffected twins	Affected twins	Unaffected twins
Birth weight, g	2627	2649	2624	2625	2632	2650
Birth length, cm	48.37	48.41	48.60	48.17	48.40	48.44
Apgar score	9.81	9.68	9.80	9.75	9.80	9.67
Female sex	52.3	47.4	53.4	53.4	53.1	47.8

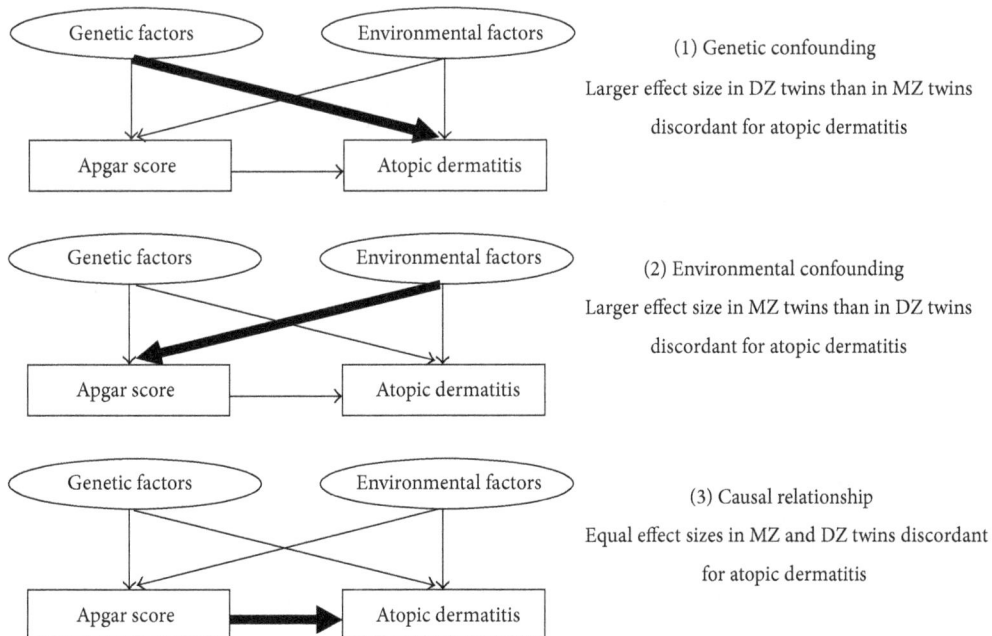

FIGURE 1: Possible association between Apgar score and atopic dermatitis predicted by the cotwin control method.

TABLE 3: Significant risk factors for atopic dermatitis in 907 twin pairs, 3–9 years of age, discordant for atopic dermatitis.

| | All twin pairs | | MZ twin pairs | | DZ twin pairs | | $OR_{MZ} = OR_{DZ}$ |
	OR (95% CI)	P value	OR (95% CI)	P value	OR (95% CI)	P value	P value[1]
Birth weight	1.02 (0.81–1.28)	0.884	0.96 (0.12–7.86)	0.972	0.98 (0.77–1.24)	0.880	NS
Birth length	1.00 (0.08–13.03)	1.00	8.31 (N/A)	0.854	1.62 (0.11–22.01)	0.758	NS
Apgar score	1.23 (1.06–1.44)	0.008	1.19 (0.60–2.34)	0.615	1.21 (1.04–1.42)	0.015	NS
Female sex	1.31 (1.06–1.61)	0.012			1.31 (1.07–1.61)	0.011	NS

Only statistically significant predictors for atopic dermatitis are presented in the table (adjusted for birth weight, birth length).
[1]Test for heterogeneity between odds ratios for MZ and DZ twin pairs.
NS: nonsignificant.

4. Discussion

In this nationwide cohort of Danish twin pairs discordant for atopic dermatitis, a high Apgar score and female sex were significant determinants of atopic dermatitis, whereas birth weight and birth length were not significantly related to disease development.

Apgar score is a clinical test performed on a newborn one and five minutes after birth. It is a composite measure of breathing effort, heart rate, muscle tone, reflexes, and skin colour and is an indicator of the newborn's need for medical attention shortly after birth. A detrimental effect of high Apgar score on the risk of atopic dermatitis is, to our knowledge, a novel finding that needs to be confirmed in subsequent studies. Among Finnish children low Apgar score increased the risk of asthma [20, 21]. Contrary to this, Apgar score was not related to asthma [22] or hay fever [23] in Finnish twin children and did not interact with in vitro fertilization on the risk of asthma in children born after assisted reproduction [24]. Moreover, Gilman et al. found no significant association between Apgar score and maternal smoking [25]. It is somewhat counterintuitive that it is the twin with the highest Apgar score that has the highest risk of later development of atopic dermatitis. However, previous studies have found a harmful effect on atopic dermatitis of other birth-related factors linked to high Apgar score such as increased fetal growth [9], high socioeconomic status (SES) [26, 27], and nonsmoking of the mother [9, 10]. Particularly, Lundholm et al. examined the association between fetal growth and atopic diseases and found that the rate of atopic dermatitis increased with higher levels of the mother's education and furthermore that children of mothers who did not smoke during pregnancy also had slightly higher rates of atopic dermatitis compared with children of mothers who smoked during pregnancy [9]. Furthermore, a Dutch study showed that smoking during pregnancy resulted in decreased birth weight and that women of low SES give birth to lighter babies [28]. These findings are inline with the assumption that atopic dermatitis is a disease affecting apparently robust children from high SES families. Because the affected (atopic) and the unaffected twin were matched on exposure status in our paired analysis, the observed positive association between atopic dermatitis and Apgar score is adjusted for confounding due to SES, parental smoking, and gestational age. Taken together, multiple factors are involved in the development of atopic dermatitis, particularly, genetics, fetal programming, and environmental effects, which makes it difficult to deduce which risk factors represent direct effects and which represent mediatory effects. The equal effect sizes in MZ and DZ twins for Apgar score in cotwin control analysis suggest a direct effect of one or more of the factors attributable to the Apgar score in relation to atopic dermatitis.

The prevalence of atopic dermatitis was higher in girls than in boys in the present study. Other studies contradict this, concluding that boys have a higher prevalence of atopic dermatitis and yet other studies find no significant difference between the prevalence of atopic dermatitis in boys and girls. Notably, a study from Taiwan found that the prevalence of atopic dermatitis in females is lower than in males before the age of 8 years but subsequently becomes higher [29], whereas studies from Japan and Italy show no significant difference in the prevalence of atopic dermatitis in boys and girls [30, 31]. A recent study of another (comparable) Scandinavian population from Sweden found a female preponderance of atopic dermatitis (14.5% in girls versus 9.4% in boys) [32].

We found an overall higher prevalence of atopic dermatitis among the entire group of MZ twins than among the group of DZ twins. This finding could be due to confounding from factors in the MZ group not present in the DZ group, for example, a larger susceptibility gene pool among MZ twins or a more unfavorable intrauterine environment in MZ than in DZ twins. Also, these could be factors such as differences in the MZ and DZ families in terms of smoking and SES, but evidence in support of this theory is lacking.

The large population size with identification of 907 twin pairs discordant for atopic dermatitis and the high response rate are strengths of this study, although the number of discordant MZ pairs was quite small (58 in total). We had complete ascertainment of all live-born twins in Denmark between 1993 and 2000 and cross-linked these data to data from the Danish Birth Registry combining information from two independent sources. Data on perinatal risk factors were obtained by professional midwifes' records, which increased the validity of the data. Contrary to this, the diagnosis of atopic dermatitis was self-reported by the parents of the twins, which could have induced recall and reporting bias. Moreover, the question used to diagnose atopic dermatitis has not been systematically validated. Another limitation alludes to the differing age at ascertainment of the eczema diagnosis, which may have influenced the results. However, age was automatically eliminated as possible confounder in the cotwin control analysis model since it was the same for the two twins within the pair.

The fact that we studied twins may have had implications for the generalisability of the results to the population as a whole. Particularly, twins differ from singletons in a number of ways related to prenatal and early life that potentially could affect the risk of atopic dermatitis differentially in twins. These factors, which may be related to gestation, intrauterine environment, and mode of delivery, could also be expected to influence the variation in Apgar score. However, in a matched case-control study of 112 infant twins and singletons from the United States 5-minute Apgar score was not different in twins compared with singletons when matched for gestational age and mode of delivery [33], suggesting that results in relation to Apgar score can be extrapolated to the general singleton population. Still, we acknowledge that there may be unmeasured factors in our sample that could have interfered with our conclusions.

We conclude that a high Apgar score may be linked to development of atopic dermatitis. Although this finding agrees with the theory that robust babies of high SES are at increased risk of atopic dermatitis, this has not been previously documented and awaits support from future studies.

References

[1] C. A. Akdis, M. Akdis, T. Bieber et al., "Diagnosis and treatment of atopic dermatitis in children and adults: European Academy of Allergology and Clinical Immunology/American Academy of Allergy, Asthma and Immunology/PRACTALL consensus report," *Allergy*, vol. 61, no. 8, pp. 969–987, 2006.

[2] R. A. H. M. van den Oord and A. Sheikh, "Filaggrin gene defects and risk of developing allergic sensitisation and allergic disorders: systematic review and meta-analysis," *British Medical Journal*, vol. 339, Article ID b2433, 2009.

[3] L. Paternoster, M. Standl, C. M. Chen et al., "Meta-analysis of genome-wide association studies identifies three new risk loci for atopic dermatitis," *Nature Genetics*, vol. 44, pp. 187–192, 2011.

[4] L. Stensen, S. F. Thomsen, and V. Backer, "Change in prevalence of atopic dermatitis between 1986 and 2001 among children," *Allergy and Asthma Proceedings*, vol. 29, no. 4, pp. 392–396, 2008.

[5] T. K. Ninan and G. Russell, "Respiratory symptoms and atopy in Aberdeen schoolchildren: evidence from two surveys 25 years apart," *British Medical Journal*, vol. 304, no. 6831, pp. 873–875, 1992.

[6] M. I. Asher, S. Montefort, B. Björkstén et al., "Worldwide time trends in the prevalence of symptoms of asthma, allergic rhinoconjunctivitis, and eczema in childhood: ISAAC Phases One and Three repeat multicountry cross-sectional surveys," *The Lancet*, vol. 368, no. 9537, pp. 733–743, 2006.

[7] C. G. Carson, L. B. Halkjaer, S. M. Jensen, and H. Bisgaard, "Alcohol intake in pregnancy increases the child's risk of atopic dermatitis. The COPSAC prospective birth cohort study of a high risk population," *PLoS ONE*, vol. 7, Article ID e42710, 2012.

[8] A. Linneberg, J. Petersen, M. Grønbæk, and C. S. Benn, "Alcohol during pregnancy and atopic dermatitis in the offspring," *Clinical and Experimental Allergy*, vol. 34, no. 11, pp. 1678–1683, 2004.

[9] C. Lundholm, A. K. Örtqvist, P. Lichtenstein, S. Cnattingius, and C. Almqvist, "Impaired fetal growth decreases the risk of childhood atopic eczema: a Swedish twin study," *Clinical and Experimental Allergy*, vol. 40, no. 7, pp. 1044–1053, 2010.

[10] A. Linneberg, J. B. Simonsen, J. Petersen, L. G. Stensballe, and C. S. Benn, "Differential effects of risk factors on infant wheeze and atopic dermatitis emphasize a different etiology," *Journal of Allergy and Clinical Immunology*, vol. 117, no. 1, pp. 184–189, 2006.

[11] D. J. Purvis, J. M. D. Thompson, P. M. Clark et al., "Risk factors for atopic dermatitis in New Zealand children at 3.5 year of age," *British Journal of Dermatology*, vol. 152, no. 4, pp. 742–749, 2005.

[12] C. S. Benn, J. Wohlfahrt, P. Aaby et al., "Breastfeeding and risk of atopic dermatitis, by parental history of allergy, during the first 18 months of life," *American Journal of Epidemiology*, vol. 160, no. 3, pp. 217–223, 2004.

[13] J. F. Ludvigsson, M. Mostrom, J. Ludvigsson, and K. Duchen, "Exclusive breastfeeding and risk of atopic dermatitis in some 8300 infants," *Pediatric Allergy and Immunology*, vol. 16, no. 3, pp. 201–208, 2005.

[14] P. Leadbitter, N. Pearce, S. Cheng et al., "Relationship between fetal growth and the development of asthma and atopy in childhood," *Thorax*, vol. 54, no. 10, pp. 905–910, 1999.

[15] A. Sevelsted and H. Bisgaard, "Neonatal size in term children is associated with asthma at age 7, but not with atopic dermatitis or allergic sensitization," *Allergy*, vol. 67, no. 5, pp. 670–675, 2012.

[16] M. M. Moore, S. L. Rifas-Shiman, J. W. Rich-Edwards et al., "Perinatal predictors of atopic dermatitis occurring in the first six months of life," *Pediatrics*, vol. 113, no. 3, pp. 468–474, 2004.

[17] C. D. Mallen, S. Mottram, G. Wynne-Jones, and E. Thomas, "Birth-related exposures and asthma and allergy in adulthood: a population-based cross-sectional study of young adults in North Staffordshire," *Journal of Asthma*, vol. 45, no. 4, pp. 309–312, 2008.

[18] L. Christiansen, H. Frederiksen, K. Schousboe et al., "Age- and sex-differences in the validity of questionnaire-based zygosity in twins," *Twin Research*, vol. 6, no. 4, pp. 275–278, 2003.

[19] D. L. Duffy, "The co-twin control study," in *Advances in Twin and Sib-Pair Analysis*, T. D. Inspector, H. Snieder, and A. J. MacGregor, Eds., Greenwich Medical Media, 2000.

[20] B. Xu, J. Pekkanen, and M.-R. Järvelin, "Obstetric complications and asthma in childhood," *Journal of Asthma*, vol. 37, no. 7, pp. 589–594, 2000.

[21] J. Metsälä, A. Kilkkinen, M. Kaila et al., "Perinatal factors and the risk of asthma in childhood—a population-based register study in Finland," *American Journal of Epidemiology*, vol. 168, no. 2, pp. 170–178, 2008.

[22] M. Räsänen, J. Kaprio, T. Laitinen, T. Winter, M. Koskenvuo, and L. A. Laitinen, "Perinatal risk factors for asthma in Finnish adolescent twins," *Thorax*, vol. 55, no. 1, pp. 25–31, 2000.

[23] M. Räsänen, J. Kaprio, T. Laitinen, T. Winter, M. Koskenvuo, and L. A. Laitinen, "Perinatal risk factors for hay fever—a study among 2550 Finnish twin families," *Twin Research*, vol. 4, no. 5, pp. 392–399, 2001.

[24] B. Källén, O. Finnström, K. G. Nygren, and P. Otterblad Olausson, "Asthma in Swedish children conceived by in vitro fertilisation," *Archives of Disease in Childhood*, 2012.

[25] S. E. Gilman, H. Gardener, and S. L. Buka, "Maternal smoking during pregnancy and children's cognitive and physical development: a causal risk factor?" *American Journal of Epidemiology*, vol. 168, no. 5, pp. 522–531, 2008.

[26] S. P. DaVeiga, "Epidemiology of atopic dermatitis: a review," *Allergy and Asthma Proceedings*, vol. 33, pp. 227–234, 2012.

[27] R. Schmitz, K. Atzpodien, and M. Schlaud, "Prevalence and risk factors of atopic diseases in German children and adolescents," *Pediatric Allergy and Immunology*, vol. 23, pp. 716–723, 2012.

[28] L. M. Silva, P. W. Jansen, E. A. P. Steegers et al., "Mother's educational level and fetal growth: the genesis of health inequalities," *International Journal of Epidemiology*, vol. 39, no. 5, pp. 1250–1261, 2010.

[29] C.-Y. Hwang, Y.-J. Chen, M.-W. Lin et al., "Prevalence of atopic dermatitis, allergic rhinitis and asthma in Taiwan: a national study 2000 to 2007," *Acta Dermato-Venereologica*, vol. 90, no. 6, pp. 589–594, 2010.

[30] H. Saeki, H. Iizuka, Y. Mori et al., "Prevalence of atopic dermatitis in Japanese elementary schoolchildren," *British Journal of Dermatology*, vol. 152, no. 1, pp. 110–114, 2005.

[31] L. Naldi, F. Parazzini, and S. Gallus, "Prevalence of atopic dermatitis in Italian schoolchildren: factors affecting its variation," *Acta Dermato-Venereologica*, vol. 89, pp. 122–125, 2009.

[32] N. Ballardini, I. Kull, C. Söderhäll, G. Lilja, M. Wickman, and C. F. Wahlgren, "Eczema severity in preadolescent children and its relation to sex, filaggrin mutations, asthma, rhinitis, aggravating factors and topical treatment: a report from the BAMSE birth cohort," *British Journal of Dermatology*, vol. 168, pp. 588–594, 2013.

[33] S. A. Friedman, E. Schiff, L. Kao et al., "Do twins mature earlier than singletons? Results from a matched cohort study," *American Journal of Obstetrics and Gynecology*, vol. 176, no. 6, pp. 1193–1199, 1997.

25

Exploring Perceptions and Experiences of Food Allergy among New Canadians from Asia

Stephanie K. Lu,[1] **Susan J. Elliott,**[1] **and Ann E. Clarke**[2]

[1] *School of Public Health and Health Systems, University of Waterloo, 200 University Avenue West, Waterloo, ON, Canada N2L 3G1*
[2] *Department of Medicine, University of Calgary, Calgary, AB, Canada T2N 1N4*

Correspondence should be addressed to Stephanie K. Lu; s4lu@uwaterloo.ca

Academic Editor: William E. Berger

Introduction. In Canada, perceived prevalence of food allergy surpasses systematic estimates. Canadian immigrants have been found more likely to rate the risk of food allergy as "high" compared to nonimmigrants. *Methods.* Qualitative interviews were conducted with 3 key informants and 18 allergic individuals of East and Southeast Asian descent in order to capture their lived experience with food allergies. *Results.* Participants found food allergies to be more common in Canada than in Asia. Participants also agreed that having a food allergy is more manageable in Canada as a result of the policy environment (e.g., food labelling and school policies). In addition, participants had dealt with skepticism and disbelief about their food allergy in Asia, resulting in social exclusion and impacting quality of life. *Discussion.* Findings demonstrate the need to recognize the varied impacts and experiences of food allergy among new Canadians, given that immigrants represent a large and growing proportion of the Canadian population.

1. Introduction

Food allergy policies in public places and stories in the popular press are evidence of the rising awareness of food allergies as an important public health risk [1]. In its most severe form, IgE-mediated food allergies can lead to anaphylaxis, which is potentially fatal. Internationally, food allergy prevalence varies widely with age and geography. For example, self-reported prevalence in the US is 9.1% (8% for children) and 5.3% for respondents with a physician diagnosis [2, 3]. In Canada, overall prevalence rates are around 7% [4]. The Canadian estimates, however, were based on a nonrepresentative sample that underrepresented vulnerable populations (i.e., low income families, immigrants, and Aboriginal Peoples) [5, 6]; a second national survey undertaken to address this limitation indicated that the prevalence of self-reported food allergy for immigrants who have lived in Canada for less than 10 years (herein referred to as "new Canadians") was substantially lower than their Canadian born counterparts: 3.2% [7]. These researchers also investigated perceived prevalence of food allergy in the same populations and found that perceived prevalence was observed to surpass systematic estimates by up to 30% [8].

The gap between perceived and actual risk of food allergy suggests that the public's perception of true risk of allergy is, in fact, inflated [9]. Moreover, new Canadians were found more likely to rate the risk of food allergy as "high" compared to nonimmigrants or immigrants who have lived in Canada for over 10 years [9], despite the substantial differences in measured prevalence.

In light of the above, this paper used a qualitative research design to unpack the perceptions and experiences of new Canadians directly affected by food allergy by addressing the following objectives: (1) to understand how new Canadians perceive food allergies and their associated risks and (2) to investigate how new Canadians manage and cope with food allergies.

2. Methods

Waterloo Region, Ontario, Canada, was chosen as the research site as it is one of the fastest-growing areas in the province with the 9th highest proportion of visible minorities of all Census Metropolitan Areas across Canada [10].

Qualitative methods were chosen in order to privilege the voices of those affected. Qualitative methods have been used with several populations at risk of anaphylaxis: children [11–13], adolescents [14, 15], their parents [13, 14, 16], allergists [17], and the general public [18, 19].

In-depth interviews were conducted in two stages. First, key informants (an allergist, public health nutritionist, and public health planner) recruited through telephone and e-mail were interviewed in person (averaging 30 minutes) as representatives of key constituencies able to provide an information-rich connection to the research topic [20], as well as access to the wider food allergies community. Service providers and health workers have been shown to be rich and largely untapped sources of information with important insights to issues of health and migration [21]. Each interview covered topics specific to the key informant's observations and knowledge of food allergies from their professional work experience.

Second, in-depth interviews with affected individuals were conducted with new Canadians who either had a physician-diagnosed food allergy of their own or were a parent of a food allergic child. The focus was on individuals of East and Southeast Asian descent as 50% of the immigrant participants in the Canadian national prevalence survey were born in an Asian country [4, 5]. East and Southeast Asians are also two of the most common visible minorities in Waterloo Region [10]. Participants (n = 18) were recruited using Kijiji (an online network for posting local classified advertisements), the interviewed key informants, and contacts made with local cultural centres. Interviews averaged 30 minutes in length and were conducted (Nov. 2012 to Jan. 2013) until saturation was reached (i.e., until no new themes emerged from the interviews) [22]. Participants were also asked to complete a short demographic survey to gather additional information on their food allergy and length of time in Canada. 78% of the sample was female and 72% of all participants were under 30 years old (Table 1). Just over half the participants have lived in Canada for less than 10 years (n = 10). The most common self-reported allergen was shellfish (n = 12) and the majority of participants were over 5 years old when their allergy was diagnosed (n = 15).

Each interview was conducted by the primary author and audio-recorded for transcription and subsequent thematic analysis using QSR International's NVivo 9. A theme code set was created both deductively (based on the research objectives and interview guides) and inductively (themes emerging from the interview transcripts). Coding was assessed for inter- and intra-rater reliability [22], achieving 81% agreement with a second coder at the graduate level. Key themes that were identified were those that appeared with the greatest frequency as discrete units of text in the interview transcripts. Ethics clearance was received from the University of Waterloo.

3. Results

3.1. Key Informants. Three key themes emerged from the key informant interviews, the first being appropriate and informed diagnosis. New Canadians are concerned with receiving confirmation of their allergy and getting reassurance that their problem is not life-threatening. While the

TABLE 1: Participant characteristics (n = 18).

Participant characteristics		Number of participants (%)
Gender	Male	4 (22)
	Female	14 (78)
Age group	18–21	4 (22)
	22–25	7 (39)
	26–30	2 (11)
	31–40	3 (17)
	41–50	2 (11)
Birth place	China	5 (28)
	Hong Kong	3 (17)
	Malaysia	1 (5)
	Philippines	4 (22)
	Thailand	2 (11)
	Vietnam	1 (5)
	Other[a]	2 (11)
Years lived in Canada	0–5	6 (33)
	6–10	4 (22)
	11–20	6 (33)
	21+	2 (11)
Allergic person in household	Self	14 (78)
	Child	4 (22)
Allergy[b]	Peanut	6 (33)
	Shellfish (including lobster, shrimp, and prawns)	12 (67)
	Fish	5 (27)
	Fruit (including lychee, durian, blueberries, and mango)	4 (22)
	Beans	2 (11)
	Egg	2 (11)
	Wheat	1 (5)
	Milk	1 (5)
Age of diagnosis (years)	0-1	2 (11)
	2–5	1 (5)
	6–10	3 (17)
	11–15	7 (39)
	16–20	5 (28)

[a]Participant was raised, but not born, in East or Southeast Asia.
[b]Sum is not equal to number of participants due to multiple responses.

diagnosis process is straightforward, it can be difficult to educate new Canadians about how to avoid a reaction as well as the importance of using epinephrine in the form of an Epi-Pen:

> Understanding what the issue is, is tough enough for patients that have grown up in Canada. To really appreciate and understand what a food

allergy is, what it involves, and the potential risks, I think for immigrants it is even tougher because in most countries where they have immigrated from, allergy didn't exist. Or if it did exist, it was a really, really small issue. (Key Informant 1)

The second theme that emerged is the challenge of shaping a safe school environment for food allergic children. Placing bans on foods in schools can be very restrictive, making it difficult for people to find food alternatives, especially if cost is a concern. A restrictive diet can also make it more difficult to ensure that children are meeting nutritional needs:

It becomes very restrictive for the students who aren't allergic. So it is really concerning when foods are starting to be banned from the classroom, because soon, if there are more and more allergic students, many foods will be banned and it's very hard for people to find those foods and for there to be foods that are within the right price range, especially for people with lower income. So this is a major issue, and we really strive towards educating that it should be an allergy *safe* environment as opposed to an allergy *free* environment, because it really, in our opinion, is almost impossible to do that. (Key Informant 2)

Furthermore, studies have shown that food allergic children have been known to experience stigma and/or social exclusion, particularly in the school setting. How allergic children are being perceived by their peers, especially if an incident gets reported in the media, was raised by key informants:

I was really disturbed by the fact that you know [a story about an allergic child] was in the paper, and it was naming the school and the age of the child and the parent, so people know who this child is… I don't think it is fair to anyone involved, but it is definitely not fair to the child and we don't want to be causing that, so I just want to make it as normal as possible for them. (Key Informant 2)

3.2. Food Allergic New Canadians. Four key themes emerged from interviews with affected individuals: perceived prevalence, perceived etiology, management and coping, and quality of life. Initially, however, participants were asked to describe the emotions and feelings they experienced when they had their first allergic reaction. Many were surprised or even shocked to learn of their allergy ($n = 12$):

Yeah, I was actually quite surprised and so were my parents because we had been around people with allergies before, like my friends and stuff, but none of them had such a severe reaction… And especially because it was so unexpected

at such a young age. I don't know, it is not common, so yeah, surprised was one thing. Scared was another. (Participant 15: *female raised in Singapore and Japan, <5 years in Canada, allergic to peanut and shellfish*)

Participants also felt disappointment ($n = 7$) and even sadness ($n = 1$) when they were diagnosed because they either found it difficult to give up a kind of food they liked or were upset that previous allergic reactions could have been prevented:

I would just feel sad, like I just think that it is a kind of sickness. I just feel it is a misfortune right, why do we have a son that has food allergy? Why other people don't have such problem, right? I just feel it is sad. I just kind of accept the fact. I have to face it, right? (Participant 4: *female from China, <10 years in Canada, son is allergic to peanuts and beans*)

One of the predominant perceptions regarding food allergies is that prevalence is lower in Asia than it is in North America [23]. Current evidence supports this perception, although it is speculated that rates of prevalence in more modernized regions of Asia, such as Hong Kong, are comparable to rates in North America [24, 25]. This perception was also held by participants, as 83% of them thought that food allergies were less common in their birth place:

Well I realized especially like in grade four and grade five, all my friends could not eat peanuts, so we couldn't even bring peanuts to school, so that is when I realized, oh food allergies are pretty common here in Canada. Whereas I never really thought about it back in the Philippines. (Participant 7: *male from Philippines, <20 years in Canada, allergic to shrimp and shellfish*)

It is a lot rarer in China. Over here there is a lot of emphasis [on it], like one of the first things you learn in school is don't bring any peanuts. You don't find that in China. (Participant 12: *female from China, <20 years in Canada, allergic to shrimp and prawns*)

78% of participants could not speculate on the cause of their allergy. However, when asked to speculate on the etiology of food allergy more generally, they cited examples related to diet, genetics, and the hygiene hypothesis. For example:

It might be because Chinese people eat everything, so from their ancestry they kind of don't have those allergies, because they start to eat anything like from years ago, but here people only eat certain kinds of food. They don't eat animals, like dogs and stuff, and so it is really hard to say. I don't know. (Participant 14: *female from China, <5 years in Canada, allergic to peanuts, beans, fish, and shrimp*)

TABLE 2: Obstacles to managing food allergy in birth place.

Obstacle	Number of participants (% of the total)	Mentions (% of the total)
Different eating habits	3 (17)	4 (18)
Different attitudes towards food	2 (11)	2 (9)
Less accommodative (in restaurants, schools, etc.)	7 (39)	9 (41)
Different health safety standards	5 (28)	6 (27)
Cost	1 (5)	1 (5)
Total	18 (100)	22 (100)

TABLE 3: Impact of food allergy on quality of life in Canada.

Impact level	Number of participants (% of the total)	Mentions (% of the total)
Negligible	7 (39)	18 (46)
Noticeable	11 (61)	14 (36)
Significant	3 (17)	7 (18)
Total	18[a] (100)	39 (100)

[a]This is not equal to the sum of the numbers in the column due to multiple responses.

Participants also found it harder to manage their allergy in their birth place (Table 2). Participants attributed this difference to lower levels of awareness and, subsequently, less respect and understanding of their needs for accommodation.

Food allergy impacts the quality of life of not only the allergic individual, but also their family. 39% of respondents reported that the impact of the food allergy on their quality of life was "negligible" (Table 3); that is, they adapted quickly to their food allergy and never felt any serious disappointment from being allergic. More participants (61%) felt that their allergy had a "noticeable" impact on their quality of life as it took some time to accept the allergy and learn how to manage everyday life. The allergy often went from being a nuisance to just a fact of life. Three participants reported being significantly impacted by the allergy; two had multiple allergies and one had tried various remedies, both Chinese and Western medicines, to alleviate symptoms. A third who reported significant quality of life impacts had been teased by family and friends:

> My parents started helping me to treat my allergy back when I was fifteen or sixteen. I started eating this one particular thing called bird's nest. It is like a drink that is similar to ginseng. It is supposed to make your metabolism better. Every day I was drinking it. I wouldn't say for sure that I got better because of it. (Participant 1: *female from Hong Kong, <10 years in Canada, allergic to lychee and lobster*)

> My mom, she is not allergic to anything, so she is always like "why are you allergic?" There is a phrase that she says [often]. She always says my sister will eat anything she cooks, but I am always the weird kid that [she] always has to be careful with, [because there are] so many limitations to the food that I eat. So it is just kind of annoying at times. (Participant 3: *male raised in Hong Kong, <20 years in Canada, allergic to shellfish and peanut*)

The presence of a strong support system can make a positive difference in coping. 72% of participants said their family and friends are supportive because they understand the severity of their allergy and are willing to make accommodations (Table 4). However, 39% of participants reported that their family was initially skeptical of their food allergy:

> A lot of people are skeptical. My relatives [will say something] like "are you sure that you are allergic to it?" "Maybe you should try without knowing it and see if it is a psychological thing." But I actually proved it to them many times that I am allergic. It is actually about my physical reaction. (Participant 3: *male raised in Hong Kong, <20 years in Canada, allergic to shellfish and peanut*)

Participants had to "prove" their allergy to their relatives by showing their physical reaction when they consumed an allergen.

Misinformed perceptions about oral immunotherapy were also raised, as participants had experienced situations in which they were encouraged by family members to eat an allergen. The thinking was that regular exposure to the allergen would eventually cure them of their condition:

> [My dad] is like just keep eating, because whenever there were shrimps or like at home, my dad would always kind of force me to eat it, and he would be just like "oh it is all in your head. You can like overcome it if you just slowly like try to build immunity against it"... But I kind of didn't want to do it, just because I was afraid of getting a reaction. (Participant 7: *male from Philippines, <20 years in Canada, allergic to shrimp and shellfish*)

Interestingly, some participants had no prior knowledge of what a food allergy was, even if they had one, until they came to Canada:

> R (R refers to the question asked by the researcher): When you were growing up were you familiar with what food allergies are? P (P refers to the participant's response): No, I actually wasn't. I didn't even know anyone who had allergies. It was only when I came to Canada that I had heard that people have allergies to peanuts and stuff like that. I didn't know how severe it can

TABLE 4: Family and friends' attitudes towards food allergy.

	Family		Friends	
Attitude	Number of participants (% of the total)	Mentions (% of the total)	Number of participants (% of the total)	Mentions (% of the total)
Surprise	4 (22)	7 (14)	1 (22)	1 (3)
Skeptical	7 (39)	8 (16)	3 (17)	4 (13)
Scared	2 (11)	2 (4)	0	0
Quick acceptance	4 (22)	4 (8)	3 (17)	3 (10)
Slow acceptance	5 (28)	8 (16)	2 (11)	2 (6)
Disappointment	0	0	1 (6)	1 (3)
Supportive/cautious	13 (72)	19 (39)	13 (72)	20 (65)
Other	1 (6)	1 (2)	0	0
Total	18^a (100)	49 (100)	18^a (100)	31 (100)

^{a}This is not equal to the sum of the numbers in the column due to multiple responses.

get, that people can actually get it, and so forth. (Participant 11: *male from Thailand, <20 years in Canada, allergic to fish and shellfish*)

Further, even if they were familiar, there was no mechanism in their native language to describe it. For example, 28% of participants could say "food allergy" in Chinese (Mandarin and Cantonese), but there was no equivalent Chinese term for "anaphylaxis." The same observation was made by participants who spoke Malay, Thai, and Japanese. It was speculated by some participants that familiarity with food allergies in Asia may increase over time, but at this point it has not been recognized as a medical condition, at least not in the general population.

A key aspect of managing and coping with food allergies is information. Approximately 56% of participants said that their physician was their go-to source for information. Three of the four mothers with an allergic child identified their allergist as being extremely helpful. Community and public health services were mentioned less frequently (14% of total mentions).

Personal internet research was the preferred method for learning more about food allergies with 67% of participants having conducted internet searches at least once:

> ...thank god we have internet. A lot of information is on the internet. We have spent lots of time doing that... I can't remember the website I went to, but I do a lot of research. I try to dig into why he has this allergy. I have spent tons of time trying to figure that out. Unfortunately, I haven't found out why. (Participant 4: *female from China, <10 years in Canada, son is allergic to peanuts and beans*)

4. Discussion

Shellfish was the most common self-reported allergen amongst participants (Table 1). This finding is consistent with studies from Asia where shellfish allergy predominates. In contrast, the risk of peanut and tree nut allergy is much higher in individuals from Western countries [5, 26–28]. While the influence of birth place in development of shellfish allergy is still unknown, it is likely that multiple environmental factors are contributing to this phenomenon, including gender, living environment (urban versus rural), and age of intake [5]. Researchers are only beginning to find potential links between age of fish intake and allergic disease that may also be the case of shellfish allergy [28, 29]. These links are further complicated by genetic predisposition [30].

Interestingly, twelve participants were 10 years or older when diagnosed (Table 1). This is in sharp contrast to the high rates of allergic children in North America who are diagnosed at a much younger age (between 2 and 4 years) [3]. While reasons for this are unclear, contributing factors may include a lower level of awareness in new Canadians and limited availability of epinephrine autoinjectors in Asia [30, 31]. In countries such as the Philippines, Epi-Pens are not even available due to cost constraints [30]. Limited accessibility to health care in parts of Asia may partially explain why several participants never opted to have their food allergy confirmed by a doctor, a challenge to determining prevalence based on self-report.

These findings support the hypothesis that new Canadians may have a lower level of awareness of food allergies and, hence, their inflated perception of risk. The difference in their level of awareness was evident in discussions that touched on their first allergic experience, the etiology of food allergies, and the lack of policies in their birth place to protect them in public places. Furthermore, similar findings have been found in the reverse situation; parents of expatriate children with a food allergy in Singapore reported that differences in food preparation and food labeling in Asia caused the greatest rise in stress levels after moving to Singapore [32]. Most schools in Asia do not take precautionary measures to protect food allergic children and legislature on food labeling is rare [32]. By understanding factors that influence risk perception such as familiarity and personal ability to affect risk, policy makers can anticipate how the public will respond [33].

Furthermore, health professionals should be aware that there is a wide variation in the quality of information on food allergy distributed to patients when diagnosed overseas, if they receive any information at all. The internet was the preferred source of information reported. Hence, health professionals and leaders in food allergy advocacy should be encouraged to tailor comprehensive, online resources that are accessible to new Canadians.

In terms of management and coping, participants relied on food labels and prior experience with allergens to stay safe. Unsupervised oral immunotherapy, however, emerged as an unexpected theme. This is concerning as oral immunotherapy is not yet widely accepted as a treatment [34, 35]. Moreover, this practice put participants in an uncomfortable situation, which could have possibly led to accidental exposure and/or issues of management anxiety.

Social isolation/exclusion also emerged as participants who had lived with their food allergy in Asia expressed frustration as they fended for themselves, especially if they were the only one in their social circle with a food allergy.

Qualitative research studies are by definition constrained by sample size but allow for a deeper exploration of lived experience. The reliance on self-reported food allergy in this study is typical of research in this field but does present a potential bias on the part of respondents. Further, not all countries in East and Southeast Asia were represented in the sample, so transferability of research findings to other regions may not be possible. Given the level of diversity within Asia itself, we recognize that the treatment of our participants as a homogenous group is a limitation of this study.

5. Conclusions

These findings indicate that food allergy among new Canadians is an important (and potentially growing) public health issue deserving of attention, given the reported impacts on social isolation/exclusion and quality of life, as well as the dearth of resources available. This exploratory research raises several issues deserving of more research: health literacy levels in immigrant populations, the wider variety of allergens that immigrants may be reacting to, and further research to understand the impacts of food allergies in other ethnocultural groups in Canada as immigrants represent a large and growing proportion of the Canadian population. Subsequently, further research will be needed to inform and facilitate change at the policy level in order to protect allergic individuals in Canada and abroad.

Conflict of Interests

The authors declare that there is no conflict of interests regarding the publication of this paper.

Authors' Contribution

Each author named in this submission has contributed to the completion of this paper and agrees to its submission.

Acknowledgments

Research is funded by Allergy, Genes, and Environment (AllerGen) Network of Centres of Excellence. The authors thank the participants of this study, as well as Daniel Harrington at the University of Toronto, and Leia Minaker and Kristin Brown at the University of Waterloo for their assistance.

References

[1] C. Rachul and T. Caulfield, "Food allergy policy and the popular press: perspectives from Canadian newspapers," *Journal of Asthma and Allergy Educators*, vol. 2, no. 6, pp. 282–287, 2011.

[2] K. A. Vierk, K. M. Koehler, S. B. Fein, D. A. Street, and C. Park, "Prevalence of self-reported food allergy in American adults and use of food labels," *Journal of Allergy and Clinical Immunology*, vol. 119, no. 6, pp. 1504–1510, 2007.

[3] R. S. Gupta, E. E. Springston, M. R. Warrier et al., "The prevalence, severity, and distribution of childhood food allergy in the United States," *Pediatrics*, vol. 128, no. 1, pp. e9–e17, 2011.

[4] L. Soller, M. Ben-Shoshan, D. W. Harrington et al., "Overall prevalence of self-reported food allergy in Canada," *Journal of Allergy and Clinical Immunology*, vol. 130, no. 4, pp. 986–988, 2012.

[5] M. Ben-Shoshan, D. W. Harrington, L. Soller et al., "Demographic predictors of peanut, tree nut, fish, shellfish, and sesame allergy in Canada," *Journal of Allergy*, vol. 2012, Article ID 858306, 6 pages, 2012.

[6] M. Ben-Shoshan, D. W. Harrington, L. Soller et al., "A population-based study on peanut, tree nut, fish, shellfish, and sesame allergy prevalence in Canada," *Journal of Allergy and Clinical Immunology*, vol. 125, no. 6, pp. 1327–1335, 2010.

[7] L. Soller, M. Ben-Shoshan, D. W. Harringtan et al., "Prevalence and predictors of food allergy in Canada: a focus on vulnerable populations," *Journal of Allergy and Clinical Immunology*. In press.

[8] D. W. Harrington, S. J. Elliott, and A. E. Clarke, "Frames, claims and audiences: construction of food allergies in the Canadian media," *Public Understanding of Science*, vol. 21, no. 6, pp. 724–739, 2012.

[9] D. W. Harrington, S. J. Elliott, A. E. Clarke, M. Ben-Shoshan, and S. Godefroy, "Exploring the determinants of the perceived risk of food allergies in Canada," *Human and Ecological Risk Assessment*, vol. 18, no. 6, pp. 1338–1358, 2012.

[10] Region of Waterloo, "Immigrants in Waterloo Region," 2009, http://chd.region.waterloo.on.ca/en/researchResourcesPublications/resources/Immigrants_Status.pdf.

[11] N. J. Avery, R. M. King, S. Knight, and J. O. Hourihane, "Assessment of quality of life in children with peanut allergy," *Pediatric Allergy and Immunology*, vol. 14, no. 5, pp. 378–382, 2003.

[12] N. E. Fenton, S. J. Elliott, L. Cicutto, A. E. Clarke, L. Harada, and E. McPhee, "Illustrating risk: anaphylaxis through the eyes of the food-allergic child," *Society for Risk Analysis*, vol. 31, no. 1, pp. 171–183, 2011.

[13] W. Hu, I. Kerridge, and A. Kemp, "Risk, rationality, and regret: responding to the uncertainty of childhood food anaphylaxis," *Medical Humanities*, vol. 31, no. 1, pp. 12–16, 2005.

[14] N. Akeson, A. Worth, and A. Sheikh, "The psychosocial impact of anaphylaxis on young people and their parents," *Clinical and Experimental Allergy*, vol. 37, no. 8, pp. 1213–1220, 2007.

[15] M. A. Sampson, A. Muñoz-Furlong, and S. H. Sicherer, "Risk-taking and coping strategies of adolescents and young adults with food allergy," *Journal of Allergy and Clinical Immunology*, vol. 117, no. 6, pp. 1440–1445, 2006.

[16] D. Mandell, R. Curtis, M. Gold, and S. Hardie, "Anaphylaxis: how do you live with it?" *Health and Social Work*, vol. 30, no. 4, pp. 325–335, 2005.

[17] Y. S. Xu, S. B. Waserman, S. Waserman, L. Connors, K. Stawiarski, and M. Kastner, "Food allergy management from the perspective of patients or caregivers, and allergists: a qualitative study," *Allergy, Asthma & Clinical Immunology*, vol. 6, no. 1, article 30, 2010.

[18] R. S. Gupta, J. S. Kim, J. A. Barnathan, L. B. Amsden, L. S. Tummala, and J. L. Holl, "Food allergy knowledge, attitudes and beliefs: focus groups of parents, physicians and the general public," *BMC Pediatrics*, vol. 8, article 36, 2008.

[19] B. Sora, A. Boulay, R. Sala et al., "A characterization of peanut consumption in four countries: results from focus groups and their implications for peanut allergy prevalence," *International Journal of Consumer Studies*, vol. 33, no. 6, pp. 676–683, 2009.

[20] B. F. Crabtree and W. L. Miller, Eds., *Doing Qualitative Research*, Sage, Thousand Oaks, Calif, USA, 2nd edition, 1999.

[21] S. J. Elliott and J. Gillie, "Moving experiences: a qualitative analysis of health and migration," *Health and Place*, vol. 4, no. 4, pp. 327–339, 1998.

[22] M. B. Miles and A. M. Huberman, *Qualitative Data Analysis: An Extended Sourcebook*, Sage, Thousand Oaks, Calif, USA, 2nd edition, 1994.

[23] I. F. A. Gerez, B. W. Lee, H. P. van Bever, and L. P. Shek, "Allergies in Asia: differences in prevalence and management compared with Western populations," *Expert Review of Clinical Immunology*, vol. 6, no. 2, pp. 279–289, 2010.

[24] T. F. Leung, E. Yung, Y. S. Wong, C. W. K. Lam, and G. W. K. Wong, "Parent-reported adverse food reactions in Hong Kong Chinese pre-schoolers: epidemiology, clinical spectrum and risk factors," *Pediatric Allergy and Immunology*, vol. 20, no. 4, pp. 339–346, 2009.

[25] M. H. K. Ho, S. L. Lee, W. H. S. Wong, P. Ip, and Y. L. Lau, "Prevalence of self-reported food allergy in Hong Kong children and teens—a population survey," *Asian Pacific Journal of Allergy and Immunology*, vol. 30, no. 4, pp. 275–284, 2012.

[26] D. L. Goh, Y. N. Lau, F. T. Chew, L. P. Shek, and B. W. Lee, "Pattern of food-induced anaphylaxis in children of an Asian community," *Allergy*, vol. 54, no. 1, pp. 84–86, 1999.

[27] P. Hajeb and J. Selamat, "A contemporary review of seafood allergy," *Clinical Reviews in Allergy and Immunology*, vol. 42, no. 3, pp. 365–385, 2012.

[28] J. C. Kiefte-de Jong, J. H. de Vries, O. H. Franco et al., "Fish consumption in infancy and asthma-like symptoms at preschool age," *Pediatrics*, vol. 130, no. 6, pp. 1060–1068, 2012.

[29] T. Oien, O. Storrø, and R. Johnsen, "Do early intake of fish and fish oil protect against eczema and doctor-diagnosed asthma at 2 years of age? A cohort study," *Journal of Epidemiology and Community Health*, vol. 64, no. 2, pp. 124–129, 2010.

[30] L. P. C. Shek, E. A. Cabrera-Morales, S. E. Soh et al., "A population-based questionnaire survey on the prevalence of peanut, tree nut, and shellfish allergy in 2 Asian populations," *Journal of Allergy and Clinical Immunology*, vol. 126, no. 2, pp. 324.e7–331.e7, 2010.

[31] E. H. Tham, S. Y. Tay, D. L. C. Lim et al., "Epinephrine auto-injector prescriptions as a reflection of the pattern of anaphylaxis in an Asian population," *Allergy and Asthma Proceedings*, vol. 29, no. 2, pp. 211–215, 2008.

[32] H. Sivaraj, M. Rajakulendran, B. W. Lee, and L. Shek, "Challenges faced by expatriate children with food allergy in an Asian country," *Annals of Allergy, Asthma & Immunology*, vol. 105, no. 4, pp. 323–324, 2010.

[33] R. E. Kasperson, O. Renn, P. Slovic et al., "The social amplification of risk: a conceptual framework," *Risk Analysis*, vol. 8, no. 2, pp. 177–187, 1988.

[34] M. Ben-Shoshan and A. E. Clarke, "Anaphylaxis: past, present and future," *Allergy*, vol. 66, no. 1, pp. 1–14, 2011.

[35] R. Q. Chaudhry and J. J. Oppenheimer, "Update on food allergy in adults," *Current Allergy and Asthma Reports*, vol. 12, no. 4, pp. 311–320, 2012.

26

Thermal Water Applications in the Treatment of Upper Respiratory Tract Diseases: A Systematic Review and Meta-Analysis

Sarah Keller, Volker König, and Ralph Mösges

Institute of Medical Statistics, Informatics and Epidemiology (IMSIE), University Hospital of Cologne, 50924 Cologne, Germany

Correspondence should be addressed to Ralph Mösges; ralph@moesges.de

Academic Editor: Desiderio Passali

Background. Thermal water inhalations and irrigations have a long tradition in the treatment of airway diseases. Currently there exists no systematic review or meta-analysis on the effectiveness of thermal water treatment in upper respiratory tract diseases. *Methods.* A systematic search in the databases of MEDLINE, EMBASE, CENTRAL, ISI Web of Science, and MedPilot was accomplished. *Results.* Eight evaluable outcome parameters from 13 prospective clinical studies were identified for 840 patients. Mucociliary clearance time improves significantly ($P < 0.01$) for the pooled thermal water subgroup and the sulphurous subgroup after 2 weeks (-6.69/minutes) and after 90 days (-8.33/minutes), not for isotonic sodium chloride solution (ISCS). Nasal resistance improved significantly after 2 weeks (Radon, ISCS, and placebo), after 30 days (sulphur and ISCS), and after 90 days (sulphur). Nasal flow improved significantly with the pooled thermal water, radon alone, and ISCS subgroups. For the IgE parameter only sulphurous thermal water ($P < 0.01$) and ISCS ($P > 0.01$) were analyzable. Adverse events of minor character were only reported for sulphurous treatment (19/370). *Conclusion.* Thermal water applications with radon or sulphur can be recommended as additional nonpharmacological treatment in upper airway diseases. Also in comparison to isotonic saline solution it shows significant improvements and should be investigated further.

1. Introduction

Upper airway diseases compass acute and chronic conditions. In this study, we focus on recurrent upper respiratory tract infections (RURT), allergic rhinitis (AR), nonallergic rhinitis (NAR), and acute and chronic rhinosinusitis (ARS/CRS) with and without nasal polyps. These disorders are extremely common and present in all ages, all ethnic populations, and all countries [1]. Apart from their high socioeconomic burden [2], "comorbidities are common and increase the complexity of the management and costs" [1].

Rhinitis is a symptomatic inflammation of the nasal mucosa including nasal symptoms like rhinorrhea, nasal obstruction, nasal itching, and sneezing [3]. The most common form of noninfectious rhinitis is AR with immunoglobulin E- (IgE-) mediated immune response after allergen exposure [1]. Nonallergic rhinitis shows periodic or perennial symptoms, which are not IgE-dependent such as infectious

or vasomotor rhinitis [4]. Infectious rhinitis has either viral, bacterial, or other infectious agents origin [3] and affects millions of people annually [5].

Rhinitis and sinusitis mostly coexist and have been proposed as *rhinosinusitis* [6]. The European Position Paper on Rhinosinusitis and Polyps *EPOS* 2012 [7] defines rhinosinusitis as an inflammation of the nose and paranasal sinuses characterised by two or more symptoms, one of which should be either nasal blockage/obstruction/congestion or nasal discharge. Further, either endoscopic or CT proof is obligatory. Acute and chronic rhinosinusitis are distinguished in length of illness and grade of decay of symptoms. It is characterised by a duration of more than 12 weeks without complete resolution of symptoms and affects approximately 5–15% of the general population [7–9].

State-of-the-art documents ARIA [3] and EPOS [7] provide evidence-based treatment guidelines where "anti-inflammatory medication represents the first-line treatment"

[10]. Along with steroid/pharmacological treatment, EPOS [7] recommends nasal saline irrigation as additional first-line treatment in acute and chronic rhinosinusitis and after sinonasal surgery [7]. Some reviews also state nasal irrigation as adjunctive treatment for allergic rhinitis, acute upper respiratory tract infections, and rhinitis of pregnancy [11–13]. Data for nasal inhalation is limited; EPOS [7] mentions inhalation treatment only in acute rhinosinusitis without evidence. Other guidelines from the German Society of Otorhinolaryngology have an open suggestion for inhalation in rhinosinusitis for symptomatic relief [14].

The current treatment regimens for CRS and AR are effective in the majority of patients, but there are a number of patients still suffering from symptoms [10]. Especially under chronic conditions with long-term drug consumption like glucocorticosteroids, many patients hesitate to take medicine. A publication by Kaschke points out that 64% of AR patients have steroid phobia [15]. It is observed that more and more patients inquire about nonpharmacological therapy approaches in the treatment of rhinosinusitis [16]. Possible approaches besides the proven saline irrigation could be the use of thermal water irrigations and inhalations.

Concerning medical spending, a study by Bhattacharyya points out that the annual costs for medication to treat CRS with intranasal steroids, nonsedating antihistamines, and antibiotic therapy were $213, $227, and $335 in 2003 [2]. Averaging the annual cost of sinus medications including over-the-counter remedies, nasal steroid sprays, and antibiotics, the calculations of Gliklich and Metson result in $1220 per patient [17].

In the United States the medical spending for AR almost doubled from $6.1 billion in 2000 to $11.2 billion in 2005 [18]. Nasal saline irrigation in AR patients helps to reduce medicine consumption by an average of 2.99% [19]. Thermal water applications present an inexpensive nonpharmacological adjunction as well and could therefore further reduce the medicine consumption and costs.

Thermal water treatment belongs to Balneology. Balneology (lat. *balneum*: bath) is the science of natural curative waters, curative gases, and peloides and their use in the treatment of diseases not only as baths, inhalations, or irrigations but also as drinking cures or mud packs [20]. Thermal inhalations and irrigations are century-old practices and already the Romans appreciated the health-promoting effects of different thermal sources.

According to German regulations, natural curative waters are characterised by a minimum content of 1 g dissolved minerals per liter. The designation "thermal water" requires a temperature of a minimum of 20°C when emerging from the spring [21]. Among the many different types of thermal waters our focus is on sulphurous and radon waters. Sulphurous water and its therapeutical use belong to the oldest forms of balneology. It is said to break disulphide bonds of the mucin and activate breathing and blood circulation and helps to reduce inflammation [20, 22, 23]. Radon is a radioactive gas which emits alpha rays. Its very low content in thermal sources has biopositive effects which stimulate cellular activity [24].

Several studies show significant results in thermal water treatment with inhalation or irrigation treatment [25–29]. Up to now no systematic review or meta-analysis on thermal water application in upper airway diseases exists.

2. Materials and Methods

A comprehensive search in the databases of MEDLINE (Medical Literature Analysis and Retrieval System Online), CENTRAL (Cochrane Central Register of Controlled Trials), EMBASE (Excerpta Medica Database), Web of Science, and MedPilot was conducted. In the systematic search the terms "thermal water," "Spa therapy," "thermal water inhalations," and "Spa treatment" were combined with the terms "rhinitis," "rhinosinusitis," "allergic rhinitis," "chronic rhinitis," and "nasal irrigation" with the Boolean operator "and" in all fields. Furthermore, the terms "Radon Spa therapy," "Balneotherapy," "Sulphurous Water," "Bromide Water," "Iodic Water," "Salty Water," and "Radon Water" were linked through "and" with "rhinitis" or "rhinosinusitis." No limitation was made in language, publication date, and duration of the study or the demographic data of patients. Literature published up to and including 27 February 2014 was included.

The inclusion criteria for this meta-analysis were as follows: clinical studies conducted with thermal water for the upper airway diseases, allergic, chronic, or acute rhinosinusitis, at least three or more points on the modified JADAD scale [30], and the presence of the complete statistical data sets consisting of mean deviation, standard deviation, and sample size (if appropriate, calculation using standard error or the upper and lower quartile) at defined follow-up time points.

The following outcome parameters were examined in this study: the mucociliary clearance time (MCT), nasal respiratory flow (Flow), nasal resistance (R), immunoglobulin values A, E, G, and M, and adverse events (AE).

3. Data Collection and Analysis

The search described above initially resulted in 2113 matches. Duplicates and studies that were either nonclinical or disease-specific not relevant for this analysis were excluded so that the abstracts of 50 remaining studies were examined. Another 15 could be excluded after the perusal of the abstract. 35 studies were investigated in full-text which led to the exclusion of another seven studies due to divergent treatment modalities [22, 31, 32], mismatching disease patterns [33, 34], unavailability [35], or the conduction of the study with animals [36].

The remaining 28 articles were evaluated by two independent reviewers with the modified Jadad Scale by Oremus et al. [30]. It amplifies the original 3-item Jadad Scale [37] consisting of randomization, blinding, and study dropouts by adding inclusion/exclusion criteria, side effects, and statistical methods. Additionally, it features two bonus points for appropriate randomisation method and double-blinding. If this does not apply, these points are deducted. The minimum score is 0 points; the maximum score is 8 points.

We set a minimal score of at least three points to establish a qualitative homogeneity essential for our meta-analysis. Thus another 15 studies were excluded [38–52] and 13 studies remained for our analysis. Four of those are in Italian and nine in English.

The different thermal waters used in the studies included were pooled concerning their different substances. This resulted in two main groups: sulphurous water with nine studies [25–28, 53–57] and radon water with two studies [29, 58]. Salt-bromine-iodine water [59] and hypermineral chloride sodium water [60] were used once. We also pooled a common thermal water group to compare it to isotonic sodium chloride solution (ISCS) and placebo. Figure 1 shows a flowchart of the literature identification process. Tables 1 and 2 show the included studies in a systemic overview.

3.1. Statistical Methods. The statistical calculations were performed using the statistic software Comprehensive Meta-Analysis Version 2.2.064 (Biostat, Inc.). The study values for the identified outcome parameters were sorted according to the time of measurement (baseline, 12 days, 2 weeks, 30 days, and 90 days). Studies with the same parameter and different (follow-up) times of measurement, of 12 and 14 days, were combined to one-time measurement (2 weeks). All points of measurements of the different studies were summarised and analysed using the random-effect model. The mean and, respectively, the standard error of the mean are depicted in the figures (Figures 2–5). In the following analysis we assumed a significance if the P value was less than or equal to 5% ($P \leq 0.05$). For clarification, significant improvements/changes are marked with * in Tables 4–7. For some identified parameters data were available from one study only and therefore had to be excluded from the meta-analysis but are, for the sake of completeness, included in the figures with an interrupted line.

4. Results

In total, 13 studies published between 1998 and 2013 have been included in this analysis.

All forms of applications were pooled. The specific form of application and the number of patients is depicted in Table 3. An aerosol therapy is categorised under inhalations. Altogether, 430 patients received irrigations and 557 patients inhalations.

4.1. Study Design. All studies feature a prospective study design. Five studies are randomised, controlled, and double-blind [25–28, 54]; other three studies are randomised and controlled [56, 59, 60]; one study is controlled and double-blind [29]; one is only double-blind [55]. The remaining studies are not randomised, blinded, or controlled [53, 57, 58]. ISCS was used for the control groups, drinking water or distilled water for placebo groups. The duration of the studies varies between 12 days and 6 months.

4.2. Selection of Patients. A total number of 840 patients aged between 2 and 100 years took part in these studies, 510 of them received an application with thermal water, 285 were treated with ISCS [25–28, 56, 59], 20 inhaled drinking water [29], and 25 inhaled distilled water [54].

4.3. Mucociliary Clearance Time. MCT was examined in seven studies with 422 patients in total (Table 4). Thermal water (radon, sulphur, and salt-bromine-iodine) applications showed a significant improvement of MCT compared to baseline at both points of measurement (Figure 2). The measurement for ISCS compared to baseline showed no significance after two weeks but after 90 days in the followup. Only one study was conducted with placebo which did not show any significance neither did radon water applications ($P = 0.059$). Sulphurous water applications showed significant lower values after two weeks compared to the baseline value ($P < 0.01$) and are also significant lower after 90 days compared to the baseline values ($P < 0.01$).

In an internal comparison between the ISCS group and the sulphurous water group we had nonsignificant initial situations ($P = 0.211$), but after 2 weeks and 90 days the outcome differed significantly ($P < 0.01$). The ISCS and the radon group already differed significantly in baseline values ($P < 0.05$) and had almost parallel curves.

Figure 2 illustrates all values calculated in the meta-analysis and noted in Table 4.

4.4. Nasal Resistance. Nasal resistance was measured in six of the included trials with a total number of 347 patients (Table 5). Thermal water treatment was not significant after two weeks but after 30 and 90 days compared to baseline. ISCS treatment showed significance after two weeks and 30 days compared to baseline, but after 90 days there was no significance. This graph (Figure 3, ISCS graph) showed a very erratic curve due to the very heterogeneous study design and the different points of measurement of the three studies included. Both the treatment with placebo and the treatment with radon water showed significance after two weeks. The treatment with sulphurous water showed significance after 30 ($P < 0.01$) and 90 days ($P < 0.05$) but not after two weeks ($P = 0.118$).

4.5. Nasal Flow. The nasal flow was specified in three of the included trials with 117 patients (Table 6). All of these patients received inhalation and aerosol therapy. Figure 4 shows all included studies, using this outcome parameter, the dotted lines for placebo and sulphur indicate single studies. Compared to baseline, the combined thermal water group ($P < 0.05$), as well as the radon ($P < 0.05$) and the sulphurous water group ($P < 0.01$), showed significant improvement after two weeks, whereas drinking water application ($P = 0.425$) showed no improvement or significance.

4.6. Immunoglobulins E, A, G, and M. Immunoglobulin concentrations in the blood were examined in two of the included trials [25, 26] with a total number of 180 patients. Both studies compared sulphurous water treatment to ISCS treatment. Distribution of the number of patients (90 patients per group) was equal in both studies.

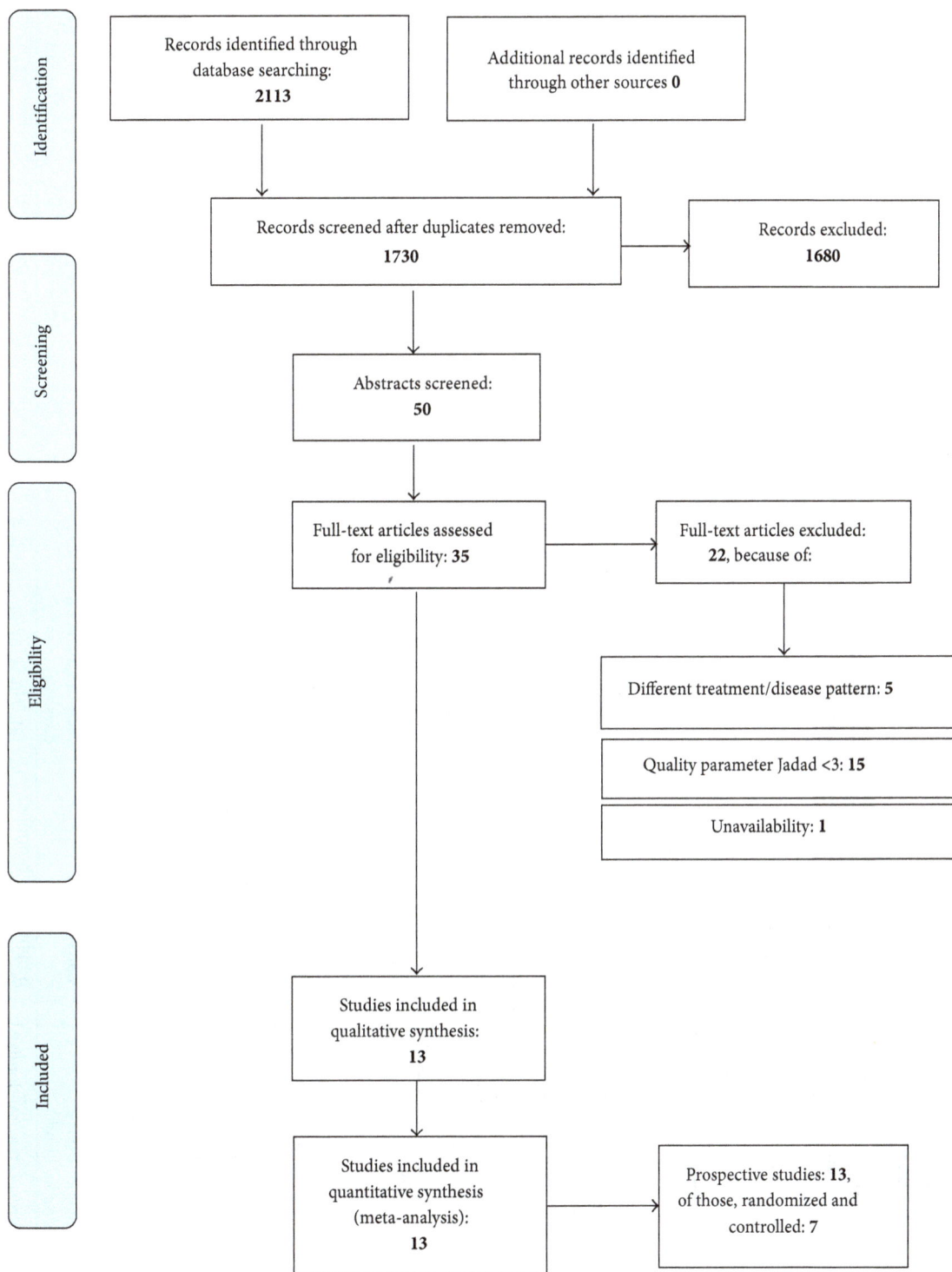

FIGURE 1: Flow chart. Source: PRISMA 2009 Flow chart [61], augmented with exclusions and types of included studies.

4.7. IgE. Figure 5 illustrates the meta-analysis outcome for IgE. Both groups started from a comparable initial position. Sulphurous water treatment rose significantly ($P < 0.01$) at both measurement points 12 and 90 days compared to baseline in contrast to ISCS treatment which was neither significant after 12 days ($P = 0.442$) nor after 90 days ($P = 0.567$).

4.8. IgA, G, and M. No significant differences could be revealed in the analysis of the immunoglobulins A, G,

Table 1: Included studies.

Author	Year	Study design	Thermal water/control	Application	Adverse events	MCT	Flow	Resistance	IgA	IgE	IgG	IgM
De Luca et al. [53]	2006	Prospective, nonrandomized, noncontrolled	Sulphur/—	Inhalation 1x daily 10 min for 12 days	X	X						
Marullo and Abramo [29]	2000	Prospective, nonrandomized, controlled, double-blind	Radon/Tap water	Inhalation 10 min, Aerosol 10 min, 1x daily for 12 days	X	X	X	X				
Miraglia del Giudice et al. [60]	2011	Prospective, randomized, controlled	Hypermineral chloride sodium water/ISCS	Aerosol 15 days a month for 3 months/ ISCS daily for 3 months	X							
Ottaviano et al. [27]	2012	Prospective, randomized, controlled, double-blind	Sulphur-Arsenic-Ferrous water diluted to 10% solution with distilled water/ISCS	Irrigation 1x daily 20 mL for 1 month	X			X				
Ottaviano et al. [28]	2011	Prospective, randomized, controlled, double-blind	Sulphur-Salt-Bromine-Iodine/ISCS	Irrigation 4x daily 5 mL for 1 month	X			X				
Passali et al. [58]	2013	Prospective, nonrandomized, noncontrolled	Radon/—	Inhalation, Aerosol, each 10 min 1x daily for 14 days	X	X	X	X				
Passali et al. [59]	2008	Prospective, randomized, controlled	Salt-Bromine-Iodine/ISCS	Inhalation 10 min, Aerosol 10 min, Irrigation 5 min 1x daily for 14 days	X	X						
Passariello et al. [57]	2012	Prospective, nonrandomized, noncontrolled	Sulphate-Sodium-Chloride/—	Aerosol 15 min 1x daily for 15 days	X							
Salami et al. [26]	2010	Prospective, randomized, controlled, double-blind	Sulphur/ISCS	Inhalation, 10 min Irrigation 6 min 1x daily for 12 days	X	X		X	X	X	X	
Salami et al. [25]	2008	Prospective, randomized, controlled, double-blind	Sulphur/ISCS	Inhalation 10 min 1x daily for 12 days	X	X			X	X	X	
Staffieri et al. [56]	2008	Prospective, randomized, controlled	Sulphur-Arsenic-Ferrous water diluted to 10% solution with distilled water/ISCS	Irrigation 4x daily 20 mL for 6 months	X							
Staffieri and Abramo [55]	2007	Prospective, nonrandomized, noncontrolled, double-blind	Sulphur-Arsenic-Ferrous water/—	Inhalation, Aerosol each 10 min, 1x daily for 12 days	X	X	X	X				
Staffieri et al. [54]	1998	Prospective, randomized, controlled, double-blind	Sulphur-Salt-Bromine-Iodine/distilled water	Inhalation, 10 min, Aerosol 10 min 1x daily for 12 days	X							

TABLE 2: Systematic presentation of the studies included.

Author	Year	Jadad score	Number of patients thermal water/control	Age span/average age	Duration of treatment	Measurement time points	Inclusion criteria	Exclusion criteria
De Luca et al. [53]	2006	3	40/—	74–100/86,5	12 days	Baseline Follow-Up: Day 12	(i) Presence of chronic rhinitis or chronic rhinosinusitis (ii) Allergic or vasomotor nasal hyperactivity (iii) Chronic laryngitis (iv) Chronic pharyngitis	(i) Acute pathologies in ENT region (ii) Steroids, mucolytics, antihistamine, NSAIDs, vasoconstrictive drugs or antibiotics in the last 30 days (iii) Autoimmune disease (iv) Patients with malignant neoplasms, surgical intervention, and/or radio chemotherapy
Marullo and Abramo [29]	2000	3	27/20	15–81/52.4	12 days	Baseline Follow-Up: Day 12	(i) At least 3 confirmed episodes of sinonasal infection in the previous 12 months (ii) Evidence of chronic sinonasal inflammation at objective otorhinolaryngologic evaluation	(i) Vasoconstrictive drugs, local and systemic steroids, NSAIDs, antihistamine, and mucolytics in the last 2 months (ii) Patients who for various reasons were not able to ensure the conclusion of the study (iii) Patients who present anterior rhinoscopy
Miraglia del Giudice et al. [60]	2011	5	20/20	6–14/	15 days a month for 3 months	Baseline Follow-Up: Week 12, 14	(i) Age from 6 to 14 (ii) History of seasonal moderate to severe allergic rhinitis for at least 2 years (iii) Positive skin prick test to Parietaria pollen (iv) History of mild intermittent asthma	(i) Antihistamines, intranasal, bronchial, or systemic corticosteroids, cromolyn sodium, and leukotriene modifiers in the previous 6 weeks (ii) sinus and/or upper or lower respiratory tract infection, persistent asthma, nasal surgery within the last year, respiratory tract abnormalities, and systemic diseases
Ottaviano et al. [27]	2012	5	35/35	18–65/ not specified	12 weeks	Baseline Follow-Up: Day 30, 90	(i) Age from 18 to 65 (ii) Nonallergic chronic rhinitis (iii) Cigarette smoking habit for at least 5 years	Autoimmune diseases, cystic fibrosis, and diabetes
Ottaviano et al. [28]	2011	8	40/40	18–65/ not specified	1 month	Baseline Follow-Up: Day 30	(i) Age from 18 to 65 (ii) Nonallergic chronic rhinosinusitis	Autoimmune diseases, cystic fibrosis, and diabetes
Passali et al. [58]	2013	3	33/—	12 years and older/ not specified	14 days	Baseline Follow-Up: Day 14	(i) Nasal obstruction evaluated by a 10-point Visual Analog Scale (1: nasal airways completely free; 10: nasal airway completely blocked) higher than 7 in the previous 2 months (ii) Chronic rhinosinusitis, persistent allergic rhinitis, vasomotor rhinitis with inferior turbinate hypertrophy	(i) Acute viral rhinitis (ii) Obstructive polyposis (iii) Nasal steroid, vasoconstrictive drug therapies or systemic NSAIDs, oral steroids and mucolytic treatment in the previous 2 months

TABLE 2: Continued.

Author	Year	Jadad score	Number of patients thermal water/control	Age span/average age	Duration of treatment	Measurement time points	Inclusion criteria	Exclusion criteria
Passali et al. [59]	2008	3	60/60	15–65/not specified	14 days	Baseline Follow-Up: Day 14	Chronic rhinosinusitis with/or nasal polyposis of 1 second degree of the Lund-Mackay-Classification [62]	Not specified
Passariello et al. [57]	2012	3	60/—	2–12/3.4 ± 1	15 days	Baseline Follow-Up: Day 15	(i) Age from 2 to12 (ii) CRS (iii) One or more of the following sinonasal symptoms: nasal discharge, congestion, obstruction, postnasal drip, daytime cough, and foul breath (iv) Failed courses of antibiotics, saline irrigation, nasal steroids, or antihistamine (v) Persistent symptoms for ≥1 month	(i) Steroids, nonsteroidal anti-inflammatory drugs, antihistamines, and vasoconstrictors in the previous 4 weeks (ii) Primary diagnosis of obstructive sleep apnea syndrome caused by tonsillar hyperplasia (iii) Chronic diseases, immunodeficiency, and neurological impairment (iv) Varicose veins of the nasal septum, and suspect ciliary abnormalities (v) Previous sinonasal surgery (vi) Malformation of the upper airway sinonasal osteogenesis, tumors, and obstructive lesions (vii) History of facial trauma that distorted the sinus anatomy
Salami et al. [26]	2010	5	40/40	26–58/46.4	12 days	Baseline Follow-Up: Day 12, 90	CRS without polyps	(i) Immunostimulant or immunosuppressive agents in the previous 6 months (ii) Genetic and congenital condition: cystic fibrosis and primary ciliary dyskinesia (iii) Nasal polys (iv) Positive allergy testing (v) Anatomic abnormalities (severe septal deviation among others) (vi) Acquired mucociliary dysfunction (vii) Neoplasms (viii) Acute contemporary bacterial and/or viral rhinosinusitis, middle ear, and respiratory tract (ix) Bronchopulmonary disease (x) Nasal trauma (xi) Smoker (xii) Previous nasal and sinus surgery

TABLE 2: Continued.

Author	Year	Jadad score	Number of patients thermal water/control	Age span/average age	Duration of treatment	Measurement time points	Inclusion criteria	Exclusion criteria
Salami et al. [25]	2008	7	50/50	6–14/9	12 days	Baseline Follow-Up: Day 12, 90	At least 3 acute episodes of upper respiratory tract infections in the last year	(i) Immunostimulant or immunosuppressive agents in the previous 6 months (ii) Previous adenoidectomy and/or tonsillectomy (iii) Anatomic anomalies (iv) Other acute infections (v) Allergic rhinitis (vi) Congenital immunodeficiency's (vii) Pulmonary disease
Staffieri et al. [56]	2008	5	40/40	18–65/not specified	6 months	Baseline Follow-Up: Day 30, 90, 180	(i) Age from 18 to 65 (ii) CRS not responding to medical treatment (iii) No contraindications to general anaesthesia and FESS	(i) Autoimmune disease (ii) Cystic fibrosis (iii) Diabetes (iv) Sinonasal inverted papilloma or sinonasal malignancy
Staffieri and Abramo [55]	2007	4	37/—	40/not specified	12 days	Baseline Follow-Up: Day 12	(i) At least 3 confirmed episodes of sinonasal infection in the previous 12 months (ii) Evidence of chronic sinonasal inflammation at otorhinolaryngologic endoscopic evaluation	Nasal steroid, vasoconstrictive drug therapies or systemic NSAIDs, and steroid or mucolytic treatments in the previous 2 months
Staffieri et al. [54]	1998	3	25/25	18–83/50.5	12 days	Baseline Follow-Up: Day 12	Chronic rhinopharyngotubaric inflammation	Not specified

TABLE 3: Type of application.

Application	Inhalation	Inhalation + aerosol	Irrigation	Inhalation + irrigation	Inhalation + aerosol + irrigation	Aerosol
Number of patients	140	117	230	80	120	100
Study	De Luca et al. [53] Salami et al. [25]	Marullo and Abramo [29] Passali et al. [58] Staffieri and Abramo [55] Staffieri et al. [54]	Ottaviano et al. [27] Ottaviano et al. [28] Staffieri et al. [56]	Salami et al. [26]	Passali et al. [59]	Miraglia del Giudice et al. [60] Passariello et al. [57]

TABLE 4: Results of MCT.

	Patients	MCTt	CI 95%	P value
Thermal water (sulphur + salt-bromine-iodine + radon)				
Baseline	265	19.67020883	[17.40; 21.94]	
2 weeks	265	12.98258754	[11.34; 14.63]	<0.01*
90 days	90	11.34482778	[10.91; 11.78]	<0.01*
ISCS				
Baseline	137	21.81138859	[18.19; 25.05]	
2 weeks	137	18.54655442	[17.09; 20.01]	0.107
90 days	90	17.60438587	[17.17; 18.04]	<0.05*
Placebo				
Baseline	20	19.8	[17.78; 21.82]	
2 weeks	20	18.5	[15.65; 21.35]	0.465
Radon				
Baseline	60	15.84974132	[11.85; 19.85]	
2 weeks	60	11.95305164	[11.33; 12.58]	0.059
Sulphur				
Baseline	205	19.43087224	[18.89; 19.97]	
2 weeks	205	12.57267757	[10.30; 14.85]	<0.01*
90 days	90	11.34482778	[10.91; 11.78]	<0.01*

*Significant in comparison to baseline ($P < 0.05$).

TABLE 5: Results of nasal resistance.

	Patients	NasRes	CI 95%	P value
Thermal (sulphur +radon)				
Baseline	212	0,442260114	[0.26; 0.62]	
2 weeks	137	0.257467503	[0.22; 0.30]	0.051
30 days	66	0.113901251	[0.05; 0.18]	<0.01*
90 days	64	0.159927083	[0.003; 0.32]	<0.05*
ISCS				
Baseline	115	0.516633	[0.13; 0.90]	
2 weeks	40	1.28	[1.16; 1.40]	<0.01
30 days	62	0.124408602	[0.10; 0.15]	<0.05
90 days	68	0.617283393	[−0.36; 1.60]	0.851
Placebo				
Baseline	20	0.23	[0.19; 0.27]	
2 weeks	20	0.19	[0.17; 0.21]	<0.05*
Radon				
Baseline	60	0.364606147	[0.33; 0.40]	
2 weeks	60	0.240700629	[0.15; 0.33]	<0.05*
Sulphur				
Baseline	152	0.495021367	[0.22; 0.77]	
2 weeks	77	0.272182942	[0.26; 0.29]	0.118
30 days	66	0.113901251	[0.05; 0.18]	<0.01*
90 days	64	0.159927083	[0.003; 0.32]	<0.05*

*Significant in comparison to baseline ($P < 0.05$).

TABLE 6: Results of nasal flow.

	Patients	NasFlow	CI 95%	P value
Thermal (sulphur + radon)				
Baseline	97	604.1	[513.68; 694.45]	
12–14 days	97	721.5	[697.18; 745.84)	<0.05*
Placebo				
Baseline	20	714.3	[664.13; 764.47]	
12–14 days	20	687.5	[644.79; 730.21]	0.425
Radon				
Baseline	60	633.4	[540.95; 725.90]	
12–14 days	60	738.8	[703.64; 773.89]	<0.05*
Sulphur				
Baseline	37	558.4	[526.53; 590.27]	
12–14 days	37	705.6	[671.86; 739.34]	<0.01*

*Significant in comparison to baseline ($P < 0.05$).

and M, neither beyond the subgroups between ISCS and sulphur nor in the individual groups between the baseline and the maximal treatment duration of 90 days.

4.9. Adverse Events. All adverse events that occurred during the studies in the entire patient population were extracted and illustrated in forest plots. In total, 19 patients out of 840 treated patients suffered from study related adverse events.

All adverse events occurred under the treatment with sulphurous water: 13 patients experienced mild nasal irritation and a sensation of burning after application and five suffered from very limited epistaxis, one from an aggravation of the symptoms, and one from dermatological hypersensitivity. No adverse events are reported for the treatment with another thermal water, ISCS, or placebo.

For sulphurous water, 19 adverse events occurred in a total group of 370 patients. This led to an adverse event rate of

TABLE 7: Results of IgE.

	Patients	IgE	CI 95%	P value
Sulphur				
Baseline	90	105.11	[98.53; 111.69]	
12 days	90	75.65	[70.13; 81.18]	<0.01*
90 days	90	74.79	[69.38; 80.19]	<0.01*
ISCS				
Baseline	90	101.69	[94.03; 109.35]	
12 days	90	97.10	[88.22; 105.98]	0.442
90 days	90	98.30	[89.60; 107.00]	0.567

*Significant in comparison to baseline ($P < 0.05$).

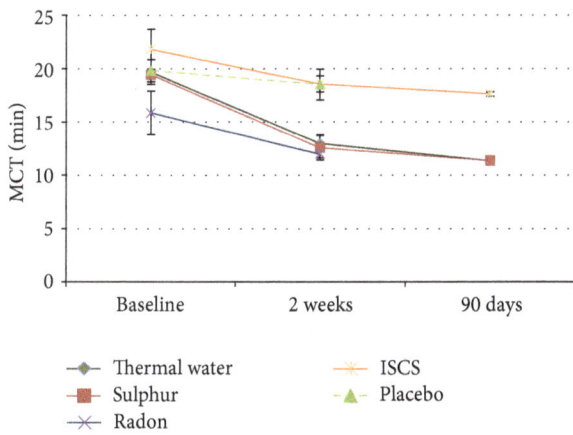

FIGURE 2: Mucociliary clearance time.

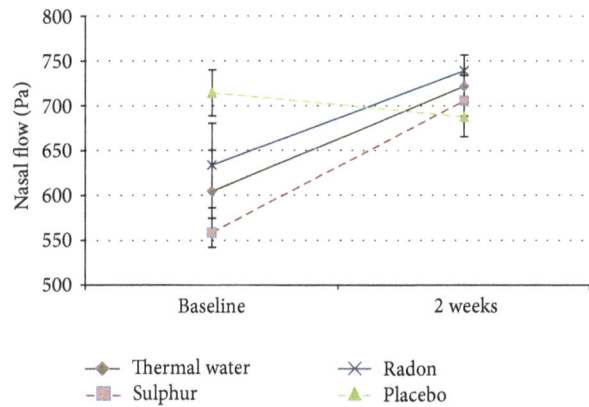

FIGURE 4: Nasal flow. Dotted lines present single studies.

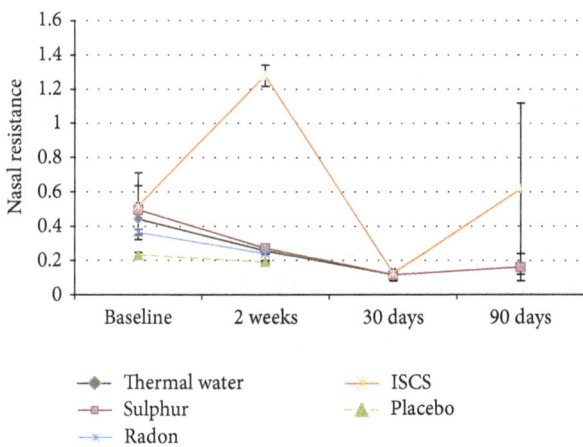

FIGURE 3: Nasal resistance.

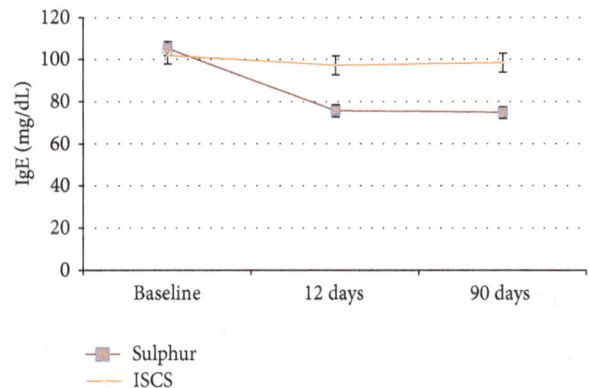

FIGURE 5: IgE in serum.

5. Discussion

This review and its appertaining meta-analysis is the first systematic approach to thermal water treatment in upper respiratory tract diseases. For the identified outcome parameters some significant improvements could be found in the treatment with thermal water irrigation and inhalation.

In order to ensure methodological quality of the included trials, two independent reviewers applied the modified Jadad Scale to every study with a minimal score of 3.

11.9%. The assumed rate of adverse events ranged from 7.8 to 17.6% (Figure 6).

By pooling all thermal water subgroups we received a total number of 510 treated patients with 19 adverse events. This led to an adverse event rate of 9.8% with an assumed range from 6.6 to 14.4% (Figure 7).

Study name	Event rate	Lower limit	Upper limit	Total	Event rate and 95% CI
De_Luca et al._2006	0.125	0.053	0.267	5/40	
Ottaviano et al._2011	0.275	0.159	0.432	11/40	
Ottaviano et al._2012	0.014	0.001	0.187	0/35	
Salami et al._2008	0.010	0.001	0.138	0/50	
Salami et al._2010	0.012	0.001	0.167	0/40	
Staffieri et al._1998	0.019	0.001	0.244	0/25	
Staffieri and Abramo_2007	0.013	0.001	0.178	0/37	
Staffieri et al._2008	0.075	0.024	0.208	3/40	
Passariello et al._2012	0.008	0.000	0.113	0/63	
	0.119	**0.078**	**0.176**		

Statistics for each study

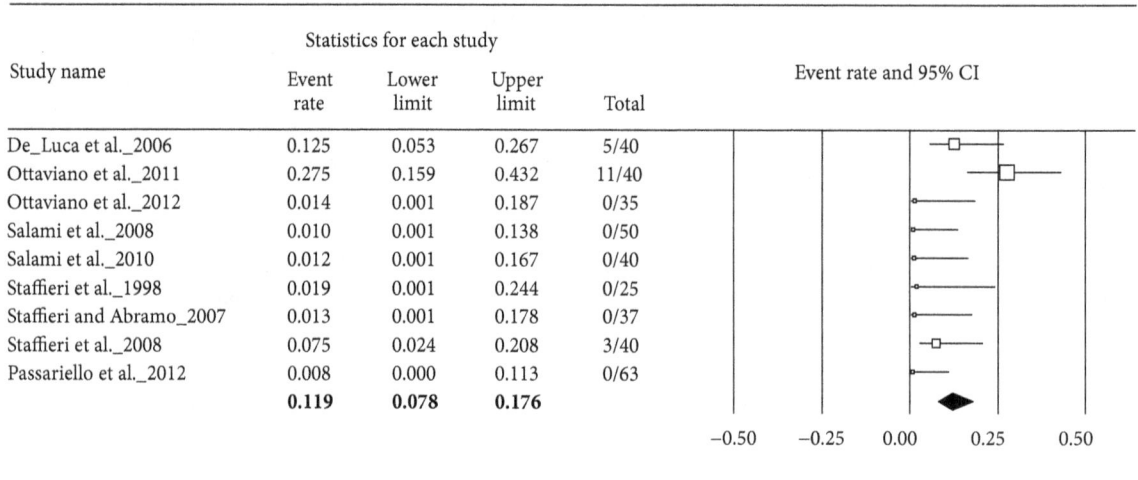

FIGURE 6: Adverse events for sulphurous water.

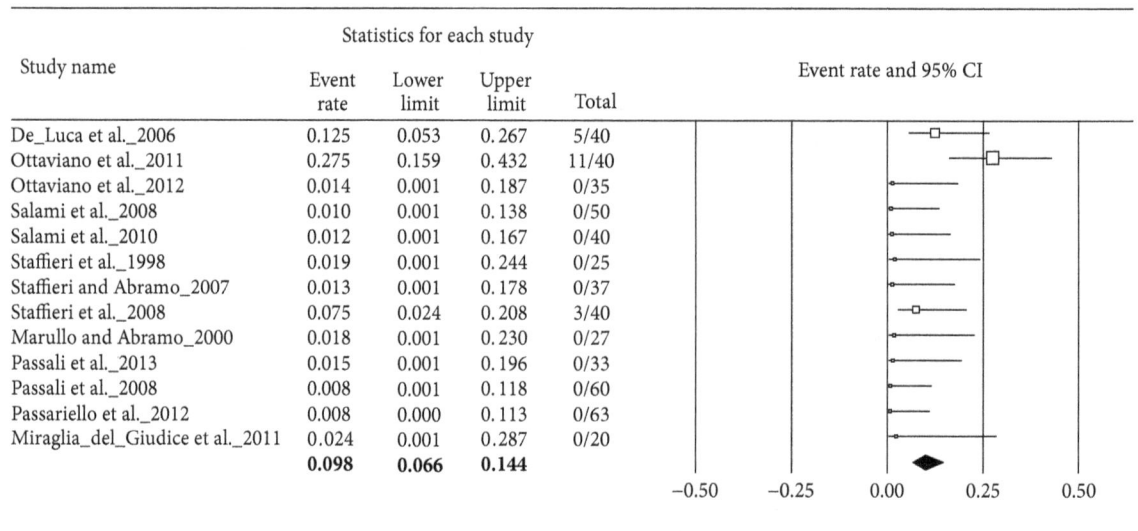

Study name	Event rate	Lower limit	Upper limit	Total	Event rate and 95% CI
De_Luca et al._2006	0.125	0.053	0.267	5/40	
Ottaviano et al._2011	0.275	0.159	0.432	11/40	
Ottaviano et al._2012	0.014	0.001	0.187	0/35	
Salami et al._2008	0.010	0.001	0.138	0/50	
Salami et al._2010	0.012	0.001	0.167	0/40	
Staffieri et al._1998	0.019	0.001	0.244	0/25	
Staffieri and Abramo_2007	0.013	0.001	0.178	0/37	
Staffieri et al._2008	0.075	0.024	0.208	3/40	
Marullo and Abramo_2000	0.018	0.001	0.230	0/27	
Passali et al._2013	0.015	0.001	0.196	0/33	
Passali et al._2008	0.008	0.001	0.118	0/60	
Passariello et al._2012	0.008	0.000	0.113	0/63	
Miraglia_del_Giudice et al._2011	0.024	0.001	0.287	0/20	
	0.098	**0.066**	**0.144**		

Statistics for each study

FIGURE 7: Adverse events for thermal water.

Further this meta-analysis is calculated by the "random effects" model, which takes possible heterogeneity more into consideration than the "fixed effect" model. The confidence intervals are broader and thus capture the true value of the meta-analysis. Where relative overestimation of smaller studies can result in greater inaccuracy, this is a more conservative and cautious estimation. It constitutes a higher risk for bias of the results [63].

In addition, we pooled the clinical pictures of allergic, acute, and chronic rhinosinusitis as well as studies with children, adults, and elderly people. In two studies patients with minimally invasive functional endoscopic sinus surgery (FESS) before treatment were included. This can be assumed as selection bias for this meta-analysis. Furthermore, only published studies were included in this meta-analysis. Thus, publication bias may occur.

Besides irrigation, also inhalation therapy was used in the different studies. Both treatments reduced inflammatory mediators in nasal secretions [64]. Nasal irrigation had a direct physical cleansing effect by flushing out thick mucus, crusts, debris, allergens, and air pollutants [65]. In a review by Hermelingmeier et al. the conclusion drawn is that there is no clear data available naming the most advantageous form of application in nasal saline irrigation [19].

The present meta-analysis shows a significant advantage of mucociliary clearance changes with thermal water in comparison to isotonic saline solution. This leads to a more detailed view of the results of thermal water applications found in this meta-analysis.

The MCT parameter comprises the best set of data in our meta-analysis with seven included studies and 422 patients. Mucociliary clearance is an important defence mechanism for both upper and lower airways and "its impairment[…] predisposes to chronic infection of the nose, paranasal sinuses and the respiratory tree" [66]. The average MCT values range below 15 minutes with a test duration of less than

1 hour [67]. In this meta-analysis a significant improvement of the mucociliary clearance could be determined in thermal water applications. Hereby, the transport time could be reduced from 19.67 minutes initially to 12.98 minutes after two weeks and to 11.34 minutes after 90 days. Especially the application of sulphurous water showed a high significance ($P < 0.001$) after the two-week treatment period. At the same time the treatment with radon thermal water ($P = 0.059$) only just lacked a significant improvement ($P = 0.059$).

The literature available for these two subgroups was $5 : 2$ with only 60 patients in the radon group which might have had an influence on the significance. In contrast to the thermal water group, the ISCS group only showed significance after 90 days of treatment. In turn the literature available was quite strong with 4 studies and a total of 205 patients.

Based on Marullo's study only it was not possible to conduct a meta-analysis and draw a valid conclusion on the use of placebo [29]. The meta-analysis of the mucociliary clearance time showed a significant benefit especially of the pooled thermal water treatment and sulphurous water over ISCS.

The "nasal resistance is the resistance offered by the nasal cavity to inspired air" [68] and it is measured in Pascal (Pa). All studies used for this analysis already resulted in significant changes after two weeks of treatment with radon thermal water. ISCS differed significantly after two weeks and after 30 days of treatment. The meta-analysis revealed significant variations in the three pooled ISCS studies. Especially the study of Salami et al. displayed a high deviation from the baseline of 13.1 Pa, which was reduced to 1.28 Pa after two weeks and remained rather high after 90 days of treatment with 1.12 Pa.

Opposed to these findings were those of the two other studies of this pool [27, 28], which began with much lower baseline values of 0.14 and 0.17 Pa and had different followups. Therefore these led to an unsteady curve and limited the possibility of a serious interpretation of the healing process. Nevertheless, each of these three studies showed a reduction of the nasal resistance.

The treatment with sulphurous water showed good results throughout the whole treatment period of 90 days. The results were even better after 30 and 90 days than at the beginning, which allows for the assumption that a more permanent improvement is gained here.

Based on this meta-analysis we can assume that radon water application shows significant improvement in nasal flow. The data is quite limited with the results of only one study for placebo and one for sulphurous treatment, so that we cannot compare it to the pooled results.

The use of radon thermal water as well as the entire thermal water subgroup showed a significant improvement in the nasal flow after two weeks of treatment.

In our meta-analysis of IgE, sulphurous water treatment was highly significant after 12 and 90 days. ISCS treatment showed no significance. The present IgE results were measured in patients with chronic inflammatory conditions, where eosinophil cells in the mucus are increased [69]. Reduction of eosinophil cells after thermal water treatment was also reported in Passali et al. [58] and significantly

decreased in Staffieri and Abramo [55]. Hypereosinophilia is related to high levels of serum concentrations of IgE [26, 70]. The IgE concentration which decreased significantly after the application with sulphurous water confirmed beneficial effects on chronic inflammatory disorders. Sulphurous water helps to clean the nasal mucosa from irritations and reduces immune responses at a local level [25, 71]. These results support the assumption that sulphurous water has an anti-inflammatory effect.

IgA, IgG, and IgM values in the blood did not increase significantly neither with sulphurous water nor with ISCS. Unfortunately the literature available on the secretory IgA, which is secreted across the mucosa and plays a significant role in specific immune defence by preventing or blocking the adhesion of bacteria and defending the mucous membranes from common infection [72, 73], was not sufficient for a statistical analysis. Similarly, comparable studies investigating the IgM and IgG in the mucosa were missing.

Generally speaking, thermal water application is a safe treatment. Adverse events occurred in 19 out of 510 thermal water treatments and mainly consisted of mild nasal irritation, a sensation of local burning after application, and very limited epistaxis. All of these adverse events occurred under the treatment with sulphurous water. Neither for radon water, ISCS, nor placebo treatment adverse events were reported. It should be noted that both the studies by Staffieri et al. [56] and Ottaviano et al. [28] were conducted in a postoperative setting, which makes the occurrence of such adverse events more likely. Further, the study by De Luca et al. [53] was conducted with elderly people between 72 and 100 years.

6. Conclusion

Nasal application of thermal water results in a significant improvement of MCT, nasal flow, nasal resistance, and IgE concentration. The systematic review and the meta-analysis demonstrate an advantage of thermal water treatment over isotonic saline solution and placebo. Even though this aspect needs to be investigated further with randomised controlled trials in bigger cohorts and longer follow-up periods, it was shown that the application with thermal water can serve as additional nonpharmacological alternative.

Abbreviations

AE: Adverse events
AR: Allergic rhinitis
ARIA: Allergic rhinitis and its impact on asthma
ARS: Acute rhinosinusitis
CRS: Chronic rhinosinusitis
EPOS: European Position Paper on
        Rhinosinusitis and Polyps
FESS: Functional endoscopic sinus surgery
Flow: Nasal respiratory flow
Ig: Immunoglobulin
ISCS: Isotonic sodium chloride solution
MCT: Mucociliary clearing time
NAR: Nonallergic rhinitis
Pa: Pascal

R: Resistance
RURT: Recurrent upper airway infections.

Conflict of Interests

Sarah Keller, Volker König, and Ralph Mösges report no conflict of interests concerning this paper.

Authors' Contribution

All authors have contributed to, seen, and approved the paper.

Acknowledgment

The authors would like to thank Marie-Josefine Joisten, M.A., for her editorial assistance.

References

[1] J. Bousquet, C. Bachert, G. W. Canonica et al., "Unmet needs in severe chronic upper airway disease (SCUAD)," *Journal of Allergy and Clinical Immunology*, vol. 124, no. 3, pp. 428–433, 2009.

[2] N. Bhattacharyya, "The economic burden and symptom manifestations of chronic rhinosinusitis," *American Journal of Rhinology*, vol. 17, no. 1, pp. 27–32, 2003.

[3] J. Bousquet, P. van Cauwenberge, and N. Khaltaev, "Allergic rhinitis and its impact on asthma," *Journal of Allergy and Clinical Immunology*, vol. 108, supplement 5, pp. S147–334, 2001.

[4] D. V. Wallace, M. S. Dykewicz, D. I. Bernstein et al., "The diagnosis and management of rhinitis: an updated practice parameter," *Journal of Allergy and Clinical Immunology*, vol. 122, supplement 2, pp. S1–S84, 2008.

[5] M. A. Sande and J. M. Gwaltney, "Acute community-acquired bacterial sinusitis: continuing challenges and current management," *Clinical Infectious Diseases*, vol. 39, supplement 3, pp. S151–S158, 2004.

[6] M. Thomas, B. Yawn, D. Price, V. Lund, J. Mullol, and W. Fokkens, "EPOS primary care guidelines: European Position Paper on the primary care diagnosis and management of Rhinosinusitis and Nasal Polyps 2007—a summary," *Primary Care Respiratory Journal*, vol. 17, no. 2, pp. 79–89, 2008.

[7] W. J. Fokkens, V. Lund, J. Mullol et al., "EPOS, 2012: European position paper on rhinosinusitis and nasal polyps 2012. A summary for otorhinolaryngologists," *Rhinology*, vol. 50, no. 1, pp. 1–12, 2012.

[8] D. Hastan, W. J. Fokkens, C. Bachert et al., "Chronic rhinosinusitis in Europe—an underestimated disease. A GA2LEN study," *Allergy*, vol. 66, no. 9, pp. 1216–1223, 2011.

[9] V. Benson and M. A. Marano, "Current estimates from the National Health Interview Survey, 1995," *Vital and Health Statistics. Series 10, Data from the National Health Survey*, no. 199, pp. 1–428, 1998.

[10] P. W. Hellings, W. J. Fokkens, C. Akdis et al., "Uncontrolled allergic rhinitis and chronic rhinosinusitis: where do we stand today?" *Allergy*, vol. 68, no. 1, pp. 1–7, 2013.

[11] D. Rabago and A. Zgierska, "Saline nasal irrigation for upper respiratory conditions," *American Family Physician*, vol. 80, no. 10, pp. 1117–1119, 2009.

[12] J. C. Kassel, D. King, and G. K. Spurling, "Saline nasal irrigation for acute upper respiratory tract infections," *Cochrane Database of Systematic Reviews*, no. 3, Article ID CD006821, 2010.

[13] R. Harvey, S. A. Hannan, L. Badia, and G. Scadding, "Nasal saline irrigations for the symptoms of chronic rhinosinusitis," *Cochrane Database of Systematic Reviews*, no. 3, Article ID CD006394, 2007.

[14] B. A. Stuck, C. Bachert, P. Federspil et al., "Rhinosinusitis guidelines-unabridged version: S2 guidelines from the German Society of Otorhinolaryngology, Head and Neck Surgery," *HNO*, vol. 60, no. 2, pp. 141–162, 2012.

[15] O. Kaschke, "Auswirkungen einer Steroidphobie in Deutschland auf die Therapie mit topischen Glukokortikoiden," *MedReport*, vol. 32, article 10, 2008.

[16] N. Achilles and R. Mösges, "Nasal saline irrigations for the symptoms of acute and chronic rhinosinusitis," *Current Allergy and Asthma Reports*, vol. 13, no. 2, pp. 229–235, 2013.

[17] R. E. Gliklich and R. Metson, "Economic implications of chronic sinusitis," *Otolaryngology—Head and Neck Surgery*, vol. 118, no. 3, part 1, pp. 344–349, 1998.

[18] M. S. Blaiss, "Allergic rhinitis: direct and indirect costs," *Allergy and Asthma Proceedings*, vol. 31, no. 5, pp. 375–380, 2010.

[19] K. E. Hermelingmeier, R. K. Weber, M. Hellmich, C. P. Heubach, and R. Mösges, "Nasal irrigation as an adjunctive treatment in allergic rhinitis: a systematic review and meta-analysis," *American Journal of Rhinology and Allergy*, vol. 26, no. 5, pp. e119–e125, 2012.

[20] G. Hildebrandt and C. Gutenbrunner, "Balneologie," in *Handbuch der Balneologie und Medizinischen Klimatologie*, pp. 187–476, Springer, 1998.

[21] W. Fresenius and H. Kußmaul, "Einführung in Chemie und Charakteristik der Heilwässer un Peloide," in *Die deutschen Kurorte und ihre natürlichen Heilmittel*, Flöttmann, 2004, http://www.baederkalender.de/broschuere/11/Einfuehrung-in-Chemie-und-Charakteristik-der-Heilwaesser-und-Peloide.

[22] M. Costantino, E. Lampa, and G. Nappi, "Effectiveness of sulphur spa therapy with politzer in the treatment of rhinogenic deafness," *Acta Otorhinolaryngologica Italica*, vol. 26, no. 1, pp. 7–13, 2006.

[23] P. C. Braga, G. Sambataro, M. Dal Sasso, M. Culici, M. Alfieri, and G. Nappi, "Antioxidant effect of sulphurous thermal water on human neutrophil bursts: chemiluminescence evaluation," *Respiration*, vol. 75, no. 2, pp. 193–201, 2008.

[24] P. Deetjen, "Radon-Balneotherapie—neue Aspekte," *Physikalische Medizin Rehabilitationsmedizin Kurortmedizin*, vol. 2, no. 3, pp. 100–103, 2008.

[25] A. Salami, M. Dellepiane, B. Crippa et al., "Sulphurous water inhalations in the prophylaxis of recurrent upper respiratory tract infections," *International Journal of Pediatric Otorhinolaryngology*, vol. 72, no. 11, pp. 1717–1722, 2008.

[26] A. Salami, M. Dellepiane, F. Strinati, L. Guastini, and R. Mora, "Sulphurous thermal water inhalations in the treatment of chronic rhinosinusitis," *Rhinology*, vol. 48, no. 1, pp. 71–76, 2010.

[27] G. Ottaviano, G. Marioni, L. Giacomelli et al., "Smoking and chronic rhinitis: effects of nasal irrigations with sulfurous-arsenical-ferruginous thermal water. A prospective, randomized, double-blind study," *American Journal of Otolaryngology—Head and Neck Medicine and Surgery*, vol. 33, no. 6, pp. 657–662, 2012.

[28] G. Ottaviano, G. Marioni, C. Staffieri et al., "Effects of sulfurous, salty, bromic, iodic thermal water nasal irrigations in

nonallergic chronic rhinosinusitis: a prospective, randomized, double-blind, clinical, and cytological study," *American Journal of Otolaryngology—Head and Neck Medicine and Surgery*, vol. 32, no. 3, pp. 235–239, 2011.

[29] T. Marullo and A. Abramo, "Effects of one cycle of inhalation crenotherapy with radioactive fluoridated oligomineral," *Acta Otorhinolaryngologica Italica*, vol. 20, supplement 63, no. 4, pp. 1–13, 2000.

[30] M. Oremus, C. Wolfson, A. Perrault, L. Demers, F. Momoli, and Y. Moride, "Interrater reliability of the modified Jadad quality scale for systematic reviews of Alzheimer's disease drug trials," *Dementia and Geriatric Cognitive Disorders*, vol. 12, no. 3, pp. 232–236, 2001.

[31] K. Obtułowicz, J. Składzień, J. Michalak, J. Gawlik, and I. Wróblewska, "The efficacy of subterranean therapy in the salt chamber of Kinga Spa in Wieliczka for patients suffering from allergic rhinitis," *Przeglad Lekarski*, vol. 56, no. 12, pp. 760–762, 1999.

[32] M. Costantino, "The rhinogenic deafness and SPA therapy: clinical-experimental study," *Clinica Terapeutica*, vol. 159, no. 5, pp. 311–315, 2008.

[33] A. V. Pagliari, F. Klinger, V. Bandi, B. P. Banzatti, M. Rosmarini, and M. Klinger, "Efficacy of thermal sulphurous water after functional septo-rhinoplasty," *Medicina Clinica e Termale*, vol. 20, no. 64, pp. 21–23, 2008.

[34] G. Nappi, C. de Vita, M. M. Masciocchi, and S. de Luca, "A clinical study of the use of sulphurous water "Madonna Assunta" as a treatment of rhinogenous deafness," *Medicina Clinica e Termale*, vol. 12, no. 44-45, pp. 103–109, 1998.

[35] A. Varricchio, M. Giuliano, M. Capasso et al., "Salso-sulphide thermal water in the prevention of recurrent respiratory infections in children," *International Journal of Immunopathology and Pharmacology*, vol. 26, no. 4, pp. 941–952, 2013.

[36] D.-H. Kim and S. W. Yeo, "Effects of normal saline and selenium-enriched hot spring water on experimentally induced rhinosinusitis in rats," *International Journal of Pediatric Otorhinolaryngology*, vol. 77, no. 1, pp. 117–122, 2013.

[37] A. R. Jadad, R. A. Moore, D. Carroll et al., "Assessing the quality of reports of randomized clinical trials: is blinding necessary?" *Controlled Clinical Trials*, vol. 17, no. 1, pp. 1–12, 1996.

[38] G. Nappi, D. Passali, and S. de Luca, "A case-control study of the inhalatory therapy in nasal respiratory activity at Grotta Giusti Spa," *Medicina Clinica e Termale*, vol. 19, no. 61, pp. 74–78, 2006.

[39] D. Pagani, E. Galliera, G. Dogliotti et al., "Carbon dioxide-enriched water inhalation in patients with allergic rhinitis and its relationship with nasal fluid cytokine/chemokine release," *Archives of Medical Research*, vol. 42, no. 4, pp. 329–333, 2011.

[40] D. Passali, M. Lauriello, G. C. Passali et al., "Clinical evaluation of the efficacy of Salsomaggiore (Italy) thermal water in the treatment of rhinosinusal pathologies," *Clinica Terapeutica*, vol. 159, no. 3, pp. 181–188, 2008.

[41] A. Vassallo, L. Califano, and G. Villari, "Clinical study on 40 cases of inflammatory pathologies of upper respiratory and digestive tract treated by inhalatory crenotherapy," *Clinica Terapeutica*, vol. 160, no. 1, pp. 17–20, 2009.

[42] M. Bregant, "Combined thermal-surgical therapeutic approach in vasomotor rhinitis," *Medicina Clinica e Termale*, vol. 19, no. 60, pp. 24–26, 2006.

[43] R. Jean, M. Fourot-Bauzon, and P. Perrin, "Cures thermales en pneumo-allergologie et en ORL pédiatriques," *Expansion Scientifique Publications*, vol. 39, no. 5, pp. 293–299, 1992.

[44] G. Fenu, A. Carai, A. C. Montella et al., "Effects of isotonic salso-bromo-iodine thermal water after sinunasal surgery: a preliminary morphological study," *Journal of Alternative and Complementary Medicine*, vol. 16, no. 4, pp. 341–343, 2010.

[45] T. Marullo and A. Abramo, "Effects of sulphur-arsenic-ferrous water treatment on specific chronic phloglosis of the upper respiratory tract," *Acta Otorhinolaryngologica Italica*, vol. 19, supplement 61, no. 4, pp. 5–14, 1999.

[46] M. Costantino, G. Nappi, S. de Luca, F. Rossi, and E. Lampa, "Efficacy of inhalation crenotherapy with oligomineral radioactive water on ORL: clinic-experimental study," *Medicina Clinica e Termale*, vol. 13, no. 47, pp. 211–219, 2001.

[47] E. de Nobili and V. G. Tiepolo, "Comparative evaluation of efficacy of crenotherapeutic Politzer with sulphurous water versus crenotherapeutic Politzer and autoinsufflation (Otovent) in patients with tubaric dysfunction and secretory otitis media," *Medicina Clinica e Termale*, vol. 20, no. 64, pp. 30–34, 2008.

[48] S. Ragusa, G. Caruso, and T. Bensi, "Efficacy of sulphurous Spa therapy on inflammatory chronic disease of VADS," *Medicina Clinica e Termale*, vol. 14, no. 50-51, pp. 377–387, 2002.

[49] M. Costantino, F. Rossi, and E. Lampa, "Inhalant therapy with sulphur water in ORL: clinical-experimental study," *Clinica Terapeutica*, vol. 154, no. 6, pp. 395–400, 2003.

[50] G. Nappi, I. G. Carrubba, and S. de Luca, "Spa therapy influence on nasal mucociliary transport in patients with rhinosinusitis," *Medicina Clinica e Termale*, vol. 14, no. 49, pp. 305–313, 2002.

[51] L. Pollastrini, G. Cristalli, and A. Abramo, "The treatment of a chronic inflammation of the upper respiratory airways by inhalation thermal therapy with sulfur-sulfate-bicarbonate-alkaline-earth metal water: rhinomanometric study and the study of the mucociliary transport," *Acta Otorhinolaryngologica Italica*, vol. 16, supplement 55, no. 6, pp. 85–90, 1996.

[52] G. Cristalli, A. Abramo, and L. Pollastrini, "Treatment of chronic inflammation of the upper respiratory airways by inhalation thermal therapy with sulfur-sulfate-bicarbonate-carbonate-alkaline earth mineral water: a study of nasal cytology," *Acta Otorhinolaryngologica Italica*, vol. 16, supplement 55, no. 6, pp. 91–94, 1996.

[53] S. De Luca, D. Antonaci, and G. Nappi, "Efficacy of inhalatory Spa therapy for upper respiratory tract pathologies with sulphurous water of Tabiano Spa in Hospital far from Spa Centre," *Medicina Clinica e Termale*, vol. 19, no. 62-63, pp. 107–115, 2006.

[54] A. Staffieri, C. Miani, A. M. Bergamin, P. Arcangeli, and P. Canzi, "Effect of sulfur salt-bromine-iodine thermal waters on albumin and IgA concentrations in nasal secretions," *Acta Otorhinolaryngologica Italica*, vol. 18, no. 4, pp. 233–238, 1998.

[55] A. Staffieri and A. Abramo, "Sulphurous-arsenical-ferruginous (thermal) water inhalations reduce nasal respiratory resistance and improve mucociliary clearance in patients with chronic sinonasal disease: preliminary outcomes," *Acta Oto-Laryngologica*, vol. 127, no. 6, pp. 613–617, 2007.

[56] A. Staffieri, F. Marino, C. Staffieri et al., "The effects of sulfurous-arsenical-ferruginous thermal water nasal irrigation in wound healing after functional endoscopic sinus surgery for chronic rhinosinusitis: a prospective randomized study," *American Journal of Otolaryngology—Head and Neck Medicine and Surgery*, vol. 29, no. 4, pp. 223–229, 2008.

[57] A. Passariello, M. di Costanzo, G. Terrin et al., "Crenotherapy modulates the expression of proinflammatory cytokines and immunoregulatory peptides in nasal secretions of children with chronic rhinosinusitis," *American Journal of Rhinology and Allergy*, vol. 26, no. 1, pp. e15–e19, 2012.

[58] D. Passali, E. de Corso, S. Platzgummer et al., "Spa therapy of upper respiratory tract inflammations," *European Archives of Oto-Rhino-Laryngology—Head Neck Surg*, vol. 270, no. 2, pp. 565–570, 2013.

[59] F. M. Passali, A. Crisanti, G. C. Passali et al., "Efficacy of inhalation therapy with water of Salsomaggiore (Italy) in chronic and recurrent nasosinusal inflammation treatment," *Clinica Terapeutica*, vol. 159, no. 3, pp. 175–180, 2008.

[60] M. Miraglia del Giudice, F. Decimo, N. Maiello et al., "Effectiveness of ischia thermal water nasal aerosol in children with seasonal allergic rhinitis: a randomized and controlled study," *International Journal of Immunopathology and Pharmacology*, vol. 24, no. 4, pp. 1103–1109, 2011.

[61] D. Moher, A. Liberati, J. Tetzlaff, and D. G. Altman, "Preferred reporting items for systematic reviews and meta-analyses: the PRISMA statement," *Annals of Internal Medicine*, vol. 151, no. 4, pp. 264–269, W64, 2009.

[62] V. J. Lund and I. S. Mackay, "Staging in rhinosinusitus," *Rhinology*, vol. 31, no. 4, pp. 183–184, 1993.

[63] A. Timmer and B. Richter, "Systematische Übersichtsarbeiten zu Fragen der Therapie und Prävention. Teil 3-Wie werden die Ergebnisse zusammengefasst und dargestellt?" *Arzenimitteltherapie*, vol. 26, no. 10, pp. 299–303, 2008.

[64] J. W. Georgitis, "Nasal hyperthermia and simple irrigation for perennial rhinitis: changes in inflammatory mediators," *Chest*, vol. 106, no. 5, pp. 1487–1492, 1994.

[65] O. Michel, "Nasal irritation in case of rhinosinusitis," *Laryngo-Rhino-Otologie*, vol. 85, no. 6, pp. 448–460, 2006.

[66] G. M. Corbo, A. Foresi, P. Bonfitto, A. Mugnano, N. Agabiti, and P. J. Cole, "Measurement of nasal mucociliary clearance," *Archives of Disease in Childhood*, vol. 64, no. 4, pp. 546–550, 1989.

[67] P. W. Hellings, G. Scadding, I. Alobid et al., "Executive summary of European Task Force document on diagnostic tools in rhinology," *Rhinology*, vol. 50, no. 4, pp. 339–352, 2012.

[68] B. Thiagarajan, "Nasal resistance its importance and measurement," *ENT Scholar*, vol. 1, no. 3, 2012.

[69] R. Jankowski, M. Persoons, B. Foliguet, L. Coffinet, C. Thomas, and B. Verient-Montaut, "Eosinophil count in nasal secretions of subjects with or without nasal symptoms," *Rhinology*, vol. 38, no. 1, pp. 23–32, 2000.

[70] S. K. Wise, C. N. Ahn, D. M. R. Lathers, R. M. Mulligan, and R. J. Schlosser, "Antigen-specific IgE in sinus mucosa of allergic fungal rhinosinusitis patients," *American Journal of Rhinology*, vol. 22, no. 5, pp. 451–456, 2008.

[71] H. Garn and H. Renz, "Epidemiological and immunological evidence for the hygiene hypothesis," *Immunobiology*, vol. 212, no. 6, pp. 441–452, 2007.

[72] L. Bellussi, J. Cambi, and D. Passali, "Functional maturation of nasal mucosa: role of secretory immunoglobulin A (SIgA)," *Multidisciplinary Respiratory Medicine*, vol. 8, no. 1, article 46, 2013.

[73] Y. Kurono, G. Mogi, and T. Fujiyoshi, "Secretory IgA and bacterial adherence to nasal mucosal cells," *Annals of Otology, Rhinology and Laryngology*, vol. 98, no. 4, part 1, pp. 273–277, 1989.

27

Hypersensitivity and the Working Environment for Allergy Nurses in Sweden

Pia Kalm-Stephens,[1] Therese Sterner,[2] Kerstin Kronholm Diab,[3] and Greta Smedje[4]

[1] *Department of Women's and Children's Health, Uppsala University, 751 85 Uppsala, Sweden*
[2] *Division of Woman, Child and Reproduction, Department of Pediatrics, Skåne University Hospital, 205 02 Lund, Sweden*
[3] *Occupational and Environmental Medicine, University and Regional Laboratories Region Skåne, 205 02 Lund, Sweden*
[4] *Department of Medical Sciences/Occupational and Environmental Medicine, Uppsala University, 751 85 Uppsala, Sweden*

Correspondence should be addressed to Pia Kalm-Stephens; pia.kalm-stephens@akademiska.se

Academic Editor: Ting Fan Leung

Background. Allergy nurses are exposed to allergens and respiratory irritants, and there are no national guidelines addressing personnel safety when working with these agents. *Objective.* To investigate the prevalence of allergies, asthma, and hypersensitivity symptoms among allergy nurses and the use of protective equipment and measures when working with allergen concentrates and respiratory irritants. *Methods.* A questionnaire survey was performed among the members of the Swedish Association of Allergy Nurses. *Results.* Diagnosed asthma was reported by 17%, while 18% had allergy to pets, 28% had allergy to pollens, and 26% reported nasal symptoms. Fifty-one percent reported a history of asthma, allergic diseases, or hypersensitivity symptoms in their family. Exhaust ventilation was used by 24% during skin prick tests, 17% during allergen specific immunotherapy, and 33% when performing methacholine challenge tests. Tightly closed containers for disposable waste were used by 58% during skin prick tests, by 60% during immunotherapy, and by 40% during Pc provocation tests. *Conclusion.* Allergy nurses had a tendency to increased prevalence of lower respiratory symptoms, asthma, and allergic rhinitis and more than half of the nurses had a family history of asthma, allergic diseases, or hypersensitivity symptoms. Additional studies are needed to evaluate the validity of these results.

1. Introduction

Allergy nurses work with various tests aimed at diagnosing allergic diseases and other hypersensitivity disorders. Common tests are skin prick test (SPT), where different allergens are used, penicillin (Pc) provocation tests, and tests with various respiratory irritants, such as methacholine (MCH). Many allergy nurses also perform allergen specific immunotherapy (ASIT) by injecting the allergen concentrates. In the clinical working situation with the patients, it is common to be exposed to drops of allergen extracts and to dried allergen on extract bottles and tissues used when performing SPT and ASIT. All these exposures may potentially lead to effects on the health of the nurses. Efforts have been made to improve the working environment in some clinics, using fume or downdraft hoods for diagnostic tests, whereas such preventive and safety measures are missing in other clinics.

There are no existing national guidelines for these specific tests concerning safety for the allergy nurses and local recommendations may vary.

Four main risk factors have been identified for developing occupational asthma (OA): the causative factor of exposure to an agent at work, the predisposing factors of atopy and genetic predisposition, and the contributing factor of cigarette smoking. Rhinoconjunctivitis is more likely to appear before the onset of IgE associated OA, and IgE sensitization and OA are most likely to develop in the first years of exposure [1].

Within the Swedish Association of Allergy Nurses (ASTA), discussions have been carried out concerning deficiencies in the working environment and there have been reports of members that have become sensitized or developed respiratory symptoms at work but there are few studies on this issue. Previously, there was a case report concerning two nurses in Sweden, who often conducted MCH tests and who developed an increased bronchial hyperreactivity related to their work [2]. In 1991, ASTA conducted a questionnaire survey among all members, studying the correlation between asthma and bronchial provocation tests. Among the 259 (80%) respondents, 27% were working with MCH and 15% with histamine tests. Among those who performed the MCH tests, 31% reported respiratory symptoms associated with the test situation and 4% (3 subjects) reported the development of asthma during the time they had been working with such tests [3]. In cooperation with the Department of Occupational Medicine in Gothenburg, Sweden, further analysis was carried out. No evidence for a relationship between MCH tests and development of new asthma was found, but it was concluded that individuals with bronchial hyperreactivity could experience respiratory problems associated with testing, especially if they did not use respiratory protection [4].

There are a few international studies that indicate higher frequencies of asthma and bronchial hyperreactivity among "respiratory therapists (RT)" [5, 6]. An RT works to prevent, treat, and assist in the diagnosis of respiratory diseases and asthma is one of several assignments for the RT. The studies indicate that cleaning of instruments, such as bronchoscopes, in glutaraldehyde and administration of certain antiviral agents in aerosol form are the main risk factors [7, 8]. Furthermore, a higher incidence of asthma among nurses has been reported in some studies [9–12]. The principal risks recognized are the handling of detergents and disinfectants, the use of latex gloves, and the administration of certain drugs in aerosol form. All these studies are only partially relevant for nurses working in Sweden with asthma and allergy, since their main exposures are allergen extracts and respiratory irritants when performing, for example, SPT, ASIT, and MCH provocation tests and specific safety guidelines concerning work exposure to allergens, except for a recently published case report describing a compounding technician, with a known allergy to timothy grass, who experienced anaphylaxis after a needle stick from a stock bottle of timothy grass extract while preparing immunotherapy vials [13]. The authors of this case report established that this raises a new question of occupational safety for allergy immunotherapy extract-compounding personnel safety not previously discussed in the allergy literature. They also considered a need for pre-employment and regular screening for allergen sensitivity in these employees. In February 2010, ASTA organized a workshop on this subject and it was decided to perform a questionnaire survey among its members for the purpose of gathering information about these issues as a primary orientation to further discussions.

1.1. Study Objectives. The aims of the current study were to

(i) investigate the prevalence of allergies, asthma, and hypersensitivity symptoms among the members of ASTA;

(ii) investigate the use of protective equipment and measures when working with allergen concentrates and respiratory irritants;

(iii) gather data for further discussion concerning the working environment.

2. Methods

Data were collected using a web-based questionnaire that contained 40 questions addressing personal characteristics, work situation, protection at work, and hypersensitivity symptoms. The questions on work situation and protection at work were constructed by the project group, while questions on hypersensitivity symptoms were taken from validated questionnaires, particularly those used in the European Community Respiratory Health Survey (ECRHS) II [14]. Furthermore, one question concerned heredity (parents or siblings) for asthma and allergies. All questions were presented with fixed alternative answers. The questions used in the questionnaire to evaluate hypersensitivity symptoms are presented in Table 1. Similar symptoms were compiled in groups and these group definitions (Table 1) are used in the presentation of the results.

ASTA is an organization with members from most parts of Sweden and represents a great majority of nurses working with asthma and allergy in Sweden. It includes nurses working both in primary care and in hospitals.

Webropol, a web-based survey tool provided by the County Council of Uppsala, Sweden, was used to gather the data. An e-mail was sent out in February 2011 to all ASTA members containing information about the study and a link to the survey. A paper questionnaire was provided to a few members without an e-mail address. In both cases, three reminders were sent out. After the data collection was completed, an Excel file with all the data was compiled and the data were subsequently deleted from the Webropol server. The study was approved by the Regional Ethical Review Board in Uppsala, Sweden.

Most of the data are descriptive in character, since the purpose of the study was to describe certain aspects of allergy nurses' health and working environment. The alternative answers to the questions concerning frequencies of performing SPT, Pc, and MCH provocation tests were classified into five groups: never, less than once a week, 1–5 times a week, 6–10 times a week, and more than 10 times a week. Data were compiled into two groups: ≤5 times a week and >5 times a week in order to identify nurses who had low or high exposure to these agents and to establish larger groups. Subjects that had been working with specific tasks for different periods of time (0–2 years, 3–5 years, 6–10 years, and more than 10 years) were also compiled into two groups: nurses who had worked ≤5 years and >5 years, for the same reasons as mentioned above. Five years was chosen as suitable cut-off time to be able to include possible new onset asthma, allergies, and hypersensitivity symptoms that would appear after some years in the profession. Differences in symptoms between groups were analyzed by χ^2 Test, and a significance level of 5%.

There was no control group in this study but symptom prevalences among the allergy nurses were compared with

TABLE 1: Questions used for evaluating hypersensitivity symptoms and definitions used in the presentation of the results.

Questions	Definitions
Did you have wheezing or whistling in chest at any time in the last 12 months? Have you been woken up by an attack of shortness of breath at any time in the last 12 months? Did you have dry cough at night without having a cold or upper respiratory infection in the last 12 months?	Lower respiratory symptoms
Do you have a doctor diagnosed asthma?	Asthma
Do you get hyperreactive airways in contact with cigarette smoke, fumes, strong odours, and so forth?	Hyperreactivity
Do you have any nasal allergies, including hay fever?	Allergic rhinitis
Have you ever had a problem with sneezing or a runny or a blocked nose when you did not have a cold or the flu? Has this nose problem been accompanied by itchy eyes?	Nasal symptoms
Have you ever had an itchy rash that was coming and going for at least 6 months? Have you had this itchy rash in the last 12 months?	Eczema
Do you have allergies to furry pets? Do you have allergies to pollens? Do you have allergies to dust mites? Do you have allergies to mold?	Airborne allergy

data on women aged 30–67 years old from the general population collected by the Swedish part (Stockholm, Gothenburg, Umeå, and Uppsala) of the GA2LEN survey [15].

3. Results

The questionnaire was sent to 585 nurses belonging to ASTA: 570 via e-mail and 15 via paper mail. After three reminders, 418 had answered, resulting in a participation rate of 71%. The average age of responders was 53 years (range 30–67 years) and 98% were female. 71% reported that they had never smoked regularly, 28% were previously smokers, and 0.5% were current smokers.

Fifty-eight percent of the responders worked in primary care, 41% in hospitals, and 1% in both. Thirty-four percent worked with children, 37% with adults, and 29% with both children and adults. Forty-four percent worked with asthma and allergy approximately one day a week and 27% worked two to four days a week while 29% worked almost exclusively with asthma and allergy. A majority, 56%, had worked with asthma and allergy for more than ten years, and 75% for more than five years. Among the requested tasks, SPT was the most common task performed, followed by Pc provocation tests and ASIT (Figure 1). MCH provocation test was the most common test among various hyperreactivity provocations, being performed by 11% (Figure 1).

3.1. Symptoms. Asthma diagnosed by a doctor was reported by 17% of the responders to the questionnaire, while 18% had allergy to furry pets and 28% to pollens and 31% reported allergic rhinitis. Thirty-four percent reported bronchial hyperreactivity to cigarette smoke, fumes, strong odors, and so forth. Lower respiratory symptoms in the last 12 months, when not having a cold, were reported by in total 48%. Symptoms of wheezing were reported by 21%, shortness of breath by 7%, and dry cough at night by 24%. Itchy rash was reported by 15%, while 26% had nasal symptoms such as sneezing or a runny or a blocked nose and itchy eyes without having a cold or the flu. Fifty-one percent

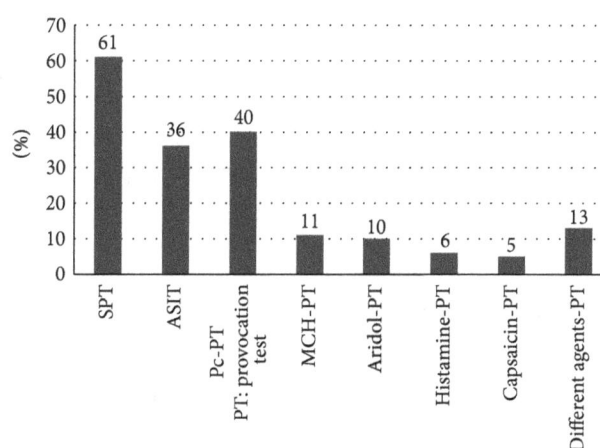

FIGURE 1: Specific working tasks of nurses in ASTA (%); $n = 256$.

acknowledged that they had a history of asthma, allergic diseases, or hypersensitivity symptoms in their family.

3.1.1. Work-Related Symptoms. Thirty-three members (8%) reported that they had asthma, allergies, or hypersensitivity symptoms related to their working situation. Of these, asthma or some kind of respiratory symptoms was reported by 28 subjects. Twenty-one subjects reported allergic rhinitis and 25 nurses were bothered by nasal symptoms. Two subjects had been out of work for more than ten days during the last six months due to colds or bronchial problems. Of the 28 nurses who reported work-related asthma or some kind of respiratory symptoms, 19 developed these symptoms after entering the profession. Two-thirds of the nurses, who had reported work-related symptoms, had a family history of asthma, allergic diseases, or hypersensitivity disorders.

All ASTA members were also asked about when their hyperreactivity, respiratory, or asthma symptoms first appeared. Fifty-seven percent of the responders reported that the symptoms occurred after some years in the profession, while 43% indicated that they had their symptoms before

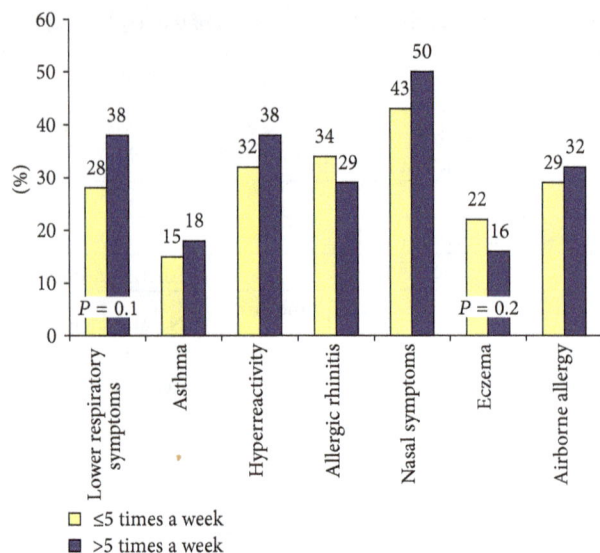

FIGURE 2: Prevalence (%) of symptoms in nurses who have worked with SPT ≤5 times a week and >5 times a week; $n = 256$.

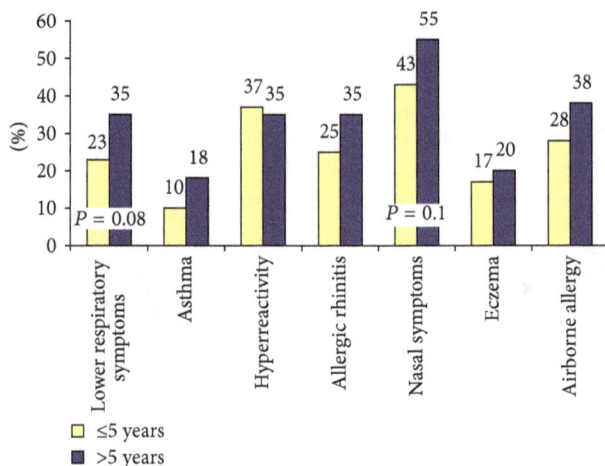

FIGURE 3: Prevalence (%) of symptoms in nurses who have worked with SPT for ≤5 years and for >5 years; $n = 256$.

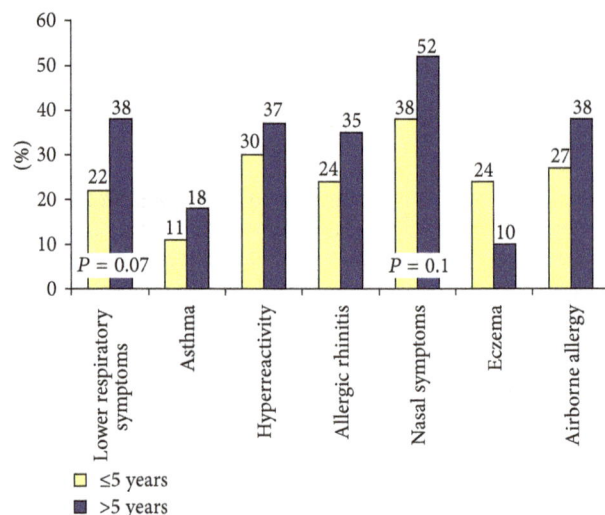

FIGURE 4: Prevalence (%) of symptoms in nurses who have worked with Pc provocations for ≤5 years and for >5 years; $n = 157$.

entering the profession. In the case of allergic rhinitis or nasal symptoms, 37% reported no symptoms prior to the work as an allergy nurse. The same results were seen in the group that reported work-related eczema.

3.2. Diagnostic Tests

3.2.1. Skin Prick Test and Symptoms. Lower respiratory symptoms during the last 12 months were reported by 38% of those who performed SPT more than five times a week compared with 28% for those who did fewer tests although not significant in χ^2 Test (Figure 2). However, there was a tendency to reverse results regarding allergic rhinitis, where 29% of those who performed SPT more than five times a week reported symptoms, compared with 34% for those who worked with SPT less frequently, $P = 0.3$ in the χ^2 Test.

There was a tendency that the nurses in ASTA who had worked with SPT for more than five years, being 65% of those who performed SPT, experienced more symptoms than those who had worked for a shorter period, although the differences were not statistically significant in the χ^2 Test (Figure 3).

3.2.2. Pc Provocation Test and Symptoms. Pc provocations were performed by 40% of the respondents and 59% of these reported some kind of symptoms. There was no difference in the prevalence of lower respiratory symptoms in nurses who performed Pc tests less than once a week compared with those who worked with this test one to five times a week. Nobody worked with Pc provocation tests more than 5 times a week. However, there was a tendency that those who had performed Pc provocation tests for more than five years reported more lower respiratory symptoms, allergic rhinitis, nasal symptoms, and airborne allergy, although the differences were not statistically significant in the χ^2 Test (Figure 4).

3.2.3. MCH Provocation Test and Symptoms. MCH provocation tests were performed by 44 (11%) of the ASTA members and 25 performed this task more than once a week. In the latter group, 10 nurses reported that they had asthma, hyperreactive airways, or lower respiratory symptoms and for seven subjects the symptoms had developed after they had started work as allergy nurses. Nasal symptoms were reported by 14 of the nurses who performed this test more than once a week (25) and 8 reported allergic rhinitis. Eighty percent of these nurses reported either airway or nasal symptoms, or both. A large majority, 38 of the 44 nurses who performed MCH provocation tests, had worked with this test for more than 5 years. Nasal and lower respiratory symptoms are common among nurses who have worked with MCH provocation test for more than five years but due to few nurses in the groups, the differences are not statistically significant in the χ^2 Test (Figure 5).

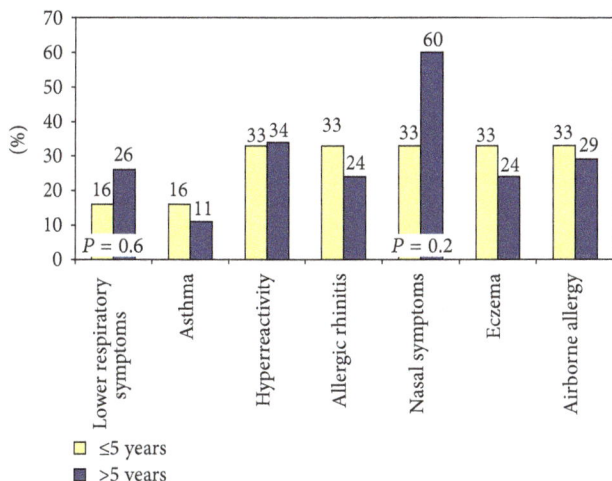

FIGURE 5: Prevalence (%) of symptoms in nurses who have worked with MCH provocations for ≤5 years and for >5 years; $n = 44$.

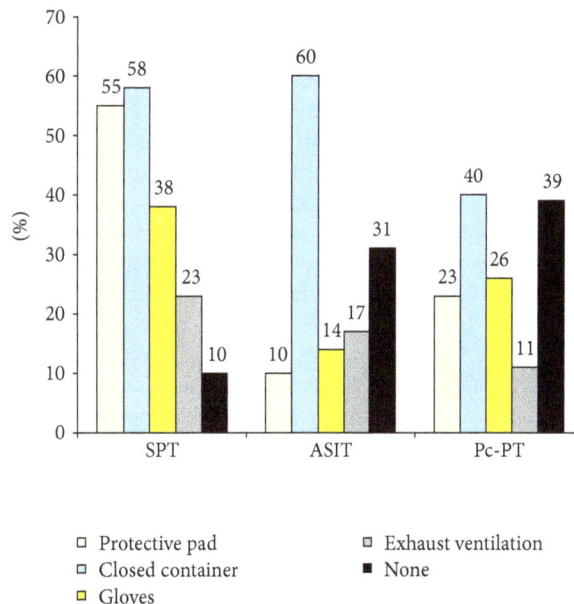

FIGURE 6: Protective equipment used during different work tasks (%); $n = 256$.

3.3. Protective Measures.

The use of protective equipment during SPT, ASIT, and Pc provocation tests varied, as is shown in Figure 6. A closed container is a container with a lid aimed to stop evaporation from used materials containing allergens and respiratory irritants, and a protective pad is a paper mat used to create a clean working area. Approximately, a third of the responders did not take any protective measures when performing ASIT and Pc provocation tests. Protective equipment during MCH provocation tests was primarily aimed at the presence of respiratory irritants. Most of the responders, (73%) used a separate room or space with additional ventilation and the remainder mainly used the fume hood or downdraft hood. Thirteen percent used gloves and 4% respiratory protection devices. For MCH provocation tests, nobody reported that no protective measures were taken.

4. Discussion

The results show that asthma and hypersensitivity symptoms are common among the members of ASTA, that most of the subjects have been in the profession for a long time, and that over half of the nurses have a family history of asthma, allergy, or hypersensitivity symptoms. In order to make a preliminary evaluation of the results concerning asthma allergies and hypersensitivity symptoms, a comparison has been done with the prevalence in the Swedish general population [14, 16]. A general population is judged to be neutral and unexposed to these agents and working tasks. Since almost all respondents in the present ASTA survey were women, a comparison with data from the Swedish part of the GA2LEN survey for women, from 2008, was chosen to be the most suitable [15]. The prevalence among ASTA's members seems to be slightly higher for most symptoms (Figure 7).

About one-third of the responders to the questionnaire reported that they become hyperreactive in contact with cigarette smoke and so forth. Another Swedish survey on the

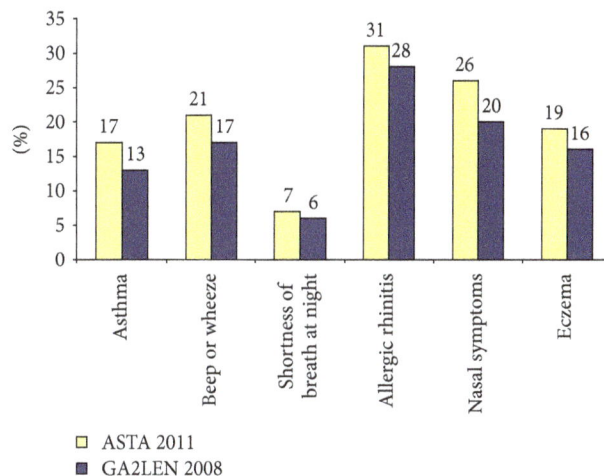

FIGURE 7: Prevalence of asthma and respiratory symptoms in ASTA's members and in the Swedish part of the GA2LEN study; $n = 14000$.

general population showed a prevalence among women of the same magnitude, 31% [17].

The high proportion of allergy nurses with a family history of asthma, allergy, or hypersensitivity symptoms suggests that there might be a biased selection of individuals entering the profession. If this is the case, it is very important that the working environment is adapted to their special needs. There are regulations to protect employees in the working environment. In addition to the general Work Environment Act [18], the Swedish Work Environment Authority has also issued provisions on Systematic Work Environment Management 2001:01 [19], Workplace Design, AFS 2009:02 [20], and the Chemical Working Environment, AFS 2011:19 [21]. The employer is responsible for establishing a working environment that does not expose workers to health risks and to investigate the working environment regularly to assess such risks. For example, hazardous chemicals that may occur at work should be identified and working conditions at such sites need to be planned to minimize the exposure. The working premises should have ventilation so that air quality in the breathing zone is satisfactory and air pollution generated in the operations should be effectively removed. However, the rules are very general. Exposures, such as allergens and substances for respiratory provocations, which are relevant to allergy nurses, are not discussed explicitly. Furthermore, the professionals in health care have established recommendations for performing these tasks, but there appear to be few recommendations in such methodology manuals and so forth concerning how these substances should be handled from an occupational perspective.

The present survey found that the use of protective measures varied between different working tasks. The proportion of lack of use of any protection was the highest (39%) for those working with Pc provocations, compared with 10% for those working with SPT. There was also a higher proportion who reported symptoms among those who carried out the Pc provocation tests (59%), compared with that for SPT (52%). The highest risk for symptoms (80%) seemed to be caused by performing MCH tests more regularly, even though protection measures, in many cases, had been used. The reason why nurses have not used protection measures might be linked to the fact that occupational safety for allergy nurses has not been discussed in a sufficient way, neither in the clinical settings nor in the scientific literature.

Health problems linked to the working situation cannot have been a major concern for a majority of the ASTA members, since 56% had been in the profession for ten years or more. It may be difficult to establish a connection between work and perceived symptoms when the symptoms are the same as those perceived by the general population. The specific knowledge owned by allergy nurses may have had an impact on their assessment of their own hyperreactive symptoms. However, 8% considered that they had developed allergies or hypersensitivity disorders as a result of their work and 4.5% (19 nurses) reported that their respiratory problems had started after initiating work with allergens or provocations. The number of new cases of asthma among women in the general population has been estimated to be approximately 1.8/1000 person-years and the number of new cases of rhinitis to be approximately 7/1000 person-years [22, 23]. On the basis of these figures, 0.7 new cases of asthma and 2.8 new cases of rhinitis per year could be predicted in a group of 400 women. We do not know exactly for how long time the nurses had worked with asthma and allergy, but more than half of them had worked for more than 10 years. If we assume an average experience of 15 years, the number of new cases of asthma would be 11, while at 20 years of experience it would be 14 new cases. The corresponding figures for rhinitis would be 42 or 56 new cases. Based on these conceptual calculations, the number of responders, who reported that they had new hypersensitivity symptoms which they attribute to their work, is not significantly higher than the incidence of new symptoms in the general population. Nevertheless, the frequency of those reporting current symptoms was higher than in the general population. Furthermore, we found an increase in symptoms among those having performed provocation tests for a longer period.

4.1. Method Discussion. The validated questions taken from ECHRS II have been suitable for the purpose of this study, but the questions on work tasks that were constructed for this study could have been more specific. The classification concerning frequencies of work tasks was somewhat arbitrary and might have influenced the outcome of the results. However, when comparing symptoms in groups with different number of years in service, the use of different cut-points gave similar results (a tendency to increased symptoms with numbers of years in service). The participation rate was 71% which should be satisfactory but only 29% of the respondents worked exclusively with asthma and allergy and 44% worked just one day a week. Consequently, a large proportion of the studied group had a regular but not a high exposure to allergens and respiratory irritants. There might also be a "healthy worker effect," since the study was only directed towards present members of ASTA, thus not giving any information from nurses who have left the profession and ASTA. However, the purpose of the study was to give some general descriptive information of an issue which has not been previously highlighted.

5. Conclusions

Among the members of ASTA, there is a tendency towards increased prevalence of lower respiratory symptoms, asthma, allergic rhinitis, nasal symptoms, and eczema and more than half of the nurses had a family history of these diseases and symptoms. With this knowledge, it is of great importance to be observant of the work environment and of hypersensitivity disorders in the nurses. Preventive work environment efforts have largely been made concerning MCH provocations. The results of this study imply that further work should also be carried out to establish recommendations concerning protective measures for allergen management and other tasks. Additional studies are needed to evaluate the validity of these results and to be able to answer more specific questions concerning causal relationship between the working conditions and the occurrence of respiratory and allergic symptoms.

Conflict of Interests

The authors declare that there is no conflict of interests regarding the publication of this paper.

Acknowledgments

The authors thank the ASTA Board for professional advice and general support for the study and the ASTA association for financial support with the help of a study grant. They also would like to thank an anonymous reviewer for the useful comments that have improved the paper.

References

[1] P. J. Nicholson, P. Cullinan, A. J. Newman Taylor, P. S. Burge, and C. Boyle, "Evidence based guidelines for the prevention, identification, and management of occupational asthma," *Occupational and Environmental Medicine*, vol. 62, no. 5, pp. 290–299, 2005.

[2] R. Lundgren, M. Soderberg, L. Rosenhall, and E. Norrman, "Development of increased airway responsiveness in two nurses performing methacholine and histamine challenge tests," *Allergy*, vol. 47, no. 2, pp. 188–189, 1992.

[3] B. Balder, E. Bergmann, A. M. Ericson, and I. L. Henriksson, "Work environment survey of asthma and allergen diagnostics," *Hygiea*, vol. 101, no. 2, p. 99, 1992 (Swedish).

[4] J. Brisman, B. Balder, and S. Hagberg, *Aerosol Leakage at Methacholine Testing*, Department of Occupational Medicine, Gothenburg, Sweden, 1996, (Swedish).

[5] D. C. Christiani and D. G. Kern, "Asthma risk and occupation as a respiratory therapist," *American Review of Respiratory Disease*, vol. 148, no. 3, pp. 671–674, 1993.

[6] D. G. Kern and H. Frumkin, "Asthma in respiratory therapists," *Annals of Internal Medicine*, vol. 110, no. 10, pp. 767–773, 1989.

[7] H. Dimich-Ward, M. L. Wymer, and M. Chan-Yeung, "Respiratory health survey of respiratory therapists," *Chest*, vol. 126, no. 4, pp. 1048–1053, 2004.

[8] H. Dimich-Ward, P. G. Camp, and S. M. Kennedy, "Gender differences in respiratory symptoms-Does occupation matter?" *Environmental Research*, vol. 101, no. 2, pp. 175–183, 2006.

[9] A. A. Arif, G. L. Delclos, and C. Serra, "Occupational exposures and asthma among nursing professionals," *Occupational and Environmental Medicine*, vol. 66, no. 4, pp. 274–278, 2009.

[10] G. L. Delclos, D. Gimeno, A. A. Arif et al., "Occupational risk factors and asthma among health care professionals," *American Journal of Respiratory and Critical Care Medicine*, vol. 175, no. 7, pp. 667–675, 2007.

[11] M. Kogevinas, J.-P. Zock, D. Jarvis et al., "Exposure to substances in the workplace and new-onset asthma: an international prospective population-based study (ECRHS-II)," *The Lancet*, vol. 370, no. 9584, pp. 336–341, 2007.

[12] M. C. Mirabelli, J.-P. Zock, E. Plana et al., "Occupational risk factors for asthma among nurses and related healthcare professionals in an international study," *Occupational and Environmental Medicine*, vol. 64, no. 7, pp. 474–479, 2007.

[13] M. L. Bandino and M. S. Tankersley, "Anaphylaxis in an allergy immunotherapy extract-compounding technician after an extract needle stick," *Journal of Allergy and Clinical Immunology*, vol. 129, no. 1, pp. 250–251, 2012.

[14] European Community Respiratory Health Survey II Steering Committee, "The European Community Respiratory Health Survey II," *European Respiratory Journal*, vol. 20, no. 5, pp. 1071–1079, 2002.

[15] F. Sundbom, E. Lindberg, A. Bjerg et al., "Asthma symtoms and nasal congestion as independent risk factors for insomnia in a general population. Results from the GA2LEN survey," *Allergy*, vol. 68, no. 2, pp. 213–219, 2013.

[16] A. Bjerg, L. Ekerljung, R. Middelveld et al., "Increased prevalence of symptoms of rhinitis but not of asthma between 1990 and 2008 in Swedish adults: comparisons of the ECRHS and GA2LEN surveys," *PLoS ONE*, vol. 6, no. 2, Article ID e16082, 2011.

[17] "Questionnaire survey of the residents' perceived indoor environment and health—results from the BETSI project," Swedish National Board of Housing, Building and Planning, 2009 (Swedish).

[18] *Work Environment Act with Comments*, Swedish Work Environment Authority, Stockholm, Sweden, 2011.

[19] *Provision; Systematic Work 2001:1*, Swedish Work Environment Authority, Stockholm, Sweden, 2001.

[20] *Provision; Workplace Design 2009:2*, Swedish Work Environment Authority, Stockholm, Sweden, 2001.

[21] *Provision; Chemical Work Hazards. 2011:19*, Swedish Work Environment Authorithy, Stockholm, Sweden, 2011.

[22] K. Torén, L. Ekerljung, J.-L. Kim et al., "Adult-onset asthma in west Sweden—incidence, sex differences and impact of occupational exposures," *Respiratory Medicine*, vol. 105, no. 11, pp. 1622–1628, 2011.

[23] U. Nihlén, L. Greiff, P. Montnémery et al., "Incidence and remission of self-reported allergic rhinitis symptoms in adults," *Allergy*, vol. 61, no. 11, pp. 1299–1304, 2006.

Permissions

List of Contributors

Carmen Cuéllar and Marta Rodero
Departamento de Parasitología, Facultad de Farmacia,Universidad Complutense, 28040Madrid, Spain

Ana Valls, Consolación de Frutos and Alvaro Daschner
Servicio de Alergia, Instituto de Investigación Sanitaria, Hospital Universitario de la Princesa, C/Diego de León 62, 28006 Madrid, Spain

Ashley A. Foster
Department of Emergency Medicine, University of California, San Francisco, San Francisco, CA, USA

Ronna L. Campbell and Jana L. Anderson
Department of Emergency Medicine, Mayo Clinic, Rochester, MN, USA

Sangil Lee
Department of Emergency Medicine, Mayo Clinic Health System in Mankato, Mankato, MN, USA

Nayot Suetrong
Department of Medicine, Faculty of Medicine, Chulalongkorn University, Bangkok 10330, Thailand

Jettanong Klaewsongkram
Division of Allergy and Clinical Immunology, Department of Medicine, Faculty of Medicine, and Allergy and Clinical Immunology Research Group, Chulalongkorn University, Bangkok 10330,Thailand

Michael J. Coffey, Barbara Torretti and PeterMancuso
Division of Pulmonary and Critical Care Medicine, University of Michigan Medical Center, Ann Arbor, MI 48109, USA

Uwe Sonnemann
Private Health Centre, Institute for ENT Elmshorn, Hermann-Ehlers-Weg 4, 25337 Elmshorn, Germany

Marcus Möller
Joint Practice for ENT,Willy-Brandt Straße 2, 21335 Lüneburg, Germany

Andreas Bilstein
Bitop AG, Stockumer Straße 28, 58453Witten, Germany

Uwe Sonnemann
Private Health Centre, Institute for ENT Elmshorn, Hermann-Ehlers-Weg 4, 25337 Elmshorn, Germany

Olaf Scherner and NinaWerkhäuser
Bitop AG, Stockumer Street 28, 58453Witten, Germany

Samuel Kyei
Discipline of Optometry, School of Health Sciences, College of Health, University of KwaZulu-Natal, Durban 4041, South Africa
Department of Optometry, School of Allied Health Sciences, University of Cape Coast, Cape Coast, Ghana

George Asumeng Koffuor
Discipline of Optometry, School of Health Sciences, College of Health, University of KwaZulu-Natal, Durban 4041, South Africa
Department of Pharmacology, Faculty of Pharmacy and Pharmaceutical Sciences, Kwame Nkrumah University of Science and Technology, Kumasi, Ghana

Paul Ramkissoon
Discipline of Optometry, School of Health Sciences, College of Health, University of KwaZulu-Natal, Durban 4041, South Africa

Samuel Abokyi and Eric Addo Wiredu
Department of Optometry, School of Allied Health Sciences, University of Cape Coast, Cape Coast, Ghana

Osei Owusu-Afriyie
Department of Pathology, Komfo Anokye Teaching Hospital, Kumasi, Ghana

Leia M. Minaker
School of Public Health and Health Systems, University ofWaterloo LHN 1711, 200 University AvenueWest, Waterloo, ON, Canada N2L 3G1

Susan J. Elliott
Faculty of Applied Health Sciences, University ofWaterloo BMH 3115, 200 University AvenueWest,Waterloo, ON, Canada N2L 3G1

Ann Clarke
Department of Medicine, McGill University, Room 101, Lady Meredith House, 1110 Pine AvenueWest, Montreal, QC, Canada H3A 1A3

Prasad Muley
Department of Paediatrics, S.B.K.S MIRC, Sumandeep Vidyapeeth, Vadodara, Gujarat 391760, India

Monali Shah
Department of Periodontics, K.M.S DCH, Sumandeep Vidyapeeth, Vadodara, Gujarat 391760, India

ArtiMuley
Department of Medicine, S.B.K.S MIRC, Sumandeep Vidyapeeth, Vadodara, Gujarat 391760, India

Andrea Eichel and Ralph Mösges
Institute of Medical Statistics, Informatics and Epidemiology, Faculty of Medicine, University of Cologne, Lindenburger Allee 42, 50931 Cologne, Germany

Andreas Bilstein and Nina Werkhäuser
Bitop AG, Stockumer Straße 28, 58453Witten, Germany

Nina Werkhäuser and Andreas Bilstein
Bitop AG, Stockumer Straße 28, 58453Witten, Germany

Uwe Sonnemann
Private Health Centre, Institute for ENT Elmshorn, Hermann-Ehlers-Weg 4, 25337 Elmshorn, Germany

Ina Gouteva and Kija Shah-Hosseini
Institute of Medical Statistics, Informatics and Epidemiology, University Hospital of Cologne, Lindenburger Allee 42, 50931 Cologne, Germany

Peter Meiser
Ursapharm Arzneimittel GmbH, Industriestraße 35, 66129 Saarbrücken, Germany

Volker König and Ralph Mösges
Institute of Medical Statistics, Informatics and Epidemiology, University of Cologne, 50924 Cologne, Germany

Norah G. Verbout, Leandro Benedito, Alison S. Williams, David I. Kasahara, Allison P.Wurmbrand, Huiqing Si and Stephanie A. Shore
Department of Environmental Health, Harvard School of Public Health, 665 Huntington Avenue, Boston, MA 02115, USA

Andrew J. Halayko
Departments of Physiology and Internal Medicine, University of Manitoba,Winnipeg, MB, Canada R3A 1R9

Christopher Hug
Children's Hospital, Boston, MA 02115, USA

Mohammad-Hosein Shamsbiranvand and Ali Khodadadi
Cancer Research Center of Ahvaz Jundishapur University of Medical Sciences, Ahvaz, Iran
Department of Immunology, Faculty of Medicine, Ahvaz Jundishapur University of Medical Sciences, Ahvaz 6135715794, Iran

Mohammad-Ali Assarehzadegan and Akram Amini
Department of Immunology, Faculty of Medicine, Ahvaz Jundishapur University of Medical Sciences, Ahvaz 6135715794, Iran

Seyed Hamid Borsi
Department of Internal Medicine, Faculty of Medicine, Ahvaz Jundishapur University of Medical Sciences, Ahvaz, Iran

Anna Eitenmüller, Lisa Piano, Myriam Böhm, Kija Shah-Hosseini, and Ralph Mösges
Institute of Medical Statistics, Informatics and Epidemiology, University of Cologne, 50924 Cologne, Germany

Andreas Glowania
Ear, Nose andThroat Department, General Hospital Hietzing, 1130 Vienna, Austria

Oliver Pfaar and Ludger Klimek
Center for Rhinology and Allergology, 65183Wiesbaden, Germany

Atqah AbdulWahab
Department of Pediatrics, Hamad Medical Corporation, P.O. Box 3050, Doha, Qatar Weill Cornell Medical College, Doha, Qatar

Muna M. Maarafiya and Ashraf Soliman
Department of Pediatrics, Hamad Medical Corporation, P.O. Box 3050, Doha, Qatar

Noura B. M. Younes
Laboratory Medicine and Pathology, Hamad Medical Corporation, P.O. Box 3050, Doha, Qatar

Prem Chandra
Medical Research Center, Hamad Medical Corporation, P.O. Box 3050, Doha, Qatar

Laura Keglowich, Jun Zhong, Nicola Miglino and Pieter Borger
Department of Biomedicine, University Hospital Basel, Hebelstrasse 20, 4031 Basel, Switzerland

Michael Tamm
Department of Pulmonology, University Hospital Basel, Petersgraben 2, 4031 Basel, Switzerland

Klaus Unfried, Matthias Kroker, Andrea Autengruber, and Ulrich Sydlik
IUF Leibniz Research Institute for Environmental Medicine, Auf 'm Hennekamp 50, 40225 Düsseldorf, Germany

Marijan Gotić
Department of Material Chemistry, Ruđer Bosković Institute, Bijenička cesta 54, 10000 Zagreb, Croatia

Bettina Hauswald, Christina Dill, Jürgen Boxberger, Thomas Zahnert, and YuryM. Yarin
Clinic of Otorhinolaryngology, Department of Medicine, University Hospital Dresden, Fetscherstraße 74, 01307 Dresden, Germany

Eberhard Kuhlisch
Institute for Medical Informatics and Biometry, Department of Medicine, University Hospital Dresden, Fetscherstraße 74, 01307 Dresden, Germany

Larissa Carvalho Costa, Erica Rodrigues Rezende and Gesmar Rodrigues Silva Segundo
Pediatrics Department, Federal University of Uberlândia, Campus Umuarama, Avenida Para 1720, 38400-920 Uberlândia, MG, Brazil

Karin C. Ringsberg
Nordic School of Public Health, 402 42 Gothenburg, Sweden
Sahlgrenska Academy, University of Gothenburg, 413 90 Gothenburg, Sweden

Paula Bjärneman and Olle Löwhagen
Sahlgrenska Academy, University of Gothenburg, 413 90 Gothenburg, Sweden

Ronny Larsson and ElisabethWallström
Kungsten Health Care Centre, 414 74 Gothenburg, Sweden

H. Alkhouri, V. Cha, K. Tong and J.M. Hughes
Faculty of Pharmacy, The University of Sydney, Sydney, NSW2006, Australia

L. M. Moir and C. L. Armour
Discipline of Pharmacology andWoolcock Institute of Medical Research, The University of Sydney, Sydney, NSW2006, Australia

Vibeke Naeser, Niklas Kahr and Vibeke Backer
Department of Respiratory Medicine, Bispebjerg Hospital, 2400 Copenhagen, Denmark

Lone Graff Stensballe
Danish Epidemiology Science Centre, Statens Serum Institut, 2300 Copenhagen, Denmark

Kirsten Ohm Kyvik
Institute of Regional Health Services Research & Odense Patient Data Explorative Network, University of Southern Denmark, 5000 Odense, Denmark

Axel Skytthe
The Danish Twin Registry, University of Southern Denmark, 5000 Odense, Denmark

Charlotte Giwercman Carson
Danish Pediatric Asthma Center, Gentofte Hospital, 2900 Hellerup, Denmark

Simon Francis Thomsen
Department of Dermato-Allergology, Gentofte Hospital, 2900 Hellerup, Denmark

Stephanie K. Lu and Susan J. Elliott
School of Public Health and Health Systems, University ofWaterloo, 200 University Avenue West,Waterloo, ON, Canada N2L 3G1

Ann E. Clarke
Department of Medicine, University of Calgary, Calgary, AB, Canada T2N 1N4

Sarah Keller, Volker König and Ralph Mösges
Institute of Medical Statistics, Informatics and Epidemiology (IMSIE), University Hospital of Cologne, 50924 Cologne, Germany

Pia Kalm-Stephens
Department ofWomen's and Children's Health, Uppsala University, 751 85 Uppsala, Sweden

Therese Sterner
Division ofWoman, Child and Reproduction, Department of Pediatrics, Skåne University Hospital, 205 02 Lund, Sweden

Kerstin Kronholm Diab
Occupational and Environmental Medicine, University and Regional Laboratories Region Skåne, 205 02 Lund, Sweden

Greta Smedje
Department of Medical Sciences/Occupational and Environmental Medicine, Uppsala University, 751 85 Uppsala, Sweden